I0057347

New Frontiers in Respiratory Infections Research

New Frontiers in Respiratory Infections Research

Edited by Mike Rudd

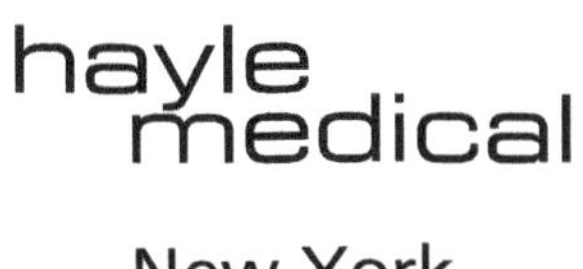

New York

Hayle Medical,
750 Third Avenue, 9th Floor,
New York, NY 10017, USA

Visit us on the World Wide Web at:
www.haylemedical.com

ISBN: 978-1-63241-755-8

Cataloging-in-Publication Data

New frontiers in respiratory infections research / edited by Mike Rudd.
p. cm.
Includes bibliographical references and index.
ISBN 978-1-63241-755-8
1. Respiratory infections. 2. Respiratory infections--Research.
3. Respiratory organs--Diseases. I. Rudd, Mike.

RC740 .N49 2019
616.2--dc23

Table of Contents

Preface ... IX

Chapter 1 **Human Coronaviruses Associated with Upper Respiratory Tract Infections in Three Rural Areas of Ghana** ... 1
Michael Owusu, Augustina Annan, Victor Max Corman, Richard Larbi, Priscilla Anti, Jan Felix Drexler, Olivia Agbenyega, Yaw Adu-Sarkodie and Christian Drosten

Chapter 2 **Quantification of Shared Air: A Social and Environmental Determinant of Airborne Disease Transmission** ... 11
Robin Wood, Carl Morrow, Samuel Ginsberg, Elizabeth Piccoli, Darryl Kalil, Angelina Sassi, Rochelle P. Walensky and Jason R. Andrews

Chapter 3 **Latent Tuberculosis Infection and Occupational Protection among Health Care Workers in Two Types of Public Hospitals** ... 19
Feng Zhou, Li Zhang, Lei Gao, Yibin Hao, Xianli Zhao, Jianmin Liu, Jie Lu, Xiangwei Li, Yu Yang, Junguo Chen and Ying Deng

Chapter 4 **Quantifying Age-Related Rates of Social Contact using Diaries in a Rural Coastal Population** ... 27
Moses Chapa Kiti, Timothy Muiruri Kinyanjui, Dorothy Chelagat Koech, Patrick Kiio Munywoki, Graham Francis Medley and David James Nokes

Chapter 5 **IL-21 Promotes Late Activator APC-Mediated T Follicular Helper Cell Differentiation in Experimental Pulmonary Virus Infection** ... 36
Jae-Kwang Yoo and Thomas J. Braciale

Chapter 6 **Absence of Detectable Influenza RNA Transmitted via Aerosol during Various Human Respiratory Activities** ... 50
Julian W. Tang, Caroline X. Gao, Benjamin J. Cowling, Gerald C. Koh, Daniel Chu, Cherie Heilbronn, Belinda Lloyd, Jovan Pantelic, Andre D. Nicolle, Christian A. Klettner, J. S. Malik Peiris, Chandra Sekhar, David K. W. Cheong, Kwok Wai Tham, Evelyn S. C. Koay, Wendy Tsui, Alfred Kwong, Kitty Chan and Yuguo Li

Chapter 7 **Correlation of *Klebsiella pneumoniae* Comparative Genetic Analyses with Virulence Profiles in a Murine Respiratory Disease Model** ... 59
Ramy A. Fodah, Jacob B. Scott, Hok-Hei Tam, Pearlly Yan, Tia L. Pfeffer, Ralf Bundschuh and Jonathan M. Warawa

Chapter 8 **GBA2-Encoded β-Glucosidase Activity is Involved in the Inflammatory Response to *Pseudomonas aeruginosa*** ... 70
Nicoletta Loberto, Maela Tebon, Ilaria Lampronti, Nicola Marchetti, Massimo Aureli, Rosaria Bassi, Maria Grazia Giri, Valentino Bezzerri, Valentina Lovato, Cinzia Cantù, Silvia Munari, Seng H. Cheng, Alberto Cavazzini, Roberto Gambari, Sandro Sonnino, Giulio Cabrini and Maria Cristina Dechecchi

Chapter 9 **Transcription Analysis of the Porcine Alveolar Macrophage Response to *Mycoplasma hyopneumoniae*** 83
Li Bin, Du Luping, Sun Bing, Yu Zhengyu, Liu Maojun, Feng Zhixin, Wei Yanna, Wang Haiyan, Shao Guoqing and He Kongwang

Chapter 10 **Integrative Model of the Immune Response to a Pulmonary Macrophage Infection: What Determines the Infection Duration?** 92
Natacha Go, Caroline Bidot, Catherine Belloc and Suzanne Touzeau

Chapter 11 **Modeling the Dynamics and Migratory Pathways of Virus-Specific Antibody-Secreting Cell Populations in Primary Influenza Infection** 110
Hongyu Miao, Mark Y. Sangster, Alexandra M. Livingstone, Shannon P. Hilchey, Le Zhang, David J. Topham, Tim R. Mosmann, Jeanne Holden-Wiltse, Alan S. Perelson, Hulin Wu and Martin S. Zand

Chapter 12 **The Effect of TIP on Pneumovirus-Induced Pulmonary Edema in Mice** 122
Elske van den Berg, Reinout A. Bem, Albert P. Bos, Rene Lutter and Job B. M. van Woensel

Chapter 13 **Infection with Host-Range Mutant Adenovirus 5 Suppresses Innate Immunity and Induces Systemic CD4+ T Cell Activation in Rhesus Macaques** 129
Huma Qureshi, Meritxell Genescà, Linda Fritts, Michael B. McChesney, Marjorie Robert-Guroff and Christopher J. Miller

Chapter 14 **Increased Risk of Dementia in Patients Exposed to Nitrogen Dioxide and Carbon Monoxide: A Population-Based Retrospective Cohort Study** 138
Kuang-Hsi Chang, Mei-Yin Chang, Chih-Hsin Muo, Trong-Neng Wu, Chiu-Ying Chen and Chia-Hung Kao

Chapter 15 **Avian Influenza A H7N9 Virus Induces Severe Pneumonia in Mice without Prior Adaptation and Responds to a Combination of Zanamivir and COX-2 Inhibitor** 146
Can Li, Chuangen Li, Anna J. X. Zhang, Kelvin K. W. To, Andrew C. Y. Lee, Houshun Zhu, Hazel W. L. Wu, Jasper F. W. Chan, Honglin Chen, Ivan F. N. Hung, Lanjuan Li and Kwok-Yung Yuen

Chapter 16 **Spatial Analysis on Hepatitis C Virus Infection in Mainland China: From 2005 to 2011** 158
Lu Wang, Jiannan Xing, Fangfang Chen, Ruixue Yan, Lin Ge, Qianqian Qin, Liyan Wang, Zhengwei Ding, Wei Guo and Ning Wang

Chapter 17 **Modes of Transmission of Influenza B Virus in Households** 165
Benjamin J. Cowling, Dennis K. M. Ip, Vicky J. Fang, Piyarat Suntarattiwong, Sonja J. Olsen, Jens Levy, Timothy M. Uyeki, Gabriel M. Leung, J. S. Malik Peiris, Tawee Chotpitayasunondh, Hiroshi Nishiura and J. Mark Simmerman

Chapter 18 **Comorbidities and Disease Severity as Risk Factors for Carbapenem-Resistant *Klebsiella pneumonia* Colonization: Report of an Experience in an Internal Medicine Unit** 173
Antonio Nouvenne, Andrea Ticinesi, Fulvio Lauretani, Marcello Maggio, Giuseppe Lippi, Loredana Guida, Ilaria Morelli, Erminia Ridolo, Loris Borghi and Tiziana Meschi

Chapter 19 **Immune Biomarkers Predictive of Respiratory Viral Infection in Elderly Nursing Home Residents** ... 181
Jennie Johnstone, Robin Parsons, Fernando Botelho, Jamie Millar, Shelly McNeil, Tamas Fulop, Janet McElhaney, Melissa K. Andrew, Stephen D.Walter, P. J. Devereaux, Mehrnoush Malekesmaeili, Ryan R. Brinkman, James Mahony, Jonathan Bramson and Mark Loeb

Chapter 20 **Mortality among People with Severe Mental Disorders who Reach Old Age: A Longitudinal Study of a Community-Representative Sample of 37892 Men** ... 191
Osvaldo P. Almeida, Graeme J. Hankey, Bu B. Yeap, Jonathan Golledge, Paul E. Norman and Leon Flicker

Chapter 21 **Is there Still Room for Novel Viral Pathogens in Pediatric Respiratory Tract Infections?** ... 202
Blanca Taboada, Marco A. Espinoza, Pavel Isa, Fernando E. Aponte, María A. Arias-Ortiz, Jesús Monge-Martínez, Rubén Rodríguez-Vázquez, Fidel Díaz-Hernández, Fernando Zárate-Vidal, Rosa María Wong-Chew, Verónica Firo-Reyes, Carlos N. del Río-Almendárez, Jesús Gaitán-Meza, Alberto Villaseñ or-Sierra, Gerardo Martínez-Aguilar, Ma. del Carmen Salas-Mier, Daniel E. Noyola, Luis F. Pérez-Gónzalez, Susana López, José I. Santos-Preciado and Carlos F. Arias

Chapter 22 **c-di-GMP Enhances Protective Innate Immunity in a Murine Model of Pertussis** ... 216
Shokrollah Elahi, Jill Van Kessel, Tedele G. Kiros, Stacy Strom, Yoshihiro Hayakawa, Mamoru Hyodo, Lorne A. Babiuk and Volker Gerdts

Chapter 23 **Real-Time Bioluminescence Imaging of Mixed Mycobacterial Infections** ... 224
MiHee Chang, Katri P. Anttonen, Suat L. G. Cirillo, Kevin P. Francis and Jeffrey D. Cirillo

Permissions

List of Contributors

Index

Preface

All the infectious diseases related to the respiratory tract can be categorized as respiratory tract infection. Such type of infection can be divided into two types, namely, upper respiratory tract infection and lower respiratory tract infection. The upper respiratory tract consists of the nose, larynx, pharynx and sinuses. Some of the common types of infection associated with it include sinusitis, tonsillitis, influenza, common cold, laryngitis and pharyngitis. The lower respiratory tract consists of the lungs, trachea, bronchioles and the bronchial tubes. The common infections associated with the lower respiratory tract are bronchitis, influenza and pneumonia. The topics included in this book on respiratory infections are of utmost significance and bound to provide incredible insights to readers. It will also provide interesting topics for research which interested readers can take up. This book on respiratory infections is a collective contribution of a renowned group of international experts.

Significant researches are present in this book. Intensive efforts have been employed by authors to make this book an outstanding discourse. This book contains the enlightening chapters which have been written on the basis of significant researches done by the experts.

Finally, I would also like to thank all the members involved in this book for being a team and meeting all the deadlines for the submission of their respective works. I would also like to thank my friends and family for being supportive in my efforts.

Editor

Human Coronaviruses Associated with Upper Respiratory Tract Infections in Three Rural Areas of Ghana

Michael Owusu[1], Augustina Annan[1], Victor Max Corman[2], Richard Larbi[1], Priscilla Anti[3], Jan Felix Drexler[2], Olivia Agbenyega[3], Yaw Adu-Sarkodie[4], Christian Drosten[2]*

1 Kumasi Centre for Collaborative Research in Tropical Medicine, Kwame Nkrumah University of Science and Technology, Kumasi, Ghana, **2** Institute of Virology, University of Bonn Medical Centre, Bonn, Germany, **3** Institute of Renewable and Natural Resources, Kwame Nkrumah University of Science and Technology, Kumasi, Ghana, **4** Department of Clinical Microbiology, Kwame Nkrumah University of Science and Technology, Kumasi, Ghana

Abstract

Background: Acute respiratory tract infections (ARI) are the leading cause of morbidity and mortality in developing countries, especially in Africa. This study sought to determine whether human coronaviruses (HCoVs) are associated with upper respiratory tract infections among older children and adults in Ghana.

Methods: We conducted a case control study among older children and adults in three rural areas of Ghana using asymptomatic subjects as controls. Nasal/Nasopharyngeal swabs were tested for Middle East respiratory syndrome coronavirus (MERS-CoV), HCoV-22E, HCoV-OC43, HCoV-NL63 and HCoV-HKU1 using Reverse Transcriptase Real-Time Polymerase Chain Reaction.

Results: Out of 1,213 subjects recruited, 150 (12.4%) were positive for one or more viruses. Of these, single virus detections occurred in 146 subjects (12.0%) and multiple detections occurred in 4 (0.3%). Compared with control subjects, infections with HCoV-229E (OR = 5.15, 95%CI = 2.24–11.78), HCoV-OC43 (OR = 6.16, 95%CI = 1.77–21.65) and combine HCoVs (OR = 2.36, 95%CI = 1.5 = 3.72) were associated with upper respiratory tract infections. HCoVs were found to be seasonally dependent with significant detections in the harmattan season (mainly HCoV-229E) and wet season (mainly HCoV-NL63). A comparison of the obtained sequences resulted in no differences to sequences already published in GenBank.

Conclusion: HCoVs could play significant role in causing upper respiratory tract infections among adults and older children in rural areas of Ghana.

Editor: Krzysztof Pyrc, Faculty of Biochemistry Biophysics and Biotechnology, Jagiellonian University, Poland

Funding: This work was funded by the Deutsche Forschungsgemeinschaft under grant No DR 772/3-1, to YAS and CD. The funders had no role in study design, data collection and analysis, decision to publish, or preparation of the manuscript.

Competing Interests: The authors have declared that no competing interests exist.

* Email: drosten@virology-bonn.de

Background

Acute respiratory tract infections (ARI) are a leading cause of morbidity and mortality among young children and adults in developing countries, especially Africa [1–3]. The majority of ARI are of viral origin including respiratory syncytial virus (RSV), Influenza viruses, Rhinoviruses, Parainfluenza viruses, Human metapneumovirus and human coronaviruses (HCoVs) [4–7]. Coronaviruses (CoVs) are enveloped RNA viruses and belong to the family *Coronaviridae* and subfamily *Coronavirinae*. CoVs are positive strand viruses with genome sizes ranging from 27–33 kilobases (kb). They are classified into four genera named *Alphacoronavirus*, *Betacoronavirus*, *Gammacoronavirus* and *Deltacoronavirus* [8]. HCoV-NL63 and HCoV-229E belong to the alphacoronaviruses while HCoV-OC43, HCoV-HKU1, and the severe acute respiratory syndrome coronavirus (SARS-CoV) belong to the betacoronaviruses [8]. A recent HCoV that was first identified in the Middle East region is termed Middle East respiratory syndrome coronavirus (MERS-CoV) and belongs to the genus *Betacoronavirus* [9]. Despite the detection of MERS-CoV-related sequences in bats worldwide and neutralising antibodies against MERS-CoV in camels, the evolutionary source of this novel HCoV still remains unclear [10–17].

The evolving trend in the emergence of new strains of HCoVs coupled with an increase in advanced molecular techniques has revived the interest of researchers in finding the epidemiologic association between respiratory diseases and HCoV infection. Some studies in developed countries have reported HCoV-OC43 and HCoV-229E to be responsible for up to 10% of upper respiratory tract infections [18,19] whereas others identified these viruses along with HCoV-NL63 and HCoV-HKU1 to be more prevalent in severe respiratory tract infections of immunocompromised individuals, institutional elderly subjects and infants [20–23]. Severe infections and deaths have been associated with MERS-CoV infections [17,24–27]. Other studies on the contrary identified HCoVs to be quite common in healthy individuals thus raising questions about its association with respiratory illness [28,29]. Finally, even though HCoVs are believed to be most relevant in young children, the contribution of these viruses to

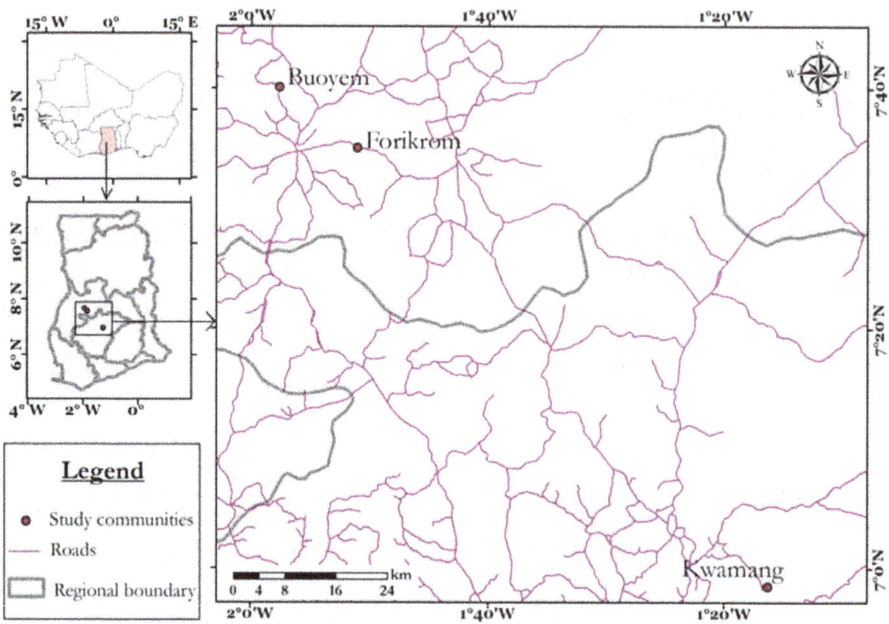

Figure 1. Geographical location of study areas in Ghana. The study communities are represented by three red dots. The geographic coordinates on the horizontal and vertical regions of the bar show the latitude and longitude coordinates. The red lines show the roads the link the respectively communities.

disease in older children and adults still needs to be addressed worldwide [30].

Knowledge of the contribution of HCoVs to the burden of respiratory tract infections in rural areas of Africa is rare. Rural regions are considered as the focus of morbidity and mortality associated with infectious diseases due to the poor hygienic practices and the lack of quality healthcare systems. Information on the aetiologies of disease in these areas will therefore help to reduce disease burden. However, even in developed countries most studies are hospital based and lack healthy humans as control groups [6,7,31].

This study aims to provide information on the association of HCoVs with upper respiratory tract infections in remote rural areas of Ghana with additional focus on seasonal variation and the spectrum of circulating HCoV strains.

Materials and Methods

Ethics statement

The study protocol was approved by the Committee for Human Research, Publications and Ethics of KATH and School of Medical Sciences, KNUST, Kumasi, Ashanti region, Ghana (Ethical clearance reference: CHRPE 49/09). We first explained the study protocol captured on the "Participant Information Leaflet and Consent Form" to every subject who was enrolled in the study. This was done in the local language of the subjects. Once they agreed, we asked them to thumbprint the consent form attached to the participant leaflet form for subjects who were illiterates. For those who were literates, we asked them to sign the consent forms.

Written informed consent was obtained for data and sample collection for all subjects. For subjects less than 18 years of age, written informed consent was obtained from parents or guardians and assent from the minors.

Study Area

The study was performed in three rural areas of Ghana, namely Buoyem, Kwamang and Forikrom communities, from September 2011 to September 2012. **Figure 1** shows the geographic location of all three communities. Buoyem and Forikrom communities are located in the Techiman municipality of the Brong Ahafo Region of Ghana. The Techiman municipality is among the 22 administrative districts in the region [32]. It shares common boundaries with the Wenchi district to the northwest and Nkoranza district to the southeast. The municipality has a total land surface of 669.7 Km^2 with climate and vegetation that promotes the production of food. Kwamang community is in the Sekyere Central district of the Ashanti Region of Ghana. The community is part of 5 sub-districts of Sekyere Central and forms one third of the total land size of the district [32].

Population Characteristics

The population of Techiman municipality based on the 2010 population census is 206,856 [33]. The projected population of Forikrom and Buoyem are 3,800 and 3,900 individuals respectively [34]. The Techiman municipality has a population density of 318 people per Km^2 with several ethnic groups [32]. The population of Sekyere Central district is 71,232 and the projected population of Kwamang is 8,000 [34]. The population density of the district is 64 people per Km^2 [35].

Study design

We conducted an unmatched case control study to identify the association between HCoVs and upper respiratory tract infection. Subjects were identified as cases if they presented with symptoms of upper respiratory illness with rapid onset of any of the following conditions: cough, sneezing, runny nose and nasal congestion. Subjects were selected as controls if they did not present with any symptom of upper respiratory illness for at least 8 days prior to recruitment. Subjects were excluded if they were less than 10 years

Table 1. Primers used for PCR Testing.

Virus Type	Forward Primers 5'----->3'	Reverse Primer 5'------>3'	Probe	Target Region	Usage	Reference
HCoV-229E	CAGTCAAATGG GCTGATGCA	AAAGGGCTATAAA GAGAATAAGGTATT CT	JOE-CCCTGACGACCACGT TGTGGTTCA-BHQ1	Nucleoprotein	RT-PCR	[18]
	F1-GTGCTTAGTCTT GTTAGGAGTGG	TCACGAACTGTCTT AGGTAGTGC	N/A	Spike	Sequencing	This study
	F2-GTAAGTTGCTTG TAAGGGGTAAT G		N/A	Spike	Sequencing	This study
HCoV-OC43	CGATGAGGCTAT TCCGACTAGGT	CCTTCCTGAGCCTT CAATATAGTAACC	FAM-TCCGCCTGGCACGGT ACTCCCT-BHQ1	Necleoprotein	RT-PCR	[18]
	F1-ACTAGGCTGCAT GATGCTTAGA	CACATATTATACTG GCAAACAGA	N/A	Spike	Sequencing	This study
	F2-GCATGATGCTTA GACCATAATCT		N/A	Spike	Sequencing	This study
HCoV-NL63	GACCAAAGCACTGAA-TAACATTT TCC	ACCTAATAAGCCTC TTTCTCAACCC	FAM-ATGTTATTCAGTGCT TTGGTCCTCGTGAT-BHQ1	Necleoprotein	RT-PCR	[29]
	F1-GTGTGGTGACAT TCACAGTAACG	GTGTGGTGACATTC ACAGTAACG	N/A	Spike	Sequencing	This study
	F2-GAGTTTGATTAA GAGTGGTAGGT		N/A	Spike	Sequencing	This study
HCoV-HKU1	CCTTGCGAATGA ATGTGCT	TTGCATCACCACTG CTAGTACCAC	JOE-TGTGTGGCGGTTGCT ATTATGTTAAGCCTG-BHQ1	Replicase 1b	RT-PCR	[29]
	F1-TTGCCTACAACA TTAGCTGTTA	CCACGTTCTTGATA AAAATGAAAATAC	N/A	Spike	Sequencing	This study
	F2-CAACATTAGCTG TTATAGGTGAT		N/A	Spike	Sequencing	This study
MERS-CoV	GCAACGCGCGA TTCAGTT	GCCTCTACACGGGA CCCATA	FAM-CTCTTCACATAATCG C CCCGAGCTCG-TAMRA	Envelope	RT-PCR	[36]

F1 and F2: First and second round forward primers for sequencing of samples, one reverse primer for both rounds.
NA: Not applicable.

old, had a history of epistaxis or refused clinical samples to be collected.

For a random selection of the study participants, the communities were divided into four quadrants using major roads. Social centres at each quadrant were selected at random and every other adjacent house starting from the social centre was marked and subjects were selected. Once the communities got well informed about the study, radio announcements were used to call individuals to major community centres where recruitment was continued.

Recruitment of subjects was done on seasonal basis. There are two major seasons in the study areas; the wet and harmattan season. The harmattan is characterised by dry wind carrying dust from the Sahara desert while the wet has mainly heavy rains with high humidity. The periods in-between these seasons (pre-harmattan and interim) are characterised by hot temperatures and minor rains. Major recruitments were made in the pre-harmattan season (September, October, November), harmattan season (December, January, February) and wet season (May, June, July). Minor sampling was done in the pre- wet season (March, April). Cases were recruited in each season alongside controls. Demographic information was collected from all subjects using structured questionnaires. The questionnaires were written in English and interpreted to subjects in their local dialects.

Clinical Sampling

Nasopharyngeal specimens were taken with flocked swabs (Copan, Italy) from subjects by gently inserting the swab up the nostril towards the pharynx until resistance was felt and was then rotated 3 times to obtain epithelial cells. In cases where subjects objected to nasopharyngeal sampling, nasal swabs were taken. From field observations, nasopharyngeal swabs were taken from about 90% of all study subjects. The swabs were stored in 1.5 ml RNAlater (Qiagen, Hilden, Germany) and transported to the laboratory where they were frozen at −20°C until testing.

Laboratory Methods

Viral RNA was extracted from the samples using the spin protocol of the QIAamp Viral RNA Mini Kit (Qiagen, Hilden, Germany) as described by the manufacturer and extended with an

Table 2. Demographic characteristics of study subjects.

	Control groups	Case groups
Variables	**n = 620**	**n = 593**
Study communities		
Buoyem n (%)	194 (31.3)	208 (35.1)
Forikrom n (%)	162 (26.1)	195 (32.9)
Kwamang n (%)	264 (42.6)	190 (32)
Gender (Female) n (%)	360 (58.2)	334 (56.3)
Age n % (IQR)	40 (24.5–54)	35 (20–52)
Occupation		
High social contact n (%)	260 (41.9)	264 (44.5)
Low social contact n (%)	360 (58.1)	329 (55.5)
Type of Accommodation		
Crowded accommodation n (%)	408 (66.2)	397 (67.7)
Non-crowded accommodation n (%)	208 (33.8)	189 (32.3)

additional centrifugation step for 5 min at 20,000×g to dispose all residues of washing buffer before elution. Samples were eluted in 100 µl of pre-warmed 80°C AVE buffer.

Real-time reverse transcription polymerase chain reaction (RT-PCR) was performed for the detection of five HCoVs; HCoV-229E, HCoV-OC43, HCoV-NL63, HCoV-HKU1 and MERS-CoV. Testing of samples was performed by pooling in batches of five to ten samples. Singleplex RT-PCR was used for detection of MERS-CoV as described elsewhere [36] while the other four HCoVs were detected with multiplex RT-PCR.

For Multiplex RT-PCR testing of HCoV-NL63 and HCoV-HKU1, a 25 µl reaction was set up containing 5 µl of RNA, 1 µl of 10 mM dNTP mix (Qiagen), 5 µl of OneStep 5x buffer (Qiagen), 1 µl of Enzyme Mix (Qiagen), 600 nM of each forward and reverse primers for HCoV-NL63, 400 nM of each forward and reverse primers for HCoV-HKU1, 200 nM probe for each virus and 7 µl of RNASE free water. HCoV-229E and HCoV-OC43 multiplex RT-PCR testing was similarly performed as described above except that 400 nM of each forward and reverse primers for HCoV-229E and HCoV-OC43 and 200 nM of the respective probes were used. The amplification procedure comprised reverse transcription at 55°C for 20 min followed by initial denaturation at 94°C for 3 min and 45 cycles of 94°C for 15 s and 58°C for 30 s.

The sequences of primers and probes for each assay are shown in **Table 1** as described elsewhere [18,29,36]. All PCR's were performed using light cycler 480 II (Roche, Germany).

Controls and Standards

All runs included RNase free water as a negative control and quantified in-vitro transcripts of each virus as positive control. The in-vitro transcripts were prepared as described previously [36]. Briefly, target amplicons were TA cloned. Plasmids were purified and reamplified using vector specific oligonucleotides and then finally *in vitro* transcribed using a T7 promoter (Ambion Mega-script kit, Invitrogen). Ten-fold dilutions of the RNA transcripts were prepared using RNase free water containing 10 µg/ml of carrier RNA. Standard curves were generated from serial dilutions of the in-vitro transcripts. Two controls with concentrations of 10^2 and 10^3 copies per reaction were included in each PCR run for HCoV-NL63, HCoV-OC43 and HCoV-HKU1. For MERS-CoV assay, concentrations of 10^1 and 10^2 copies per reaction were used. All positive samples were quantified using the positive controls and connected external standard curves.

Sequencing of positive HCoVs using Heminested PCR

For all positive samples, PCRs were done to amplify the first 500 base pairs of the spike gene using primers listed in **Table 1**. For the first round of PCR, a 25 µl reaction was set up containing 5 µl of RNA, 12.5 µl of 2 X reaction buffer (Invitrogen; containing 0.4 mM of each dNTP and 3.2 mM MgSO4), 1 µl of reverse transcriptase/Taq mixture from the kit, 0.4 µl of a 50 mM $MgSO_4$, 1 µg of non-acetylated bovine serum albumin (Roche) and 400 nM of each primer. The amplification procedure comprised 15 min at 50°C; 3 min at 95°C; 10 cycles of 15 s at 94°C, 15 s starting at 60°C with a decrease of 0.5°C per cycle, and 40 s at 72°C; and 40 cycles of 15 s at 95°C, 30 s at 56°C, and 40 s at 72°C. A second-round reaction was set up from the first round using 5 µl of 10 X reaction buffer (Invitrogen), 2.5 µl of a 50 mM $MgCl_2$ solution, 200 nM of dNTP, 400 nM of each forward and reverse primer and 0.2 µl of platinum Taq DNA Polymerase. Thermal cycling was performed at 95°C for 3 min and 45 cycles of 95°C for 15 s, 56°C for 15 s and 72°C for 40 s, followed by a 2 min extension step at 72°C. All obtained PCR products were sequenced and compared to GenBank via the BLAST Algorithm as well as aligned together with reference sequences from the GenBank.

Data Analysis

All data obtained from the communities were recorded using EPI INFO version 5 (CDC, Atlanta) and imported into Microsoft Excel. Subsequent analysis was performed using R statistical software version 2.15.2 [37]. Categorical variables and their association with respiratory agents were analysed using the Fischer's exact test. Continuous variables were expressed as medians with their inter-quartile ranges (IQR). A non-parametric K-sample test on the equality of medians was used to evaluate the differences in the medians of the various subgroups of the continuous variables. The association of HCoVs with upper respiratory tract infection was assessed by fitting five logistic regression models controlling for age group, age as a continuous variable and study communities. Results were expressed as

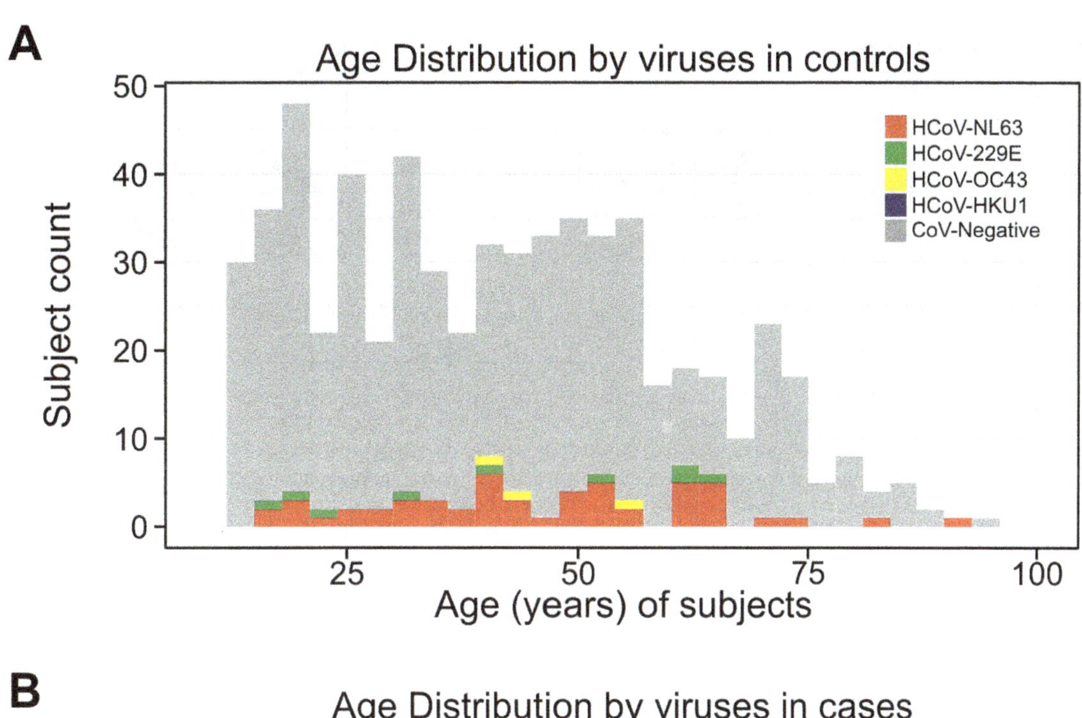

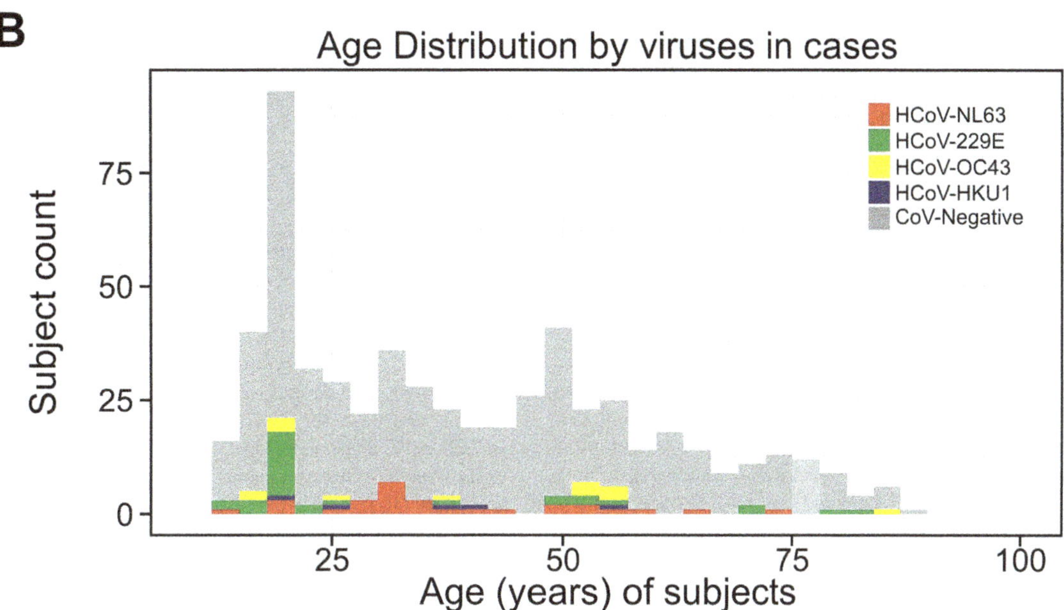

Figure 2. Virus distribution among age categories of cases and controls. The x-axis represents the age groups and y-axis shows the number of subjects. Grey bars represent the total number of samples per age group, coloured bars the virus-positive samples. Colour coding is according to virus species as indicated in the legend.

Table 3. Viruses detected in cases and controls.

Viruses	Control groups	Case groups	Total	p-value
	n = 620	n = 593	n = 1213	
HCoV-229E [n (%)]	9 (1.5)	36 (6.1)	45 (3.7)	**0.001**
HCoV-HKU1 [n (%)]	0 (0)	5 (0.8)	5 (0.4)	0.065
HCoV-NL63 [n (%)]	53 (8.5)	30 (5.1)	83 (6.8)	**0.022**
HCoV-OC43 [n (%)]	3 (0.5)	18 (3)	21 (1.7)	**0.001**
Overall HCoV [n (%)]	65 (10.5)	81 (13.7)	146 (12)	0.107

Table 4. Viruses detected in concentrations above 100 copies per RT-PCR reaction.

Viruses	Control group	Case group	Total	p-value
	n = 620	n = 593	1213	
HCoV-229E n (%)	7 (1.1)	35 (5.9)	42 (3.5)	**0.001**
HCoV-HKU1 n (%)	0 (0)	3 (0.5)	3 (0.2)	0.23
HCoV-NL63 n (%)	20 (3.2)	20 (3.4)	40 (3.3)	1
HCoV-OC43 n (%)	3 (0.5)	17(2.9)	20 (1.6)	**0.002**
Overall HCoVs n (%)	30 (4.8)	68 (11.5)	98 (8.1)	**0.001**

adjusted odd ratios and 95% confidence interval (CI). Graphs were plotted using ggplot2 package [38] and R base plots. For all analysis, a two-sided p-value of less than 0.05 was considered significant.

Results

Reproducibility of HCoV assays

To determine the reproducibility of the human Coronavirus RT-PCR assays used in this study, we included two in-vitro transcripts with a defined RNA concentration of 100 copies per reaction in each RT-PCR run. The mean and standard deviations specified as m (s.d) of the real-time PCR signal crossing points for HCoV-HKU1, HCoV-NL63, HCoV-OC43, MERS-CoV and HCoV-229E were respectively determined to be 31.27 (0.24), 33.61 (0.34), 35.06 (0.6), 33.85 (0.94) and 36.31 (1.12). It was concluded that all assays provided high sensitivity and reliable performance.

Characteristics of Study Subjects

A total of 1213 subjects were recruited during the study period. Major recruitments were done in the pre-harmattan (385, 32%), harmattan (215, 18%) and wet seasons (516, 43%), and minor recruitment was done in the pre-wet season (97, 8%). Overall four 487 (40%) were enrolled in 2011 and 726 (60%) were enrolled in 2012. Of the 1213 subjects recruited, 620 (51.1%) were controls and 593 (48.9%) were cases. Table 2 shows the demographic description of cases and controls. The occupation of subjects was classified into one group with a high rate of social interactions and a second group with a lesser rate of interactions. Occupations with high social contact include health workers, dressmakers, students, teachers, hairdressers, traders, drivers and food vendors. The second group comprised farmers, hunters, traditional authorities and carpenters.

Human Coronavirus Epidemiology

The present study identified four HCoVs (HCoV-229E, HCoV-OC43, HCoV-NL63 and HCoV-HKU1). No sample was positive for the recently emerged MERS-CoV. The overall detection of HCoVs was 12.4% (150/1213). Single virus detections occurred in 146 samples (12.0%) and multiple detections occurred in 4 samples (0.3%). The most prevalent virus identified was HCoV-NL63 (82 detections, 6.8%) followed by HCoV-229E (41, 3.4%), HCoV-OC43 (18, 1.5%) then HCoV-HKU1 (5, 0.4%). Three samples were positive (0.2%) for HCoV-OC43 and HCoV-229E and one sample for HCoV-NL63 and HCoV-229E.

Virus distribution in cases and controls

As shown in **Figure 2**, a comparison of the age distribution of the different viruses detected in case and control groups revealed HCoV-229E to be more frequent in cases with age below 20 years whereas HCoV-NL63 was common in the middle age group. Among control subjects, HCoV-NL63 was found to occur almost equally in all ages. We did not find a significant difference (p = 0.43) comparing overall virus detection rates in all subjects with ages from 10 to 40 years (54.1%; 84/146) and those above 40 years (61%; 42.1).

HCoVs were detected in 65 (10.5%; 65/629) controls and 81 (13.7%; 81/593) cases. Notably, this difference was not statistically significant (p = 0.11). The most common virus among cases and controls were HCoV-229E (36, 6.1%) and HCoV-NL63 (53, 8.5%), respectively (**Table 3**). HCoV-229E and HCoV-OC43 were more frequently encountered in cases than in controls whereas HCoV-NL63 was more common in control subjects. The results for all virus detections in cases and controls did not change significantly when cases showing co-infections with multiple CoV were excluded from the analysis.

High HCoV detection rates in control subjects were compatible with prolonged excretion of very low levels of viral RNA after convalescence. As these detections would reduce the clinical utility of RT-PCR diagnostics, the analysis was repeated excluding all cases showing viral loads of 100 or less copies per reaction. The modified dataset is presented in **Table 4**. Except for HCoV-NL63 and -HKU1, virus detection rates were now higher in cases as compared to controls. Also the overall detection rate for all HCoVs including HCoV-NL63 and -HKU1 was higher among cases compared to control subjects (p = 0.001).

Using the dataset from which cases containing less than 100 copies per reaction had been eliminated, quantitative results were compared between cases and controls. Virus loads of HCoV-229E showed no significant difference between cases and controls. Cases yielded an average of 27,400 RNA copies per RT-PCR reaction (interquartile range (IQR) $6.4\times10^2-2.4\times10^7$) while controls had 197,000 copies per PCR reaction on average (IQR = $4110–1.28\times10^6$). The trend was similar for cases and controls with HCoV-OC43 detection (115,000 copies per PCR reaction; IQR = $412–7.5\times10^5$ vs. 5,480 copies per PCR reactions; IQR = $3270–3.47\times10^7$). HCoV-NL63 median concentration was however significantly higher in cases compared to controls (2.41×10^6 copies per PCR reaction; IQR = $1.96\times10^4-2.3\times10^6$ vs. 1,876.5 copies per PCR reaction; IQR = $387.2–8.6\times10^4$, p = 0.003). Low detection rates for HCoV-HKU1 did not warrant a quantitative comparison for this virus. Due to the differences in HCoV-NL63 virus loads, the virus load of cases and controls were analysed in different communities. **Figure 3 A** shows that there

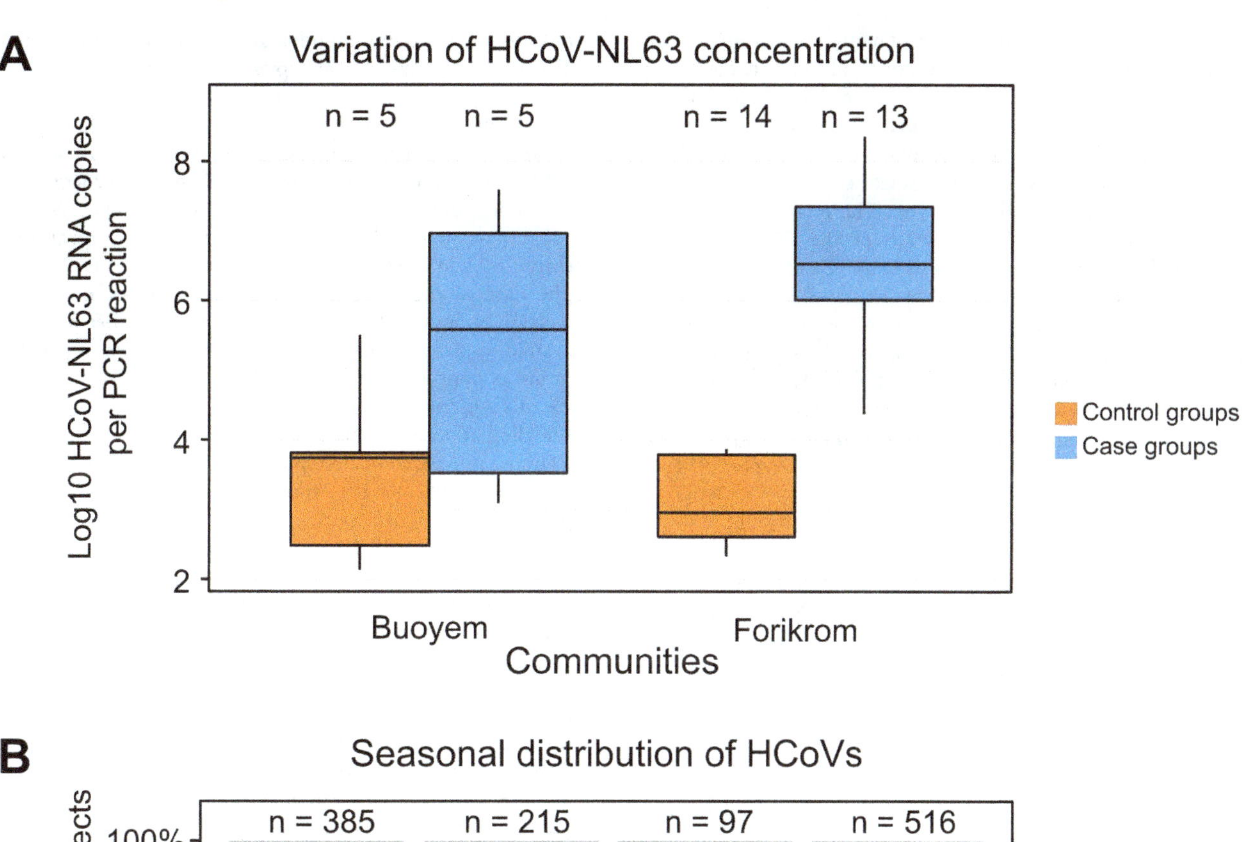

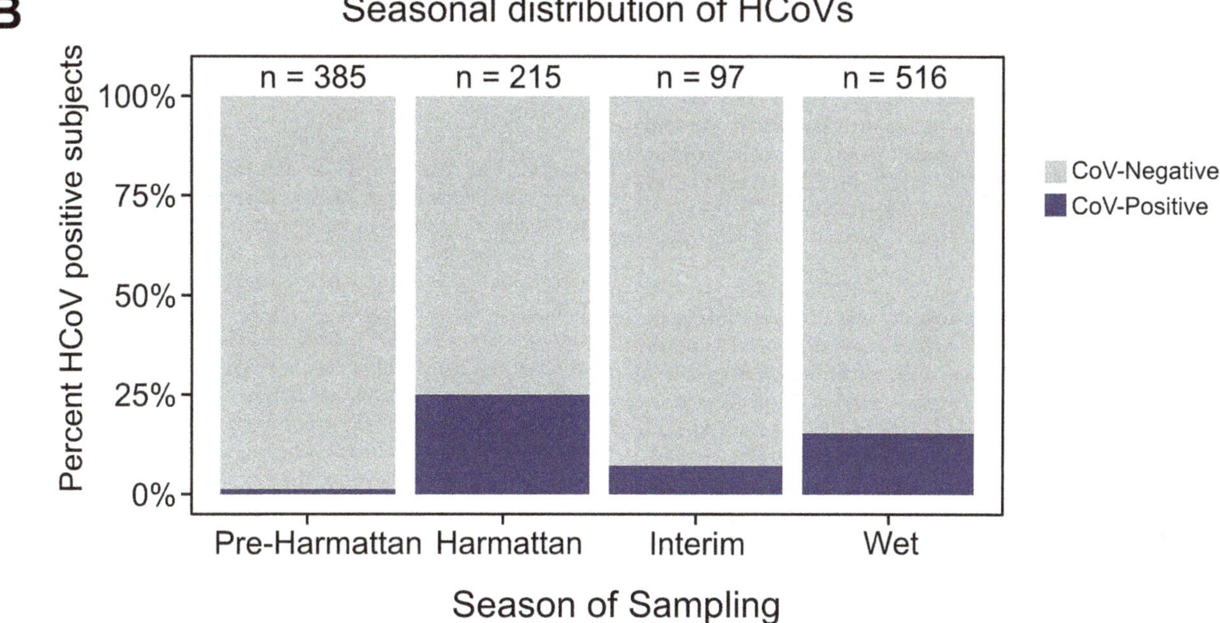

Figure 3. Seasonal distribution and concentration variation of HCoVs. A: Variation of HCoV-NL63 Concentration. The study areas are represented on the x-axis and the y-axis shows the log10 of HCoV-NL63 concentration in copies per RT-PCR reaction. Data for Kwamang is not shown because of the low numbers detected. Significant differences in viral loads between healthy and control subjects were detected for only the Forikrom community. B: Seasonal distribution of HCoVs. The x-axis shows the various seasons and the "n" value on top of each bar represents the number of subjects recruited in each season. The y-axis shows the percentage of subjects positive for HCoVs.

was a significant difference (higher in cases compared to controls) in Forikrom (p = 0.005) but not in the other study areas.

Seasonal distribution of HCoVs

The present study also investigated the seasonal variation of HCoVs in all study communities (**Figure 3 B**). High proportions of HCoVs were identified in the harmattan season (54/215, 25.1%) compared to the wet (80/516, 15.5%) seasons (p = 0.003). The increase of detection of HCoVs in the harmattan season was also significant compared to detections in the pre-harmattan season (1.3%, p<0.01) and the interim season (7.2%, p<0.0004). The most frequent viruses detected in the harmattan and wet seasons were HCoV-229E and HCoV-NL63, respectively. HCoV-OC43 and HCoV-HKU1 were almost equally distributed throughout the year.

To further explore the frequency of virus circulation among subjects with high or low social interactions, all subjects consisting of cases and controls were regrouped into low social contact groups (689/1,213; 56.8%) and high social contact groups 524;(43.2%) based on their occupations. HCoVs were identified in 88 (12.8%) individuals in the low social contact group and 58 (11.1%) in the high social contact group. There was no significant difference (p = 0.42) in the proportion of the overall HCoVs detected in the two groups. A comparison of the individual HCoVs however showed high proportions of HCoV-229E in the high social contact group (26/524; 5.0%) compared to the low social contact group (15/689; 2.2%). The difference in proportions of HCoV-229E was significant (p = 0.01). All other HCoV detections were not significant between the groups except HCoV-NL63, which was slightly higher (p = 0.04) in the low social group (56/689; 8.1%) compared to the high social group (26/524; 5.0%).

Sequence typing

To determine whether HCoVs circulating in rural Africa were similar to viruses encountered in the northern hemisphere, a representative sample of the encountered viruses were sequenced. Sequencing of a variable part of the viral spike protein gene was successful for 53 out of 146 samples (36.3%). Of the 53, 12 (22.6%) were HCoV-OC43, 14 (26.4%) were HCoV-NL63, 24 (45.3%) were HCoV-229e and 3 (5.7%) were HCoV-HKU1. A comparison of the all sequences to sequences published in GenBank identified no relevant differences against previously described viruses. In contrast, sequences resembling the homologous spike gene portions of bat-associated HCoV-229E-related coronaviruses previously described by our group in animals sampled in the study area were not detected in any sample [39,40]. All sequences have been deposited in the GenBank under the accession numbers KJ768612–KJ768646 and KJ796450–KJ796467.

Discussion

HCoVs contribute significantly to the burden of upper respiratory tract infections. Therefore most developed countries have investigated the molecular and epidemiological profile of these viruses. On the contrary, information from developing countries, particularly in tropical areas of sub-Saharan Africa is scarce. The few published data were mostly from hospitalised subjects under five years and without the inclusion of control subjects. We performed a case-control study in sub-Saharan Africa that reports the detection of HCoVs in older children and adults with and without upper respiratory tract infection.

Our study resulted in the detection of 146 (12.4% of tested specimens) HCoVs occurring in both cases and controls. A comparison of viruses in cases and controls showed higher detections of HCoV-229E and HCoV-OC43 among cases compared to controls. These findings are similar to previous reports that identified HCoV-229E and HCoV-OC43 as being commonly associated with upper respiratory tract infections [18,41]. These differences did not change significantly when low viral loads of less than 100 copies per RT-PCR reaction were excluded from the analysis. Robustness of results against the exclusion of low-copy samples is important, as RT-PCR suffers from inconsistencies at the lower end of the detection range, in particular if carried out in settings with only a basic level of training and technology, such as in this study. Caveats include the potential of contamination of test tubes with low copy numbers of target RNA template. Moreover, test sensitivity can vary greatly at the lower end of the detection range, which is why we have demonstrated for our methodology that more useful results are achieved at levels above 100 copies per reaction.

In this light it is interesting that HCoV-NL63 was found to occur at almost equal rates in cases and controls. This observation was previously reported among young children [28] and could possibly suggest the virus may have an insignificant role in causing ARI among adults and older children. However, our results have to be interpreted with caution because some control subjects positive for HCoV-NL63 might have had yet subclinical infections at the time of recruitment. This scenario cannot be ruled out, especially because HCoV-NL63 has generally been associated with mild respiratory infection. Lower levels of virus replication in controls as opposed to cases are also suggested by the diverging levels of virus concentration particularly for HCoV-NL63.

One limitation of this study could be the overestimation of viral detection rates in control subjects probably due to shedding of HCoVs following earlier symptomatic infections. The ideal approach would have been to recruit controls who had no symptoms of respiratory infection for at least one month. However the enrolment of such subjects during sampling will be difficult, especially in rural areas, where illiteracy rate is high and subjects may not be able to document or recall the occurrence of symptoms for prolonged periods. A further explanation of this overestimation might be the persistent or residual RNA fragments in the respiratory tract of adults. This phenomenon of RNA persistence was generally described for other respiratory viruses in children [42–44]. Another limitation was our inability to test other known respiratory viruses among our study subjects. Future studies could explore the role of other viruses among subject with URTI compare to control groups.

The present study did not identify the novel MERS-CoV in any subject. The reason could be that the virus was localized in some geographical areas (e.g. Middle East) and perhaps had not spread to Ghana as at the time of sampling our subjects.

In temperate countries, seasonal variations of HCoVs are discernible with most cases occurring in winter [7,28,29]. In China, detection of HCoV-OC43 is reported to increase in summer whereas HCoV-229E and HCoV-NL63 occurs mainly in autumn [45,46]. Other tropical countries like Thailand have however reported peak detections of HCoV-OC43 in winter whereas HCoV-NL63 occurred frequently in autumn [29]. In sub-Saharan African countries with unique seasonal patterns such as harmattan and wet seasons, the circulation of HCoVs tends to be different. Our study recorded high detection rates of HCoVs in the harmattan and the wet seasons compared to the other seasons. Possible explanations for this include seasonal variations in host immune status to infection [47] and changes in humidity which increase viral survival in the environment [48]. In the harmattan season for instance humidity is extremely low with heavy amount of dust that could injure the respiratory system thus exposing individuals to infection [49]. Our results may be comparable to a study in Senegal that identified HCoVs in October (rainy season) [50]. Additional investigation is needed to define the seasonality of HCoVs especially in sub-Saharan African countries with tropical climates.

A comparison of the first 500 base pairs of the spike region, which is the region with most variation in the CoV genome [51], did not show differences in the strains from our study compared to reference strains from the GenBank. We also did not find variation in strains from the different communities as well as between cases and controls. This contrasts the observation of variable sequences from the spike region of HCoV-NL63 detected in three different years in the United States of America [51]. It is conceivable that connectivity on an international scale contributes to the variability of the spectrum of prevalent viruses in communities. Such connectivity may be low in the remote communities investigated here.

Conclusion

This study has demonstrated that the same strains of HCoVs detected in the northern hemisphere circulate at high rates in a remote and rural setting in Western Africa. The general pattern of virus detection rates and virus concentrations suggest these agents to be causative for upper respiratory tract infections among older children and adults. However, in this environment with presumably low standards of personal and community hygiene, viruses are frequently detected in healthy control subjects, identifying an important caveat concerning the use of pure virological diagnostic data for clinical decision-making.

Acknowledgments

We are grateful to Monika Eschbach-Bludau, Sebastian Brünink, Tobias Bleicker at the Institute of Virology, Bonn, for technical assistance.

Author Contributions

Conceived and designed the experiments: MO AA VMC PA JFD OA YAS CD. Performed the experiments: MO VMC RL. Analyzed the data: MO AA VMC RL PA OA JFD YAS CD. Wrote the paper: MO VMC JFD YAS CD.

References

1. Denny FW, Loda FA (1986) Acute respiratory infections are the leading cause of death in children in developing countries. The American journal of tropical medicine and hygiene 35: 1–2.
2. Williams BG, Gouws E, Boschi-Pinto C, Bryce J, Dye C (2002) Estimates of world-wide distribution of child deaths from acute respiratory infections. The Lancet infectious diseases 2: 25–32.
3. Gessner BD (2011) Acute lower respiratory infection in the developing world. Expert Review of Respiratory Medicine 5: 459–463.
4. Arden KE, McErlean P, Nissen MD, Sloots TP, Mackay IM (2006) Frequent detection of human rhinoviruses, paramyxoviruses, coronaviruses, and bocavirus during acute respiratory tract infections. Journal of medical virology 78: 1232–1240.
5. Xiao NG, Zhang B, Duan ZJ, Xie ZP, Zhou QH, et al. (2012) [Viral etiology of 1165 hospitalized children with acute lower respiratory tract infection]. Zhongguo Dang Dai Er Ke Za Zhi 14: 28–32.
6. Venter M, Lassauniere R, Kresfelder TL, Westerberg Y, Visser A (2011) Contribution of common and recently described respiratory viruses to annual hospitalizations in children in South Africa. J Med Virol 83: 1458–1468.
7. Smuts H, Workman L, Zar HJ (2008) Role of human metapneumovirus, human coronavirus NL63 and human bocavirus in infants and young children with acute wheezing. J Med Virol 80: 906–912.
8. Adams MJ, Carstens EB (2012) Ratification vote on taxonomic proposals to the International Committee on Taxonomy of Viruses (2012). Arch Virol 157: 1411–1422.
9. de Groot RJ, Baker SC, Baric RS, Brown CS, Drosten C, et al. (2013) Middle East Respiratory Syndrome Coronavirus (MERS-CoV): Announcement of the Coronavirus Study Group. J Virol 87: 7790–7792.
10. Annan A, Baldwin HJ, Corman VM, Klose SM, Owusu M, et al. (2013) Human Betacoronavirus 2c EMC/2012-related Viruses in Bats, Ghana and Europe. Emerg Infect Dis 19: 456–459.
11. Lau SK, Li KS, Tsang AK, Lam CS, Ahmed S, et al. (2013) Genetic Characterization of Betacoronavirus Lineage C Viruses in Bats Reveals Marked Sequence Divergence in the Spike Protein of Pipistrellus Bat Coronavirus HKU5 in Japanese Pipistrelle: Implications for the Origin of the Novel Middle East Respiratory Syndrome Coronavirus. J Virol 87: 8638–8650.
12. Anthony SJ, Ojeda-Flores R, Rico-Chavez O, Navarrete-Macias I, Zambrana-Torrelio CM, et al. (2013) Coronaviruses in bats from Mexico. J Gen Virol 94: 1028–1038.
13. Reusken CB, Haagmans BL, Muller MA, Gutierrez C, Godeke GJ, et al. (2013) Middle East respiratory syndrome coronavirus neutralising serum antibodies in dromedary camels: a comparative serological study. Lancet Infect Dis 13: 859–866.
14. Ithete NL, Stoffberg S, Corman VM, Cottontail VM, Richards LR, et al. (2013) Close relative of human Middle East respiratory syndrome coronavirus in bat, South Africa. Emerg Infect Dis 19: 1697–1699.
15. Perera RA, Wang P, Gomaa MR, El-Shesheny R, Kandeil A, et al. (2013) Seroepidemiology for MERS coronavirus using microneutralisation and pseudoparticle virus neutralisation assays reveal a high prevalence of antibody in dromedary camels in Egypt, June 2013. Euro Surveill 18: pii = 20574.
16. Memish ZA, Mishra N, Olival KJ, Fagbo SF, Kapoor V, et al. (2013) Middle East respiratory syndrome coronavirus in bats, Saudi Arabia. Emerg Infect Dis 19.
17. The WHO MERS-CoV Research Group (2013) State of Knowledge and Data Gaps of Middle East Respiratory Syndrome Coronavirus (MERS-CoV) in Humans. PLoS Curr 5.
18. van Elden LJ, van Loon AM, van Alphen F, Hendriksen KA, Hoepelman AI, et al. (2004) Frequent detection of human coronaviruses in clinical specimens from patients with respiratory tract infection by use of a novel real-time reverse-transcriptase polymerase chain reaction. J Infect Dis 189: 652–657.
19. Mackay IM, Arden KE, Speicher DJ, O'Neil NT, McErlean PK, et al. (2012) Co-circulation of four human coronaviruses (HCoVs) in Queensland children with acute respiratory tract illnesses in 2004. Viruses 4: 637–653.
20. Vabret A, Mourez T, Gouarin S, Petitjean J, Freymuth F (2003) An outbreak of coronavirus OC43 respiratory infection in Normandy, France. Clin Infect Dis 36: 985–989.
21. Vabret A, Dina J, Gouarin S, Petitjean J, Tripey V, et al. (2008) Human (non-severe acute respiratory syndrome) coronavirus infections in hospitalised children in France. Journal of Paediatrics and Child Health 44: 176–181.
22. Falsey AR, McCann RM, Hall WJ, Criddle MM, Formica MA, et al. (1997) The "common cold" in frail older persons: impact of rhinovirus and coronavirus in a senior daycare center. J Am Geriatr Soc 45: 706–711.
23. Graat JM, Schouten EG, Heijnen ML, Kok FJ, Pallast EG, et al. (2003) A prospective, community-based study on virologic assessment among elderly people with and without symptoms of acute respiratory infection. J Clin Epidemiol 56: 1218–1223.
24. Drosten C, Seilmaier M, Corman VM, Hartmann W, Scheible G, et al. (2013) Clinical features and virological analysis of a case of Middle East respiratory syndrome coronavirus infection. Lancet Infect Dis 13: 745–751.
25. Zaki AM, van Boheemen S, Bestebroer TM, Osterhaus AD, Fouchier RA (2012) Isolation of a novel coronavirus from a man with pneumonia in Saudi Arabia. N Engl J Med 367: 1814–1820.
26. Penttinen PM, Kaasik-Aaslav K, Friaux A, Donachie A, Sudre B, et al. (2013) Taking stock of the first 133 MERS coronavirus cases globally - Is the epidemic changing? Euro Surveill 18.
27. Assiri A, Al-Tawfiq JA, Al-Rabeeah AA, Al-Rabiah FA, Al-Hajjar S, et al. (2013) Epidemiological, demographic, and clinical characteristics of 47 cases of Middle East respiratory syndrome coronavirus disease from Saudi Arabia: a descriptive study. Lancet Infect Dis 13: 752–761.
28. Prill MM, Iwane MK, Edwards KM, Williams JV, Weinberg GA, et al. (2012) Human Coronavirus in Young Children Hospitalized for Acute Respiratory Illness and Asymptomatic Controls. The Pediatric Infectious Disease Journal Publish Ahead of Print:10.1097/INF.1090b1013e31823e31807fe.
29. Dare RK, Fry AM, Chittaganpitch M, Sawanpanyalert P, Olsen SJ, et al. (2007) Human coronavirus infections in rural Thailand: a comprehensive study using real-time reverse-transcription polymerase chain reaction assays. J Infect Dis 196: 1321–1328.
30. McIntosh K (2012) Proving etiologic relationships to disease: the particular problem of human coronaviruses. Pediatr Infect Dis J 31: 241–242.
31. Njouom R, Yekwa EL, Cappy P, Vabret A, Boisier P, et al. (2012) Viral etiology of influenza-like illnesses in Cameroon, January-December 2009. J Infect Dis 206 Suppl 1: S29–35.
32. Techiman Municipal Health Directorate (2010) Annual Report. Techiman, Brong Ahafo Region. 1–27 p.
33. Ghana Statistical Service (2010) Population and Housing Census. Accra.
34. Ghana Statistical Service (2000) Population and Housing Census. Accra.
35. Sekyere Central District Assembly (2010) Sekyere Central District. Ashanti Region: Sekyere Central District Assembly.
36. Corman VM, Eckerle I, Bleicker T, Zaki A, Landt O, et al. (2012) Detection of a novel human coronavirus by real-time reverse-transcription polymerase chain reaction. Euro Surveill 17.
37. R Development Core Team (2008) A language and environment for statistical computing. R Foundation for Statistical Computing. Vienna, Austria.
38. Hadley Wickham (2009) ggplot2: elegant graphics for data analysis: Springer New York.
39. Pfefferle S, Oppong S, Drexler J, Gloza-Rausch F, Ipsen A, et al. (2009) Distant relatives of severe acute respiratory syndrome coronavirus and close relatives of human coronavirus 229E in bats, Ghana.
40. Annan A, Baldwin HJ, Corman VM, Klose SM, Owusu M, et al. (2013) Human betacoronavirus 2c EMC/2012–related viruses in bats, Ghana and Europe. Emerging infectious diseases 19: 456.
41. McIntosh K, Chao RK, Krause HE, Wasil R, Mocega HE, et al. (1974) Coronavirus Infection in Acute Lower Respiratory Tract Disease of Infants. Journal of Infectious Diseases 130: 502–507.

42. Jartti T, Lehtinen P, Vuorinen T, Koskenvuo M, Ruuskanen O (2004) Persistence of rhinovirus and enterovirus RNA after acute respiratory illness in children. J Med Virol 72: 695–699.
43. Herberhold S, Eis-Hubinger AM, Panning M (2009) Frequent detection of respiratory viruses by real-time PCR in adenoid samples from asymptomatic children. J Clin Microbiol 47: 2682–2683.
44. Sato M, Li H, Ikizler MR, Werkhaven JA, Williams JV, et al. (2009) Detection of viruses in human adenoid tissues by use of multiplex PCR. J Clin Microbiol 47: 771–773.
45. Ren L, Gonzalez R, Xu J, Xiao Y, Li Y, et al. (2011) Prevalence of human coronaviruses in adults with acute respiratory tract infections in Beijing, China. J Med Virol 83: 291–297.
46. Cui LJ, Zhang C, Zhang T, Lu RJ, Xie ZD, et al. (2011) Human Coronaviruses HCoV-NL63 and HCoV-HKU1 in Hospitalized Children with Acute Respiratory Infections in Beijing, China. Adv Virol 2011: 129134.
47. Cannell JJ, Vieth R, Umhau JC, Holick MF, Grant WB, et al. (2006) Epidemic influenza and vitamin D. Epidemiol Infect 134: 1129–1140.
48. Shaman J, Kohn M (2009) Absolute humidity modulates influenza survival, transmission, and seasonality. Proc Natl Acad Sci U S A 106: 3243–3248.
49. Adefolalu DO (1984) On bioclimatological aspects of Harmattan dust haze in Nigeria. Archives for meteorology, geophysics, and bioclimatology, Series B 33: 387–404.
50. Niang M, Diop O, Sarr F, Goudiaby D, Malou-Sompy H, et al. (2010) Viral etiology of respiratory infections in children under 5 years old living in tropical rural areas of Senegal: The EVIRA project. Journal of medical virology 82: 866–872.
51. Dominguez SR, Sims GE, Wentworth DE, Halpin RA, Robinson CC, et al. (2012) Genomic analysis of 16 Colorado human NL63 coronaviruses identifies a new genotype, high sequence diversity in the N-terminal domain of the spike gene and evidence of recombination. J Gen Virol 93: 2387–2398.

2

Quantification of Shared Air: A Social and Environmental Determinant of Airborne Disease Transmission

Robin Wood[1]*, Carl Morrow[1], Samuel Ginsberg[2], Elizabeth Piccoli[1], Darryl Kalil[1], Angelina Sassi[1], Rochelle P. Walensky[3], Jason R. Andrews[4]

1 Desmond Tutu HIV Centre, Institute of Infectious Diseases and Molecular Medicine, and Department of Medicine, University of Cape Town Faculty of Health Sciences, Cape Town, South Africa, **2** Department of Electrical Engineering, Faculty of Engineering & the Built Environment, University of Cape Town, Cape Town, South Africa, **3** Center for AIDS Research, Harvard Medical School, Boston, Massachusetts, United States of America, **4** Division of Infectious Diseases and Geographic Medicine, Stanford University School of Medicine, Stanford, California, United States of America

Abstract

Background: Tuberculosis is endemic in Cape Town, South Africa where a majority of the population become tuberculosis infected before adulthood. While social contact patterns impacting tuberculosis and other respiratory disease spread have been studied, the environmental determinants driving airborne transmission have not been quantified.

Methods: Indoor carbon dioxide levels above outdoor levels reflect the balance of exhaled breath by room occupants and ventilation. We developed a portable monitor to continuously sample carbon dioxide levels, which were combined with social contact diary records to estimate daily rebreathed litres. A pilot study established the practicality of monitor use up to 48-hours. We then estimated the daily volumes of air rebreathed by adolescents living in a crowded township.

Results: One hundred eight daily records were obtained from 63 adolescents aged between 12- and 20-years. Forty-five lived in wooden shacks and 18 in brick-built homes with a median household of 4 members (range 2–9). Mean daily volume of rebreathed air was 120.6 (standard error: 8.0) litres/day, with location contributions from household (48%), school (44%), visited households (4%), transport (0.5%) and other locations (3.4%). Independent predictors of daily rebreathed volumes included household type ($p = 0.002$), number of household occupants ($p = 0.021$), number of sleeping space occupants ($p = 0.022$) and winter season ($p < 0.001$).

Conclusions: We demonstrated the practical measurement of carbon dioxide levels to which individuals are exposed in a sequence of non-steady state indoor environments. A novel metric of rebreathed air volume reflects social and environmental factors associated with airborne infection and can identify locations with high transmission potential.

Editor: Stefano Merler, Fondazione Bruno Kessler, Italy

Funding: This work was supported by the National Institute of Allergy and Infectious Diseases [R01 AI058736 to RW, RPW, CM; R01 AI093269 to RPW, RW; U01 AI069519 and U01 AI069926 to RW; and K01 AI104411 to JRA]. The funders had no role in study design, data collection, analysis, decision to publish, or preparation of the manuscript.

Competing Interests: The authors have declared that no competing interests exist.

* Email: Robin.Wood@uct.ac.za

Introduction

South Africa has one of the highest population notification rates of tuberculosis (TB) in the world with approximately 1% of population diagnosed with TB disease each year [1,2]. The annual risk of infection of children in Cape townships has remained high for decades, [3] and currently 5% to 8% of township adolescents become TB-infected each year [4–6]. A majority of the Cape Town population therefore becomes TB-infected before adulthood [4–6]. Molecular epidemiologic evidence indicates that most infections occur outside of households [7,8]; however, the specific locations where TB transmission is occurring remain undefined.

The contribution of social deprivation to endemic TB has been debated both before and after *Mycobacterium tuberculosis* was identified as the etiologic agent causing TB [9–11]. In the 1950's, the work of Riley and Wells defined TB transmission on a purely physical basis related to the volume of air respired by a susceptible individual and the concentration of exhaled quanta capable of establishing infection [12,13]. Infectious quanta are micronuclei (<4 microns), which remain airborne and survive for prolonged periods, diffuse throughout indoor spaces and are diluted by infection-free ventilation [12,13]. In poor communities with high TB prevalence, social interactions frequently occur in crowded and poorly ventilated indoor locations resulting in high probability of TB transmission [14].

Several studies have used the Riley and Wells model to estimate TB transmission risks in specific single locations (e.g. hospital wards) [15–20]. However, estimation of contributions from multiple locations to TB infection risk is complex as the exposure time, social-mixing and ventilation differ in each location. Cape township social contacts occur in a variety of indoor locations including households, school classrooms, work places and public

Transportation [21,22]. Therefore, TB transmission risk may be determined by the quantity of infected air respired in each location.

Carbon dioxide (CO_2) is a natural tracer gas produced during normal human respiration. Exhaled breath contains approximately 40 000 parts per million (ppm) of CO_2 compared with approximately 400 ppm in outdoor air [23]. Our study location in Masiphumelele, a township located 40 km from Cape Town, had an average level of 390.8 ppm of CO_2 in 2012 (IQR: 389.5–391.47) [24]. In the absence of other sources, indoor CO_2 levels reflect exhaled breath (respiration) and air exchange (ventilation) [25,26]. Rudnick and Milton demonstrated that measuring "excess" CO_2 in indoor air can be used to estimate the fraction of air in each inhalation that has been exhaled from other room occupants, and that the "rebreathed fraction" can estimate risk of infection with airborne particles [25]. The equation derived by Rudnick and Milton expanded upon the work of Wells and Riley and used rebreathed fraction to substitute for the more difficult analysis of room ventilation and size. We postulated that the sum of rebreathed air volumes (RAV) from others during normal indoor activities would allow quantification of the social and environmental factors impacting TB transmission. We therefore developed a portable CO_2 logging device to continuously measure the levels of CO_2 to which township adolescents were exposed and to thereby determine RAV in all visited indoor locations during a 24-hour period.

Materials and Methods

CO_2 and Global Positioning System logger

A portable logger [Figure 1] was designed to measure CO_2 concentration, temperature and humidity every 60 seconds, using the COZIR *Ambient 0–1%* transducer (Gas Sensing Solutions Ltd, Glasgow, United Kingdom, http://www.cozir.com/), together with location data captured from a global positioning system (GPS) receiver and time from an onboard, independently powered clock. The logger's dimensions were 10×6×2.5 centimetres and component costs were approximately $250.

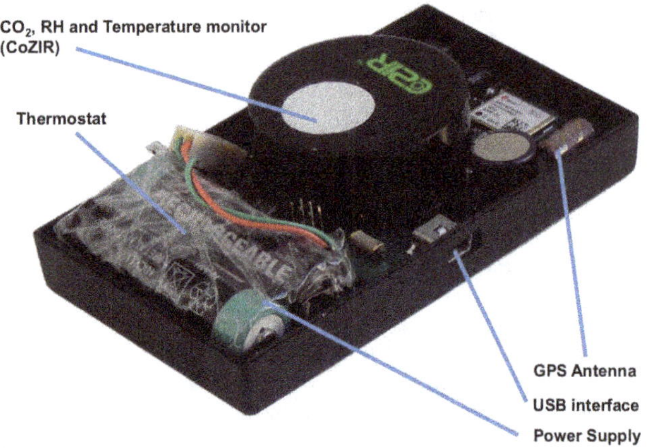

Figure 1. Portable logger to measure CO_2 concentration, temperature and humidity. An internal view of the portable personal CO_2 logger incorporated a COZIR Ambient 0–1% transducer (Gas Sensing Solutions Ltd., Glasgow, United Kingdom), GPS sensor, independent power supply and USB interface. Unit dimensions were length 10 cm, width 6 cm and depth 2.5 cm.

The data are delivered to the microcontroller device in serial digital format, which is then stored on flash memory. The microcontroller device can then retrieve flash memory data, on demand, for uploading to a computer via a Universal Serial Bus (USB) port. The logger is powered by Nickel Metal Hydride (NiMH) batteries and includes circuitry for recharging from external power sources. For safety purposes, the electronic circuitry is fused to prevent current in either discharge or charge mode from exceeding safe limits. In addition, a thermostat device has been incorporated to cut the battery from the circuit should battery temperature exceed 70 degrees Celsius. The accuracy of CO_2 measurements taken by the sensor is ±50 ppm or 3% of each reading (www.cozir.com).

Time-location diary

A time-location diary was provided to all participants to capture daily routine data including date, location type, time of arrival and departure, and numbers of individuals present for all locations visited. Each diary was filled out continuously, and a field worker clarified incomplete diary entries. The diaries were then entered into a database and were later rechecked by a research assistant. Twenty location types were aggregated to 5 major location categories for data analysis: school/work (daytime activity), transport, own home, other household, and other places. This instrument had been previously used for a social contact study in this community [19].

Air sampling

Participants underwent training on how to use and recharge the logger, and complete the diary. The logger was attached to a provided lanyard (~50 cm) or worn in a waist pocket during a 48-hour period. Participants were instructed not to breathe directly into the logger. Sets of more than 1 100 logged environmental data points recorded during any 24-hour period were used in subsequent analyses.

Pilot study

A pilot study established the practicality of carrying the logger for 48 hours, including position on person, battery recharging procedures and recording of location data in the diary. A heterogeneous sample (15 females and 2 males) with a median age of 39-years (range: 21–63 years) was recruited from the clinical, research and secretarial staff of the Desmond Tutu HIV Centre at the University of Cape Town. The subjects provided 29 daily records with an overall mean RAV of 58.6 (standard error [SE] 11.4) litres per day [Figure 2]. Volume contributions by location were highly variable; mean RAV in transport was 7.1 (SE 3.4) litres per day but with up to 85.5 litres per day recorded in public transport. The location contributions to daily-RAV were 12.4% for transport, 50.3% for own and visited households, 26.8% for workplace and 10.4% for various other locations. The pilot study population was a low TB risk group as no TB diagnoses had been made in the prior 10 years.

Adolescent study population

A high-TB risk study population of 63 adolescents (37 female, 26 male) with a median age of 17-years (range: 12–20 years) was recruited at the Desmond Tutu Youth Centre in Masiphumelele, Cape Town; a poor community where the annual TB notification rate exceeds 2000 cases per 100 000 [27].

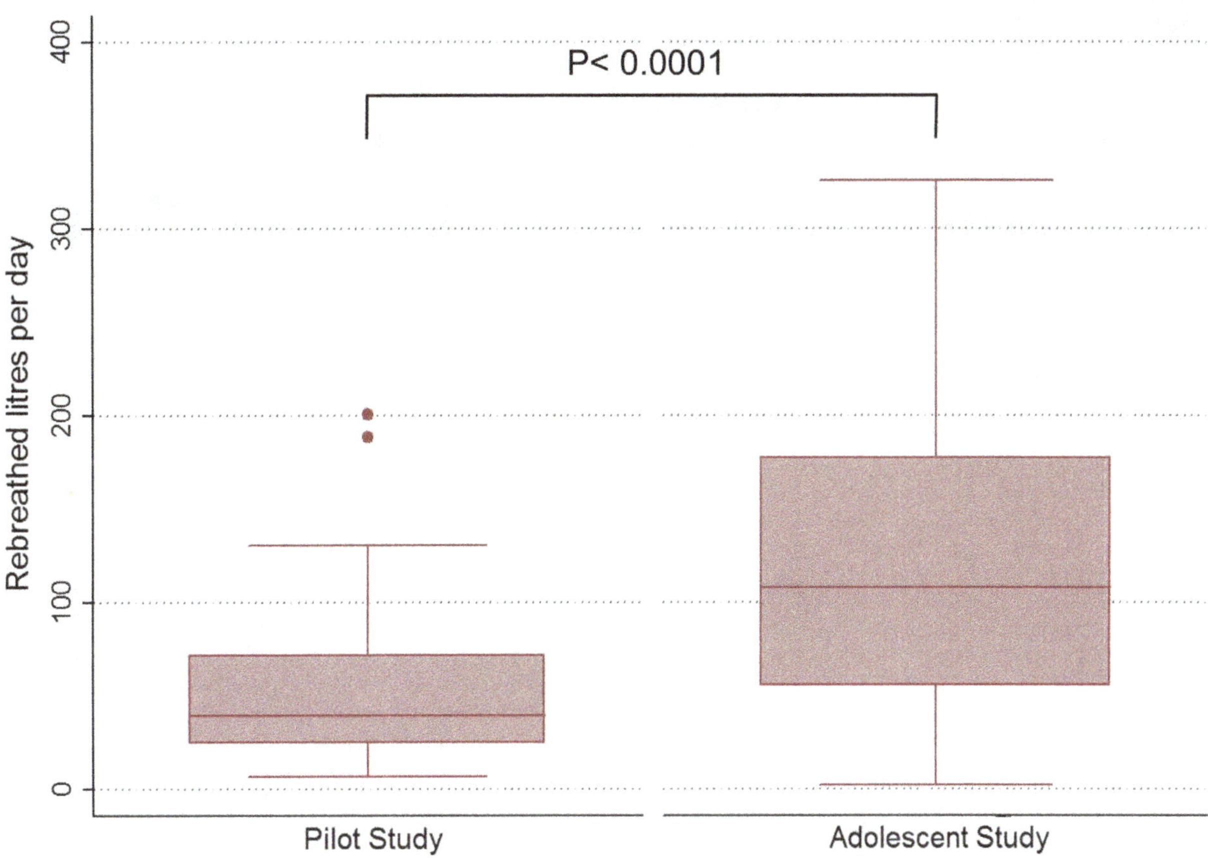

Figure 2. Daily volumes of rebreathed air in the pilot study and the adolescent study. Pilot study (left bar) shows median, inter-quartile ranges and maximum and minimum daily volumes of rebreathed air from others for 17 adults providing 29 daily records. Adolescent study (right bar) shows median, inter-quartile ranges and maximum and minimum daily volumes of rebreathed air of 108 daily records from 63 adolescents living in a high TB prevalence township. N.B. A single outlier value of 550 litres per day for the adolescent study is not shown as it exceeds the maximal value of the ordinate scale.

Data processing and analysis

The data were downloaded as text files and entered into a customised Microsoft Access database. The diary data and times were aligned with the CO_2 values and corresponding times recorded by the CO_2 logger. The time period of interest was identified and the rebreathed values were calculated against the lowest CO_2 value measured in the 24-hour time period. Small gaps in the environmental data capturing were observed and these were filled using an automated algorithm that identified gaps in the trace of more than one minute in length, averaged the starting and ending rebreathed values, multiplied the result by the period of the gap to estimate rebreathed air during the gap. This value was distributed between the beginning and end point of the gap.

Rebreathed proportions were calculated using Rudnick and Milton's equation as shown [25]:

$$f = \frac{C - Co}{Ca} \tag{1}$$

Where f is equivalent to the fraction of air that is exhaled breath, C is the observed concentration of CO_2 in the indoor air, Co is the concentration of CO_2 in the outdoor air and Ca is the concentration of CO_2 in the exhaled air (estimated from literature) [23]. In other words, the proportion of air that is being rebreathed can be estimated from the excess carbon dioxide observed in the room, divided by the concentration of carbon dioxide in exhaled breath. The outdoor CO_2 values were defined by the minimum recorded value from each 24-hour record set. For persons at low levels of physical activity, Ca was estimated to be 38,000 ppm based on a CO_2 production rate of 0.31 litres/minute and respiratory minute volume of 8.0 litres/minute [23].

The recorded number of people present in the indoor location was used to estimate the rebreathed proportion from other people:

$$fo = f \times \frac{(n-1)}{n} \tag{2}$$

Here, n is the number of people recorded at the indoor location (including the participant). RAV for each 60-second time-period was calculated from the product of fo and the minute respiratory volume, p *(8 liters per minute)*, and summed over all observations:

$$RebreathedAirVolume = \sum\nolimits_{t=1}^{j} pfo(t) \tag{3}$$

Thus, continuously recorded ambient CO_2 values [Figure 3A] can be transformed (using equations 1 and 2) into continuous

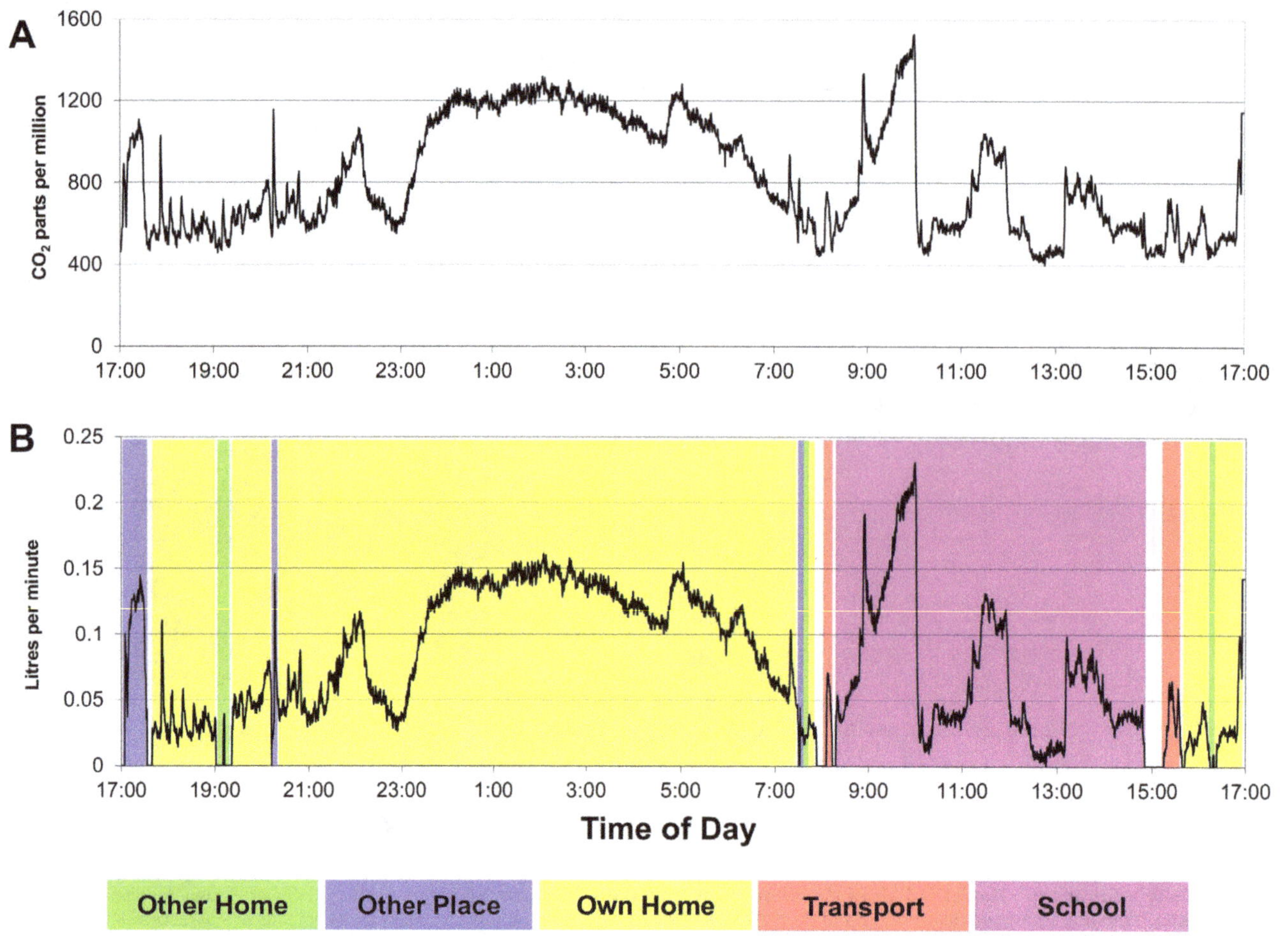

Figure 3. Figure 3 A: Ambient parts per million of CO_2 recorded at minute intervals by the logging device carried by a subject during a 24-hour period. **Figure 3 B**: Litres per minute of rebreathed air with additional allocation to specific locations. Litres per minute of rebreathed air were calculated for a 24-hour period (transformation from ambient CO_2 levels in Figure 2A) and additionally allocated to specific locations using diary and GPS information. The volume of rebreathed shared air is represented by the area under the curve for each location visited and the daily rebreathed volume is the sum of all volumes at all locations visited.

measures of rebreathed (shared) air at different visited locations [Figure 3B]. The RAV for any time-period was the sum of the 60-second rebreathed volumes accruing in that time period equal to the area under the curve of rebreathed air for the time-period of interest [Figure 3B].

We examined determinants of RAV through linear, mixed-effects, multilevel bivariate and multivariate models, including age, sex, housing type (shack/brick), season, and the number of individuals in household and sleeping space. To account for correlation in multiple, nested observations of the same individual on different days, we used a two-level model with individuals and observations. Season was dichotomized into colder months (May-October) and warmer months (November-April).[28] Because rebreathed litres were non-normally distributed, we log-transformed rebreathed litres, which reduced the skewness and kurtosis and improved the normality of the regression residuals. We further examined residual plots for the predicted, transformed dependent variables. For multivariable analyses, we used Allen-Cady, modified backward selection procedure. In this procedure, we pre-specified forced variables for inclusion (age and sex) and then used a threshold p-value of 0.20 for removal of variables of least importance. Ultimately, all considered variables were found to be under this p-value threshold and were retained [29]. We calculated conditional goodness-of-fit for the mixed-effects model using the approach of Nakagawa and Schielzeth [30]. We also used a multilevel model as above to compare rebreathed litres between adults (pilot study) and students. Statistical analyses were performed using Stata 11.0 (StataCorp, College Station, Texas, USA).

Ethics Statement

For adults, written informed consent for participation in the study was obtained while for minors, written informed assent was obtained along with written informed consent from a parent or guardian. The Human Research Ethics Committee of the Faculty of Health Sciences at the University of Cape Town approved the study.

Results

Township adolescent study

Subjects were all residents of the township, and 45 (71%) lived in a wooden shack and 18 (29%) in brick-built house. The median household size was 4 individuals (range: 4–9) and the median number of individuals sharing sleeping quarters was 2 (range: 1–5). Subjects recorded a total of 108 daily records with a median

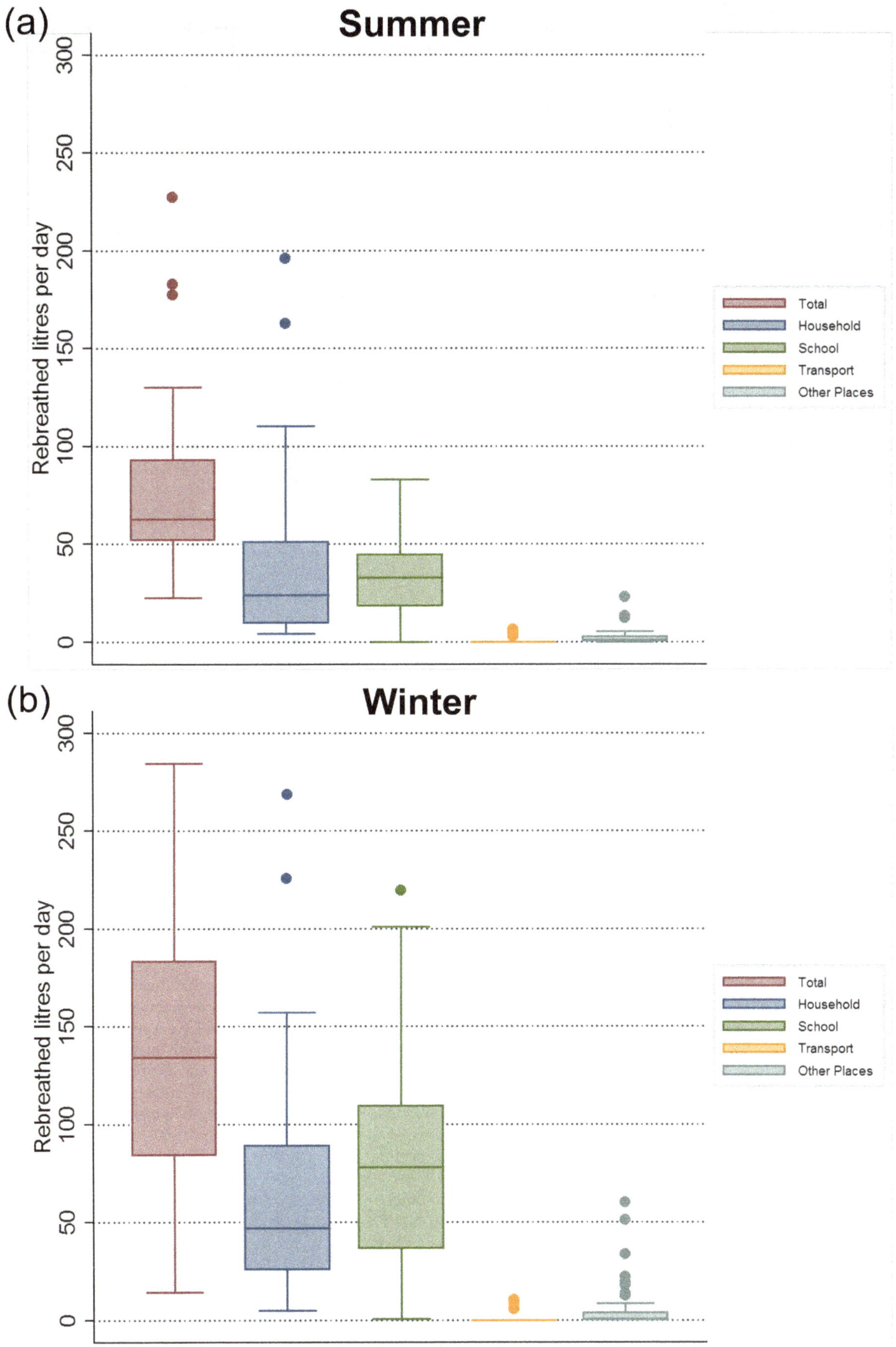
(a)
Summer
Rebreathed litres per day
0
50
100
150
200
250
300
Total
Household
School
Transport
Other Places
(b)
Winter
Rebreathed litres per day
0
50
100
150
200
250
300
Total
Household
School
Transport
Other Places

Figure 4. Figure 4 A: Volumes of rebreathed air recorded in summer months. The figure shows median, inter-quartile ranges and maximum and minimum volumes of rebreathed air from others for 28 weekdays recorded between November and April together with volume contributions from households, school attendance, transport and various other locations. **Figure 4 B**: Volumes of rebreathed air recorded in winter months. The figure shows median, inter-quartile ranges and maximum and minimum volumes of rebreathed air from others for 63 weekdays recorded between May and October together with volume contributions from households, school attendance, transport and various other locations. N.B. Two outlier values of 395 and 550 litres per day for total volumes and a single outlier of 395 for household volumes are not shown as they exceed the maximal value of the ordinate scale.

volume of air rebreathed from others of 120.6 [standard error (SE) 8.0] litres per day [Figure 2] with location contributions from own household (48%), school (44%), visited households (4%), transport (0.5%) and other locations (3.5%). While all participants rebreathed air in households every day [59.5 (SE 7.3) litres per day], only 81% (87/108) of recorded days included school attendance, with a mean RAV of 63.1 (SE 5.4) litres per day. Public transport contributed only 0.5% of total RAV of study participants as only 9 adolescents used public transport (12 recorded days) with a mean of 5.8 (SE 0.7) litres in transport per day.

Calculations of mean RAV per hour for each location type were conducted to determine the relative risk in each environment. A mean RAV of 11.5 litres per hour (SE 0.07) was recorded in schools, a mean RAV of 6.3 litres per hour in transport (SE 0.25), a mean RAV of 4.4 litres per hour in households (SE 0.02) and a mean RAV of 5.8 litres in other places (SE 0.09).

Twenty-four adolescents recorded 28 summer weekday records with a mean RAV of 79.2 (SE 9.2) litres per day and 39 adolescents recorded 65 winter weekday records with a mean RAV of 147.1 (SE 10.5) litres per day [Figure 4] ($p = 0.008$). The mean number of daily contacts in summer (16.9) and winter (14.34) did not differ ($p = 0.76$). However, the mean time spent indoors was higher in the winter (22.2 hours) than in the summer (19.4 hours) ($p<0.001$).

In order to establish if alternative locations visited during weekends might contribute to total rebreathed litres, 8 of the subjects completed 15 weekend daily records. Mean weekend litres per day (82.6; SE 20.7) were considerably lower than on weekdays (147.12; SE 10.55), with own (82%) and visited households (10%) the major contributing locations.

In multivariable analysis of the 108 adolescent daily records (Table 1), log RAV per day increased 8% per year of age, increased 14% per added household occupant, increased 17% per additional occupant of sleep space, was 77% higher in winter months and 43% lower in shacks compared with brick dwellings. The median and distribution of RAV at each indoor location are shown in Figure 4, demonstrating increased rebreathing of air in all locations during winter months with greatest impact on household and school. School was the major location of RAV contributing a mean of 77.6 litres per day in winter months.

Discussion

The transmission of communicable diseases is understood to be a function of social contact rates and the probability of transmission per contact. Recent studies have illuminated some of the structure and heterogeneity of social contacts [19–22], however, there have been few data on the role of the indoor environment for airborne infections which, as Wells and Riley demonstrated, is a key determinant of transmission [12,13]. Virtually all studies examining environmental risk for tuberculosis focus on households or outbreaks in single environments (e.g. commercial airliners, hospitals). However, studies from Cape Town and Lima have demonstrated that a minority of tuberculosis transmission occurs within households [7,8]. It has remained unclear where most transmission occurs in endemic settings. In this paper, we demonstrated the measurement of a simple metric—RAV— that integrates social contact and environmental data pertinent to transmission of small particle airborne infections.

We have demonstrated that it is practical to continuously measure ambient CO_2 concentrations surrounding an individual and thereby estimate the RAV rebreathed from others during normal daily activities. Our approach extends the work of Wells [12], Riley [13], and Rudnick [25] by enabling quantitation of exposure to infected air in multiple non-steady state environments. The sum of the contributions from all visited indoor locations allowed estimation of total daily RAV from others. Adolescents living in a high TB-burdened community recorded very large daily volumes of rebreathed air, such that calculated annual RAV would reach between (IQR) 20 000 to 65 000 litres. Township adolescents had higher RAV compared with our pilot study adults ($p<0.0001$).

We were able to allocate 93% of rebreathed air to 4 locations: own home, visited homes, transport and work or school. These results corroborate findings of an earlier social mixing study performed in this community in 2010, which reported that 97% of indoor time was spent in these locations. [22] Public transportation use was minimal in this largely local school-attending adolescent population for whom school and household locations contributed the majority of RAV. The daily RAVs were nearly twice as high in the colder winter months than during summer months. The contact rates were comparable between seasons and time spent indoors in winter was only 14% higher, together indicating that increased RAVs were predominantly a result of reduced ventilation, presumably because of need for heat conservation (i.e. closed windows) in cold weather. While there is presently no data on the seasonality of TB infection, our findings may be compatible to the observed seasonality of TB disease in South Africa [31].

While earlier work has examined the role of socio-demographic contact structure in tuberculosis transmission, the role of the indoor environment has not been factored into models of endemic transmission [32].

We propose that the daily RAV may be a useful surrogate marker for the social and environmental components of TB transmission that have been so long recognised but not quantified [9–11,14]. Both the number of individuals within indoor locations and the prevailing environmental ventilation conditions impacts RAV. For an airborne disease such as TB, it is biologically plausible that the total volume exchanged with others would be a major determinant for transmission and acquisition of TB infection [33], which is also consistent with the approaches of Wells [13], Riley [14], Rudnick [25], and others [15–20]. The number of secondary active cases generated by an average person with TB in a susceptible population (the basic reproductive number, R_o) is a fundamental epidemiologic driver of TB epidemics [33]. High-RAV may therefore be a major component maintaining high levels of TB transmission in endemic township populations in Southern Africa [34].

There are several limitations to our study. The major assumption underlying the use of concentrations of inspired CO_2 as a surrogate for expired air and infection risk is that the

Table 1. Predictors of total log rebreathed litres per day in an unadjusted, multilevel analysis and in a multivariable, multilevel linear regression analysis.

	Unadjusted			Adjusted		
Predictor	**ß Coefficient**	**Exp***	**p-value**	**ß Coefficient**	**Exp***	**p-value**
Age *(per year)*	0.05	1.05	0.231	0.08	1.08	0.041
Female *(vs male)*	0.13	1.14	0.468	−0.35	0.70	0.059
Winter *(vs summer)*	0.48	1.62	0.008	0.57	1.77	<0.001
Household *(number)*	0.13	1.14	0.026	0.13	1.14	0.021
Sleep space *(number)*	0.15	1.16	0.041	0.16	1.17	0.022
Shack *(vs brick house)*	−0.44	0.64	0.021	−0.56	0.57	0.002
Weekend *(vs weekday)*	−0.64	0.53	<0.001			

Multivariable model conditional goodness-of-fit: 0.73.
*Exponent of ß coefficient, indicating magnitude of change in daily rebreathed volume per unit change in predictor or binary comparator.

dispersion of CO_2 within an enclosed space reflects the dispersal of infectious particles within that space. According to Stoke's Law, which states that "the nuclei of most droplets atomized indoors shall remain in atmospheric suspension until they are breathed or vented or until they die", small particles such as TB would not be limited by settling [12]. However, CO_2 is a highly diffusible gas. CO_2 decay curves have been widely used for ventilation estimation [35]. Ambient levels of CO_2 have been long used as a measure of air quality [26], mechanical ventilation control [36] and for airborne disease modelling [25]. CO_2 concentrations were not sensitive to height of the logger in a room or whether the logger was located on a lanyard or in a waist pocket (data not shown). In order to minimize any direct exposure to exhaled air, the subjects were advised to wear the logger well away from the face and only near the waist. A further caveat to the use of the CO_2 tracer gas methodology is the assumption that humans are the sole source of CO_2 in the environments studied. We did require that participants record if there was an obvious alternative source of CO_2, such as open flame heat sources. However, other less obvious CO_2 sources such as the degradation of biological material in earthen floors could possibly impact measurements in informal dwellings [37]. Consistent with prior literature, we assumed that ventilation, rather than CO_2 absorption or other forms of removal, is the dominant driver of CO_2 removal from indoor settings [23]. The finding of lower volumes of rebreathed air in shacks compared with brick built structures is compatible with structural leakages which contribute to ventilation, and would also indicate that unsealed, earthen floors did not contribute majorly to household CO_2 levels. The proportion of RAV from others is also dependent on the accurate recording in the daily diary of person numbers in each indoor location. The precision of recording of small numbers in locations impacts results, but accuracy becomes less important with increased occupancy numbers. If a recording error resulted in 25 persons being recorded as only 20 persons or 50 persons as 40 persons, the errors in rebreathed air would be only 1% and 0.5% respectively. Additionally, the findings of these studies may not be generalizable to other population groups, as the pilot study population was a heterogeneous convenience sample, while the adolescent study was performed in an age-restricted population from a high TB transmission community. Repeated measurements from a small number of schools may underestimate the population variability of RAV. We recorded only up to two daily measurements per person, and additional studies will be required to illuminate the intra-individual variability in rebreathed litres. Finally, the mixed-effect multivariable linear regression analysis was intended to be hypothesis-generating in this study. We had a limited sample size of 93 observations from 63 individuals for the full model. While the design effect was small, there is a possibility of over-fitting, and larger studies are needed to validate these findings.

Conclusions

In summary, we have demonstrated the practical measurement of CO_2 over time in a sequence of non-steady state indoor environments, which, combined with data on number of room occupants, enabled the estimation of daily RAV from others. This approach enables comparison of composite social and environmental risk between individuals, settings, and exploration of the determinants of risk (e.g., season). In adolescents residing in a high burden community, this revealed marked variability in RAV between individuals and locations. Future work will be needed to validate this metric by assessing its ability to predict tuberculosis and other respiratory infection risk, which will require larger studies. Continuous monitoring of CO_2 and subsequent quantification of rebreathed air has great potential as a tool to inform public health interventions targeted at reducing the transmission of airborne respiratory diseases.

Author Contributions

Conceived and designed the experiments: RW CM SG. Performed the experiments: CM SG EP DK AS. Analyzed the data: CM EP DK AS JRA. Contributed to the writing of the manuscript: RW CM SG DK AS RPW JRA.

References

1. World Health Organization (2012) Global Tuberculosis Report 2012. Geneva, Switzerland: WHO; available at http://www.who.int/tb/publications/global_report/gtbr12_main.pdf (15 October 2013, date last accessed).
2. Wood R, Lawn SD, Caldwell J, Kaplan R, Middelkoop K, et al. (2011) Burden of new and recurrent tuberculosis in a major South African city stratified by age and HIV status. PLoS ONE 6(10):e25098.
3. Kritzinger FE, den Boon S, Verver S, Enarson DA, Lombard CJ, et al. (2009) No decrease in annual risk of tuberculosis infection in endemic area in Cape Town, South Africa. Trop Med Int Health 14(2):136–42.
4. Middelkoop K, Bekker LG, Myer L, Dawson R, Wood R (2008) Rates of tuberculosis transmission to children and adolescents in a community with a high prevalence of HIV infection among adults. Clin Infect Dis 47(3):349–55.
5. Wood R, Liang H, Wu H, Middelkoop K, Oni T, et al. (2010) Changing prevalence of TB infection with increasing age in high-TB burden townships in South Africa. Int J Tuberc Lung Dis 14(4):406–12.
6. Middelkoop K, Bekker L-G, Liang H, Aquino LD, Sebastian E, et al. (2011) Force of tuberculosis infection among adolescents in a high HIV and TB prevalence community: a cross-sectional observation study. BMC Infect Dis 11: 156.
7. Verver S, Warren RM, Munch Z, Richardson M, van der Spuy GD, et al. (2004) Proportion of tuberculosis transmission that takes place in households in a high-incidence area. Lancet 363(9404):212–14.
8. Brooks-Pollock E, Becerra MC, Goldstein E, Cohen T, Murray MB (2011) Epidemiologic inference from the distribution of tuberculosis cases in households in Lima, Peru. J Infect Dis 203(11):1582–89.
9. Murphy S, Egger M (2002) Studies of the social causes of tuberculosis in Germany before the First World War: extracts from Mosse and Tugendreich's landmark book. Int J Epidemiol 31(4):742–49.
10. Reider HL (1999) Socialization patterns are key to the transmission dynamics of tuberculosis. Int J Tuberc Lung Dis 3(3):177–78.
11. Ho MJ (2004) Sociocultural aspects of tuberculosis: a literature review and a case study of immigrant tuberculosis. Soc Sci Med 59(4):753–762.
12. Wells WF (1955 Airborne contagion and air hygiene: an ecological study of droplet infections. Cambridge (MA): Harvard University Press.
13. Riley RL, Wells WF, Mills CC, Nyka W, McLean RL (1957) Air hygiene in tuberculosis: quantitative studies of infectivity and control in a pilot ward. Am Rev Tuberc 75(3):420–31.
14. Chapman JS, Dyerly MD (1964) Social and other factors in intrafamilial transmission of tuberculosis. Am Rev Respir Dis 90: 48–60.
15. Cantazaro A (1982) Nosocomial tuberculosis. Am Rev Respir Dis 125(5):559–62.
16. Ko G, Thompson KM, Nardell EA (2004) Estimations of tuberculosis risk on a commercial airliner. Risk Anal 24(2):379–88.
17. Noakes CJ, Sleigh PA (2009) Mathematical models for assessing the role of airflow on the risk of airborne infection in hospital wards. J R Soc Interface 6: 791–800.
18. Furuya H, Nagamine M, Watanabe T (2009) Use of a mathematical model to estimate tuberculosis transmission risk in an Internet café. Environ Health Prev Med 14(2):96–102.
19. Wood R, Johnstone-Robertson S, Uys P, Hargrove J, Middelkoop K, et al. (2010) Tuberculosis transmission to young children in a South African community: modeling household and community infection risks. Clin Infect Dis 51(4):401–8.
20. Johnstone-Robertson S, Lawn SD, Welte A, Bekker L-G, Wood R (2011) Tuberculosis in a South African prison - a transmission modeling analysis. S Afr Med J 101(11):809–13.
21. Johnstone-Robertson S, Mark D, Morrow C, Middelkoop K, Bekker L-G, et al. (2011) Social mixing patterns within a South African township community: implications for respiratory disease transmission and control. Am J Epidemiol 174(11):1246–55.
22. Wood R, Racow K, Bekker L-G, Morrow C, Middelkoop K, et al. (2012) Indoor social networks in a South African township: potential contribution of location to tuberculosis transmission. PLoS One 7(6):e39246.
23. Emmerlich SJ, Persily AK (2001) State-of-the-art review of CO_2 demand controlled ventilation technology and application. National Institute of Standards and Technology; available at http://fire.nist.gov/bfrlpubs/build01/PDF/b01117.pdf (19 December 2013, date last accessed).
24. South African Weather Service (2012) CO_2 Cape Point – SAWS. Stellenbosch, South Africa: World Data Centre for Greenhouse Gases; available at http://ds.data.jma.go.jp/gmd/wdcgg/cgi-bin/wdcgg/accessdata.cgi?index = CPT134S00-SAWS¶m = 200612120113&select = parameter¶c = observation (19 December 2013, date last accessed).
25. Rudnick SN, Milton DK (2003) Risk of indoor airborne infection transmission estimated from carbon dioxide concentration. Indoor Air 13(3):237–45.
26. Chaumont F (1874) On the theory of ventilation: an attempt to establish a positive basis for the calculation of the amount of fresh air required for an inhabited airspace. Proc R Soc Lond; 23: 187–201.
27. Middelkoop K, Bekker L-G, Myer L, Johnson LF, Kloos M, et al. (2011) Antiretroviral therapy and TB notification rates in a high HIV prevalence South African community. J Acquir Immune Defic Syndr 56(3):263–69.
28. Average maximum and minimum monthly temperature for Cape Town. World weather on line; available at http://www.worldweatheronline.com/Cape-Town-weather/Western-Cape/ZA.aspx (16 October 2013, date last accessed).
29. Vittinghoff E, Glidden D, Shiboski S, McCulloch C (2004) Regression Methods in Biostatistics. New York: Springer.
30. Nakagawa S, Schielzeth H (2013) A general and simple method for obtaining R^2 from generalized linear mixed-effects models. Methods Ecol Evol 4: 133–142
31. Martineau AR, Nhamoyebonde S, Oni T, Rangaka MX, Marais S, et al. (2011) Reciprocal seasonal variation in vitamin D status and tuberculosis notifications in Cape Town, South Africa. Proc Natl Acad Sci U S A 108(47):19013–17.
32. Guzzetta G, Ajelli M, Yang Z, Merler S, Furlanello C, et al. (2011) Modeling socio-demography to capture tuberculosis transmission dynamics in a low burden setting. J Theor Bio 289: 197–205
33. Reider HL (1999) Epidemiological basis of tuberculosis control. Paris: International Union Against Tuberculosis and Lung Disease.
34. Wood R, Lawn SD, Johnstone-Robertson S, Bekker L-G (2011) Tuberculosis control has failed in South Africa - time to reappraise strategy. S Afr Med J 101(2):111–14.
35. American Society for Testing and Materials (1998) Standard Guide for Using Indoor Carbon Dioxide Concentrations to Evaluate Indoor Air Quality and Ventilation. West Conshohoken, PA: American Society for Testing and Materials. D6245–98.
36. Menzies R, Schwartzman K, Loo V, Pasztor J (1995) Measuring ventilation of patient care areas in hospitals. Description of a new protocol. Am J Respir Crit Care Med 152(6):1992–99.
37. Raich JW, Schleslinger WH (1992) The global carbon dioxide flux in soil respiration and its relationship to vegetation and climate. Tellus 44(2):81–99.

3

Latent Tuberculosis Infection and Occupational Protection among Health Care Workers in Two Types of Public Hospitals in China

Feng Zhou[1,2], Li Zhang[2], Lei Gao[3], Yibin Hao[4], Xianli Zhao[5], Jianmin Liu[5], Jie Lu[6], Xiangwei Li[3], Yu Yang[3], Junguo Chen[1]*, Ying Deng[2]*

1 Third Military Medical University, Chongqing, China, **2** Beijing Center for Disease Prevention and Control, Beijing Research Center of Preventive Medicine, Beijing, China, **3** MOH Key Laboratory of Systems Biology of Pathogens, Institute of Pathogen Biology, Chinese Academy of Medical Sciences and Peking Union Medical College, Beijing, China, **4** Zhengzhou Central Hospital, Zhengzhou, China, **5** Henan Provincial Infectious Disease Hospital, Zhengzhou, China, **6** School of Public Health, Zhengzhou University, Zhengzhou, China

Abstract

Objective: To determine the impact factors of latent tuberculosis infection (LTBI) and the knowledge of TB prevention and treatment policy among health care workers (HCWs) in different types of hospitals and explore the strategies for improving TB prevention and control in medical institutions in China.

Methods: A cross-sectional study was carried out to evaluate the risk of TB infection and personnel occupational protection among HCWs who directly engage in medical duties in one of two public hospitals. Each potential participant completed a structured questionnaire and performed a tuberculin skin test (TST). Factors associated with LTBI were identified by logistic regression analysis.

Results: Seven hundred twelve HCWs completed questionnaires and 74.3% (n = 529) took the TST or had previous positive results. The TST-positive prevalence was 58.0% (n = 127) in the infectious disease hospital and 33.9% (n = 105) in the non-TB hospital. The duration of employment in the healthcare profession (6–10 years vs. ≤5 years [OR = 1.89; 95% CI = 1.10, 3.25] and>10 vs. ≤5[OR = 1.80; 95% CI = 1.20, 2.68]), type of hospital (OR = 2.40; 95% CI = 1.59, 3.62), and ever-employment in a HIV clinic or ward (OR = 1.87; 95% CI = 1.08, 3.26)were significantly associated with LTBI. The main reasons for an unwillingness to accept TST were previous positive TST results (70.2%) and concerns about skin reaction (31.9%).

Conclusion: A high prevalence of TB infections was observed among HCWs working in high-risk settings and with long professional experiences in Henan Province in China. Comprehensive guidelines should be developed for different types of medical institutions to reduce TB transmission and ensure the health of HCWs.

Editor: Julian W. Tang, Alberta Provincial Laboratory for Public Health/University of Alberta, Canada

Funding: This work was supported by the grants from the Institute of Pathogen Biology, Chinese Academy of Medical Science (IPB2011IPB104). The funders had no role in study design, data collection and analysis, decision to publish, or preparation of the manuscript.

Competing Interests: The authors have declared that no competing interests exist.

* Email: cqchenjunguo@sina.com (JC); ydeng2014@sina.com (YD)

Introduction

According to the Global Tuberculosis Report from the World Health Organization (WHO), tuberculosis (TB) remains a major global health problem. In 2011, 1.4 million people died of TB, and after the human immunodeficiency virus (HIV),TB ranks as the second leading cause of death from an infectious disease worldwide [1]. The occupational risk of TB among health care workers was demonstrated in the pre-antibiotic era [2,3]. Indeed, TB infection is a common problem in healthcare facilities [3]. With the emergence of extensively drug-resistant TB, efforts have refocused on TB infection control in healthcare facilities and occupational protection among health care workers (HCWs). The WHO issued a policy on TB infection control in health care facilities in 2009 [4]. Many high-income countries have offered detailed recommendations for latent TB infection (LTBI) screening and preventive therapy among HCWs in their TB guidelines [5]. In these countries, serial surveillance of LTBI and occupational infection control measures have been implemented as regular tasks in the TB infection control programs, and as a result, TB infections have clearly declined in number [6]; however, the situation is very different in low- and middle-income countries because of the high TB burden and limited resources [7,8,9,10]. Most TB control programs in low- and middle-income countries have focused on case detection and treatment using the DOTS strategy. A systematic review of 51 studies showed that the prevalence of LTBI and the annual incidence of TB disease in HCWs ranged from 33% to 79%and 69 to 5,780 per 100,000 in low- and middle-income countries, respectively [11].

China is one of 22 high-TB burden countries with the second largest number of cases [1]. In 2000, a nationwide survey found that 45% of Chinese had TB infections [12]. Reports from several medical institutions have shown that the average prevalence of TB infections has ranged from 49.0% to 60.4% among HCWs using a single-step TST (5 international units; 0.1 ml) [13,14]. Vaccination against TB with Bacillus Calmette-Guerin (BCG) is routinely offered to Chinese newborns. It has been reported that TST reactions ≥5 mm occur in 69% of the HCWs in Inner Mongolia, China [15]. China has established a TB prevention, treatment, and control system. All types of hospitals or community health service centers have the responsibility of finding, reporting, and referring suspected patients. Local TB centers or designated infectious disease hospitals are responsible for the diagnosis and treatment of TB patients. Local centers for disease prevention and control (CDC) or centers for TB prevention and control are in charge of epidemiologic investigations, data collection, and patient follow-up [16];however, there are no special guidelines for preventing the spread of TB in health care facilities. LTBI surveillance and risk assessment in medical institutions has not been established in China [17]. According to the Fourth National Survey, 91.2% of pulmonary TB patients are first detected in general hospitals [12]. Therefore, general hospitals should pay attention to TB infection control and occupational protection. The aim of our study was to investigate the impact factors of LTBI and the knowledge of TB prevention and treatment policy among HCWs in different types of hospitals and explore the strategies of improving TB prevention and control in medical institutions in China.

Methods

Study design and settings

A cross-sectional study was carried out to assess the risk of TB infection and the levels of personnel occupational protection among HCWs who directly engage in medical duties. The following two hospitals were involved in our survey: 1) Zhengzhou Central Hospital is a non-TB, tertiary public and general hospital with 1,400 beds and approximately 1600 HCWs; and 2) Henan Provincial Infectious Disease Hospital is an infectious disease and tertiary public infectious disease hospital with 600 beds and approximately 702 HCWs. Henan Provincial Infectious Disease Hospital is responsible for TB diagnosis, treatment, and management, and is located in Zhengzhou City. TB patients with severe complications who are referred from other cities or prefectures in Henan Province are also admitted to Henan Provincial Infectious Disease Hospital. TB patients are not admitted to Zhengzhou Central Hospital. Patients with suspected TB infections in this hospital will be referred to Henan Provincial Infectious Disease Hospital.

Participants

The sample size was determined by the number of HCWs who were directly involved in medical duties in the infectious disease hospital because our goal was to assess the influence of medical work and personnel occupational protection of HCWs on TB infection. According to the name list of this hospital, 482 HCWs in the infectious disease hospital were identified to be potential participants for our survey. The categories of departments included outpatient clinics, intensive care units, emergency, internal medicine, infectious disease, Chinese medicine, radiology, stomatology departments, and the laboratory. An equivalent number of medical staff was randomly extracted from each medical department according to the work certification number in a non-TB hospital. All of the HCWs who engaged in medical duties for more than 6 months in these two hospitals were eligible for the personal TB infection risk survey. Each HCW was recruited by their department supervisor and encouraged to complete a self-administrated and standard-structured questionnaire. A TST was performed on all potential participants unless they declined to take or were not available during the study period. The study was approved by the Ethics Committees of the Institute of Pathogen Biology, Chinese Academy of Medical Sciences & Peking Union Medical College. All HCWs provided written informed consent before recruitment.

Data collection and TST

HCWs were recruited between January and December 2011. A structured questionnaire was used for risk assessment of TB infection among HCWs, including sociodemographic characteristics (e.g., age, gender, ethnicity, education, period of professional work, and employed position), knowledge of TB prevention and control, history of professional work, clinical work, and personal occupational protection. We performed a single-step TST using 5 international units (IU; 0.1 ml) of tuberculin (Chengdu Institute of Biological Products, Chengdu, China), which produces tuberculin from *Mycobacterium bovis* BCG. The TST was administered using the Mantoux method by experienced nurses, and participants returned 48–72 hours after TST placement to obtain results, which were confirmed independently by two clinicians. The diameter of induration size was measured using a standardized ruler and the results were averaged. As the popular BCG vaccination in China, LTBI was determined using a TST induration ≥10 mm as a cut-off point for TST positivity and no TB history was reported by participants in this study. TST-positive participants were required to have an X-ray examination to rule out TB.

Statistical analysis

Questionnaires were double-entered and compared with EpiData software (EpiData 3.02 for Windows; The EpiData Association, Odense, Denmark). After cleaning, the data were then converted and analyzed using the Statistical Analysis System (SAS 9.2 for Windows; SAS Institute Inc., Cary, NC, USA).

The associations between TB infection and the sociodemographic characteristics, experiences of medical duties, and personal occupational protection, including mask use, washing hands, BCG vaccination, occupational protection training, and physical examination were estimated using univariate logistic regression models. Variables related to LTBI ($P<0.05$) in the univariate analyses were included in a multiple logistic regression model using stepwise selection of the variables. The knowledge and practices of personal occupational protection in two hospitals was analyzed using Cochran-Mantel-Haenszel test.

Results

A total of 731 eligible HCWs signed the informed consent and completed the questionnaires (333 from a non-TB hospital and 398 from the infectious disease hospital) between January and December 2011. Five hundred fifty-six of the 731 HCWs completed TSTs or had records of previous positive TST results. Twenty-seven of the 731 HCWs had a history of TB (five from the non-TB hospital and 22 from the infectious disease hospital). Finally, 529 HCWs were used for the risk analyses (310 from the non-TB hospital and 219 from the infectious disease hospital). The age of the participants ranged from 18 to 71 years, with a mean age of 31.4±9.0 years. Of the participants, 97.2% (514/529) were of Han ethnicity, 48.0% (254/529) had bachelor's degrees or higher, 30.4% (160/527) had middle or senior professional

Table 1. Associations between demographical characteristics and habit with LTBI[§].

Factors	LTBI[§] n/N[※] (%)	OR (95% CI)*	p value
Sex			
Female	188/442 (42.5)	1.00	
Male	44/87 (50.6)	1.38 (0.87, 2.19)	0.168
Age			
<30	112/289 (38.8)	1.00	
30–39	58/125 (46.4)	1.37 (0.90, 2.09)	0.147
≥40	62/111 (55.9)	2.00 (1.28, 3.12)	0.002
Han Ethnic			
No	8/15 (53.3)	1.00	
Yes	224/514 (43.6)	0.68 (0.24, 1.89)	0.456
Education status			
Under bachelor degree	104/275 (37.8)	1.00	
Bachelor degree and above	128/254 (50.4)	1.67 (1.18, 2.36)	0.004
Profession qualification			
Elementary and others	147/367 (40.1)	1.00	
middle/senior	84/160 (52.5)	1.65 (1.14, 2.40)	0.008
Monthly income (RMB)			
≤2000	114/271 (42.1)	1.00	
>2000	118/254 (46.5)	1.20 (0.85, 1.69)	0.312
Residential area			
Suburban district or rural area	71/161 (44.1)	1.00	
Downtown	161/368 (43.8)	0.99 (0.68, 1.43)	0.941
Live status			
Live by oneself or in domitary	20/53 (37.7)	1.00	
Live with family members	212/476 (44.5)	1.33 (0.74, 2.38)	0.345
Average per-capita living space			
>20 m^2	175/382 (45.8)	1.00	
≤20 m^2	53/130 (40.8)	0.81 (0.54, 1.22)	0.318
Smoking			
No	221/487 (43.3)	1.00	
Yes	21/42 (50.0)	1.31 (0.70, 2.46)	0.404
Drinking			
No	189/450 (42.0)	1.00	
Yes	43/79 (54.4)	1.65 (1.02, 2.67)	0.041
Calcium/Vitamin supplement			
No	188/414 (45.4)	1.00	
Yes	43/114 (37.7)	0.73 (0.48, 1.11)	0.144
Physical exercise (times per week)			
≥2	75/184 (40.8)	1.00	
<2	157/345 (45.5)	1.21 (0.85, 1.74)	0.295

[§]LTBI, latent tuberculosis infection.
*CI, confidential interval; OR, odds ratio.
[※]Sum may not always add up to total because of missing data.

qualifications, 90.0% (476/529) lived with family members, and 7.9% (42/529) used cigarettes. Of the participants, 47.3% (167/353) reported having received a BCG vaccination at birth. The TST induration size (mean ± S.D. [mm]) in each hospital was as follows: infectious hospital = 11.9±6.7 mm; and non-TB hospital = 5.2±6.7 mm. The nearest PPD testing was conducted one year ago. The TST results suggested that 43.9% (n = 232) were TST-positive (58.0% in the infectious disease hospital and 33.9% in the non-TB hospital using a TST induration ≥10 mm as a cut-off point; and 75.8% in the infectious disease hospital and 43.9%

Table 2. Associations between medical works and professional protection strategy with LTBI[§].

Factors	LTBI[§] n/N[※](%)	OR (95% CI)*	p value
Duration of healthcare profession (years)			
≤5	88/251 (35.1)	1.0	
6–10	43/81 (53.1)	2.10 (1.26,3.48)	0.004
>10	101/197 (51.3)	1.95 (1.33, 2.85)	0.001
Type of hospital			
General hospital	105/310 (33.9)	1.0	
Infectious disease hospital	127/219 (58.0)	2.70(1.89, 3.85)	<0.001
Department of hospital work			
Clinical systems	180/418 (43.1)	1	
Ancillary clinical systems	52/111 (46.8)	1.17 (0.77, 1.77)	0.475
Had ever worked in TB clinic or ward			
No	147/377 (39.0)	1.00	
Yes	83/139 (59.7)	2.32 (1.56, 3.45)	<0.001
Had ever worked in HIV clinic or ward			
No	170/429 (39.6)	1.00	
Yes	60/87 (69.0)	3.39 (2.07, 5.55)	<0.001
Contact with blood or other body fluid in work			
No or seldom	113/270 (41.9)	1.00	
Sometime or frequent	119/259 (45.9)	1.18 (0.84, 1.67)	0.343
Work hours everyday			
≤8	119/276 (43.1)	1.00	
>8	111/240 (46.3)	1.14 (0.80, 1.61)	0.475
Consistent mask use in professional work			
No	68/157 (43.3)	1.00	
Yes	128/281 (45.6)	1.10 (0.74, 1.63)	0.651
Kind of masks used in medical work			
mask	135/296 (45.6)	1.00	
Surgical mask	59/131 (45.0)	0.98 (0.65, 1.48)	0.913
N95 respirator	2/7 (28.6)	0.48 (0.09, 2.50)	0.381
Wash hands			
No	52/110 (47.3)	1.00	
Wash hands every time	180/418 (43.1)	0.84 (0.55, 1.29)	0.429
Attending regular physical examination every time			
No	15/47 (31.9)	1.00	
Yes	217/480 (45.2)	1.76 (0.93, 3.34)	0.083
Attending infection control training			
No	17/42 (40.5)	1.00	
Yes	215/487 (44.1)	1.16 (0.61, 2.21)	0.646
Self-reported using BCG			
No	14/43 (32.6)	1.00	
Yes	167/353 (47.3)	1.86 (0.95, 3.64)	0.070
Unknown	50/132 (37.9)	1.26 (0.61, 2.62)	0.530
Intimate contact with TB patients			
No/Unknown	98/274 (35.8)	1.00	
Yes	134/255 (52.5)	1.99 (1.40, 2.82)	<0.001
Knowledge of TB prevention and control			
Unknown	129/309 (41.7)	1.00	
Known	101/218 (46.3)	1.21 (0.85, 1.71)	0.296

Table 2. Cont.

Factors	LTBI[§] n/N[※](%)	OR (95% CI)*	p value
Policy of TB treatment and care			
Unknown	94/247 (38.1)	1.00	
Known	136/280 (48.6)	1.54 (1.09, 2.18)	0.015

[§]LTBI, latent tuberculosis infection.
*CI, confidential interval; OR, odds ratio.
[※]Sum may not always add up to total because of missing data.

in the non-TB hospital using a TST induration ≥6 mm as a cut-off point). There was no PPD boosting phenomenon in either hospital. All 232 TST-positive HCWs performed chest X-rays and one TB case was diagnosed. Age, education status, professional qualification, and alcohol consumption were associated with TST-positivity based on univariate analyses (Table 1). One tuberculosis case was diagnosed.

Among 529 HCWs, the duration of medical duties ranged from 0.5 to 55.5 years, with a mean duration of 9.7±9.1 years. Of the HCWs, 26.9% (139/516) reported a history of working in TB wards, and 48.2% (255/529) reported intimate contact with TB patients. Univariate analyses suggested that HCWs who worked in TB clinic or wards and HIV clinic or wards, had intimate contact with TB patients, the type of hospital, knowledge of TB treatment and care policy, and the duration of employment as a healthcare professional were associated with TB infection (Table 2).

The variables associated with TB infection in the univariate analyses ($P<0.05$) were included in a multivariate logistic regression model. The duration of employment as a healthcare professional (6–10 years vs. ≤5 years [OR = 1.89; 95% CI = 1.10, 3.25]; >10 vs. ≤5[OR = 1.80; 95% CI = 1.20, 2.68]), types of hospital (OR = 2.40; 95% CI = 1.59, 3.62), and ever-employment in a HIV clinic or ward (OR = 1.87; 95% CI = 1.08, 3.26)were associated significantly with TB infection (Table 3).

Subset analysis of knowledge about TB and practices of airborne infection control with the LTBI were stratified by employment duration. The depth of knowledge of TB prevention and control and the policy of TB treatment and care, consistent mask use, surgical mask or N95 respirator use, attending physical examination, and infection control training were significantly different between the two types of hospitals ($P<0.05$) after stratifying the duration of health care professional work. A longer duration of health care professional work tended to decrease the frequency of mask use (Table 4).

Among 712 HCWs who completed questionnaires, 94 provided reasons for declining a TST; 91.5% (86/94) worked in the infectious disease hospital. Previous positive TST results were the most important reason for declining a TST in 70.2% (66/94) of the HCWs. The next most frequent reason for declining a TST was concerns about skin reactions, such as blisters, necrosis, and lymphadenitis in 31.9% (30/94) of the HCWs. Finally, the third most frequent reason for declining a TST was receiving a TST in the past 3 months and anxiety about the psychological burden in 16.0% (15/94) of the HCWs (Table 5).

Discussion

Our study investigated LTBIs using TSTs and the potential impact factors among HCWs who are directly engaged in clinical work in two types of public hospitals in China. Among 529 study participants, TST positivity existed in 58.0% of the HCWs in the infectious disease hospital and 33.9% of the HCWs in the non-TB hospital. Ever-employment in a HIV clinic or ward, duration of employment in the healthcare profession, and types of hospitals were identified as significant predictors for LTBIs. The depth of knowledge of TB prevention and control and the policy of TB treatment and care, consistent mask use, surgical mask or N95 respirator use, attending physical examination, and infection control training were significantly different in the two types of hospitals. A longer duration of health care professional work tended to decrease the frequency of mask use.

Epidemiologic studies of TB infection have been conducted among HCWs using TSTs in many developing countries. A review by Menzie indicated that the median prevalence of LTBI in

Table 3. The associations of LTBI[§] with potential factors in multivariate logistic regression model.

Factors	Multivariate OR (95% CI)*	p value
Duration of healthcare profession (years)		
6–10 vs. ≤5	1.89 (1.10, 3.25)	0.021
>10 vs. ≤5	1.80 (1.20, 2.68)	0.004
Type of hospital		
Infectious disease hospital vs. general hospital	2.40 (1.59, 3.62)	<0.001
Had ever worked in HIV clinic or ward		
Yes vs. No.	1.87 (1.08, 3.26)	0.026

[§]LTBI, latent tuberculosis infection.
*CI, confidential interval; OR, odds ratio.

Table 4. Knowledge about TB and Practice of Airborne Infection Control with the LTBI, stratified by job-duration.

	Non-TB hospital	Infectious Disease Hospital	p value
Factors	n/N*(%)	n/N*(%)	
Known the knowledge of TB prevention and control			
≤5	44/156 (28.2)	39/99 (39.4)	
6–10	17/45 (37.8)	18/37 (46.7)	
>10	56/117 (47.9)	47/84 (56.0)	0.019
Consistent mask use in professional work			
≤5	71/116 (61.2)	82/96 (85.4)	
6–10	13/31 (41.9)	27/35 (77.1)	
>10	30/84 (35.7)	58/81 (71.6)	<0.001
Use surgical mask or N95 respirator in medical work			
≤5	17/115 (14.8)	52/94 (55.3)	
6–10	8/31 (25.8)	15/35 (42.9)	
>10	10/84 (11.9)	36/80 (45.0)	<0.001
Wash hands every time			
≤5	123/156 (78.9)	82/96 (85.4)	
6–10	41/45 (91.1)	27/35 (77.1)	
>10	88/116 (75.9)	67/84 (79.8)	0.794
Attending regular physical examination every time			
≤5	119/154 (77.3)	97/99 (98.0)	
6–10	40/45 (88.9)	37/37 (100.0)	
>10	109/117 (93.2)	84/84 (100.0)	<0.001
Attending infection control training			
≤5	130/156 (83.3)	96/99 (97.0)	
6–10	39/45 (86.7)	37/37 (100.0)	
>10	111/117 (94.9)	82/84 (97.6)	<0.001
Known the policy of TB treatment and care			
≤5	58/156 (37.2)	63/99 (63.6)	
6–10	23/45 (51.1)	28/37 (75.7)	
>10	56/117 (47.9)	57/84 (67.9)	<0.001

*Sum may not always add up to total because of missing data.

HCWs was 63%, and varied between33% and79% in low- and middle-income countries [18]. Recent reports from three areas of China also showed a high prevalence of LTBI in HCWs (range33.6%–55.6%) who worked in TB centers or hospitals that admitted TB patients using a TST induration ≥10 mm as a cut-off point or T-SPOT [15,19,20]. In our study, the prevalence of LTBIs in a non-TB hospital was similar to a previous report in the general population group ≥15 years of age (45%) when using a TST induration ≥6 mm as a cut-off point [12]. Although it was difficult to classify the source of TB exposure because of the lack of data of LTBI prevalence in the past few years in China, TB infection control still should be emphasized in some departments of non-TB hospitals, such as the clinical laboratory, radiology department, and intensive care unit [21]. In the TB prevention

Table 5. Reasons for refusal TST among HCWs (N = 94).

Reasons	Percentage (%)
Previous positive TST results	70.2
Worried about positive reaction	31.9
Did TST in the past 3 months	16.0
Anxious about psychological burden	16.0
Requirement for two visits	9.6
Think oneself can't be infected	4.3

and control system in Henan, provincial infectious disease hospitals are responsible for diagnosis and treatment of various critical infectious disease patients. We noted a slightly higher prevalence of LTBI (58% vs. 51.4%) in the infectious disease hospital compared with a previous study conducted among HCWs working in TB centers in Henan province [19]. This finding maybe induced by the high risk of TB infection when there is frequent contact with complicated TB cases or various infectious diseases with TB co-infections. HCWs play an important role in TB hospital infection control, but few hospitals pay attention to monitoring the status of TB infections among HCWs using TST or other developed diagnostic tests, such as TB-IGRAs (quantitative diagnostic kit for Mycobacterium tuberculosis IFN-γrelease assay) in China. X-rays are commonly used for detecting active TB during regular physical examinations. Further studies should be conducted to collect useful information to support and develop a detailed guideline for occupational prevention and hospital infection control of TB infection in different types of Chinese medical facilities.

More years of medical work have been demonstrated to bean important factor in TB infection among HCWs [18]. We found that the duration of medical work greater than 5 years had a higher risk of TB infection. Mask use was underemphasized in HCWs with a longer duration of medical work in the groups of longer job-duration. TB infection assessment and occupational protection should be of concern in these groups of HCWs.

A previous study reported no N95 respirator was available for HCWs working in TB centers in Henan Province [19]. We found that N95 respirators were still very rarely used in the two types of hospitals in our study. A protective respirator is recommended for use when HCWs directly contact active TB patients in the Guide to the Implementation of Chinese Tuberculosis Control Program [22]; however, many hospitals do not put these suggestions into effect. Therefore, improving the supplemental use of protective respirators should be considered by hospital administration. Subset analysis results also pointed out that the level of knowledge of TB and treatment care policy were low in the two hospitals, especially in the non-TB hospital. The knowledge and policy about TB and personal practice of infection control should be improved in hospitals.

TB is the most common opportunistic infection in HIV/AIDS patients. Our previous review showed that HIV/TB co-infection was 22.8% among AIDS patients in mainland China [23]. Thus, the departments with frequent contact or admission of AIDS patients may have a high risk of hospital infection. TB infection in HCWs who provided services to HIV-infected patients has been reported many years ago [24]. In this study we also found that HCWs who had ever-worked in a HIV/AIDS clinic or ward had a higher prevalence of LTBIs. Interventions that were effective in reducing nosocomial transmission of multidrug-resistant TB in HIV wards have been recommended in 1990 by the CDC in the United States [6]. TB infection control in a HIV ward should also be highlighted in Chinese guidelines. Infection control and health education should be strengthened in some high-risk departments within the hospital.

Serial tests of LTBI are effective occupational protection strategies. China has not recommended routine screening for LTBIs in hospitals and two-step TSTs. The infectious disease hospital in our study has conducted TSTs among HCWs during annual physical examinations for 3years.The non-TB hospital has never conducted TSTs among their HCWs. Considering the acceptance of serial tests and the possible effect of previous TSTs, the TST in our study was combined with the hospital annual physical examination. Even so, some participants still worried about TSTs and declined repeat testing. A description of the reasons for declining TSTs showed skin tests and side effects affected the acceptance of TSTs, especially among HCWs in the infectious disease hospital. Compared with TSTs, IGRAs have been shown to be an institutional cost-saving method and results in higher compliance rates [25,26]. Guidelines from some countries have recommended IGRAs for serial testing of LTBIs among HCWs [5]. Two commercial systems (T-SPOT.TB, Oxford Immunote Ltd., Oxford, UK and QuantiFERON-TB Gold, Cellestis, Carnegie, Australia) are very expensive in China and therefore unavailable to the general population. Developing guidelines of monitoring LTBIs among Chinese HCWs is urgent. The acceptance of serial testing, the specificity of results, and the cost of tests should be considered.

Several limitations of this study should be kept in mind. First, our study participants do not represent the general HCWs due to the potential limitation of hospital selection and enrollment methods. Second, some bias induced by refusal of TSTs should be considered when interpreting our results. Third, TSTs cannot clearly identify the infection status as current or past infections and are affected by popular BCG vaccinations in China. Potential bias caused by such misclassification cannot be excluded. Fourth, the cross-sectional study design has its limitation on association analysis. Therefore, our results need confirmation by a further large-scale case-control or cohort study.

In conclusion, a high prevalence of TB infection was observed among HCWs working in a high-risk setting and with long professional experience in Henan province in China. The knowledge and policy about TB and personal practice of infection control should be improved in hospitals. Comprehensive guidelines should be developed to ensure the health of HCWs and reduce TB transmission in medical institutions.

Acknowledgments

We thank staffs from Henan infectious disease hospital, Zhengzhou central hospital and students of Zhengzhou University for their great efforts on enrollment of study participants, TST administration, data entry and quality control.

Author Contributions

Conceived and designed the experiments: FZ LG JC. Performed the experiments: YH XZ J. Li XL YY. Analyzed the data: FZ J. Lu LZ. Contributed reagents/materials/analysis tools: XL YY. Wrote the paper: FZ. Reviewed manuscript: JC YD.

References

1. World Health Organization (2010) Global tuberculosis report 2010. WHO/HTM/TB/20107 Geneva, Switzerland: WHO.
2. Fennelly KP, Iseman MD (1999) Health care workers and tuberculosis: the battle of a century. Int J Tuberc Lung Dis 3: 363–364.
3. Sepkowitz KA (1996) Tuberculin skin testing and the health care worker: lessons of the Prophit Survey. Tuber Lung Dis 77: 81–85.
4. World Health Organization (2009) WHO policy on TB infection control in health-care facilities, congregate settings and households. . WHO/HTM/TB/2009419 Geneva, Switzerland: WHO.
5. Denkinger CM, Dheda K, Pai M (2011) Guidelines on interferon-gamma release assays for tuberculosis infection: concordance, discordance or confusion? Clin Microbiol Infect 17: 806–814.

6. Harries AD, Maher D, Nunn P (1997) Practical and affordable measures for the protection of health care workers from tuberculosis in low-income countries. Bull World Health Organ 75: 477–489.
7. Franco C, Zanetta DM (2006) Assessing occupational exposure as risk for tuberculous infection at a teaching hospital in Sao Paulo, Brazil. Int J Tuberc Lung Dis 10: 384–389.
8. Kassim S, Zuber P, Wiktor SZ, Diomande FV, Coulibaly IM, et al. (2000) Tuberculin skin testing to assess the occupational risk of Mycobacterium tuberculosis infection among health care workers in Abidjan, Cote d'Ivoire. Int J Tuberc Lung Dis 4: 321–326.
9. Kayanja HK, Debanne S, King C, Whalen CC (2005) Tuberculosis infection among health care workers in Kampala, Uganda. Int J Tuberc Lung Dis 9: 686–688.
10. Lien LT, Hang NT, Kobayashi N, Yanai H, Toyota E, et al. (2009) Prevalence and risk factors for tuberculosis infection among hospital workers in Hanoi, Viet Nam. PLoS One 4: e6798.
11. Joshi R, Reingold AL, Menzies D, Pai M (2006) Tuberculosis among health-care workers in low- and middle-income countries: a systematic review. PLoS Med 3: e494.
12. National Technical Steering Group of the Epidemiological Sampling Survey for Tuberculosis (2002) Report on fourth national epidemiological sampling survey of tuberculosis. . Chin J Tuberc Respir Dis 25: 5.
13. Wang GJ, Ma SW, Zhen XA, Meng LT, Xu JY, et al. (2007) A survey on the infection rate of tuberculosis among employees of the antituberculosis institutions in Henan province, China. Zhonghua Liu Xing Bing Xue Za Zhi 28: 980–983.
14. Li JM, Lu W, Li HF, Liu FH, Wang CR (2006) Survey of risk of Tuberculosis Infection in Hospital Workers. Chinese Journal of Public Health 22: 488.
15. He GX, Wang LX, Chai SJ, Klena JD, Cheng SM, et al. (2012) Risk factors associated with tuberculosis infection among health care workers in Inner Mongolia, China. Int J Tuberc Lung Dis 16: 1485–1491.
16. Chinese Ministry of Health (2013) Administrative Measures for Prevention and Control of Tuberculosis (2013).
17. Chai SJ, Mattingly DC, Varma JK (2013) Protecting health care workers from tuberculosis in China: a review of policy and practice in China and the United States. Health Policy Plan 28: 100–109.
18. Menzies D, Joshi R, Pai M (2007) Risk of tuberculosis infection and disease associated with work in health care settings. Int J Tuberc Lung Dis 11: 593–605.
19. He GX, van denHof S, van der Werf MJ, Wang GJ, Ma SW, et al. (2010) Infection control and the burden of tuberculosis infection and disease in health care workers in china: a cross-sectional study. BMC Infect Dis 10: 313.
20. Zhang X, Jia H, Liu F, Pan L, Xing A, et al. (2013) Prevalence and Risk Factors for Latent Tuberculosis Infection among Health Care Workers in China: A Cross-Sectional Study. PLoS One 8: e66412.
21. Zhou F, Hao YB, Wang XN, Lu J, Chen JG (2013) Tubercle bacillus Infection and occupational protection among health care workers in Central Hospital. Zhongguo Yu Fang Yi Xue Za Zhi 14: 905–909.
22. CDC, Ministry of Health of the People' Republic of China (2008) Guide to the implementation of Chinese tuberculosis control program. Beijing Peking Union Medical College Press.
23. Gao L, Zhou F, Li X, Jin Q (2010) HIV/TB co-infection in mainland China: a meta-analysis. PLoS One 5: e10736.
24. Zahnow K, Matts JP, Hillman D, Finley E, Brown LS Jr., et al. (1998) Rates of tuberculosis infection in healthcare workers providing services to HIV-infected populations. Terry Beirn Community Programs for Clinical Research on AIDS. Infect Control Hosp Epidemiol 19: 829–835.
25. Wrighton-Smith P, Sneed L, Humphrey F, Tao X, Bernacki E (2012) Screening health care workers with interferon-gamma release assay versus tuberculin skin test: impact on costs and adherence to testing (the SWITCH study). J Occup Environ Med 54: 806–815.
26. Pai M, Gokhale K, Joshi R, Dogra S, Kalantri S, et al. (2005) Mycobacterium tuberculosis infection in health care workers in rural India: comparison of a whole-blood interferon gamma assay with tuberculin skin testing. JAMA 293: 2746–2755.

4

Quantifying Age-Related Rates of Social Contact Using Diaries in a Rural Coastal Population of Kenya

Moses Chapa Kiti[1]*, Timothy Muiruri Kinyanjui[1,2], Dorothy Chelagat Koech[1], Patrick Kiio Munywoki[1], Graham Francis Medley[3], David James Nokes[1,3]

1 KEMRI-Wellcome Trust Research Programme, Kilifi, Kenya, **2** Mathematics and WIDER, University of Warwick, Coventry, United Kingdom, **3** School of Life Sciences and WIDER, University of Warwick, Coventry, United Kingdom

Abstract

Background: Improved understanding and quantification of social contact patterns that govern the transmission dynamics of respiratory viral infections has utility in the design of preventative and control measures such as vaccination and social distancing. The objective of this study was to quantify an age-specific matrix of contact rates for a predominantly rural low-income population that would support transmission dynamic modeling of respiratory viruses.

Methods and Findings: From the population register of the Kilifi Health and Demographic Surveillance System, coastal Kenya, 150 individuals per age group (<1, 1–5, 6–15, 16–19, 20–49, 50 and above, in years) were selected by stratified random sampling and requested to complete a day long paper diary of physical contacts (e.g. touch or embrace). The sample was stratified by residence (rural-to-semiurban), month (August 2011 to January 2012, spanning seasonal changes in socio-cultural activities), and day of week. Usable diary responses were obtained from 568 individuals (~50% of expected). The mean number of contacts per person per day was 17.7 (95% CI 16.7–18.7). Infants reported the lowest contact rates (mean 13.9, 95% CI 12.1–15.7), while primary school students (6–15 years) reported the highest (mean 20.1, 95% CI 18.0–22.2). Rates of contact were higher within groups of similar age (assortative), particularly within the primary school students and adults (20–49 years). Adults and older participants (>50 years) exhibited the highest inter-generational contacts. Rural contact rates were higher than semiurban (18.8 vs 15.6, $p = 0.002$), with rural primary school students having twice as many assortative contacts as their semiurban peers.

Conclusions and Significance: This is the first age-specific contact matrix to be defined for tropical Sub-Saharan Africa and has utility in age-structured models to assess the potential impact of interventions for directly transmitted respiratory infections.

Editor: Steffen Borrmann, Kenya Medical Research Institute - Wellcome Trust Research Programme, Kenya

Funding: This work was supported by the Welcome Trust, http://www.wellcome.ac.uk/, grant numbers 084633 (DJN) and 098556 (MCK). The funders had no role in study design, data collection and analysis, decision to publish, or preparation of the manuscript.

Competing Interests: The authors have declared that no competing interests exist.

* Email: mkiti@kemri-wellcome.org

Introduction

Interventions for the prevention or control of infectious diseases are better formulated on the basis of a quantitative understanding of the determinants of the spread of infection within a population. In the case of directly transmitted respiratory viruses, such as influenza viruses and respiratory syncytial virus (RSV), transmission is effected through interaction or contact between individuals sufficiently close for virus to pass from one person to the next. It follows that the transmission dynamics of these viruses are determined by the structure and rates of such contacts between susceptible and infectious individuals in a population. Mathematical models of infectious disease transmission are recognized as important tools for exploring the potential impact of interventions [1,2]. To capture greater reality these models generally incorporate age as the key structural feature governing transmission patterns [3,4]. Increasingly the models designed for the study of respiratory infections utilize direct estimates of contact rates within and between age groups of a population by which to determine who acquires infection from whom [3,5–8].

The source of direct estimates of contacts is usually the self-completed diary and follows the early work by Edmunds *et al* [9]. A sample of the population under study is selected to complete a record of each of the contacts made by the participant with other individuals on a chosen day. These diaries usually aim to collect data on the age of the participant and the ages of all individuals contacted, stratified by the intensity of the contact encounter (usually conversation and touch) [10], the frequency of contact with the same individual or the total duration of this pair-wise contact in the day, the location or context in which the interaction occurs [11,12], and the day of the week [13,14]. There are inherent problems with diary collected data including failure to record all contacts and difficulty in comprehending the process of completion. Measures taken to minimize resultant error and bias include recap interviews on collection of diaries and provision of a 'shadow' to record the contact data for very young or illiterate participants [7].

Contact diary data reflect the social, behavioural and demographic characteristics of the study population, which may vary from location to location. Specifically, there will be variation between locations in population density, age structure, household occupancy, work practices, schooling, religious gatherings and transport, all of which may have a bearing on the patterns and rates of contact and hence the spread of respiratory infection. The majority of contact diary-based studies have been conducted in developed countries, and only two have been in low income settings, one in an informal urban settlement in South Africa [7] and the other in a semi-rural community in Vietnam [8]. Given all of the above there is a need to characterize contact patterns more widely, particularly in low income communities where least is known.

We aimed to define and quantify an age-specific matrix of rates of contact between individuals within a rural Kenyan population for the purpose of generating data suitable for the mathematical modelling of the transmission dynamics of respiratory syncytial virus by which to assess the impact of vaccine intervention strategies.

Methods

Study area

The study was conducted in 5 locations in the northern part of the Kilifi Health and Demographic Surveillance System (KHDSS). The locations were categorised as semiurban (Kilifi Township [denoted A] and Tezo [B]) and rural (Ngerenya [C], Roka [D] and Matsangoni [E]) as portrayed in Figure 1. The categorisation into semiurban and rural areas is similar to that used by Molyneux *et al* [15]. In March 2011 the KHDSS had a population of 261,919 with mean age of 21.8 and 21.1 years in semiurban and rural areas, respectively. Mean population density in semiurban and rural areas was 530 and 360 people/km^2, respectively. The average household size was higher in the rural compared to semiurban areas (9.2 versus 7.0, respectively) and about a fifth of the population was below 5 years of age. The KHDSS is described further by Scott *et al* [16].

Study design

Participants were chosen at random from enumeration registers for each of the five locations (in proportion to location size) and in equal number from 6 age groups assumed to approximate to key social or behavioural groups: <1 (infants), 1–5 (pre-school), 6–15 (primary school), 16–19 (secondary school), 20–49 (adults), and > 50 (elderly) years. Recruitment was staggered over a six-month period (Aug 2011 to Jan 2012). All residents who gave informed consent or for whom informed consent was given by their parents, and who were planning to stay in the KHDSS for at least three months were included.

Sample size of the study was based on an estimate of the contact rate variation (SD = 13) from an unpublished contact diary school study (n = 177) recently undertaken in the KHDSS. Using standard methods [17] a required sample size of 150 individuals in each of the six age groups (ie 900 over all age groups) was determined to give an estimate with a 95 percent confidence interval (95% CI). To account for possible non-response and errors in diary completion, this number was scaled up by 20% to give a final sample size of 1,080 individuals.

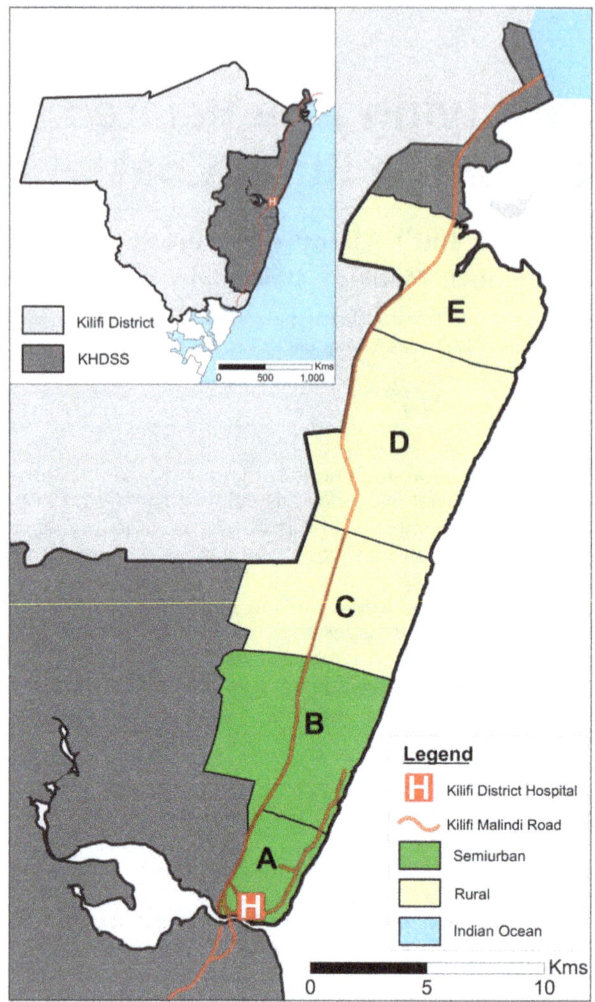

Figure 1. Map of the study area. The inset shows the location of the KHDSS in relation to the former Kilifi District (part of Kilifi County). The study area locations are conventionally categorised as semiurban (Kilifi Township [denoted A] and Tezo [B]), and rural (Ngerenya [C], Roka [D] and Matsangoni [E]).

A contact person was defined as someone with whom the participant had a direct physical encounter (a "contact"), and involved direct skin-to-skin touch such as embracing, kissing or shaking hands. Each contact was recorded only once in the diary during the day of study, and repeat encounters were recorded as tallies. Participants were expected to keep the diary for a day, defined as the period between first waking and going to bed for the night. Participants were assigned a day of the week for completing a contact diary by block randomisation.

Study implementation

Five focus group discussions were scheduled within the study area to assess the feasibility and suitability of using the diaries. The groups were composed of primary school students (class 4–8, approximate age range 10–17 y), secondary school students (form 1–4, age range 15–21 y), kindergarten teachers (age range 23–55) and separate male and female groups of Kenya Medical Research Institute (KEMRI) Community Representatives (age range 20–50 y) [18]. A pilot study was conducted in the first month among 50 participants to assess the ease of understanding the diary, and to validate an exit interview to be undertaken on collection of the diary from the participant for verification of the entries. From this, we adopted a text and pictorial diary translated from English to Swahili and Giriama (local dialect). The diaries incorporated the age-class of the persons contacted and frequency of the contacts made (Figure S1).

Each eligible participant was approached by a trained fieldworker to gain consent, train in use of the diary, select day of study, for diary collection and exit interview. All participants under 10 years old and other individuals who were unable to read and write (established by asking literacy status of individuals aged over 10 years) selected a "shadow" to record the participant's daily contacts. The shadow was someone who spent most time with the participant and would be in a position to record the contact details of the participant at regular intervals. Shadows were trained on how to keep the diary on behalf of the selected participant, and requested not to influence the normal behaviour of the participant. An alarm wrist watch was lent to each participant or shadow for the duration of study and pre-set to go off at hourly intervals providing a prompt to record recent contacts either directly in the diary or in a paper reminder table prior to transferring the data to the diary at a convenient time. One day prior to the selected day, the fieldworker visited the participant (and shadow) for training and allocation of study material (diary, pen, watch, reminder table). The fieldworkers also recorded the socio-demographic information about the participant (occupation, number of years of completed education, family composition, sleeping arrangements i.e. sharing of bedroom or bed) using a questionnaire (Figure S2).

On the appointed study day, for each different individual physically contacted, participants recorded the assumed age class of the person contacted in the diary against a unique identity (ID) code. The fieldworker revisited the participant at most 48 hours after the diary-keeping to verify the recorded details as actual events, and to fill in a questionnaire (Figure S3) on the participant's experiences, e.g. difficulty encountered, and whether all contacts were recorded or the diary induced a behaviour change such as increasing number of physical contacts. Fieldworkers also recorded whether the contact was known to the participant to assess familiarity of contacts, as well as the frequency of usual contacts with this individual (daily or almost daily, once or twice a week, once or twice a month, or less than once a month). After successful data collection, participants (and shadows) aged 18 years and over were given 3.5 US dollars as compensation for their time, while school going students were given a stationery pack containing items of similar value.

Data analysis

The primary outcome was age-specific mean number of contacts per person per day, μ_{ij} (henceforth referred to as contact rate). Let indices i and j represent age groups, such that $i,j=1,2...,6$, corresponding to <1, 1–5, 6–15, 16–19, 20–49, ≥ 50 years, respectively. Further, let N_i be the total number of participants in age group i such that $\sum_{i=1}^{6} N_i = N$, the total number of participants in the study. Let $y_{ij,k}$ be the number of contacts that participant k in age group i has with respondents in age group j. Then, the total number of contacts, denoted T_{ij} is given by $T_{ij} = \sum_{k=1}^{N_i} y_{ij,k}$. Therefore, the daily contact rate per individual of age group i with individuals of age group j is $\mu_{ij} = \frac{1}{N_i} T_{ij}$.

Differences in the mean contact rates for each covariate (gender, age group, presence of a shadow, season, residence and day of week) were assessed using analysis of variance (ANOVA). The uncertainty of the contact rate estimates was summarised by generating a 95% Confidence Interval (CI) through 2,000 non-parametric bootstraps as described by Carpenter *et al* [19]. Further analysis involved computing weights to eliminate possible selection bias within the semiurban-rural sample compared to KHDSS population (see Text S1).

Ethical review and consent

The Kenya Ethical Review Committee (KEMRI/RES/7/3/1) and the Biomedical and Social Ethics Review Committee of the University of Warwick (134-07-2011) approved the study. Written informed consent was sought from participants (and shadow) aged ≥18 years and from parents or guardians for those aged <18 years.

Results

Baseline characteristics

The study took place over the period 17th August 2011 to 31st January 2012. 1,080 individuals were randomly selected from the KHDSS register, with an additional 58 individuals randomly selected to replace those who refused to give consent. Of the 1,138 individuals no consent was obtained for 515 (45%) for the reasons detailed in Table S1. Of the 623 (55%) who agreed to participate in the study, 606 diaries were collected by the end of the study period, of which 38 were discarded due to discrepancies. The reasons for discard were primarily that participants selected several age groups per contact, or they systematically filled in the same number of contacts for all entries. Overall, data are presented for 568 (50% of 1138; 54% female) useable diaries from participants with a mean age of 23 years (range 0.1–84.9 years). See Texts S2 and S3 (raw data and data dictionary, respectively).

Table 1 provides data on some baseline characteristics of the 568 diary participants. The majority of the participants lived in Roka location (26%), with Tezo and Ngerenya providing the smallest proportion of participants. More than two-thirds had less than 4 years of education, and 349 (61%) of the total required a shadow. Half of the participants were unemployed, while a quarter were students. The majority (96%) of the participants preferred the picture to the text diaries. During the exit interview, only 8 of the participants reported having not fully understood how to keep the diary, while the most common issue raised by the shadows was the difficulty in following the selected participant wherever they went. Out of 33 participants who reported an induced behaviour change, 27 had a shadow.

The characteristics of the persons contacted by the diary participants are given in Table 2. The largest proportion of contacts was with siblings (40%) and other relatives (34%), with participants recording only 7% of contacts with parents. While 63% of contacts were with family members (parents, spouses, children and siblings), only about a third (28%) shared the same household as the participant (note that a household frequently includes more than one related family living in different dwellings but within the same compound). Additionally, a third of the contacts slept in the same room as the participants, and out of these two-thirds shared a bed with the participant. Of the total number of people contacted, only 5% were unknown. We do not present any data on the tallies of repeat encounters of contacts.

Contact rates

A total of 10,042 contacts were recorded in the diaries by the 568 participants. Each participant recorded an average of 17.7 (95% CI 16.7–18.7) contacts per day (Part A of Figure 2). We

Table 1. Baseline characteristics of 568 diary-keeping participants from Kilifi Health and Demographic Surveillance System, Kenya.

Variable		Number, n(%)
Location	Kilifi Township	110 (19.4)
	Tezo	87 (15.3)
	Ngerenya	86 (15.1)
	Roka	151 (26.6)
	Matsangoni	134 (23.6)
Number of years of education	≤4	374 (65.8)
	5–8	144 (25.4)
	9+	50 (8.9)
Diary type preference	Pictorial	545 (96.0)
	Text	23 (4.0)
Diary keeper	Participant	220 (38.7)
	Shadow[¥]	348 (61.3)
Participant's occupation[ƚ]	Student	142 (25.0)
	Employed	137 (24.1)
	Unemployed[§]	286 (50.4)
Difficulty in filling diary[ƚ]	Yes	8 (1.4)
	No	554 (97.5)

[¥]2 primary school students out of 222 participants aged <10 years required two shadows; one at home (parent) and at school (teacher).
[ƚ]Missing records as a proportion of all 568 participants: participant occupation (3, 0.5%); difficulty in filling in diary (6, 1.1%).
[§]Unemployed: these include children <6 years, unemployed participants (62% female), pre-school children and retired individuals.

Table 2. Baseline characteristics of 10,042 contacts by participants in a diary study in the Kilifi Health and Demographic Surveillance System, Kenya.

		Contacts (%)
Relationship to participant[ƚ$]	Parent	707 (7.0)
	Sibling	3,985 (39.7)
	Child	1,517 (15.1)
	Spouse	118 (1.2)
	Other relative	3,411 (34.0)
	Other	106 (1.1)
Live in same house	Yes	2,855 (28.4)
	No	7,187 (71.6)
Sleep in same room	Yes	909 (31.8)
	No	1,924 (67.4)
Sleep in same room	Yes	597 (65.7)
and share bed	No	312 (34.3)
Ever met the contact before?	Yes	9,290 (92.5)
	No	454 (4.5)
Frequency of meeting[□]	Daily	7,287 (78.4)
	Regularly	1,486 (16.0)
	Often	343 (3.7)
	Rarely	136 (1.5)

[ƚ]Missing records as a proportion of the total contacts 10,042): Relationship to participant (198, 2.0%); Sleep in same room (22, 0.8%); Ever met the contact before (298, 3.0%); Frequency of meeting (38, 0.4%).
[$]While 63% of contacts with family members (parents, spouses, children and siblings),only 28% live in the same household. Members of the same family could be living in different households and share a common compound (homestead).
[□]Frequency of meeting: daily (on a day-to-day basis); regularly (more than four times a week); often (once or twice a week); rarely (once or twice a month).

found that primary school aged children in the KHDSS had the highest contact rate (20.1, 95% CI 18.0–22.2) compared to the rest of the population, with infants and the elderly recording the lowest contact rate at 13.9 (95% CI 12.1–15.6) and 13.9 (95% CI 11.3–16.5) respectively (Part B of Figure 2, Table 3). There was strong evidence that the difference in the age specific mean contact rates was not due to chance (ANOVA F = 4.67, df = 5, p = 0.0003, Table 3). Shadows recorded fewer contacts compared to participants who kept diaries for themselves (16.3 vs 19.9 respectively, ANOVA F = 12.8, df = 1, p = 0.0004). Further analysis by age revealed that this difference was significant in ages 15–19 (p = 0.02) and 20–49 (p = 0.01) years. When stratified by residence, participants in the rural areas reported higher mean number of contacts (18.8/person/day, Part A of Figure 3) compared with their semiurban counterparts (16.5/person/day, Part B of Figure 3. ANOVA F = 9.86, df = 1, p = 0.002, Table 3). In the rural areas, significantly lower contact rates were recorded by shadows compared with participants with self-kept diaries (17.0 vs 22.4, ANOVA F = 15.5, df = 1, p = 0.0001); however, no such difference was observed in the semiurban areas. Similar analysis revealed no evidence that the mean number of contacts recorded differed by sex (p = 0.85), weekend versus weekday (p = 0.72), or season (p = 0.87) (Table 3).

Age group specific mixing patterns

Figure 2 Part C shows a heat map of mean age specific contact rates between participants in each age class ($i = 1,6$; x-axis) stratified by contacted age group ($j = 1,6$; y-axis). The corresponding data table and confidence intervals are presented in Table 4. Furthermore, Table S2 shows the age specific total contacts per day by participants with each contact age group. The effect of weighting for rural–semiurban bias in sampling on the estimated contact rates was found to negligible (not shown) and hence we present the unadjusted estimates (contact matrices in Part A and B, respectively, in Figure 3).

Figure 2 Part C highlights three key features. Overall, there is a strong diagonal element, indicating high contact rates between individuals in the same age groups (assortative mixing) relative to the average. The highest contact rates were within the 6–15 year age group (8.9, 95% CI 8.4–10.5), that is primary-to-primary school children; and adult-to-adult with 8.2 (95% CI 7.2–9.1) contacts per day. The lowest contact rates were infant-to-infant

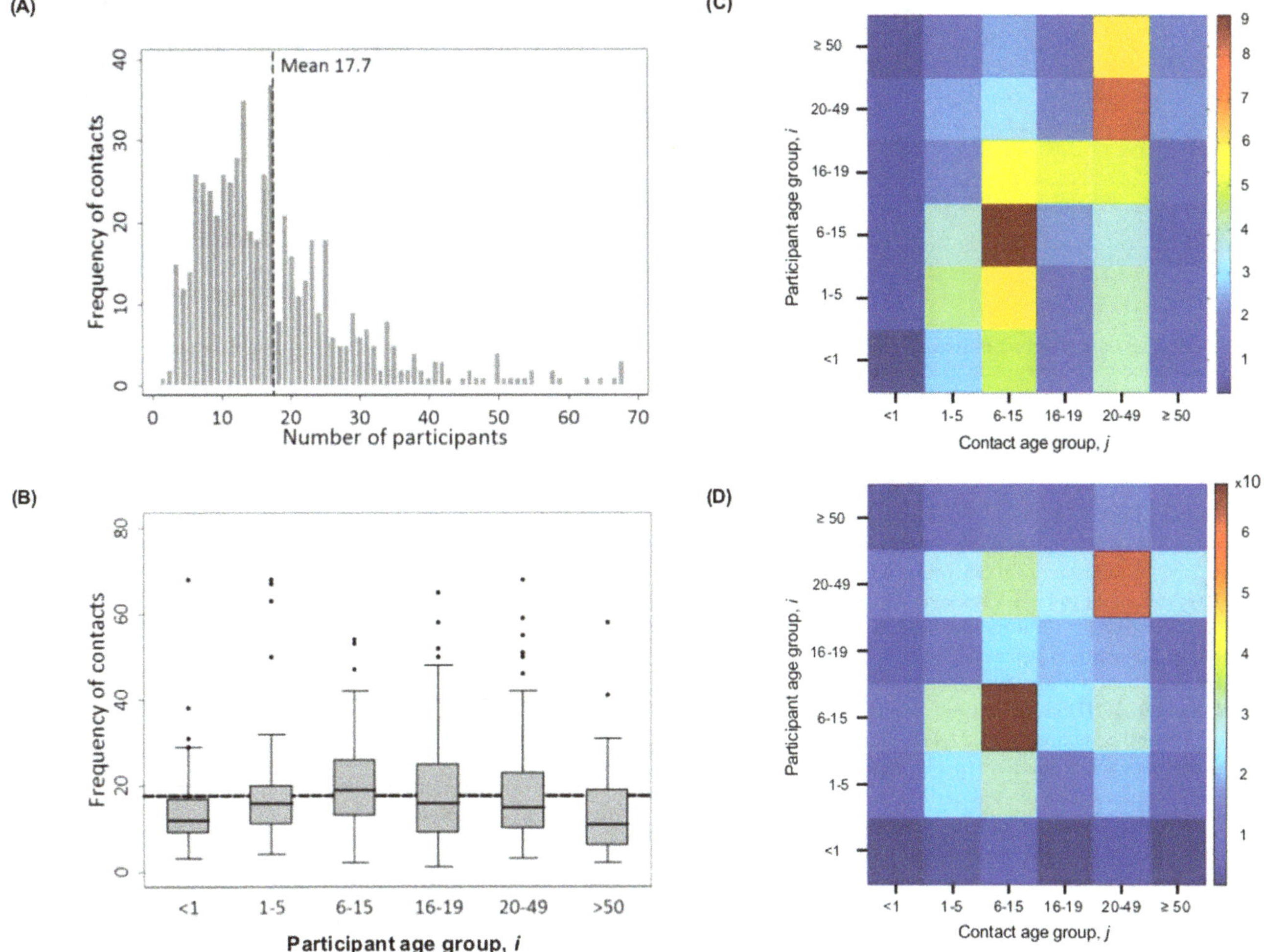

Figure 2. Contact mixing patterns. Part A: Distribution of overall number of contacts (with mean shown as a dashed line). Part B: Mean (dashed line) contact rate per person per day, with boxplots showing median (centre line) and interquartile range (IQR) of contact rates per age group per day. Part C: Contact rate surface (heat map) expressing the mean number of contacts between an individual participant in each age group i with individuals in each age group j. Part D: Population level numbers of contacts per day within and between age groups (estimated from the matrix defined in (C) scaled by the age-specific resident population size).

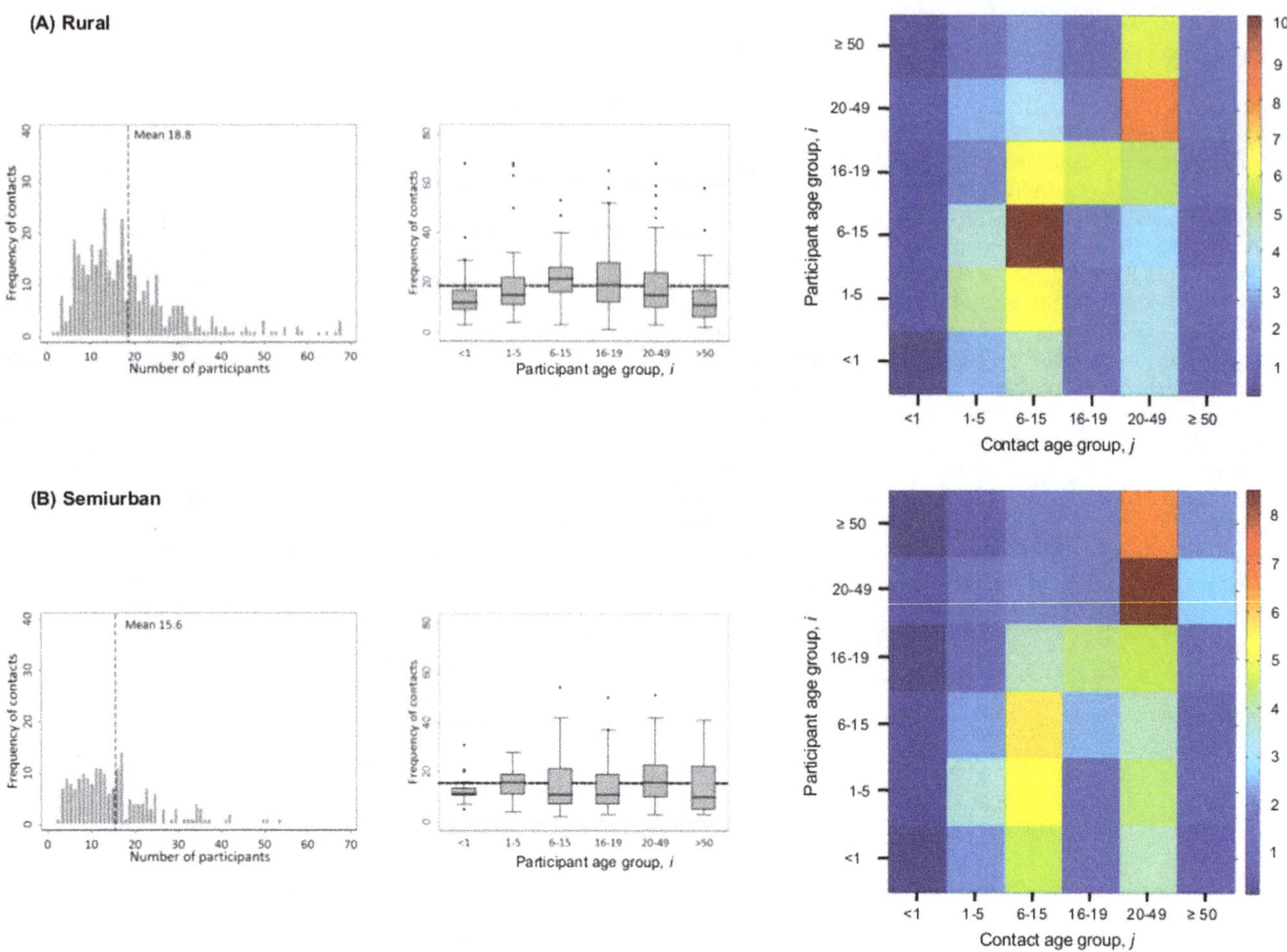

Figure 3. Age specific contact matrices. Mixing patterns for 371 participants in rural areas (Part A) and 197 participants in semiurban areas (Part B). The description of the images, from left to right, follows that in Figure 2 Parts A, B and C, respectively.

(0.2, 95% CI 0.1–0.3). Second, in general, relatively high contacts rates were recorded by participants of all ages with primary school children and with adults (20–49 years of age). Third, there is an absence of clear symmetry in mixing by reciprocal age groups. For example, the contact rate of 6–15 years old children with 16–19 year olds is estimated to be 2.3 contacts per day, whereas the rate of contact between 16–19 years olds with 6–15 years olds is over twice that at 5.5 contacts per day (Table 4). This is a reflection of the differences between age groups in actual population size. For example, within KHDSS there were 78,805 registered residents aged 5–14 years, compared with 22,440 aged 16–19 years (Table S3). Multiplying each of the rates (μ_{ij}) in Figure 2 Part C (Table 4) by the resident population of each participant age group (N_i) yields the contact matrix shown in Part D of Figure 2 that demonstrates much closer reciprocity of between age group total numbers of contacts. This figure also reveals more clearly relatively high inter-generational contact number, e.g. between school and adult age groups. Comparison of the patterns of contacts between the semiurban and rural population samples is shown in Figure 3. In the rural areas, the highest level of assortativeness is observed among people in the age range 6–14 years. In addition, high levels of mixing are observed between children aged 6–14 years and those aged 1–5 and 15–19 years. By contrast, adults in the semiurban areas have the highest assortative contact rates compared to other age groups with high between group contacts rates mainly occurring between adults and the elderly.

Discussion

We report estimates of daily physical contact rates within and between different age groups in a rural coastal Kenyan population. On average individuals made 17.7 (95% CI 16.7–18.7) contacts per person per day, with highest rates observed for primary school children aged 6–15 years (20.1, 95% CI 18.0–22.2). Assortative mixing was conspicuous, particularly amongst school-going child age group (6–19 years) and also among the adult age group (20–49 years). In addition, there was strong inter-generational mixing (presumably parents and children, or teachers and pupils), but this was most evident once differences in population size by age were accounted for (Figure 2 Part D). Contact rates were higher in rural compared to semiurban areas, with primary school children recording highest rates in the former and adults (including the elderly) recording highest rates in the latter. There was no evidence of a difference by sex, season and day of the week. These data on contact patterns and rates are important for the evaluation of empirically driven mathematical models that aim to inform prevention strategies and policies against the transmission of diseases that spread via direct contact through the respiratory route (e.g. RSV [1,3,20]) or faecal-oral route (rotavirus [21]).

Table 3. Mean number of contacts per day stratified by gender, age group (years), presence of shadow, season, residence, days of week of 568 diary participants from the Kilifi Health and Demographic Surveillance System, Kenya.

Category/Covariate		Total participants (n, %)	Mean (95% CI[‡]) number of people contacted per participant per day (D/n)	P-value
Overall		568	17.7 (16.7–18.7)	
Gender	Male	262	17.6 (16.1–19.1)	
	Female	306 (54%)	17.8 (16.5–19.0)	0.85
Participant	<1	86 (15%)	13.9 (12.0–15.7)	
age group	1–5	93 (16%)	17.6 (15.3–19.9)	
	6–15	98 (17%)	20.1 (18.0–22.2)	
	16–19	91 (16%)	19.4 (16.6–22.1)	
	20–49	139 (25%)	18.9 (16.8–21.1)	
	≥50	61 (11%)	13.9 (11.2–16.6)	0.0003
Shadow	Yes	349	16.3 (15.2–17.4)	
present	No	219 (39%)	19.9 (18.1–21.7)	0.0004
Season[$]	Dry	212	17.6 (15.9–19.3)	
	Wet	356 (63%)	17.1 (16.6–18.9)	0.87
Location[&]	Rural	371	18.8 (17.5–20.1)	
	Semiurban	197 (35%)	15.6 (14.2–16.9)	0.002
Day of week	Weekend	168	17.9 (16.2–19.7)	
	Weekday	400 (70%)	17.6 (16.4–18.7)	0.72

[‡]95% CI: 95% confidence intervals derived from 2,000 bootstraps.
[$]Season: Dry = January, August, December; Wet = September - November
[&]Location. Rural: Ngerenya, Roka, Matsangoni; Semiurban: Kilifi Township, Tezo.

We defined a contact as direct skin-to-skin touch, which has particular relevance to the transmission of RSV [22], reduces under-reporting as it is a less frequent event relative to conversation, and simplifies diary entry. The majority of earlier studies defined contacts as both conversation and skin-to-skin touch, with data being collected via self-kept paper diaries [3,6], household interviews [8,23] and web-based interfaces [10,24]. We report higher (physical only) contact rates than previous studies in urban South Africa [7] and rural Vietnam [8], which estimated both physical and non-physical contacts. Reported physical contact rates in the POLYMOD study [3] conducted in 8 European countries are also lower than those reported here. These differences could be due to the definition of a contact and the social construct (sociodemographic patterns in rural-urban areas, differences in household size, etc). This emphasizes the need for further context-specific studies and more so in developing countries where these conditions are different.

The study was designed intentionally to factor out a range of influences which might have a bearing on contact rates, through stratification by (i) time of the year to remove seasonal (dry and wet) variation from, for example, agricultural practices, (ii) location that captures differences in household occupancy and population density on the rural - semiurban continuum, and (iii) day of the week (weekend versus weekday), to avoid possible bias in behaviour over the period of a week and the context of the contact (e.g. school, household, workplace).

Similar to other studies, we report strongly assortative mixing among school children [3,5], particularly of primary school age. There is also relatively high contact rates between children of all ages and primary school-age children, and cross-generational, hence increasing the probability of spreading infection throughout the population and within the household setting [25]. This has implications for targeted vaccination as emphasised by a recent modelling exercise which predicted that vaccinating school-going children against influenza, in addition to adults, resulted in a two-fold reduction in infections per dose of vaccine compared to targeting those aged >65 years only [4]. On the other hand, in our study infants (ie aged less than 1 year) reported the lowest contact rates, presumably due to mobility limitations, although infants do spend much time carried by the mother or a sibling. This might increase contacts but potentially may not have been recorded as such in this study. Our findings are important for investigating alternative age-dependent vaccination strategies particularly because previous vaccines used in young infants, who experience the highest burden of disease [26], have experienced several obstacles summarised by Collins *et al* [27].

Higher rates of contacts were observed in rural areas compared to semiurban areas. The pattern of contact rates also differed by location type: there was strong assortative mixing rates in children aged 6–15 years and in adults 20–49 years in rural areas whereas in the semiurban area highest rates of mixing was among adults 20–49 and above. Rural areas in the KHDSS show a marked attenuation of young adults, particularly males, into the surrounding semiurban and urban centres [16] mainly for employment and education. Rural residences are also characterised by larger households and a higher proportion of children compared to semiurban areas. Fewer contacts were recorded in diaries by shadows compared with those self-kept by participants, especially for participants aged ≥15 years and those residing in rural areas. These shadows reported having to forego their daily routines to monitor the participants' contact patterns, but mainly for those participants aged less than 5 years. This suggests that older participants did not need active monitoring as they are able to recall their most recent contacts. It also suggests that in general,

Table 4. Age group specific contact rates with 95% CI[‡].

Participant age group* (years)	Contact age group*					
	<1	1–5	6–15	16–19	20–49	≥50
<1	0.2 (0.1–0.3)	2.7 (2.3–3.2)	4.6 (4.0–5.4)	1.3 (1.1–1.7)	4.0 (3.4–4.7)	1.0 (0.7–1.2)
1–5	0.5 (0.4–0.7)	4.4 (3.8–5.2)	6.0 (5.1–6.9)	1.5 (1.2–1.8)	4.1 (3.5–4.7)	1.1 (0.9–1.4)
6–15	0.6 (0.4–0.7)	3.8 (3.2–4.4)	8.9 (7.9–10.1)	2.3 (1.9–2.7)	3.6 (3.1–4.2)	0.9 (0.7–1.1)
16–19	0.5 (0.3–0.7)	2.0 (1.6–2.5)	5.5 (4.6–6.4)	5.2 (4.4–6.1)	5.0 (4.2–5.8)	1.1 (0.9–1.4)
20–49	0.7 (0.5–0.8)	2.5 (2.1–2.9)	3.1 (2.7–3.6)	2.1 (1.8–2.5)	8.2 (7.3–9.3)	2.3 (1.9–2.6)
≥50	0.4 (0.2–0.6)	1.5 (1.1–2.0)	2.5 (1.9–3.1)	1.4 (1.0–1.9)	6.0 (4.8–7.4)	2.1 (1.6–2.7)

‡Confidence intervals based on 2,000 bootstraps.
*Age group in years.

shadows did not record all contacts that a participant made. However, for older individuals, this bias was likely reduced through an exit questionnaire shortly following diary completion that aimed to elicit non-recorded contacts.

Unlike previous studies [10,13,14,28], no difference was reported in weekend versus weekday contact rates. This could be an indication of more homogenous mixing patterns throughout the week compared to developed countries. For example, the majority of the KHDSS adult population engages in informal employment and subsistence farming that entails working throughout the week. The social structure of the community also involves most of social activities occurring over the weekend, especially wedding and burial ceremonies where individuals congregate for extended periods of time. Furthermore, no differences were observed by season: a surprising result given the local migration of households to tend crops.

Limitations

Out of the 1,138 selected participants, 50% participated in the study. This resulted in disproportionate under-sampling of the semiurban setting. Exploration of the effect on contact rates by weighted analysis suggested a negligible impact. No other biases were identified arising from low participation. Replacement of all non-participants was not possible due to time constraints imposed by the monthly sampling strategy.

Data was not collected throughout the holiday period (Christmas and New Year holiday, from 23rd December 2011 to 8th January 2012). In this social context, most families congregate in their ancestral homesteads located in the rural areas over the holidays. Contact rates, therefore, do not reflect possible effects due to holiday periods, also including the effect of vacation time for school children. Over 50% of all diaries were completed with the support of a shadow. The use a third party to record contacts clearly has possible implications to the accuracy of data and comparability to records from other age groups. In general, we attempted to limit under-reporting and behavioural changes through pre-training, alarm reminders and exit interviewing. Nonetheless, a small number of the shadows reported being unable to keep track of the participants (mainly children) during the duration of the study.

Generalizability

This study was conducted along a semiurban-rural transect and spanned two climatic seasons. Kilifi has one of the highest poverty rates in Kenya, and the main seasonal economic activities are fishing, farming, agriculture and tourism [16]. Even though much of sub-Saharan Africa remains predominantly rural, such results are contextual and can only be generalized with high confidence to similar regions along the Kenyan coast where these activities are prevalent. Future studies should aim at characterizing social contact patterns across different spatial regions in Kenya and elsewhere, particularly in the urban setting which is rapidly growing.

Conclusions

In summary, we present data on contact patterns and rates in a rural coastal location in Kilifi, Kenya. We discuss the novel methods used to collect the data in sub-Saharan Africa (the use of picture diaries, shadows and reminders), as well as how the challenges encountered were minimised. Similar to earlier studies in other regions, age assortative mixing is reported. This is more pronounced in the younger age groups in rural areas, with semiurban areas indicating highest contact rates among the adults.

The age-specific contact rates estimated from this study can be used to parameterize mathematical models useful to predict the impact of different vaccination schedules.

Supporting Information

Figure S1 Sample paper diary. Participants recorded each contact person only once with a unique code, indicated their age from the groups shown, and gave a tally of repeat contacts with each person met.

Figure S2 Demographic questionnaire. This was used to collect data on participants' and shadow demographic details.

Figure S3 Sample Exit questionnaire. This was used to collect data on frequency of meeting the contact (new or common contacts).

Table S1 Reasons for refusal by location of the Kilifi HDSS, Kenya.

Table S2 Total number of age group (years)-specific contacts per person per day.

Text S1 Sample weights.

Text S2 Raw data used in analysis.

Text S3 Data dictionary.

Acknowledgments

We thank the residents of the 5 locations for participating in the study. We thank the members of the Community Advice for Specific Study Teams (CAST) in KEMRI for assisting in the focus group discussions and participation in the community engagement for this study. We would also like to thank the fieldworkers who worked tirelessly during the data collection, as well as the dedicated team of data entry clerks for data entry and management. This article is published with the permission of the Director of KEMRI.

Author Contributions

Conceived and designed the experiments: DJN GFM TMK MCK DCK PKM. Performed the experiments: MCK DCK. Analyzed the data: MCK TMK PKM. Contributed reagents/materials/analysis tools: MCK TMK PKM. Contributed to the writing of the manuscript: MCK TMK DJN PKM GFM.

References

1. Wallinga J, Teunis P, Kretzschmar M (2006) Using data on social contacts to estimate age-specific transmission parameters for respiratory-spread infectious agents. Am J Epidemiol 164: 936–944.
2. Keeling MJ, Danon L (2009) Mathematical modelling of infectious diseases. Br Med Bull 92: 33–42.
3. Mossong J, Hens N, Jit M, Beutels P, Auranen K, et al. (2008) Social contacts and mixing patterns relevant to the spreading of infectious diseases. PLoS Medicine 5.
4. Keeling MJ, White PJ (2011) Targeting vaccination against novel infections: risk, age and spatial structure for pandemic influenza in Great Britain. J R Soc Interface 8: 661–670.
5. Del Valle SY, Hymanb JM, Hethcote HW, Eubank SG (2007) Mixing patterns between age groups in social networks. Social Networks 29: 539–554.
6. Edmunds WJ, Kafatos G, Wallinga J, Mossong JR (2006) Mixing patterns and the spread of close-contact infectious diseases. Emerg Themes Epidemiol 3: 10.
7. Johnstone-Robertson SP, Mark D, Morrow C, Middelkoop K, Chiswell M, et al. (2011) Social mixing patterns within a South African township community: implications for respiratory disease transmission and control. Am J Epidemiol 174: 1246–1255.
8. Horby P, Pham QT, Hens N, Nguyen TT, Le QM, et al. (2011) Social contact patterns in Vietnam and implications for the control of infectious diseases. PLoS One 6: e16965.
9. Edmunds WJ, O'Callaghan CJ, Nokes DJ (1997) Who mixes with whom? A method to determine the contact patterns of adults that may lead to the spread of airborne infections. Proc R Soc Lond B 264: 949–957.
10. Beutels P, Shkedy Z, Aerts M, Van Damme P (2006) Social mixing patterns for transmission models of close contact infections: exploring self-evaluation and diary-based data collection through a web-based interface. Epidemiol Infect 134: 1158–1166.
11. Glass LM, Glass RJ (2008) Social contact networks for the spread of pandemic influenza in children and teenagers. BMC Public Health 8: 61.
12. McCaw JM, Forbes K, Nathan PM, Pattison PE, Robins GL, et al. (2010) Comparison of three methods for ascertainment of contact information relevant to respiratory pathogen transmission in encounter networks. BMC Infect Dis 10: 166.
13. Towers S, Chowell G (2012) Impact of weekday social contact patterns on the modeling of influenza transmission, and determination of the influenza latent period. J Theor Biol 312C: 87–95.
14. Hens N, Ayele GM, Goeyvaerts N, Aerts M, Mossong J, et al. (2009) Estimating the impact of school closure on social mixing behaviour and the transmission of close contact infections in eight European countries. BMC Infect Dis 9: 187.
15. Molyneux CS, Mung'ala-Odera V, Harpman T, Snow RW (2002) Maternal morbidity across the rural-urban divide: empirical data from coastal Kenya. Environment and Urbanization 14: 203–217.
16. Scott JA, Bauni E, Moisi JC, Ojal J, Gatakaa H, et al. (2012) Profile: The Kilifi Health and Demographic Surveillance System (KHDSS). Int J Epidemiol 41: 650–657.
17. (1992) Study size. In: Smith PG, Morrow RH, editors. Methods for Field Trials of Interventions Against Tropical Diseases - A "toolbox". New York: Oxford University Press. pp. 42–70.
18. Kamuya DM, Marsh V, Kombe FK, Geissler PW, Molyneux SC (2013) Engaging communities to strengthen research ethics in low-income settings: selection and perceptions of members of a network of representatives in coastal Kenya. Dev World Bioeth 13: 10–20. doi: 10.1111/dewb.12014. Epub 12013 Feb 12021.
19. Carpenter J, Bithell J (2000) Bootstrap confidence intervals: when, which, what? A practical guide for medical statisticians. Stat Med 19: 1141–1164.
20. Ogunjimi B, Hens N, Goeyvaerts N, Aerts M, Van Damme P, et al. (2009) Using empirical social contact data to model person to person infectious disease transmission: an illustration for varicella. Math Biosci 218: 80–87.
21. Grimwood K, Abbott GD, Fergusson DM, Jennings LC, Allan JM (1983) Spread of rotavirus within families: a community based study. Br Med J (Clin Res Ed) 287: 575–577.
22. Hall CB, Douglas RG, Jr. (1981) Modes of transmission of respiratory syncytial virus. J Pediatr 99: 100–103.
23. Fu YC, Wang DW, Chuang JH (2012) Representative contact diaries for modeling the spread of infectious diseases in Taiwan. PLoS One 7: e45113.
24. Eames KT, Tilston NL, Brooks-Pollock E, Edmunds WJ (2012) Measured dynamic social contact patterns explain the spread of H1N1v influenza. PLoS Comput Biol 8: e1002425.
25. Munywoki PK, Koech DC, Agoti CN, Lewa C, Cane PA, et al. (2014) The Source of Respiratory Syncytial Virus Infection In Infants: A Household Cohort Study In Rural Kenya. J Infect Dis 26: 26.
26. Nair H, Nokes DJ, Gessner BD, Dherani M, Madhi SA, et al. (2010) Global burden of acute lower respiratory infections due to respiratory syncytial virus in young children: a systematic review and meta-analysis. Lancet.
27. Collins PL, Murphy BR (2007) Vaccines against Human Respiratory Syncytial Virus. In: Cane P, editor. Respiratory Syncytial Virus. Amsterdam: Elsevier. pp. 233–277.
28. Hens N, Goeyvaerts N, Aerts M, Shkedy Z, Van Damme P, et al. (2009) Mining social mixing patterns for infectious disease models based on a two-day population survey in Belgium. BMC Infect Dis 9: 5.

5

IL-21 Promotes Late Activator APC-Mediated T Follicular Helper Cell Differentiation in Experimental Pulmonary Virus Infection

Jae-Kwang Yoo[1,2], Thomas J. Braciale[2,3,4]*

1 Inflammation Research, Amgen Inc., Seattle, Washington, United States of America, **2** Beirne B. Carter Center for Immunology Research, University of Virginia, Charlottesville, Virginia, United States of America, **3** Department of Microbiology, University of Virginia, Charlottesville, Virginia, United States of America, **4** Department of Pathology, University of Virginia, Charlottesville, Virginia, United States of America

Abstract

IL-21 is a type-I cytokine that has pleiotropic immuno-modulatory effects. Primarily produced by activated T cells including NKT and T_{FH} cells, IL-21 plays a pivotal role in promoting T_{FH} differentiation through poorly understood cellular and molecular mechanisms. Here, employing a mouse model of influenza A virus (IAV) infection, we demonstrate that IL-21, initially produced by NKT cells, promotes T_{FH} differentiation by promoting the migration of late activator antigen presenting cell (LAPC), a recently identified T_{FH} inducer, from the infected lungs into the draining lymph nodes (dLN). LAPC migration from IAV-infected lung into the dLN is CXCR3-CXCL9 dependent. IL-21-induced TNF-α production by conventional T cells is critical to stimulate CXCL9 expression by DCs in the dLN, which supports LAPC migration into the dLN and ultimately facilitates T_{FH} differentiation. Our results reveal a previously unappreciated mechanism for IL-21 modulation of T_{FH} responses during respiratory virus infection.

Editor: Jörg Hermann Fritz, McGill University, Canada

Funding: This work was supported by U.S. Public Health Service grants AI-15608, HL-33391, AI-37293 and U19 AI-083024 to T.J.B. and Senior Research Training Fellowship from American Lung Association to J.K.Y. The funders had no role in study design, data collection and analysis, decision to publish, or preparation of the manuscript. Amgen Inc. provided support in the form of salary for author Jae-Kwang Yoo, but did not have any additional role in the study design, data collection and analysis, decision to publish, or preparation of the manuscript. The specific roles of this author are articulated in the author contributions section.

Competing Interests: The first author, Jae-Kwang Yoo, is currently employed by a commercial company Amgen Inc. However, there are no patents, products in development or marketed products to declare.

* Email: tjb2r@virginia.edu

Introduction

Following infection with pathogenic microorganisms, the encounter of B cells with their cognate specific Ag in secondary lymphoid organs triggers B cell activation, proliferation and differentiation ultimately resulting in germinal center (GC) formation within B cell follicles. The GC response is particularly pronounced due to the inflammatory stimulus produced by the invading microorganisms. GC B cell responses and GC formation is largely T cell dependent. Hallmarks of the GC response include BcR affinity maturation, plasma cell differentiation and the generation of memory B cells. Hence, the GC response not only contributes to pathogen clearance but also plays a pivotal role in preventing subsequent infections with the infecting microorganism [1–5]. T_{FH} T cells are recently recognized as a distinct $CD4^+$ T cell subset defined as $PD1^+CXCR5^+Bcl\text{-}6^+$. This T-cell subset has been implicated as a key regulator of the GC B cell response through the delivery of multiple soluble and cell-associated signals to GC B cells including the production of soluble factors (IL-4 and IL-21) and the display of co-stimulatory ligands and receptors (ICOS, CD28, CD40L and CD84) [4,6–10].

The factors controlling T_{FH} differentiation are not as yet fully understood, and multiple cell types and molecules have been implicated in this process [4,6]. IL-21 was initially proposed as a key soluble factor driving the differentiation of Ag-primed $CD4^+$ T cells along the T_{FH} lineage pathway [8,11], and is now recognized as promoting an optimal T_{FH} response [12,13]. However, the mechanism(s) by which IL-21 optimizes the T_{FH} response has not as yet been clearly defined.

Recently, we have identified a novel immune cell population in virus infected murine lungs with migratory properties and antigen presenting capacity, the late activator antigen presenting cell (LAPC) [14]. The $mPDCA1^+CD11c^-B220^-TcR\beta^-$ LAPCs initiate their migration out of the IAV-infected lungs into the draining lymph nodes relatively late in the course of infection (i.e., between 6–12 days post-infection (d.p.i.)) *via* CXCR3-CXCL9 dependent chemotactic pathway. In the dLN, LAPCs promote T_{FH} differentiation of Ag-activated $CD4^+$ T cells by display of ICOSL and engagement of ICOS receptor on the activated $CD4^+$ T cells [14–16]. In this report we demonstrate that IL-21, initially produced by NKT cells, promotes optimal T_{FH} differentiation by augmenting CXCR3-CXCL9 dependent LAPC migration into the dLN during influenza A virus (IAV) infection. IL-21-induced TNF-α production by conventional T cells is critical to stimulate CXCL9 expression by DCs in the dLN, which supports LAPC migration into the dLN and ultimately facilitates T_{FH} differentiation.

Materials and Methods

Mice, virus and infections

CD45.1$^+$ or CD45.2$^+$ C57BL/6 mice were purchased from National Cancer Institute (NCI). *Tnf-α*$^{-/-}$ mice were generated in the Ludwig Institute for Cancer Research, purchased from Taconic farms and bred in house. *Il-21rα*$^{-/-}$, *il-21*$^{-/-}$, and OT-II mice were bred in house. *Cd-1d*$^{-/-}$ mice were provided by M.D. Okusa (University of Virginia, Charlottesville, VA). All mice were housed in a specific pathogen–free environment and all mouse experiments were performed in accordance with protocols approved by the University of Virginia Animal Care and Use Committee. A/WSN/OVA-II virus was generously provided by Dr. David Topham (University of Rochester, Rochester, USA) [18]. For virus infection, mice were infected intranasally (i.n.) with a sub-lethal dose (0.05 LD_{50}) of influenza strain A/PR/8/34 (H1N1), A/WSN/33 (H1N1) or A/WSN/OVA-II in serum-free Iscove's medium, after anesthesia with ketamine and xylazine.

Quantitative RT-PCR

dLN cell suspensions were prepared as described [14,15]. DCs were isolated by FACS (Reflection HAPS 2) to examine *cxcl-9* expression. mRNA isolation, reverse transcription and real-time PCR were performed as previously described [19]. Data were generated with the comparative threshold cycle method, by normalizing to hypoxanthine phosphoribosyltransferase (*hprt*). The sequences of primers used in the studies are available on request.

Bone marrow chimeras

To generate mixed bone marrow (BM) chimeras containing wild type (CD45.1$^+$) and *il21-rα*$^{-/-}$ (CD45.2$^+$) BM in a 1:1 ratio, we lethally irradiated (1,100 rads) CD45.1$^+$ wild type B6 mice and reconstituted the irradiated mice with CD45.1$^+$ wild type BM (2×10^6 cells) mixed with CD45.2$^+$ *il-21rα*$^{-/-}$ BM (2×10^6 cells). After 8 weeks, using PBMC the reconstitution efficiency was determined by FACS-analysis and the successfully reconstituted mice were then infected with A/PR/8/34 IAV.

OT-II T cell transfer, infection and *ex vivo* co-culture with LAPCs

For OT-II T cell transfer into CD45.1$^+$ wild type B6 mice, cells were isolated from CD45.2$^+$ OT-II lymph nodes (LNs). A total of 5×10^6 LN cells were then transferred into CD45.1$^+$ mice by *i.v.* injection. The recipient mice were infected with A/WSN/OVA-II virus 24 hrs later. At 5 d.p.i., *in vivo* virus activated OT-II cells were isolated from the dLN by FACS. LAPCs were sorted separately at 8 d.p.i. from the dLNs of A/WSN/OVAII infected either wt or *il-21rα*$^{-/-}$ mice. Isolated day 5 *in vivo* virus activated OT-II cells were *ex vivo* co-cultured with day 8 LAPC for additional 24 hrs to assess T_{FH} differentiation by FACS-analysis.

Cell sorting

For *ex vivo* co-culture experiments, recipients of transferred OT-II T-cells or wild type mice were infected with A/WSN/OVA-II influenza. Different cell populations from the dLN were sorted by FACS (Reflection HAPS 2) based on the following markers at either 5 or 8 d.p.i.: OT-II cells, CD45.2$^+$Thy1.2$^+$CD4$^+$; LAPCs, mPDCA1$^+$CD11c$^-$B220$^-$TcRβ$^-$. For *cxcl-9* qPCR, DCs (CD11c$^+$TcRβ$^-$) were sorted from the dLN of A/PR/8/34 IAV infected wild type mice at 6 d.p.i. For *tnf-α* qPCR, both wild type (CD45.1$^+$) and *il-21rα*$^{-/-}$ (CD45.2$^+$) T cells (CD4 and CD8 T) were sorted by FACS from the dLN of A/PR/8/34 IAV-infected mixed BM chimera mice at 6 d.p.i. (CD45.1$^+$Thy1.2$^+$CD4$^+$, CD45.2$^+$Thy1.2$^+$CD4$^+$, CD45.1$^+$Thy1.2$^+$CD8$^+$, CD45.2$^+$Thy1.2$^+$CD8$^+$). For *in vivo* adoptive transfer experiments, non-T_{FH} total T cells (Thy1.2$^+$CXCR5$^-$) were isolated by FACS from the dLN of A/PR/8/34 IAV-infected wild type or *tnf-α*$^{-/-}$ mice at 6 d.p.i. and adoptively transferred by the *i.v.* route (2×10^6cells/mouse) into 6 d.p.i. A/PR/8/34 IAV-infected recipient *tnf-α*$^{-/-}$ mice.

Antibodies and FACS-analysis

All antibodies were purchased from BD Biosciences or eBioscience (unless otherwise stated): CD4 (L3T4), CD8α (53-6.7), CD11c (HL3), CD45.1 (A20), CD45.2 (104), CD90.2 (30-H12), B220/CD45R (RA3-6B2), NK1.1 (PK136), TCR-β (H57-597), IL-21 (FFA21), CXCR5 (2G8), PD-1 (RMP1-30), ICOS-L (HK5.3), TNF-α (MP6-XT22) and CXCL9 (MIG-2F5.5). αmPDCA-1 mAb (JF05-1C2.4.1) was purchased from Miltenyi Biotec. A CXCR3 specific mAb was obtained from both R&D Systems (220803) and Biolegend (CXCR3-173). αmTNF-α mAb (XT3.11) were purchased from BioXcell for *in vivo* mTNF-α blocking experiments. Flow cytometry was performed on FACS-Canto with optimal compensation set for six-color staining. The data were analyzed using FlowJo software (Tree Star, Inc.). All cytokine (IL-21 and TNF-α) and chemokine (CXCL9) expressions by dLN-derived cells were measured directly *ex vivo* without further *in vitro* re-stimulation.

In vivo migration assay

Both B6 and *il-21rα*$^{-/-}$ mice were anesthetized as described above and infected by i.n. instillation with 50 µl PBS containing 0.05 LD_{50} A/PR/8/34 virus. On day 5 p.i., mice received 50 µl of either PBS (negative control) or FITC-Dextran (40 kDa, 1 mg/ml) by i.n. instillation. At 24 hrs post-treatment, mice were sacrificed and cells were collected from the dLN. FACS-analysis was performed to examine the percent population of FITC$^+$ cells, gating on LAPCs (mPDCA-1$^+$CD11c$^-$B220$^-$TCRβ$^-$).

In vivo TNF-α blocking experiments

To examine the role of TNF-α in LAPC-mediated T_{FH} differentiation, *in vivo* TNF-α blocking experiments were performed. Briefly, B6 mice infected with 0.05LD_{50} A/PR/8/34 virus were treated (i.p.) daily with either isotype control Abs (Rat IgG) or mTNF-α blocking mAb (200 µg/day/mouse) from 4 d.p.i. till 7 d.p.i. At 8 d.p.i, the levels of CXCL9 expression in DCs, LAPC accumulation and T_{FH} differentiation in the dLN were monitored and compared between isotype Ab treated and mTNF-α blocking mAb treated mice by FACS-analysis.

IAV–specific antibody ELISA

BAL fluid was collected from IAV–infected mice on 8 d.p.i. by intra-tracheal instillation of 500 µl of sterile PBS, and anti-influenza antibody responses in the BAL fluid were measured by ELISA. Briefly, wells of 96-well plates were coated overnight at room temperature with 50 µl of either A/PR/8 or B/Lee influenza virus. The plates were washed twice with PBS supplemented with 0.05% Tween-20 (PBST) and incubated with 50 µl of 2% BSA in PBST for 1 hr at room temperature. After washing the plates with PBST, 50 µl of diluted BAL fluid was added to each well and incubated for 2 hrs at room temperature.

Bound antibodies were detected by the incubation of horseradish peroxidase (HRP)–conjugated anti–mouse IgM (1:10,000; SouthernBiotech) or total IgG (1:10,000; SouthernBiotech) antibodies. After 1 hr, the plates were washed with PBST, and 100 μl of 3,3′,5,5′-tetramethylbenzidine (TMB) substrate solution (Sigma-Aldrich) was added into each well and incubated for a further 30 minutes. The enzyme reaction was stopped by adding 100 μl of 2N H_2SO_4 and O.D. values were determined at 450 nm using a plate reader (Bio-TEK).

Statistical analysis

Unless otherwise noted, an unpaired two-tailed Student's *t*-test was used to compare two treatment groups. Groups larger than two were analyzed with one-way ANOVA (Tukey's post-test). These statistical analyses were performed using Prism3 software (for Macintosh; GraphPad Software, Inc.). Data are mean ± s.e.m. A p value of <0.05 was considered to be statistically significant.

Results

IL-21 can promote T_{FH} differentiation in $CD4^+$ T cells lacking an IL-21 receptor

To characterize T follicular helper cell response to primary IAV infection at a mucosal tissue i.e. the respiratory tract, we examined the kinetics of generation and accumulation of T_{FH} T cells in the draining mediastinal lymph nodes (dLN) of C57BL/6 mice intranasally (i.n.) infected with a sub-lethal dose ($0.05LD_{50}$) of A/PR/8/34 virus. The generation of T_{FH} T cells (i.e. $CD4^+PD1^+CXCR5^+Thy1.2^+$) was monitored in the dLN by FACS-analysis. As previously shown in BALB/c mice [16], in the uninfected mice the number of T_{FH} cells was negligible. T_{FH} T cells were first detected at 6 d.p.i. and showed the accumulation (absolute number) of T_{FH} cell in the dLN was maximum at 12 d.p.i. (Fig. 1a). The kinetics of T_{FH} expansion and contraction do differ modestly from that reported by Boyden et al. [20]. The most likely explanation for this difference is the virus infectious dose since Boyden et al. used 0.1 LD_{50} A/PR/8/34 virus.

To examine whether IL-21 is necessary for optimal T_{FH} differentiation in IAV infection, we evaluated the generation/accumulation of T_{FH} cells in the dLN of IAV infected *il-21rα* deficient (*il-21rα*$^{-/-}$), *il-21* deficient (*il-21*$^{-/-}$) and wild type (WT) mice. As reported previously [8,12,13], as early as 8 d.p.i., i.e. prior to full expansion of T_{FH} cells in the dLN, IAV-infected both *il-21rα*$^{-/-}$ and *il-21*$^{-/-}$ mice showed significantly diminished T_{FH} (PD-1^+CXCR5^+ or Bcl-6^+) generation/accumulation compared to wild type mice, both in absolute T_{FH} numbers and percentage relative to other cell types (Fig. 1b). These results suggest that in IAV infection IL-21 activity may be necessary to support optimal T_{FH} differentiation. Correlated with diminished T_{FH} response, at 8 d.p.i. IAV-infected *il21rα*$^{-/-}$ mice exhibited significantly diminished both germinal center (GC)-B cell (Fig. 1c) and anti-IAV antibody responses (Fig. 1d) compared to wild type mice.

At present, it is uncertain whether IL-21 supports T_{FH} differentiation primarily through direct engagement of the IL-21 receptor (IL-21R) on activated proliferating $CD4^+$ T cells or if other indirect mechanisms of IL-21 action also play a role [12,21]. To address this issue during IAV infection, we constructed mixed bone marrow (BM) chimera in which lethally irradiated (1,100 rads) C57BL/6 mice (WT: CD45.1^+) were reconstituted with a one-to-one mixture of BM from CD45.1^+ *il-21rα* $^{+/+}$ and CD45.2^+ *il21rα*$^{-/-}$mice. Eight weeks after the successful BM reconstitution, mice were infected with A/PR/8/34 virus and at 8 d.p.i. the abundance of wild type (CD45.1^+) and *il-21rα* $^{-/-}$ (CD45.2^+) T_{FH} in the dLN were determined (Fig. 1e). Notably, at 8 d.p.i. the ratio between wild type (CD45.1^+) and *il-21rα* $^{-/-}$ (CD45.2^+) T_{FH} was comparable to that of total $CD4^+$ T cells in the dLN. Collectively, these results suggest two possibilities: 1. That during IAV infection IL-21 may support efficient T_{FH} differentiation independently of IL-21R signaling in the responding $CD4^+$ T cells; 2. That the stimulus resulting from IL-21/IL21R interaction in a signaling competent cell type in the dLN e.g. T-cells, is necessary but can act in trans, which support T_{FH} differentiation of $CD4^+$ T cells lacking the IL-21R receptor.

The tempo of IL-21 production in the dLN of IAV-infected mice correlates with LAPC accumulation at this site

To further investigate the underlying mechanism accounting for the contribution of IL-21 to T_{FH} differentiation, we next examined the kinetics of IL-21 expression in the dLN of A/PR/8/34 virus infected C57BL/6 mice. Time course studies revealed that expression of IL-21 both at the gene and protein level is first detected at 6 d.p.i. and keep increasing untill 12 d.p.i., in keeping with the kinetics of T_{FH} accumulation in the dLN of IAV-infected mice (Fig. 1a, 2a and 2b).

IL-21 is primarily produced by activated T cells including NKT and T_{FH} cells [22–25]. We next evaluate the potential sources of IL-21 produced in the dLN of IAV-infected wt mice using IAV-infected *il-21*$^{-/-}$ mice as negative control for IL-21 staining. We analyzed cells for expression of IL-21 protein directly *ex vivo* from the dLN without re-stimulation *in vitro*. Interestingly, even though at 8 d.p.i. $CD4^+$ T cells became major cell type expressing *il-21* gene (unpublished data), at 6 d.p.i. NKT cells ($NK1.1^+TcR\beta^+CD1d^+PD1^-CXCR5^-$) were most prominent cell type producing IL-21 in the dLN of IAV-infected C57BL/6 mice (Fig. 2c). This data was further confirmed using a mouse model lacking NKT cells (*cd-1d*$^{-/-}$ mice) showing that at 6 d.p.i. both protein and gene expressions of IL-21 in the dLNs were significantly impaired in IAV-infected *cd-1d*$^{-/-}$ mice compared to wild type mice (Fig. 2d and 2e). Since IL-21 promotes T_{FH} differentiation of CD4 T cells during IAV infection and NKT cells are initial primary source of IL-21 in the dLN, we determined T_{FH} response in the dLN of IAV-infected *cd1d*$^{-/-}$ mice and found that at 8d.p.i. IAV-infected *cd-1d* $^{-/-}$ mice exhibited significantly diminished T_{FH} response compared to wild type mice (Fig. 2f). Together, these data suggest that at the early phase of T_{FH} development following IAV infection NKT cells may serve as an initial major (primary) source of IL-21 in the dLN.

Recently, we have identified a novel migratory immune cell type, LAPC, in the respiratory track of IAV-infected mice [14]. LAPCs unlike conventional APCs such as respiratory dendritic cells (DCs) migrate from the infected lung tissue into the dLN late, i.e. starting at 6 d.p.i. during IAV infection and have been demonstrated to promote the differentiation of Ag-primed activated $CD4^+$ T cells along the T_{FH} differentiation pathway [14–16]. As with IL-21 production, the kinetics of LAPC accumulation in the dLN directly parallels T_{FH} accumulation in the dLN (Fig. 1a, 2a, 2b and 2g).

IL-21 receptor signaling modulates LAPC migration from lung tissue into the dLN of IAV-infected mice

Since in the mixed bone marrow (BM) chimera the absence of the IL-21R on the responding anti-viral $CD4^+$ T cells did not diminish the generation of $CD4^+$ T_{FH} T cells in the dLN but the kinetics of IL-21 expression paralleled with LAPC accumulation in the dLNs, we considered the possibility of IL- 21 expression and

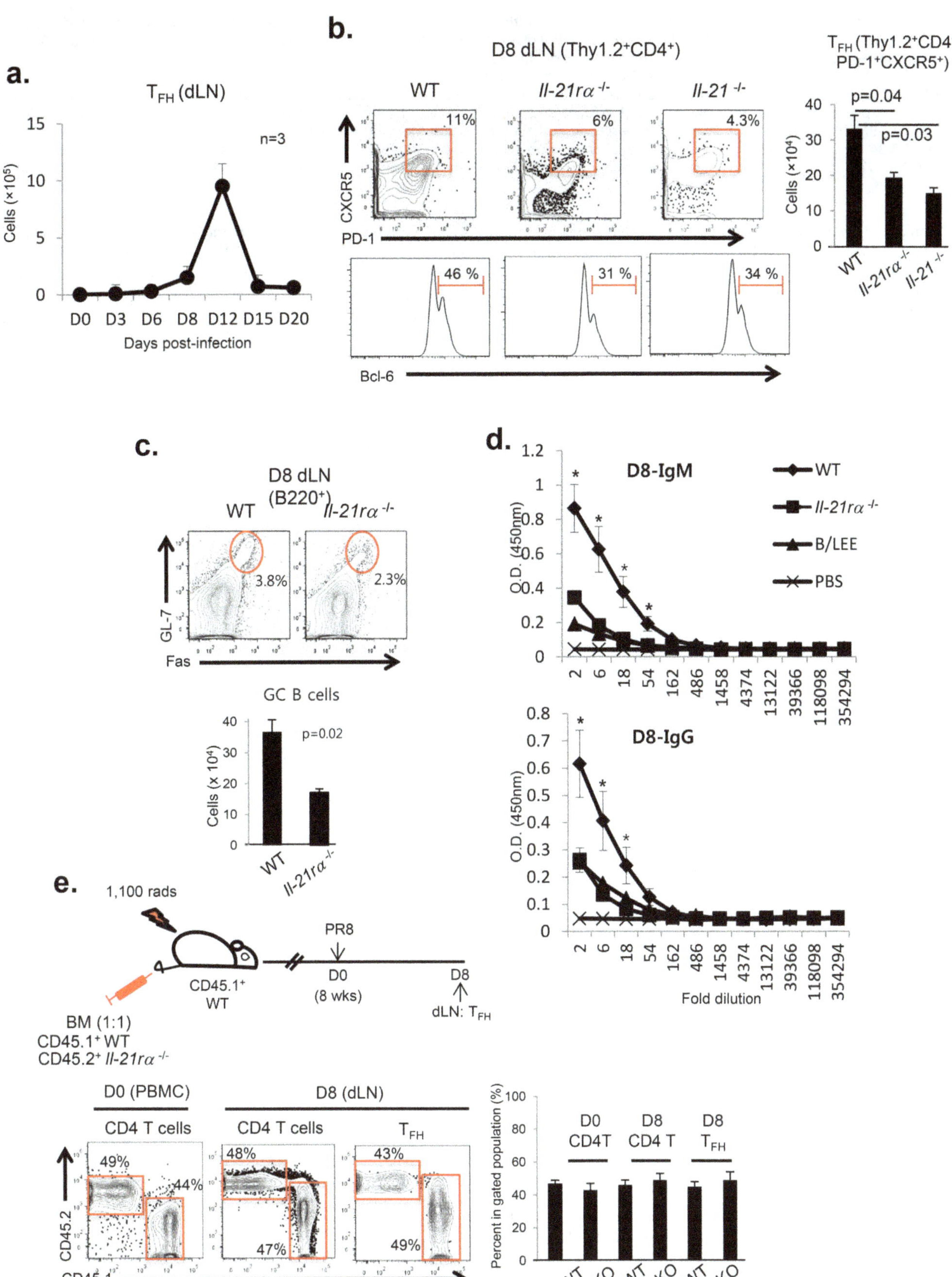

Figure 1. IL-21 can promote T_{FH} differentiation in CD4^{+} T cells lacking an IL-21 receptor. C57BL/6 (WT) (n = 51), *il-21rα* $^{-/-}$ (n = 9) and *il-21*$^{-/-}$ mice (n = 9) were infected intranasally (i.n.) with a sub-lethal dose (0.05 LD_{50}) of A/PR/8/34 virus, as described in the Materials and Methods. (**a**) The kinetics of T_{FH} accumulation in the dLNs of B6 mice was monitored by flow cytometric (FACS) analysis. The data are presented as absolute

number of T_{FH} (mean ± s.e.m.) and representative data from more than three independent experiments are shown. (**b**) The magnitude of the T_{FH} (Thy1.2$^+$CD4$^+$PD-1$^+$CXCR5$^+$ or Thy1.2$^+$CD4$^+$Bcl-6$^+$) response in the dLNs of IAV infected B6, *il-21*$^{-/-}$ and *il-21rα*$^{-/-}$ mice was determined at 8 d.p.i. by FACS-analysis. Representative data from three independent experiments are shown. The data are presented as both percentage T_{FH} cells within the total CD4$^+$ T cell population as well as absolute T_{FH} cell numbers (mean ± s.e.m.) and were analyzed by Student's *t* test. 8 d.p.i. (**c**) GC-B cells (dLN:B220$^+$Fas$^+$GL7$^+$, FACS) and (**d**) anti-influenza Ab responses (BALF: IgM and total IgG, Ab-ELISA) were determined. Representative data from two independent experiments are shown. Considered a significant difference at * (WT *vs.il-21rα*$^{-/-}$, P<0.05). (**e**) Mixed BM chimera containing wild type *and il-21rα*$^{-/-}$ BM in a 1:1 ratio were generated as described in the Materials and Methods. At 8 wks after reconstitution, mice (n = 7) were infected with A/PR/8/34 virus. At 8 d.p.i., the percentage of wild type (CD45.1) and *il-21rα*$^{-/-}$ (CD45.2) T-cells among total CD4$^+$ T cells or T_{FH} (Thy1.2$^+$CD4$^+$PD1$^+$CXCR5$^+$) cells in the dLNs were determined by FACS-analysis. Representative images of two independent experiments are shown.

LAPC migration might be linked. To examine the contribution of IL-21 in the migration of LAPCs from IAV-infected lungs into the dLN, we next evaluated the migration of LAPCs following i.n. FITC-Dextran administration and uptake of this fluorescent marker by LAPCs in IAV-infected wild type and *il-21rα*$^{-/-}$ mice. Interestingly, *il-21rα*$^{-/-}$ mice showed significantly diminished FITC positive LAPC accumulation in the dLN at 6 d.p.i. compared to wild type mice (Fig. 3a). Although we cannot formally exclude the possibility that the diminished accumulation of FITC positive LAPC from *il-21rα*$^{-/-}$ mice in the dLN at day 5–6 p.i reflects defective uptake of FITC-dextran in the lung by LAPC deficient in IL-21R signaling, diminished LAPC accumulation in the dLN of both *il-21rα*$^{-/-}$ and *il-21*$^{-/-}$ mice in terms of absolute LAPC numbers suggests that IL-21/IL-21R signaling plays a pivotal role in the migration of LAPCs from IAV-infected lungs into the dLN (Fig. 3b). Since NKT cells are the initial primary source of IL-21 in the dLN of IAV-infected mice (Fig. 2d and 2e), the mice lacking NKT cells (*cd-1d*$^{-/-}$ mice) showed significantly diminished LAPC accumulation in the dLNs comparable to that of *il-21rα*$^{-/-}$ mice at 8 d.p.i. (Fig. 3b).

To determine if the deficit in LAPC migration in mice deficient in the IL-21 receptor was attributable to a defect in the expression of this receptor by LAPC, we constructed mixed bone marrow (BM) chimeras in which mice were reconstituted with a one-to-one mixture of BM from CD45.1$^+$ *il-21rα*$^{+/+}$ and CD45.2$^+$ *il-21rα*$^{-/-}$ mice. Eight weeks after BM reconstitution, mice were infected with IAV and at 8 d.p.i. the frequency of wild type (CD45.1$^+$) and *il-21rα*$^{-/-}$ (CD45.2$^+$) LAPCs in the dLN were determined (Fig. 3c). Notably, at 8 d.p.i. the ratio of wild type (CD45.1$^+$) to *il-21rα*$^{-/-}$ (CD45.2$^+$) LAPCs was comparable and equivalent to that of total dLN cells. These results suggest that IL-21 modulates LAPC migration from infected lung tissue into the dLN independently of IL-21R signaling in LAPCs.

We recently reported that ICOS-L expression by LAPC and the engagement of ICOS on CD4$^+$ T cells is required for LAPC to promote T_{FH} differentiation [16]. We therefore wanted to determine whether IL-21 not only affects LAPC migration into the dLN but also directly enhances the capacity of LAPC to facilitate T_{FH} differentiation by up-regulating ICOS-L expression on LAPC. We found, however, that LAPCs isolated from the dLN of *il-21rα*$^{-/-}$ mice showed comparable level of ICOS-L expression to that of LAPCs from wild type mice (Fig. 3d). To further evaluate the impact of IL- 21 signaling on the ability of LAPCs to support T_{FH} differentiation, LAPC were isolated from IAV infected *il-21rα*$^{-/-}$ mice and co-cultured with activated CD4$^+$ T cells. Briefly, OVA-specific TCR transgenic CD4$^+$ OT-II T cells were isolated from naive CD45.2$^+$ OT-II mice and transferred by the intra-venous (*i.v.*) route into CD45.1$^+$ C57BL/6 mice. 24hrs later, mice were sub-lethally infected i.n. with the recombinant IAV A/WSN/OVA-II virus which expresses the OVA epitope recognized by OT-II cells. At 5 d.p.i., that is the time p.i. when the majority (>95%) of transferred OT-II T cells displayed an activated (CD44^{hi} or CD62L^{lo}) phenotype but did not as yet express the characteristic T_{FH} phenotype (PD1$^+$CXCR5$^+$) [14,16], *in vivo* activated IAV specific OT-II T cells were isolated from the dLN. These activated CD4$^+$ T cells were placed in short-term (24 hrs) culture with LAPCs isolated from the dLNs of 8 d.p.i. A/WSN/OVA-II virus infected wild type or *il-21rα* $^{-/-}$ mice. LAPC driven T_{FH} differentiation of the OT-II T cells was monitored by flow cytometry. As shown in figure 3e, LAPCs isolated from *il-21rα*$^{-/-}$ mice were comparable to their wild type counterparts in promoting T_{FH} differentiation of Ag-primed CD4$^+$T cells. This result further suggests that IL-21 does not modulate intrinsic capacity of LAPC to support T_{FH} differentiation.

IL-21 enhances CXCL9 expression by DCs in the dLN of IAV-infected mice by an IL-21R independent mechanism

LAPC in the IAV-infected lungs express CXCR3 and the migration of the cells from the lungs into the dLN is CXCL9 dependent [16]. Since IL-21 promotes LAPCs migration into the dLN, we questioned whether CXCR3 and/or CXCL9 expression was regulated by IL-21 receptor signaling during IAV infection. We observed that at the peak of LAPC accumulation in the infected lungs i.e. 6 d.p.i. when the LAPC initiate migration into the dLN [14], LAPC isolated from the lungs of infected wild type and *il21rα*$^{-/-}$ mice expressed CXCR3 at comparable levels (Fig. 4a). By contrast, the expression of CXCL9 in the 6 d.p.i. dLN, which is largely restricted to CD45$^+$ cells primarily DC (Fig. 4b and [16]), is substantially diminished in DCs from the dLN of infected *il-21rα* $^{-/-}$ mice (Fig. 4c and 4d). Importantly, compared to wild type DC, CXCL9 expression was likewise decreased in DC isolated from 6 d.p.i. dLN of infected *il-21*$^{-/-}$ mice (Fig. 4d). IAV-infected *cd-1d*$^{-/-}$ mice, deficient for the initial primary source of IL-21, NKT cell, also showed significantly diminished expression of CXCL9 in DCs comparable to that of *il-21*$^{-/-}$ mice (Fig. 4d). Of note, the gene encoding *cxcl-10,* another CXCR3 ligand, was not expressed in the dLN of wild type mice during the course of IAV infection (unpublished data).

To directly address the impact of IL-21R signaling in dLN DCs on CXCL9 expression by these cells, we employed the CD45.1$^+$ *il-21rα*$^{+/+}$ and CD45.2$^+$ *il-21rα*$^{-/-}$ mixed bone marrow (BM) chimera strategy described above (Fig. 3). After BM reconstitution, mice were infected with IAV and at 6 d.p.i. the CXCL9 expression levels by wild type (CD45.1$^+$) and *il-21rα*$^{-/-}$ (CD45.2$^+$) DCs in the dLN were determined by FACS-analysis (Fig. 4e). We found that at 6 d.p.i. the CXCL9 expression by wild type (CD45.1$^+$) and *il-21rα*$^{-/-}$ (CD45.2$^+$) DCs were comparable. This finding suggests that IL21 regulates CXCL9 production by DCs through a mechanism independent of IL-21R signaling in the chemokine producing dLN DCs.

IL-21 enhances TNF-α production by T cells in the dLN of IAV-infected mice

IL-21 can modulate a variety of the immuno-regulatory functions including IL21R signaling dependent up-regulation of TNF-α production by immune cells notably activated T cells

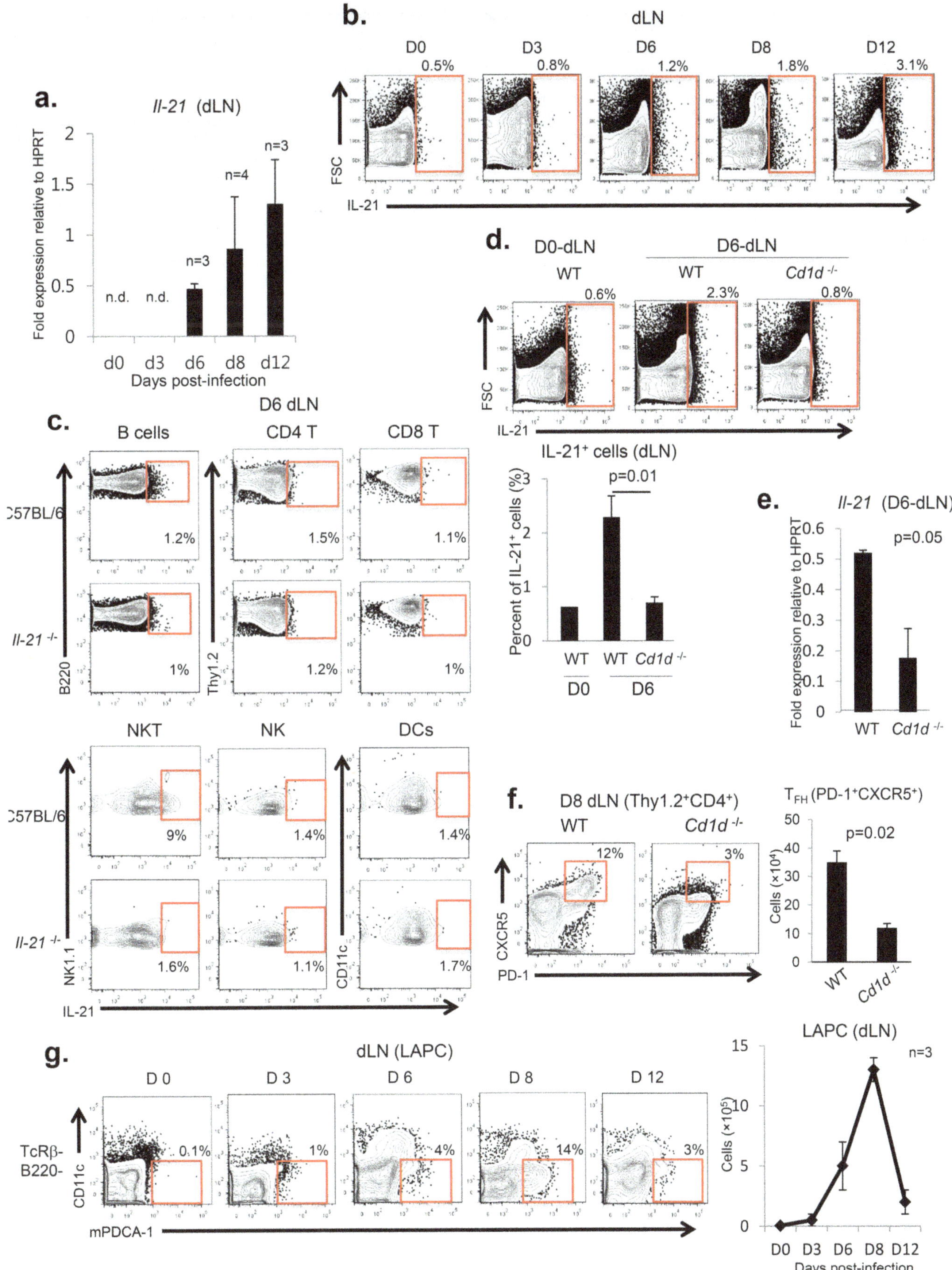

Figure 2. IL-21 expression and LAPC accumulation in the dLN of IAV-infected mice exhibit comparable kinetics. The tempo of IL-21 expression was examined by both (**a**) qPCR and (**b**) FACS-analysis in the dLNs of A/PR/8/34 virus infected C57BL/6 mice (n = 32). Representative data from three independent experiments are shown. (**c**) At 6 d.p.i., IL-21 expression was examined by FACS-analysis in each gated population isolated from the dLNs of C57BL/6 mice using IAV-infected *il-21*$^{-/-}$ mice (n = 6) as a negative control for IL-21 gating: all cells were pre-gated for live lymphocytes based on FSC/SSC profile (B cells: B220^{+} CD11c^{-}Thy1.2^{-}; CD4 T cells: CD4^{+}Thy1.2^{+}; CD8 T cells: CD8α^{+}Thy1.2^{+}; NKT cells: NK1.1^{+}TcRβ^{+}CD1d^{+}PD-1^{-}CXCR5^{-}: NK cells: NK1.1^{+}TcRβ^{-}; DCs: CD11c^{+}Thy1.2^{-}). For CD1d-tetramer and T_{FH} marker (PD-1 and CXCR5) staining, either unloaded CD1d-tetramers, isotype control Abs (Rat IgG_{2b} :RG2b) or secondary Abs (streptavidin-APC:st-APC) has been used as negative controls for CD1d-tetramer, PD-1 or CXCR5 staining, respectively. Representative data from two independent experiments are shown. C57BL/6 (n = 6) and iNKT cell deficient *cd-1d*$^{-/-}$ mice (n = 6) were infected with 0.05 LD_{50} of A/PR/8/34 virus. At 6 d.p.i. the impact of NKT cell deficiency (*cd-1d*$^{-/-}$ mice) on IL-21 production in the dLN was examined by both (**d**) FACS-analysis and (**e**) qPCR. Representative data from two independent experiments are shown. (**f**) 8 d.p.i., T_{FH} response was determined in the dLN of both wild type and *cd-1d* $^{-/-}$ mice by FACS-analysis. The data are presented as both a percentage and absolute T_{FH} numbers (mean ± s.e.m.). Representative stainings from two independent experiments are shown. (**g**) C57BL/6 mice (n = 32) were infected intranasally (i.n.) with 0.05 LD_{50} of A/PR/8/34 virus, as described in the Materials and Methods. At the indicated days after infection, the extent of LAPC (mPDCA1^{+}CD11c^{-}B220^{-}TcRβ^{-}) accumulation within the dLNs was determined by FACS-analysis. The data are presented as both a percentage of lineage^{-} i.e. TcRβ^{-} B220^{-} cells and absolute LAPC numbers (mean ± s.e.m.). Representative stainings from at least three independent experiments are shown.

[26–28]. TNF-α is well recognized as a critical regulator for immune and inflammatory cell migration into tissues through its capacity to enhance the expression of a variety of chemokines including CXCL9 [29–31]. It was therefore of interest to determine whether TNF-α was expressed in the dLN of IAV-infected mice at 6 d.p.i. and also to identify the cell type(s) producing TNF-α. This analysis revealed that TNF-α production in the dLN, analyzed by intracellular cytokine staining directly *ex vivo,* was restricted primarily to conventional T-cells (7.6% of total T cells) and to a lesser extent to NKT cells (5% of total NKT cells) (Fig. 5a). However, in terms of absolute cell number T cells are predominant producers for TNF-α in the dLN at 6 d.p.i. Both CD4^{+} and CD8^{+} T cells in the 6 d.p.i. dLN expressed TNF-α (i.e. ~7–8% of the respective T-cells subset) (Fig. 5b). It is also noteworthy that the T-cells from the corresponding dLN of IAV-infected *il-21*$^{-/-}$ mice exhibited a significantly diminished protein expression of TNF-α compared to infected wild type mice both in terms of the percentage of each subset and absolute cell numbers (Fig. 5b). To further confirm the contribution of IL-21R signaling in TNF-α expression by IAV-activated T cells, mixed BM chimeras containing wild type (CD45.1^{+}) and *il-21rα* $^{-/-}$ (CD45.2^{+}) BM in a 1:1 ratio were generated. After 8 weeks, the successfully reconstituted mice were infected with A/PR/8/34 IAV. Since TNF-α expression can be regulated both pre-and post-transcriptionally, on 6 d.p.i. both wild type (CD45.1^{+}) and *il-21rα* $^{-/-}$ (CD45.2^{+}) T cells (both CD4 and CD8 T cells) were isolated from the dLN by FACS and *tnf-α* gene expression in sorted T cells was determined by qPCR. As shown in figure.5c, *il-21rα* $^{-/-}$ T cells (both CD4 and CD8 T cells) exhibited significantly diminished *tnf-α* gene expression compared to WT-T cells (Fig. 5c). Of note, IL-21 deficiency had no impact on TNF-α production by NKT cells in the 6 d.p.i. dLN of *il-21*$^{-/-}$ mice (data not shown). However, since NKT cells are the initial primary source of IL-21 in the 6 d.p.i. dLNs, IAV-infected *cd-1d* $^{-/-}$ mice exhibited significantly diminished expression of TNF-α in conventional T cells compared to wild type mice at 6 d.p.i. (Fig. 5d). Finally, these data all together suggest that IL-21, initially produced by NKT cells, promotes TNF-α production by conventional T cells *via* IL-21R stimulation in the dLN of IAV-infected mice.

TNF-α produced by T cells promotes CXCL9-mediated LAPC migration into the dLN and subsequent T_{FH} differentiation during IAV infection

In view of the above results it was of interest first to determine if TNF-α influenced the production of CXCL9 by DCs in the dLN and thereby the migration of LAPC from the infected lungs to the dLN and subsequent T_{FH} cell accumulation. To this end IAV-infected mice were treated by i.p. with either αmTNF-α neutralizing mAbs (XT3.11) or isotype control Abs (Rat IgG) over time frame including the initial migration of LAPC into the dLN i.e. between 4 d.p.i and 7 d.p.i. (Fig. 6a). The level of CXCL9 expression by dLN DCs was evaluated directly *ex vivo* 24 hrs later by flow cytometric analysis. *In vivo* neutralization of TNF-α resulted in a significant decrease in CXCL9 production by DCs (Fig. 6b). In parallel with the decrease in CXCL9 expression, we observed that the accumulation of both LAPC and T_{FH} cells in the dLN were significantly diminished in the IAV-infected mice following TNF-α neutralization as reflected in both the absolute numbers of these two cell types and their percentage within the dLN (Fig. 6c). Next, we examined whether IAV-infected *tnf-α*$^{-/-}$ mice displayed a phenotype comparable to that of mice in which TNF-αwas neutralized *in vivo* by neutralizing αmTNF-α mAb administration and whether the transfer of TNF-α producing T cells into *tnf-α*$^{-/-}$ mice could rescue the phenotype of these mice (Fig. 7a). Indeed, compared to wild type mice IAV-infected *tnf-α*$^{-/-}$ mice showed significantly diminished CXCL9 expression in DCs (Fig. 7b). The accumulation of both LAPC and T_{FH} cells in the dLN were also significantly diminished in the IAV-infected *tnf-α*$^{-/-}$ mice (Fig. 7c). Finally, the adoptive transfer of TNF-α producing non-T_{FH} total T cells (Thy1.2^{+}CXCR5^{-}) isolated from the dLNs of IAV-infected wild type mice at 6 d.p.i. (D6 WT-T, Fig. 5a) could rescue CXCL9 expression by DCs in *tnf-α*$^{-/-}$ mice. In addition, LAPC and T_{FH} accumulation in the dLNs were restored in *tnf-α*$^{-/-}$ mice following transfer of WT-T cells to levels comparable to that of IAV-infected wild type mice (Fig. 7b and 7c). However, the adoptive transfer of *il21rα*$^{-/-}$ T cells, which exhibit significantly diminished TNF-α expression compared to WT-T cells (Fig. 5c), could not rescue the phenotype in T_{FH} accumulation of *tnf-α*$^{-/-}$ mice (data not shown). Of note, by the repeated experiments, in which the donor wild type CD4 T cells (CD45.1^{+}) were distinguished from recipient *tnf-α*$^{-/-}$ CD4 T cells (CD45.2^{+}), we confirmed that the rescue of phenotype in T_{FH} accumulation of WT-T cell supplemented *tnf-α*$^{-/-}$ mice was due to the differentiation of recipient *tnf-α*$^{-/-}$ CD4 T cells into T_{FH} cells by the help from donor WT-T cells but not solely reflect T_{FH} differentiation from transferred donor WT-T cells (data not shown). Collectively, these results suggest that IL-21-induced TNF-α production from conventional T cells enhances T_{FH} differentiation in part at least *via* modulating CXCR3-CXCL9 dependent LAPC migration into the dLN during IAV infection.

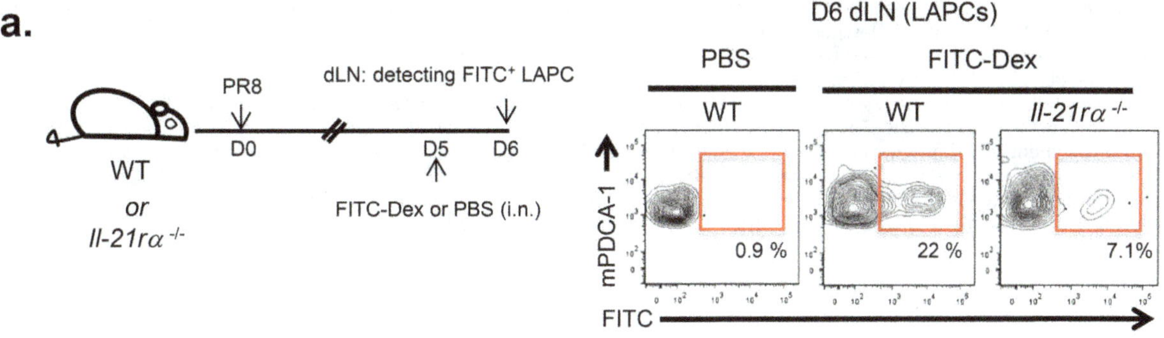

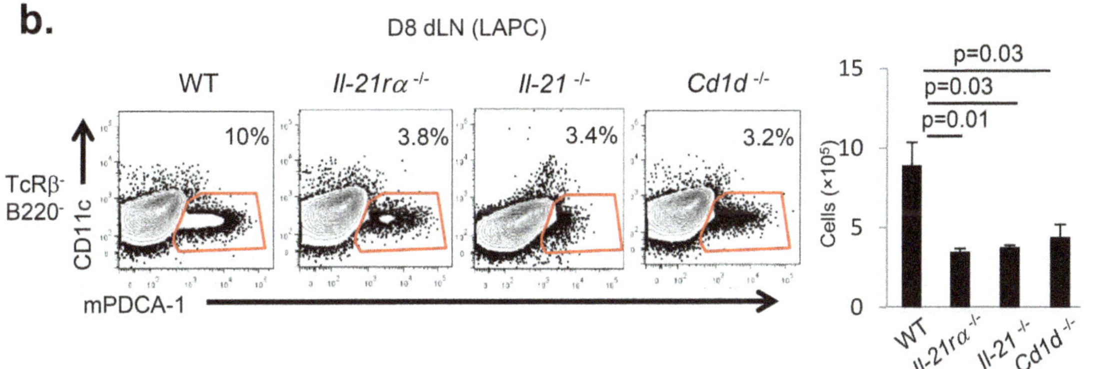

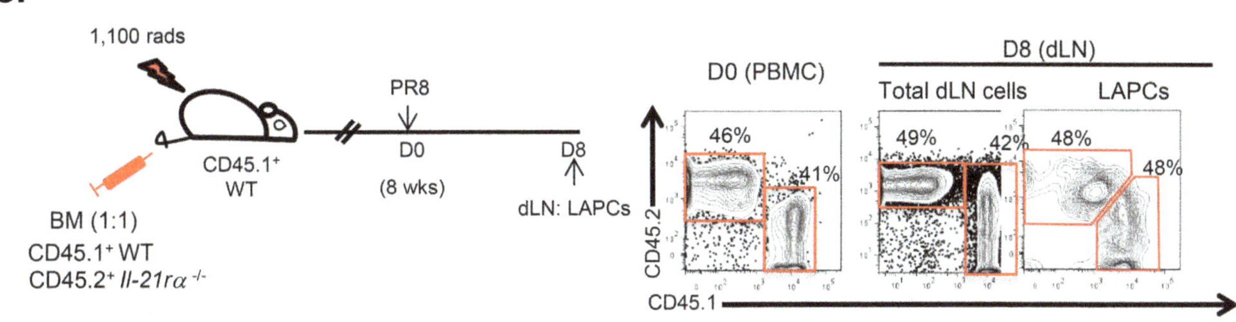

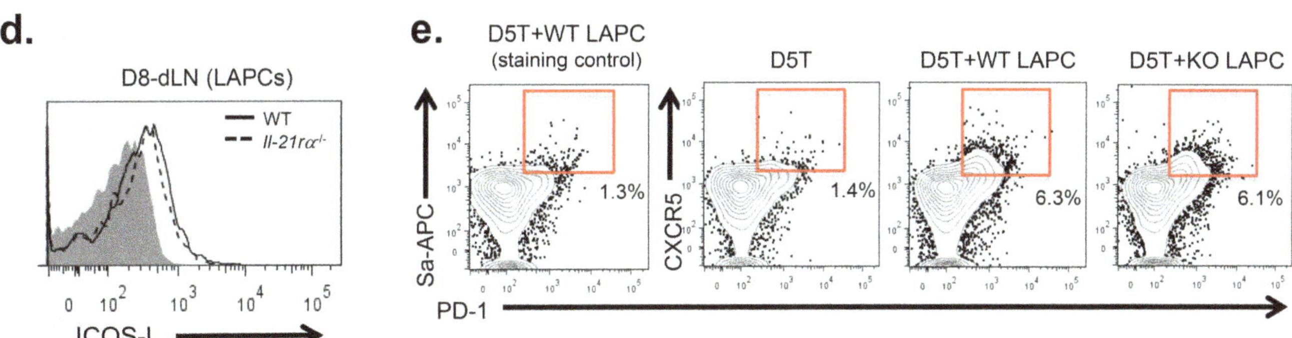

Figure 3. IL-21 modulates LAPC migration from lung tissue into the dLN of IAV-infected mice. (**a**) C57BL/6 (WT) (n = 12) *and il-21rα* $^{-/-}$ mice (n = 6) were infected with IAV, followed by FITC-Dextran administration i.n. on 5 d.p.i. 24 hrs later cells were isolated from the dLNs and the extent of LAPCs migration was determined by FACS-analysis. Numbers indicate the percentage of FITC^{+} cells within the LAPC population. Data representative of two independent experiments are shown. (**b**) At 8 d.p.i, LAPC accumulation in the dLNs was examined by FACS-analysis in C57BL/6 (WT) (n = 15), *il-21rα* $^{-/-}$(n = 15), *il21rα* $^{-/-}$ (n = 15) and *cd-1d*$^{-/-}$ mice (n = 6). The data are presented as both a percentage of lineage^{-} i.e. TcRβ^{-} B220^{-} cells and absolute LAPC numbers (mean ± s.e.m) and were analyzed by Student's *t* test. Representative data of five independent experiments

are shown. (**c**) The effect of IL-21R signaling on LAPC migration into the dLNs was evaluated in mixed BM chimera containing wild type ($CD45.1^+$) *and il-21rα*$^{-/-}$ ($CD45.2^+$) BM in a 1:1 ratio as described in the Materials and Methods. At 8 wks post reconstitution, mice (n = 7) were infected with A/PR/8/34 virus. At 8 d.p.i., the percentage of wild type (CD45.1) and *il-21rα* $^{-/-}$ (CD45.2) LAPCs among total LAPCs ($mPDCA1^+CD11c^-B220^-TcR\beta^-$) was determined in the dLNs by FACS-analysis. Representative images of three independent experiments are shown. (**d**) Both C57BL/6 (n = 6) *and il-21rα* $^{-/-}$ mice (n = 6) were infected with 0.05 LD_{50} of A/PR/8/34 virus. At 8 d.p.i., ICOSL expression on LAPCs isolated from the dLNs of C57BL/6 *and il-21rα*$^{-/-}$ mice was examined by FACS-analysis. The gray histogram represents isotype control Ab staining for ICOS-L. Representative data from two independent experiments are shown. (e) *In vivo* Ag primed OT-II cells (D5T) were generated as described in the Materials and Methods. FACS-sorted 5 d.p.i. OT-II cells (5×10^4 cells/well) (D5T) were incubated with LAPCs ($mPDCA1^+CD11c^-B220^-TcR\beta^-$) ($2.5\times10^4$ cells/well) isolated from the dLNs of A/WSN/OVA-II virus infected either C57BL/6 (wt) (n = 9) *and il-21rα* $^{-/-}$ (ko) mice (n = 18) at 8 d.p.i. 24 hrs after *ex vivo* co-culture, T_{FH} differentiation (PD-1 and CXCR5 expression) in the OT-II ($CD45.2^+Thy1.2^+CD4^+$) T-cells was evaluated by FAC-analysis. Representative data of three independent experiments are shown.

Discussion

IL-21, first identified as a product of activated human T cells, is a pleiotropic cytokine which has diverse effects on the immune response through its ability to modulate the activity of many immune cell types [23–25]. Primarily produced by activated $CD4^+$ T cell (in particular, T_{FH} effector cells), IL-21 regulates B cell responses within the B cell follicular germinal center (GC) [25]. NKT cells are an additional potential major source of IL-21 and produce even higher level of this cytokine than activated conventional $CD4^+$ T cells when appropriately stimulated [22]. As a result of engagement of IL-21Rα/c receptor complex, IL-21 promotes the survival and proliferation, as well as cytokine and chemokine production by multiple immune cell types including macrophages, B, T, NK and NKT cells [24].

Although $CD4^+$ T_{FH} effector cells are the predominant cell type producing IL-21 during the germinal center response in the dLN, in this model of respiratory virus infection, we find that NKT cells likely are a major source of IL-21 during the early phase of $CD4^+$ T_{FH} effector cell differentiation and GC formation in the dLN. Our unpublished data suggested that there is minimal IL–21 release or expression into the IAV infected lungs before day 5–6 post infection. Indeed, at later stage of infection IL–21 was present in the lung mostly derived from IAV-specific $CD4^+$ T cells entering the infected lungs from the dLN. The stimulus for IL-21 production by the NKT cells responding to IAV infection in the dLN is not as yet defined. NKT cells have been reported to produce IL-21 following antigen receptor engagement or following stimulation by TLR ligands [17,22,25]. Since the A/PR/8/34 IAV strain employed in this analysis does not efficiently replicate in the dLN of infected mice, IL-21 production as a result of stimulation of TLR on NKT cells by IAV-derived TLR ligands generated in the dLN seems unlikely. The more likely possibility is that IL-21 is produced by NKT cells following TCR-engagement in response to recognition of lipid moieties released from IAV infected cells.

IL-21 was also initially proposed as an important T cell-derived soluble factor regulating T_{FH} differentiation through engagement of the IL-21R on recently activated $CD4^+$ T cells prior to lineage commitment [8,11,13]. Subsequent reports [12,32] including our findings herein demonstrating a reduced (by ~ 50%) T_{FH} response in the dLN of IAV-infected *il-21rα*$^{-/-}$ mice (Fig. 1b) further substantiates the contribution of IL21 to T_{FH} differentiation. However, it was unclear whether IL-21 acts directly on naïve/recently activated $CD4^+$ T cells to drive T_{FH} differentiation [4,6,12]. Indeed, our analysis of T_{FH} responses in mixed BM chimeric mice indicates that when evaluated in the presence of IL-21R signaling competent T cells IL-21R deficient responding $CD4^+$ T cells are fully capable of undergoing T_{FH} differentiation (Fig. 1c). Therefore, during pulmonary IAV infection at least, there is no intrinsic signal delivered by IL-21 to the responding $CD4^+$ T cells in the dLN which is required to program the cells along the T_{FH} differentiation pathway.

Our results suggest a novel and heretofore underappreciated role of IL-21 in regulating T_{FH} differentiation that is through the production of TNF-α. IL-21 either alone or in concert with other cytokines (i.e. IL-7 or IL-15) has been demonstrated to promote TNF-α production most notably from responding T cells [26–28]. We observed that during IAV infection that the absence of TNF-α resulted in a markedly diminished T_{FH} response (Fig. 6c and 7c). In addition, the major source of TNF-α in the responding dLN were T cells whose production of this cytokine required IL-21 and the expression of the IL-21R by the responding T-cells as defective signaling through the IL-21R resulted in significantly decreased TNF-α production by the T-cells (Fig. 5a, 5b and unpublished data).

TNF-α has been demonstrated to play a central role in stimulating chemokine expression at sites of inflammation including CXCL9, which is a strong chemotactic stimulus for mononuclear cells [29–31,33–35]. We observed during IAV infection, that DCs are the major source of CXCL9 in the dLN (Fig. 4b) [16]. Of note, the absence of TNF-α mediated stimulation significantly but not completely diminished CXCL9 production by DCs isolated from the dLN of IAV-infected mice (Fig. 6b and 7b). This incomplete inhibition of CXCL9 expression may due to an effect of other soluble factors present in the dLN which are capable of regulating CXCL9 expression in the dLN, most notably, IFN- [34,35]. CXCL9 production by the dLN DCs was also significantly decreased in IAV-infected IL-21 or IL-21R deficient mice (Fig. 4c and 4d). However, in our mixed BM chimera study the absence of IL-21R expression on the dLN DC had no direct effect on CXCL9 production by these cells suggesting that the impact of IL21/IL21R signaling on CXCL9 production by the dLN DC was indirect (Fig. 4e), that is, through the effect of IL-21 on TNF-α production. Even though we cannot rule out the possibility that TNF-α works synergistically with IFN- in the dLN to induce CXCL9 expression from DCs [34,35], it is unlikely that IL-21 also modulates IFN- expression since both *il-21*$^{-/-}$ and *il-21rα*$^{-/-}$ mice showed no difference in IFN- gene expression in the dLN post-IAV infection (unpublished data).

We believe that the likely link between IL-21/IL-21R signaling, TNF-α production and T_{FH} differentiation is *via* LAPC. This antigen presenting cell type picks up vial antigen in the IAV-infected lungs, migrate from the lungs into the dLN late in the infection cycle (i.e. between 6 and 12 d.p.i.) where these cells facilitate T_{FH} differentiation of Ag-activated $CD4^+$ T cells. We recently reported that the migration of LAPC into the inflamed dLN is largely CXCR3-CXCL9 dependent [16]. In the current report we find that both IAV infected *il-21*$^{-/-}$ and *il-21rα*$^{-/-}$ mice showed significantly diminished (~ 60–70%) LAPC migration/accumulation into the dLN (Fig. 3a and 3b) and concomitantly a decreased T_{FH} response following IAV infection in spite of normal CXCR3 expression by the LAPC from the IL-21/IL-21R

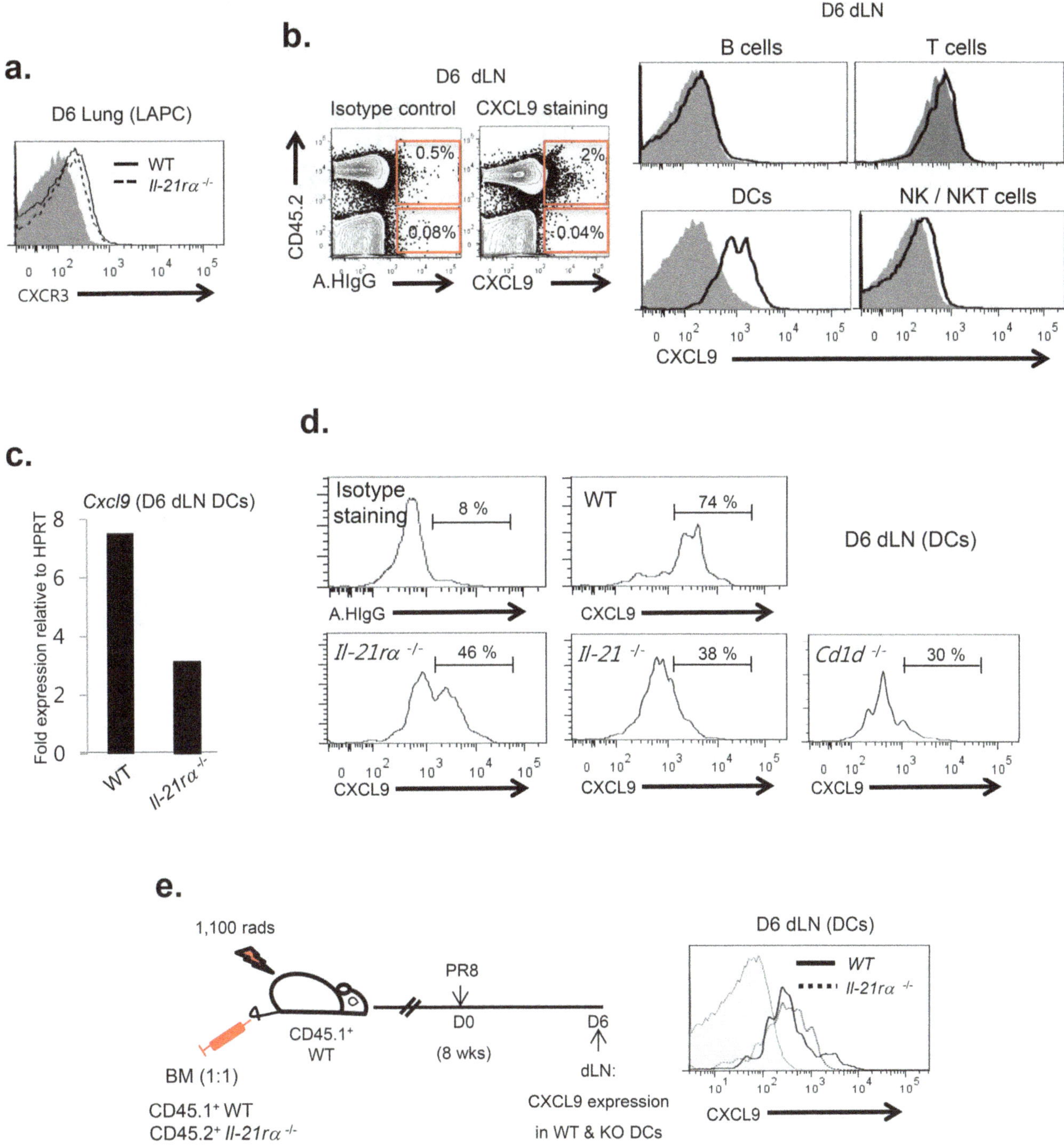

Figure 4. IL-21 enhances CXCL9 expression in IL-21R deficient dLN DCs following IAV infection. (**a**) C57BL/6 (WT) (n = 6) *and il-21rα*$^{-/-}$ mice (n = 6) were infected with 0.05 LD_{50} of A/PR/8/34 virus. At 6 d.p.i., CXCR3 expression on LAPCs isolated from the lungs of these mice was analyzed by FACS-analysis. The gray histogram represents isotype control Ab staining for CXCR3. Representative data from two independent experiments are shown. (**b**) CXCL9 expression on prominent mononuclear cell subsets was examined by FACS-analysis in each gated population (B cells: CD45.2$^+$B220$^+$ CD11c$^-$Thy1.2$^-$; T cells: CD45.2$^+$Thy1.2$^+$B220$^-$; DCs: CD45.2$^+$CD11c$^+$Thy1.2$^-$; NK/NKT cells: CD45.2$^+$NK1.1$^+$) isolated from the dLNs of 6 d.p.i. C57BL/6 mice (n = 9). The gray histogram represents isotype control Ab staining for CXCL9. Representative data from three independent experiments are shown. (**c & d**) C57BL/6 (WT) (n = 12), *il-21rα* $^{-/-}$ (n = 12), *il-21*$^{-/-}$ (n = 6) and *cd-1d*$^{-/-}$ mice (n = 6) were infected with A/PR/8/34 virus. (**c**) At 6 d.p.i., DCs were isolated by FACS-sorting from the dLNs of both C57BL/6 (WT) and *il-21rα* $^{-/-}$ mice. *Cxcl9* gene expression in these isolated DCs was evaluated by qPCR. Representative data from two independent experiments are shown. (**d**) The expression level of CXCL9 in DCs was also examined by FACS-analysis in dLN-derived DCs isolated from 6 d.p.i. C57BL/6 (WT), *il-21rα* $^{-/-}$, *il-21*$^{-/-}$ and *cd-1d* $^{-/-}$ mice. Representative data from two independent experiments are shown. (**e**) To examine whether IL-21 modulates CXCL9 production from DCs *via* IL-21R signaling in DCs, mixed BM chimera mice established using wild type (CD45.1$^+$) *and il-21rα*$^{-/-}$ (CD45.2$^+$) BM in a 1:1 ratio were generated as described in the Materials and Methods. At 8 wks after reconstitution, mice (n = 7) were infected with A/PR/8/34 virus. At 6 d.p.i., the expression level of CXCL9 in wild type and *il-21rα* $^{-/-}$ DCs (CD11c$^+$Thy1.2$^-$) was compared in the dLNs by FACS-analysis. Representative images of two independent experiments are shown.

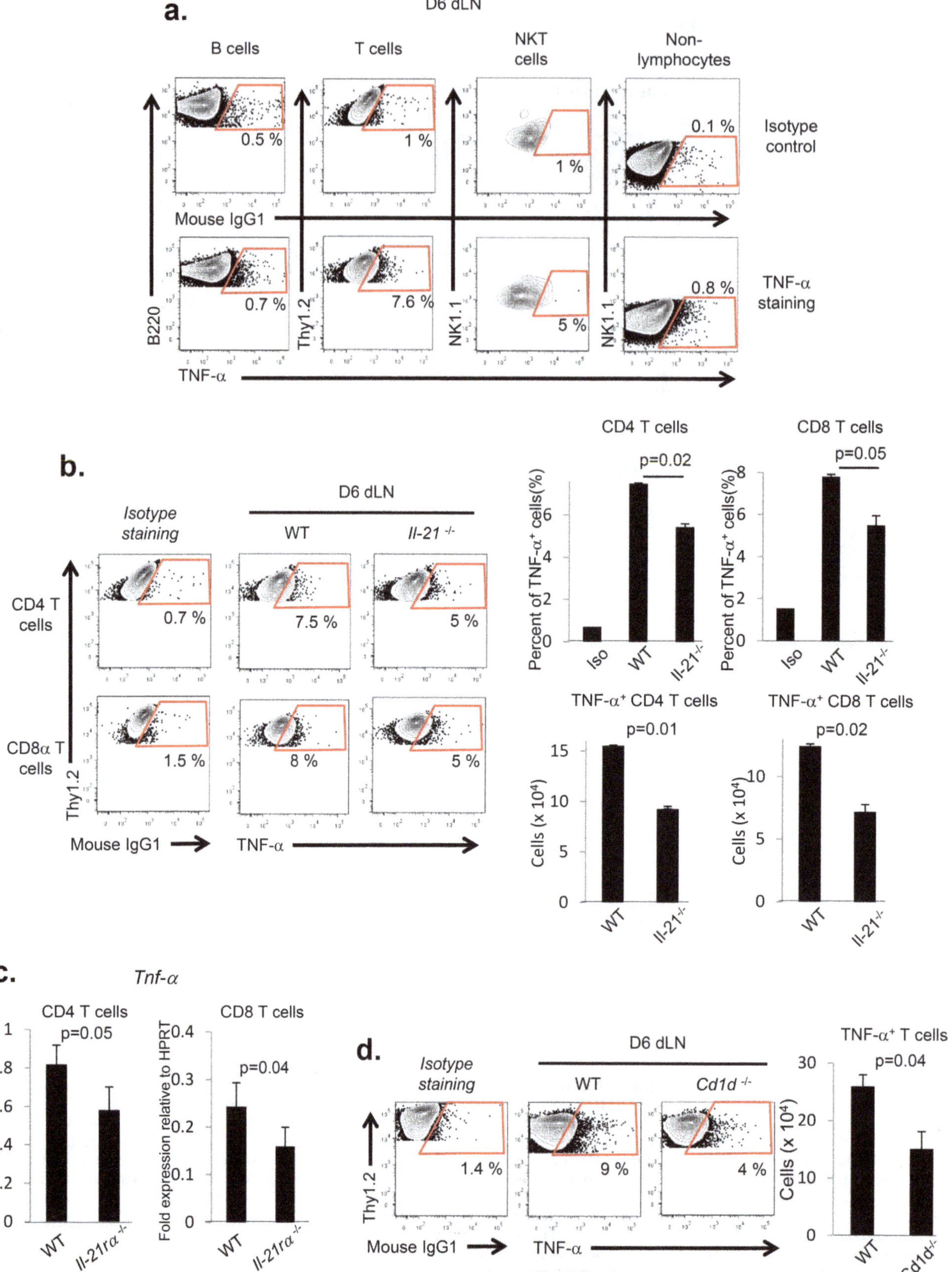

Figure 5. IL-21 stimulates TNF-α production by T cells in the dLN of IAV-infected mice. (**a**) C57BL/6 (n = 6) mice were infected with 0.05 LD_{50} of A/PR/8/34 virus. At 6 d.p.i., mTNF-α expression in gated lymphoid (B ($B220^{+}Thy1.2^{-}$), T ($B220^{-}Thy1.2^{+}$), NKT ($NK1.1^{+}TcR\beta^{+}CD1d^{+}$) and non-lymphocytes ($B220^{-}Thy1.2^{-}$) cell types isolated from the dLNs was examined by FACS-analysis. The data are representative from two independent

experiments and presented as percent mTNF-α^+ cells in the particular cell type. (**b & d**) C57BL/6 (WT) (n = 9), *il-21*$^{-/-}$(n = 9) and *cd-1d*$^{-/-}$ mice (n = 6) were infected with 0.05 LD_{50} of A/PR/8/34 virus. At 6 d.p.i., mTNF-α expression in $CD4^+$ T ($CD4^+Thy1.2^+$), $CD8^+$ T ($CD8\alpha^+Thy1.2^+$) and total T cells ($Thy1.2^+$) isolated from the dLNs of infected mice was examined by FACS-analysis. The data are presented as both percent of mTNF-α^+ cells within the T-cells subset and absolute number of mTNF-α^+ cells (mean ± s.e.m.). The data were analyzed using Student's *t* test. Representative data from three independent experiments are shown. (**c**) Mixed BM chimeras containing wild type ($CD45.1^+$) and *il-21rα* $^{-/-}$ ($CD45.2^+$) BM in a 1:1 ratio were generated. After 8 weeks, the successfully reconstituted mice were infected with A/PR/8/34 IAV. On 6 d.p.i. both wild type ($CD45.1^+$) and *il-21rα*$^{-/-}$ ($CD45.2^+$) T cells (both CD4 and CD8 T cells) were isolated from the dLN by FACS ($CD45.1^+Thy1.2^+CD4^+$, $CD45.2^+Thy1.2^+CD4^+$, $CD45.1^+Thy1.2^+CD8^+$, $CD45.2^+Thy1.2^+CD8^+$) and *tnf-α* gene expression in sorted T cells was determined by qPCR. The data were analyzed using Student's *t* test. Representative data from two independent experiments are shown.

signaling defective IAV-infected mice (Fig. 1b and 4a). Most important, the absence of TNF-α mediated stimulation *in vivo* during IAV infection, like defective IL-21/IL-21R signaling, resulted in both decreased LAPC migration into the dLN and in a diminished T_{FH} response (Fig. 6c and 7c). IL-21 also modulates B cell response which contributes to the maintenance of T_{FH} response [6]. Although B cells are poor inducers for initial T_{FH} differentiation [16], we cannot rule out the possibility that at the maintenance phase of T_{FH} response during IAV infection (after 9–10 d.p.i.) IL-21, predominantly produced by T_{FH} cells, may also contribute to T_{FH} maintenance *via* modulating B cells. Although IL–21, TNF-α and CD1d are implicated in anti-IAV T_{FH}/GC-B cell response, we found that deficiency in IL–21 or IL–21R has no effect on virus clearance or recovery from IAV infection in C57BL/6 background (unpublished data). Also, as we reported *cd-1d* deficiency does impact on IL–5 production during IAV infection but does not affect virus clearance or recovery from IAV infection in BALB/c background [36].

In conclusion, in this report we have identified a novel mechanism, by which IL21 promotes optimal T_{FH} responses in pulmonary virus infection. Our results suggests that during IAV infection IL-21 produced in the dLN early in infection i.e. 5–6 d.p.i. (most likely by NKT cells in the dLN) stimulates TNF-α production by $CD4^+$ and $CD8^+$ T cells responding to infection in the dLN. The TNF-α stimuli enhances CXCL9 production by dLN resident DCs which in turn acts as a chemotactic stimulus to

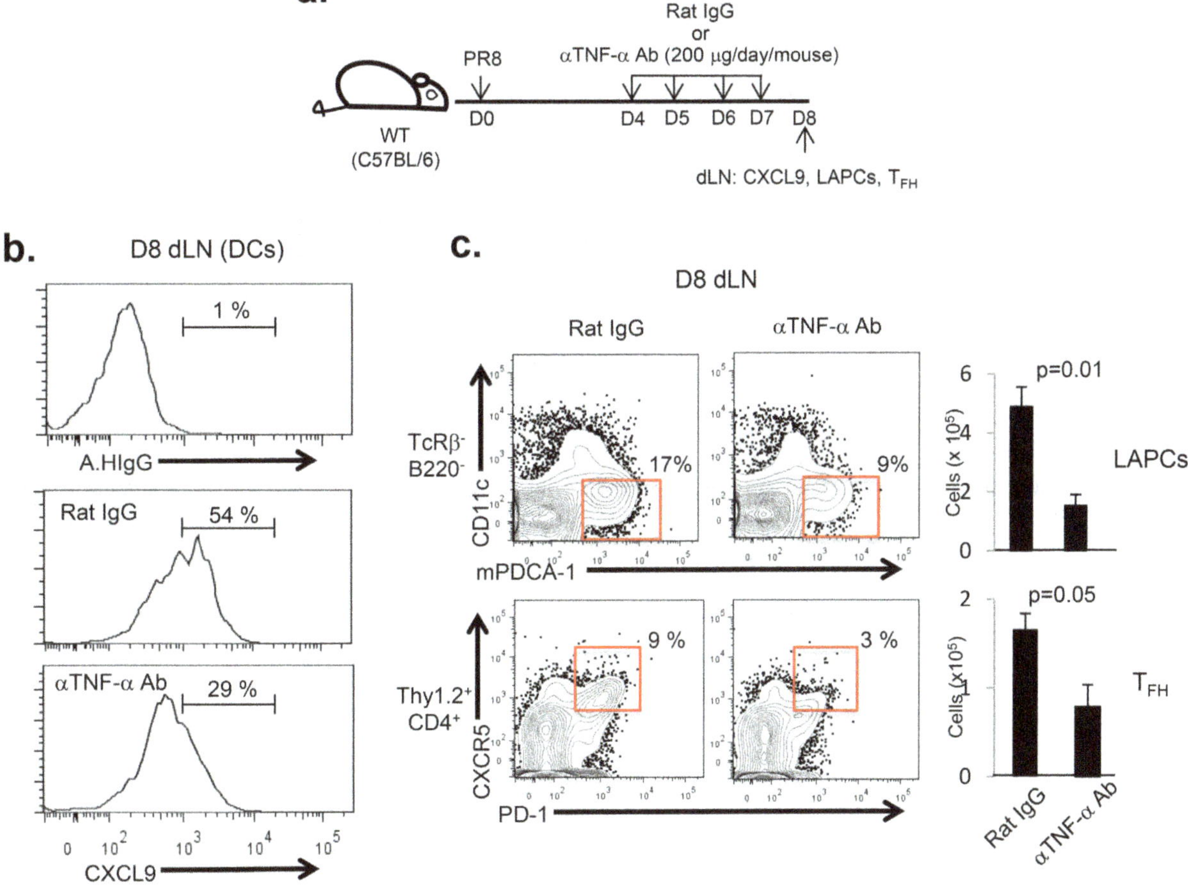

Figure 6. TNF-α promotes CXCL9-mediated LAPC migration into the dLN and subsequent T_{FH} differentiation during IAV infection. (**a**) C57BL/6 (WT) (n = 12) mice were infected with 0.05 LD_{50} of A/PR/8/34 virus. From 4 d.p.i. thru 7 d.p.i mice were treated (i.p.) with either isotype control Abs (Rat IgG) or αmTNF-α blocking mAb (XT3.11) (200 mg/day/mouse). At 8 d.p.i., (**b**) the expression level of CXCL9 was examined in DCs by FACS-analysis. (**c**) The extend of LAPC accumulation and T_{FH} differentiation in the dLN of infected mice following control Ab or αmTNF-α blocking Ab treatment were likewise evaluated by FACS-analysis. The data are presented as both percent population and absolute numbers (mean ± s.e.m.) and were analyzed by Student's *t* test. Representative data from two independent experiments are shown.

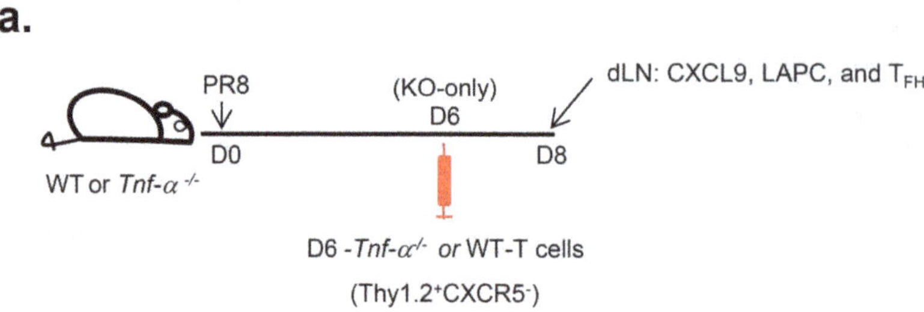

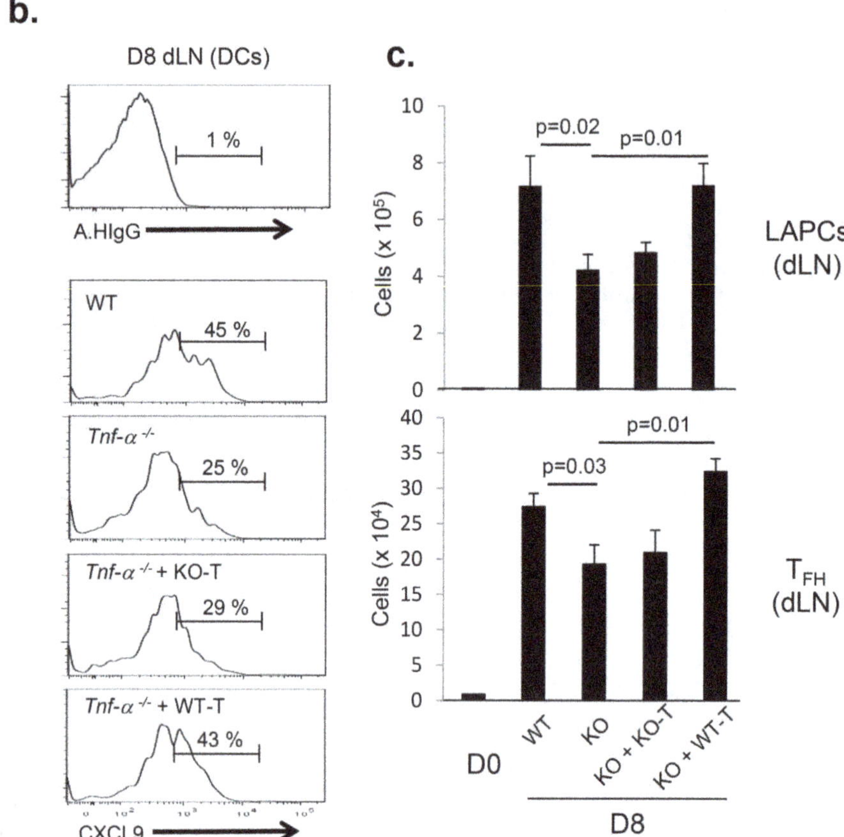

Figure 7. TNF-α producing T cells promotes CXCL9-mediated LAPC migration into the dLN and subsequent T_{FH} differentiation during IAV infection. (**a**) C57BL/6 (WT) (n = 12) and *tnf-α*$^{-/-}$ (KO) (n = 24) mice were infected with 0.05 LD_{50} of A/PR/8/34 virus. At 6 d.p.i. non-T_{FH} total T cells (Thy1.2^{+}CXCR5^{-}) were isolated from the dLN of A/PR/8/34 virus-infected either *tnf-α*$^{-/-}$ (KO-T) or C57BL/6 (WT-T) mice and adoptively transferred by the *i.v.* route (2×10^{6}cells/mouse) into A/PR/8/34 infected *tnfα*$^{-/-}$ mice (KO). At 8 d.p.i., (**b**) the expression level of CXCL9 in DCs and (**c**) the extend of LAPC accumulation and T_{FH} differentiation in the dLN of recipient mice were examined and compared with that of both WT and KO mice by FACS-analysis. The data are presented as either percent population or absolute numbers (mean ± s.e.m.) and were analyzed by Student's *t* test. Representative data from two independent experiments are shown.

promote LAPC migration into the dLN. As a result of the increased accumulation of LAPC, this antigen presenting cell can facilitate optimal differentiation of Ag-activated responding CD4^{+} T cells in the dLN into T_{FH} cells.

Acknowledgments

We thank the members of Dr. Braciale's laboratory for critical comments.

Author Contributions

Conceived and designed the experiments: JKY. Performed the experiments: JKY. Analyzed the data: JKY TJB. Contributed reagents/materials/analysis tools: JKY. Contributed to the writing of the manuscript: JKY TJB.

References

1. Baumgarth N, Herman OC, Jager GC, Brown LE, Herzenberg LA, et al. (2000) B-1 and B-2 cell-derived immunoglobulin M antibodies are nonredundant components of the protective response to influenza virus infection. J Exp Med 192: 271–280.
2. Goodnow CC, Vinuesa CG, Randall KL, Mackay F, Brink R (2010) Control systems and decision making for antibody production. Nat Immunol 11: 681–688.

3. Graham MB, Braciale TJ (1997) Resistance to and recovery from lethal influenza virus infection in B lymphocyte-deficient mice. J Exp Med 186: 2063–2068.
4. Ma CS, Deenick EK, Batten M, Tangye SG (2012) The origins, function, and regulation of T follicular helper cells. J Exp Med 209: 1241–1253.
5. Waffarn EE, Baumgarth N (2011) Protective B cell responses to flu–no fluke! J Immunol 186: 3823–3829.
6. Crotty S (2011) Follicular helper CD4 T cells (TFH). Annu Rev Immunol 29: 621–663.
7. King C, Tangye SG, Mackay CR (2008) T follicular helper (TFH) cells in normal and dysregulated immune responses. Annu Rev Immunol 26: 741–766.
8. Nurieva RI, Chung Y, Hwang D, Yang XO, Kang HS, et al. (2008) Generation of T follicular helper cells is mediated by interleukin-21 but independent of T helper 1, 2, or 17 cell lineages. Immunity 29: 138–149.
9. Vinuesa CG, Tangye SG, Moser B, Mackay CR (2005) Follicular B helper T cells in antibody responses and autoimmunity. Nat Rev Immunol 5: 853–865.
10. Yu D, Rao S, Tsai LM, Lee SK, He Y, et al. (2009) The transcriptional repressor Bcl-6 directs T follicular helper cell lineage commitment. Immunity 31: 457–468.
11. Nurieva RI, Chung Y, Martinez GJ, Yang XO, Tanaka S, et al. (2009) Bcl6 mediates the development of T follicular helper cells. Science 325: 1001–1005.
12. Eto D, Lao C, DiToro D, Barnett B, Escobar TC, et al. (2011) IL-21 and IL-6 are critical for different aspects of B cell immunity and redundantly induce optimal follicular helper CD4 T cell (Tfh) differentiation. PLoS One 6: e17739.
13. Vogelzang A, McGuire HM, Yu D, Sprent J, Mackay CR, et al. (2008) A fundamental role for interleukin-21 in the generation of T follicular helper cells. Immunity 29: 127–137.
14. Yoo JK, Galligan CL, Virtanen C, Fish EN (2010) Identification of a novel antigen-presenting cell population modulating antiinfluenza type 2 immunity. J Exp Med 207: 1435–1451.
15. Yoo JK, Baker DP, Fish EN (2010) Interferon-beta modulates type 1 immunity during influenza virus infection. Antiviral Res 88: 64–71.
16. Yoo JK, Fish EN, Braciale TJ (2012) LAPCs promote follicular helper T cell differentiation of Ag-primed CD4+ T cells during respiratory virus infection. J Exp Med 209: 1853–1867.
17. Harada M, Magara-Koyanagi K, Watarai H, Nagata Y, Ishii Y, et al. (2006) IL-21-induced Bepsilon cell apoptosis mediated by natural killer T cells suppresses IgE responses. J Exp Med 203: 2929–2937.
18. Chapman TJ, Castrucci MR, Padrick RC, Bradley LM, Topham DJ (2005) Antigen-specific and non-specific CD4+ T cell recruitment and proliferation during influenza infection. Virology 340: 296–306.
19. Sun J, Madan R, Karp CL, Braciale TJ (2009) Effector T cells control lung inflammation during acute influenza virus infection by producing IL-10. Nat Med 15: 277–284.
20. Boyden AW, Legge KL, Waldschmidt TJ (2012) Pulmonary infection with influenza A virus induces site-specific germinal center and T follicular helper cell responses. PLoS One 7: e40733.
21. Dienz O, Eaton SM, Bond JP, Neveu W, Moquin D, et al. (2009) The induction of antibody production by IL-6 is indirectly mediated by IL-21 produced by CD4+ T cells. J Exp Med 206: 69–78.
22. Coquet JM, Kyparissoudis K, Pellicci DG, Besra G, Berzins SP, et al. (2007) IL-21 is produced by NKT cells and modulates NKT cell activation and cytokine production. J Immunol 178: 2827–2834.
23. Parrish-Novak J, Dillon SR, Nelson A, Hammond A, Sprecher C, et al. (2000) Interleukin 21 and its receptor are involved in NK cell expansion and regulation of lymphocyte function. Nature 408: 57–63.
24. Skak K, Kragh M, Hausman D, Smyth MJ, Sivakumar PV (2008) Interleukin 21: combination strategies for cancer therapy. Nat Rev Drug Discov 7: 231–240.
25. Spolski R, Leonard WJ (2008) Interleukin-21: basic biology and implications for cancer and autoimmunity. Annu Rev Immunol 26: 57–79.
26. Brady J, Carotta S, Thong RP, Chan CJ, Hayakawa Y, et al. (2010) The interactions of multiple cytokines control NK cell maturation. J Immunol 185: 6679–6688.
27. Li J, Shen W, Kong K, Liu Z (2006) Interleukin-21 induces T-cell activation and proinflammatory cytokine secretion in rheumatoid arthritis. Scand J Immunol 64: 515–522.
28. Liu S, Lizee G, Lou Y, Liu C, Overwijk WW, et al. (2007) IL-21 synergizes with IL-7 to augment expansion and anti-tumor function of cytotoxic T cells. Int Immunol 19: 1213–1221.
29. Algood HM, Lin PL, Flynn JL (2005) Tumor necrosis factor and chemokine interactions in the formation and maintenance of granulomas in tuberculosis. Clin Infect Dis 41 Suppl 3: S189–193.
30. Czermak BJ, Sarma V, Bless NM, Schmal H, Friedl HP, et al. (1999) In vitro and in vivo dependency of chemokine generation on C5a and TNF-alpha. J Immunol 162: 2321–2325.
31. Janatpour MJ, Hudak S, Sathe M, Sedgwick JD, McEvoy LM (2001) Tumor necrosis factor-dependent segmental control of MIG expression by high endothelial venules in inflamed lymph nodes regulates monocyte recruitment. J Exp Med 194: 1375–1384.
32. Nguyen V, Luzina I, Rus H, Tegla C, Chen C, et al. (2012) IL-21 promotes lupus-like disease in chronic graft-versus-host disease through both CD4 T cell- and B cell-intrinsic mechanisms. J Immunol 189: 1081–1093.
33. Algood HM, Lin PL, Yankura D, Jones A, Chan J, et al. (2004) TNF influences chemokine expression of macrophages in vitro and that of CD11b+ cells in vivo during Mycobacterium tuberculosis infection. J Immunol 172: 6846–6857.
34. Antonelli A, Ferrari SM, Fallahi P, Frascerra S, Santini E, et al. (2009) Monokine induced by interferon gamma (IFNgamma) (CXCL9) and IFN-gamma inducible T-cell alpha-chemoattractant (CXCL11) involvement in Graves' disease and ophthalmopathy: modulation by peroxisome proliferator-activated receptor-gamma agonists. J Clin Endocrinol Metab 94: 1803–1809.
35. Antonelli A, Ferrari SM, Fallahi P, Ghiri E, Crescioli C, et al. (2010) Interferon-alpha, -beta and -gamma induce CXCL9 and CXCL10 secretion by human thyrocytes: modulation by peroxisome proliferator-activated receptor-gamma agonists. Cytokine 50: 260–267.
36. Gorski SA, Hahn YS, Braciale TJ (2013) Group 2 innate lymphoid cell production of IL-5 is regulated by NKT cells during influenza virus infection. PLoS Pathog 9: e1003615.

6

Absence of Detectable Influenza RNA Transmitted via Aerosol during Various Human Respiratory Activities – Experiments from Singapore and Hong Kong

Julian W. Tang[1,2,3]*, Caroline X. Gao[4,5,6], Benjamin J. Cowling[7], Gerald C. Koh[8], Daniel Chu[7], Cherie Heilbronn[5,6], Belinda Lloyd[5,6], Jovan Pantelic[9], Andre D. Nicolle[3], Christian A. Klettner[3], J. S. Malik Peiris[7], Chandra Sekhar[10], David K. W. Cheong[10], Kwok Wai Tham[10], Evelyn S. C. Koay[3,11], Wendy Tsui[12], Alfred Kwong[12], Kitty Chan[13], Yuguo Li[4]

1 Alberta Provincial Laboratory for Public Health, University of Alberta Hospital, Edmonton, Canada, **2** Department of Medical Microbiology and Immunology, University of Alberta, Edmonton, Canada, **3** Department of Laboratory Medicine, National University Hospital, Singapore, Singapore, **4** Department of Mechanical Engineering, The University of Hong Kong, Hong Kong SAR, China, **5** Turning Point Alcohol and Drug Centre, Eastern Health, Melbourne, Australia, **6** Eastern Health Clinical School, Monash University, Melbourne, Australia, **7** School of Public Health, The University of Hong Kong, Hong Kong SAR, China, **8** Saw Swee Hock School of Public Health, National University of Singapore, Singapore, Singapore, **9** Department of Mechanical Engineering, University of Maryland, Baltimore, Maryland, United States of America, **10** Department of Building, School of Design and Environment, National University of Singapore, Singapore, Singapore, **11** Department of Pathology, Yong Loo Lin School of Medicine, National University of Singapore, Singapore, Singapore, **12** Department of Family Medicine and Primary Healthcare, Hong Kong West Cluster, Hospital Authority, Hong Kong SAR, China, **13** University Health Service, The University of Hong Kong, Hong Kong SAR, China

Abstract

Two independent studies by two separate research teams (from Hong Kong and Singapore) failed to detect any influenza RNA landing on, or inhaled by, a life-like, human manikin target, after exposure to naturally influenza-infected volunteers. For the Hong Kong experiments, 9 influenza-infected volunteers were recruited to breathe, talk/count and cough, from 0.1 m and 0.5 m distance, onto a mouth-breathing manikin. Aerosolised droplets exhaled from the volunteers and entering the manikin's mouth were collected with PTFE filters and an aerosol sampler, in separate experiments. Virus detection was performed using an in-house influenza RNA reverse-transcription polymerase chain reaction (RT-PCR) assay. No influenza RNA was detected from any of the PTFE filters or air samples. For the Singapore experiments, 6 influenza-infected volunteers were asked to breathe (nasal/mouth breathing), talk (counting in English/second language), cough (from 1 m/0.1 m away) and laugh, onto a thermal, breathing manikin. The manikin's face was swabbed at specific points (around both eyes, the nostrils and the mouth) before and after exposure to each of these respiratory activities, and was cleaned between each activity with medical grade alcohol swabs. Shadowgraph imaging was used to record the generation of these respiratory aerosols from the infected volunteers and their impact onto the target manikin. No influenza RNA was detected from any of these swabs with either team's in-house diagnostic influenza assays. All the influenza-infected volunteers had diagnostic swabs taken at recruitment that confirmed influenza (A/H1, A/H3 or B) infection with high viral loads, ranging from 10^5-10^8 copies/mL (Hong Kong volunteers/assay) and 10^4–10^7 copies/mL influenza viral RNA (Singapore volunteers/assay). These findings suggest that influenza RNA may not be readily transmitted from naturally-infected human source to susceptible recipients via these natural respiratory activities, within these exposure time-frames. Various reasons are discussed in an attempt to explain these findings.

Editor: Nicole M. Bouvier, Mount Sinai School of Medicine, United States of America

Funding: Funding for the Hong Kong study was supported by the Area of Excellence Scheme of the Hong Kong University Grants Committee (grant no. AoE/M-12/06) and a RGC GRF grant (HKU7142/12). Funding for the Singapore study and support for post-doctoral research fellows ADN and CAK were provided by grants to JWT/ESCK from Singapore's National Medical Research Council (NMRC/1208/2009 and NMRC/1247/2010) and Agency for Science, Technology and Research (A*STAR: SERC 1021290099), respectively. The funders had no role in study design, data collection and analysis, decision to publish, or preparation of the manuscript.

* Email: jwtang49@hotmail.com

These authors contributed equally to this work.

Introduction

In recent years, discussions over the most clinically significant routes of influenza transmission have been extensive [1,2]. Confusion and disagreements surround the definitions of the various transmission routes including 'close contact' transmission, 'airborne' transmission and 'droplet' transmission [3–6].

Traditionally in outbreak investigations, airborne transmission has been implicated in secondary cases where direct contact with the infected source has not been documented. Close contact transmission has been used to explain secondary cases arising from documented close contact with the presumed index case [6]. However, it is important to note that even in close proximity, multiple transmission routes may all be responsible for disseminating the infection, i.e. person-to-person transmission in such situations can be potentially due to either airborne, droplet and/or direct physical contact transmission [7,8].

In the close contact exposure scenario, small droplets generated by an infectious patient can be directly inhaled and deposit in both the upper and the lower airway, whereas large droplets can be also be directly inhaled, but the majority of these will probably deposit in the upper airways only, or directly enter the recipient's eyes or even the mouth as a direct droplet infection (as opposed to self-inoculated infection) [1,9–12]. Long distance airborne transmission has been postulated to be introduced by small droplet nuclei being carried by ambient airflows, where the moisture from small droplets has mostly evaporated away [7].

The actual clinical and public health implications of these different routes of transmission in everyday situations remains controversial [1,2,6,7,9,13,14], and many researchers have been focusing on the potential for human influenza transmission during real-life activities such as breathing, talking, coughing and sneezing [15–18]. These studies have focused on characterising the number, size and content of droplets generated by such activities. Yet this data by itself is not sufficient to determine true transmissibility potential of any viruses carried in these droplets – they still need to reach a susceptible recipient and be inhaled in a sufficient infectious dose (for that individual) to cause infection and disease.

In this paper, two independent studies conducted during 2010, 2011 and 2012 by two different teams are reported, one from Hong Kong and one from Singapore. The two studies had an identical aim, to test the potential for the transmission of influenza from a naturally influenza-infected human to a life-like human manikin 'recipient' through real-life respiratory activities, such as breathing, talking, coughing sources. The outcomes of these two studies are presented together due to the similar and largely unexpected results, which showed little or no evidence of detectable influenza (RNA) transmission from the human source to the manikin recipient, with any mode of respiratory activity.

Note that the approach used in these experiments is different from several previous studies in that there is no attempt to capture all exhaled particles – the main focus of these studies is to examine how many of these potentially viral-laden particles actually reach the target manikins.

The Hong Kong study used a shop display manikin, customised for 'mouth-inhaling', to examine the quantity of influenza virus inhaled when exposed to a naturally influenza-infected human volunteer source. This study only examined the inhalation phase of a potential recipient. The Singapore study used a commercial thermal, breathing manikin with a full breathing cycle to quantify the amount of influenza virus landing on facial skin sites.

Materials and Methods

This study was approved by the Institutional Review Board of the University of Hong Kong. Signed informed consent was obtained from all participants. This ethics approval included the participation of children in this study, for whom verbal and written consent was also obtained from their parents, caregivers or guardians, as appropriate. Ethics approval for the Singapore study was granted by the Domain Specific Review Board (DSRB) of the National Healthcare Group (2009/00341) Singapore, and informed verbal and written consent was obtained from each participant in the study.

Hong Kong experiments (2010–2011)

For these experiments (performed during the 2010–2011 influenza season in Hong Kong SAR), a customised manikin was used as the model of a human recipient. A normal shop display manikin was obtained and a mouth orifice hollowed out, into which was fitted a mouth-piece connected to a pump through the back of the manikin's neck (**Figure 1**). This pump maintained a continuous inhalation flow of 12.5 L/min, to simulate the inhalation phase of human respiration. The inhalation rate of the manikin was set to twice that of natural human inhalation to create a similar inhalation flow field when both inhalation and exhalation are present. This setting arises from the following argument: if a typical human breath cycle consists of a 50:50 inhalation:exhalation ratio then the inhalation flow rate is equal to two times the tidal volume times the breathing frequency. The factor of two arises because you are only inhaling half the time, i.e. you multiply the minute ventilation by a factor of two to get the inhalation flow rate because you only spend half the breath cycle inhaling (you are exhaling for the other half) [19,20]. This also maximized SKC bio-sampler air sampling efficiency.

Once the manikin and the pump were set up, two methods were used to capture aerosolised virus produced by the naturally influenza-infected volunteers: 1) a polytetrafluoroethylene (PTFE) filter inserted into the mouth orifice of the manikin, to trap any aerosolised virus (**Figure 1A**); 2) and a commercially available air sampler (the 5 ml SKC BioSampler, SKC Inc., Eighty Four, PA USA: http://www.skcinc.com/prod/225-9594.asp) with 2 ml viral transport medium, which was attached to the mouth orifice through the back of the manikin's neck (Figures 1B and 1C). This air sampler was selected as it has been shown to perform well in collecting influenza-laden air samples effectively [21].

Each of these methods was used separately with each volunteer to capture aerosolised virus. The two methods were not used in combination with any of the volunteers. The reason for the two sampling methods was to allow the capture of large droplets that travelled ballistically as expelled from the source volunteer, transported by the source exhalation airflow (PTFE filters), as well as any smaller, droplet nuclei that were truly airborne, using the SKC BioSampler.

All the PTFE filters were kept in sealed plastic bags to prevent contamination and installed immediately prior to the experiments. Similarly, the mouth-pieces were sterilised and kept in sealed packets and only installed immediately before each experiment with the human volunteers. To capture the virus using the SKC BioSampler, a tissue culture medium (Medium 199, Life Technologies, Kowloon, Hong Kong SAR) was tested and found to be appropriate for the viral capture media. In addition, a baseline efficiency experiment was also performed to ensure that there was minimal loss of detection sensitivity using the PCR method when detecting for the presence of any viral RNA on the PTFE filter.

This study was conducted in a public hospital and a university health clinic during two distinct periods (August to September 2010 and January to February 2011). Patients over 21 years of age with influenza-like illness (ILI: any of cough, fever ≥38°C, sore throat, headache, malaise, myalgia, lethargy) in the previous three days were invited to participate in the study.

A rapid point-of-care test (QuickVue Influenza A+B rapid diagnostic test, Quidel Corp., San Diego, CA, USA: sensitivity: 0.68, specificity: 0.96) [22] was used as instructed by the

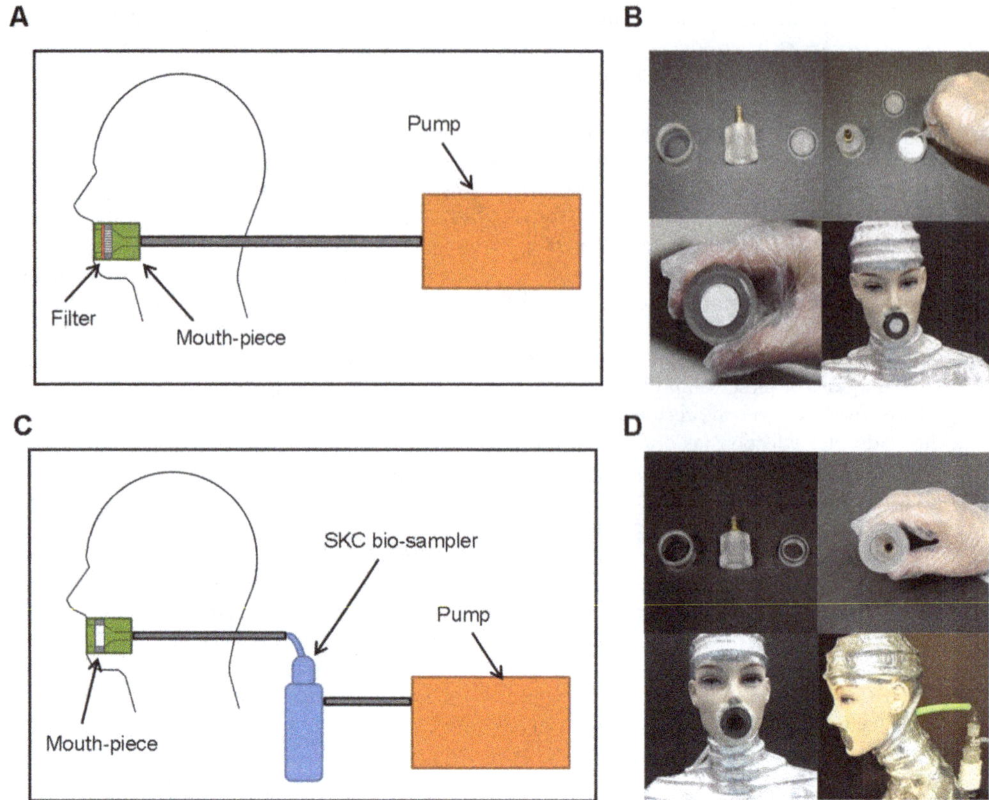

Figure 1. Airborne sampling experimental set-up (Hong Kong experiments), showing: A and B. Design of the mouthpiece with PTFE filter ('filter') in place. **C and D**. Installation of the SKC BioSampler, with the mouthpiece, in the manikin.

manufacturer as a screening test, to confirm influenza infection. Patients with positive diagnostic results were then invited for the exhaled breath sampling experiment. Nasal and throat swabs were collected into universal transport medium (UTM, Copan Diagnostics, Murietta, CA, USA) for diagnostic testing using an in-house influenza reverse transcription quantitative polymerase chain reaction (RT-qPCR) assay [23], to further confirm influenza infection and establish a baseline viral load.

Once the manikin was set up, for each sampling method, the recruited, naturally influenza-infected volunteers were asked to perform various respiratory activities (including breathing, counting, talking and coughing) when facing the customised manikin at a distance of 0.1 m and 0.5 m. The overall exposure period of the manikin target to each influenza-infected human volunteer was around 10–15 minutes. After each set of respiratory activities was conducted with the PTFE filter or the SKC BioSampler, the filter or capture media was removed and stored. The PTFE filter was first dipped in 2 mL UTM (universal viral transport medium) prior to storage. All specimens were stored at 2 to 8°C for less than 24 hours before PCR testing to determine the presence and quantity of influenza virus present.

For the PTFE filter samples, briefly, the mouthpiece filter holder was removed carefully and the filter removed. The filter was then soaked in 2 mL of UTM for 15 minutes, during which there were three episodes of vortexing for 30 seconds to transfer as much virus from the PTFE filter to the UTM for influenza RT-PCR testing. From this UTM, 140 μL was used for the RNA extraction step, without further concentration steps. This RT-PCR assay used consensus primers to target the matrix (MP) gene of the virus [23]. Calibrators were included in each run to allow a standard curve to be plotted to estimate the copy numbers in the samples. This assay had a detection limit of approximately 18,000 viral RNA copies/ml UTM.

To check the sensitivity of the PTFE capture method, samples of the PTFE filter were inoculated (by droplets of 1, 5, 25 μL volume) with different, known amounts of influenza RNA, then run through the whole extraction and RT-PCR process for influenza RNA detection. Overall, there was relatively little loss of sensitivity with the $\log_{10}$(inoculated) vs. $\log_{10}$(detected) viral loads being mostly within 10% of each other.

Singapore experiments (2011–2012)

For the Singapore experiments, otherwise healthy volunteers with an ILI were recruited from the local university student health centre clinic during the 'autumn/winter' period (September 2011 to February 2012). Successful recruits were taken directly to the experimental chamber, where they would expose a life-size, breathing, thermal manikin to various exhaled respiratory airflows. Clinical inclusion criteria included ILI with a temperature of at least 38°C. If the recruits were unable to go straight to the experimental chamber immediately after their clinic visit, they were excluded from the study. Before each experiment, a baseline nasopharyngeal swab (NPS) was taken from each participant for diagnostic testing.

A full-size, commercial thermal, breathing manikin (PT Teknik, Espergærde, Denmark: http://pt-teknik.dk/history) was used as the target for these exposure experiments. Both the manikin's thermal and breathing modes were turned on, during these exposure experiments, though only the manikin's face was to be tested for the presence of influenza RNA, after exposure to the naturally influenza-infected volunteers.

Before each exposure session, the manikin's face was cleaned with medical grade alcohol swabs and allowed to dry for 2–3 minutes. Baseline 'clean' swabs were taken from around the manikin's mouth (1 swab), nose (1 swab) and eyes (1 swab), before, then again after the manikin was exposed to the volunteer performing (Figure 2). The participant performed the following respiratory activities directly (within a 1 m distance) into the face of the manikin: nasal breathing (for 20 seconds), mouth breathing (20 s), counting slowly from one to ten in English (43 s), counting slowly from one to ten in a second language (e.g. Mandarin, German, 43 s), laughing (10 s) and coughing (10 s). Coughing was performed at both far (about ~1 m) and near (~0.1 m) distances from the manikin's face.

The airflow patterns produced during each of these exposure events were visualised and recorded using real-time shadowgraph imaging (**Figure 2, 3, Video S1**), using an experimental set-up as previously described elsewhere [24,25]. In each experiment, for a participant, one diagnostic swab from the participant and 36 facial swabs (representing pre- and post-exposure swabs from each of the eyes, nose and mouth sites), each collected in to 3 mL of UTM, from the manikin were taken for influenza testing. Testing was performed using a routine diagnostic quantitative polymerase chain reaction (qPCR) assay adapted from one already in service [26,27]. This assay had a detection limit of approximately 3000 viral RNA copies/ml UTM.

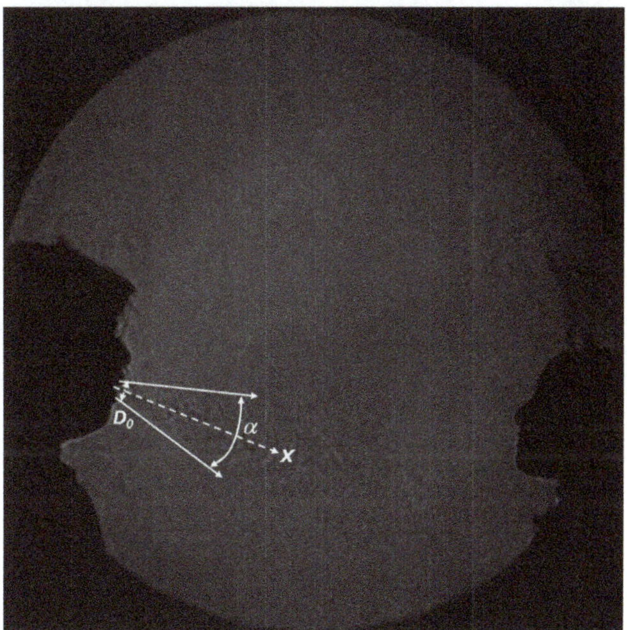

Figure 3. Example of cough shadowgraph image showing the dispersal of the exhaled puff. Parameters that affect the dispersal of this exhaled airflow include the mouth-opening diameter (D_0), propagation distance (x), and spreading angle (α) (see accompanying online Video S1 for further details of these shadowgraph images).

Results

Hong Kong experiments (2010–2011)

Results were available from 9 volunteers in total, of whom 8 were infected with influenza A and one with influenza B. Each of the volunteers either counted (and/or talked) and/or breathed and/or coughed in various combinations for varying durations. Seven of these volunteers were only 0.1 m from the recipient manikin. The last two volunteers who were exposed to the manikin when only the SKC BioSampler was being used (sampling for airborne droplet nuclei), were also exposed from a larger distance of 0.5 m. Despite the variety of source respiratory activities, the two different sampling methods and exposure distances, no influenza RNA was detected from either the PTFE filter or SKC BioSampler samples from any of the volunteer exposures (**Table 1**).

Singapore experiments (2011–2012)

Out of a total of 23 participants recruited for this study, 6 were diagnosed positive (6/23 = 26%) for influenza virus (2 seasonal A/H3N2, 1 pandemic A/H1N1pdm and 3 influenza B). Most of these volunteers presented within three days of illness onset (3 at 2 days, 1 each at 1, 3 and 6 days post-onset). Despite strongly positive diagnostic PCR results for influenza RNA (range: 4.33–6.83 $\log_{10}$) from the nasal swabs of the 6 volunteers, none of the post-exposure swabs taken from the manikin's face was found to be positive, after exposure to any of the respiratory activities. These manikin swabs were also tested for inhibitory substances to PCR by spiking them with influenza RNA positive control – no PCR inhibition was detected in any of these samples (**Table 2**).

Discussion

These experiments were conducted to further the understanding of how influenza is transmitted amongst humans. Multiple studies have been published on influenza air-sampling from the environment or human or simulated sources [15–18,28–30], as well as influenza transmission between various animal models [31,32]. Yet there have been few, if any studies focusing on the recipient end of the influenza transmission pathway. One such study by Lindsley et al [30] investigated the effect of wearing a face shield on the viral load potentially inhaled by the wearer, using a

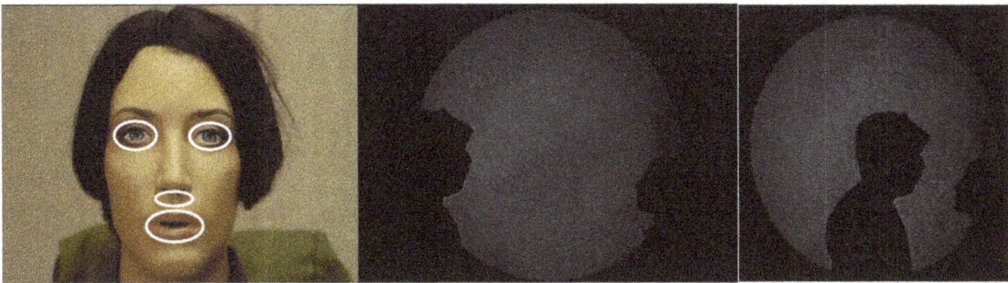

Figure 2. Singapore experimental set-up, showing: Swabbing sites for the manikins' face (A) for influenza testing. Shadowgraph images of far- (B) and near- cough (C) distances (see accompanying online Video S1 for further details of these shadowgraph images).

Table 1. Results for the Hong Kong experiments (n = 9).

Subject code no.	Influenza A/B	Age (yrs)	Sex (M/F)	Days post-onset of illness	Air sampling method	Test distance (m)	Patient 'source' activities	Influenza RNA detected in filter/sampler (cop/mL)	Influenza RNA cop/mL in source diagnostic swab
00302	A	47	M	3	PTFE filter + SKC BioSampler	0.1	Count 1–20; Cough 10 times	None	9.50×10^{7}
01402	A	42	M	3	PTFE filter + SKC BioSampler	0.1	Count 1–100; Cough 10 times	None	1.39×10^{5}
01702	A	14	F	2	PTFE filter + SKC BioSampler	0.1	Breath 1 min; Count 1–20; Cough 20 times	None	1.67×10^{5}
02602	A	17	F	3	PTFE filter + SKC BioSampler	0.1	Talk 10 min; Count 1–100; Cough 20 times	None	4.19×10^{5}
02702	A	22	F	2	PTFE filter + SKC BioSampler	0.1	Talk 10 min; Count 1–100; Cough 20 times	None	8.67×10^{6}
03802	A	49	F	3	PTFE filter + SKC BioSampler	0.1	Talk 10 min; Count 1 to 100; Cough 20 times	None	7.40×10^{6}
04102	A	57	F	2	PTFE filter + SKC BioSampler	0.1	Talk 10 min; Count 1 to 100; Cough 20 times	None	3.01×10^{6}
05602	A	62	F	2	SKC BioSampler	0.1, 0.5	Talk 10 min; Count 1 to 100; Cough 20 times	None	5.38×10^{5}
00203	B	not given	M	3	SKC BioSampler	0.1, 0.5	Talk 10 min; Count 1 to 100; Cough 20 times	None	3.70×10^{6}

Table 2. Results for Singaporean experiments (n = 6).

Subject code no.	Influenza A/subtype, or B	Age (yrs)	Sex (M/F)	Days post-onset of illness	[a]Test distance (m) – see footnote	[b]Patient 'source' activities – see footnote	Influenza RNA detected in manikin facial swabs (cop/mL)	Influenza RNA cop/mL in source diagnostic swab
1	A/H3	22	M	3	1. 1/10	See	None	1.29×10^5
2	A/H1N1pdm	22	M	2	(o0.1/10.1/1r 0.1 for additional close-up cough)	footnote*	None	2.88×10^4
3	B	23	F	6	0.1/1		None	2.14×10^4
4	A/H3	25	M	2			None	3.55×10^5
5	B	21	M	1			None	4.57×10^6
6	B	50	F	3			None	6.76×10^6

[a]0.1 m and 1 m.
[b]Nasal breathing (for 20 seconds), mouth breathing (20 s), counting slowly from one to ten in English (43 s), counting slowly from one to ten in a second language (e.g. Mandarin, German, 43 s), laughing (10 s) and coughing (10 s). Coughing was performed at both far (about ~1 m) and near (~0.1 m) distances from the manikin's face.

simulated coughing patient source and breathing healthcare worker recipient (wearing the face shield). They found that the face shield was highly effective in reducing the amount of virus potentially reaching the recipient by over 90% at separation distances of either 46 cm or 183 cm. However, continued presence in the same chamber would eventually result in a reduction of only ~80% as dispersion of the smaller, airborne particles in the room would eventually travel around the face mask to be inhaled. It was unclear what the starting aerosolised viral load was in this study.

This investigational stage of the transmission pathway might be termed: 'end-point host-exposure and sampling', i.e. what might be *actually* inhaled at the face vs. what might be *potentially* inhaled, based on the larger, air-sampled 'source' environment. The lack of any detectable influenza RNA from the swabs taken from the manikin's face (Singapore experiments) and inhaled breath (Hong Kong experiments) after exposure to infected volunteers, was initially surprising, but became more understandable in light of the study published by Milton and colleagues [18]. Again, note that the approach used in these experiments is different from several previous studies as there is no attempt to capture all exhaled particles. The main aim of these 'end-point sampling' studies is to investigate how many of these potentially viral-laden particles actually reach the target manikins.

Large droplets may be less likely to transmit influenza

In the Singapore experiments, the cycle threshold (Ct) values for the PCR positive NPS samples from the influenza positive recruits were all reasonably low (indicating the presence of a relatively high viral load) in these samples. The real-time shadowgraph video footage taken during these experiments clearly show the cough puff impinging directly onto the manikin's face in the vicinity of these swabbing sites (**Figure 2, Video S1**). Possible explanations for this might be that despite the relatively high influenza load on the NPS samples from these naturally infected recruits, the droplets expelled during these respiratory activities did not carry high numbers of viruses to transmit to the manikin's face.

More intriguingly is the possibility that the viral-laden saliva/mucous in the oral cavity is not of uniform viscosity, with the more localised immune responses in parts of the mouth (and/or oro-/naso-pharynx) increasing the local viscosity, thus allowing the lower viral load saliva/mucous of lower viscosity being preferentially expelled during respiratory activities. A review by Fabian et al. [33] suggests that salivary mucins, particularly MU7, have a high affinity for and may trap and agglutinate micro-organisms such as bacteria, fungi and viruses. Also another salivary mucin, MUC5b, has been shown to have antiviral properties, and can form hydrophilic viscoelastic gels that can increase the viscosity of saliva.

In the Hong Kong experiments, the results suggest that influenza virus cannot be detected in the inhaled breath after a source exposure from a minimum distance of 10 cm or greater, for these 15 patients. Similarly with the Singapore experiment, it is possible that the influenza virus levels in the exhalation airflows were just too low to be transmitted in detectable quantities to the recipient manikin. In these Hong Kong experiments, after the participant finished talking or coughing, large droplets were normally visible on the filters (diameters around 1–3 mm). These droplets had not evaporated by the time these filters were immersed in the transport media. Yet, influenza virus RNA was still not detectable even in these samples. The detection of little or no influenza RNA in these experiments was initially surprising, but again, maybe compatible with the results of Milton and colleagues

[18], who showed maximum copy numbers of <1000 by day 3 of illness in both coarse (>5 µm) and fine (≤5 µm) aerosol particles.

Duguid [34] suggested that large droplets are mostly generated from the anterior mouth. Influenza viruses, however, are rarely found in human saliva (Cowling et al. unpublished data) due to the antiviral substances existing in saliva [35]. Hence there is a possibility that large droplet transmission of influenza may not be important. This may also be true from a different angle. Breathing tends not to produce large droplets [28] and breathing is the most common respiratory activity in humans, so this is probably the most important human respiratory modality that would transmit influenza. Although coughing and sneezing do produce larger droplets, very little time is actually spent coughing and sneezing by most people (though admittedly the frequency of coughing and sneezing may increase with some respiratory infections), so these modalities in general, may not be most important for influenza transmission.

Dispersion of exhaled aerosols with distance may reduce the likelihood of transmission

These negative results may be also due to low virus concentration at a distance from the source caused by a dispersion effect. This is perhaps one of the more important differences between our experiment and other studies with successful virus recovery [15–18,28–29], i.e. that we did not capture the whole exhaled breath volume (regardless of modality, i.e. breathing, talking, coughing, etc.) from the sources. Hence, the total amount of viral RNA that was potentially detectable in these Hong Kong and Singapore studies may not be comparable to these other studies, and will likely be considerably less (see the estimated detectable viral loads in **Video S1**).

This explanation would also apply to the Singaporean experiments, and a qualitative visual confirmation of this dispersal effect can be seen from the shadowgraph images (**Figure 3, Video S1**). This figure also suggests the various parameters that are likely to affect the extent of the dispersal (and therefore dilution) of this exhaled airflow, including the mouth-opening diameter (D_0), mean dispersal angle (α) and propagation distance (x). Previous studies have measured these parameters in human volunteers, giving ranges for the mouth-opening diameter during coughing as $D_0 = 2.34$ cm [36], and mouth-breathing as $D_0 = 1.23$ cm [37], with a mean dispersal angle for mouth-breathing and coughing of $\alpha = 25$–$35°$ (mean 30°) [36,37]. An exact equation taking into account these parameters, together with the various air mass exchanges across the boundaries of the spreading cone due to turbulent flows, as well as the behaviour of the smaller scale airflows within the spreading cone, is beyond the scope of this article. However, it is clear from **Figure 3** (and **Video S1**) that the final numbers of droplets (and any virus that they might be carrying) arriving at the recipient's inhalation zone are likely to be considerably lower than that which left the source.

Another point to note from the shadowgraph images shown in **Figures 2 and 3 (and Video S1)** is that although the volunteers were asked to breathe, talk, cough and laugh directly towards the manikin from various distances, their natural, involuntary head movements (particularly during coughing and laughing) were not controlled in any way. These head movements, together with the dispersion factor described above, may have also acted to reduce the amount of virus landing on the manikin's face in both studies. However, these head movements were deliberately kept as natural as possible to present realistic exposure scenarios for these experiments.

Despite the sensitivity of RNA detection by the PCR method, this dispersal and accompanying dilution (with ambient air) effect may combine to make it difficult to detect any influenza RNA at the manikin - either directly landing on the facial surface (as shown in the Singapore experiments), or within the inhaled airborne particles captured by the filter or the air sampler (as shown in the Hong Kong experiments).

Totality of particle/droplet capture and durations of exposure

Another possible reason for the lack of detection of any influenza RNA is the relatively short duration of exposure: about 15 minutes in the Hong Kong and 10 seconds to a few minutes in the Singapore experiments. In addition, for the Singapore experiments, only a small rim was swabbed around the eyes, under the nose and around the mouth of the manikin, which may have reduced the amount of detectable virus in these experiments. However, to some extent, it was one of the aims of these experiments to assess what the likely influenza transmission risk would have been, given naturally occurring respiratory activities in everyday situations. Other studies have detected low levels of virus in exhaled particles from coughing and breathing in enclosed chambers for complete particle exposure/inhalation counts [15,17,28,29], with longer exposure and collection times of up to 20–30 minutes [15,29], but these are artificial experimental situations. In naturally occurring exposure scenarios, dispersion and dilution of these exhaled particles is quite normal and these experiments were designed to test how much viral RNA was detectable at the manikin's face, in spite of these dispersal and dilution factors. Two studies that investigated coughing into a closed chamber found that very little virus can be found in droplets produced by coughing (<50 viral RNA copies per cough [17], despite significant numbers of droplets being produced during coughing whilst infected with influenza (mean number 75,400/cough, median 46,400/cough, s.d. 97,300/cough, [28]). However, the diagnostic influenza viral load by qPCR from nasopharyngeal swabs collected from the infected volunteers in the former study [17] was reported as being very low (median viral copy number of 51 per sample). In this study, the diagnostic 'source' viral RNA copy numbers were much higher than this, so it might be expected that the amount of virus reaching the target manikins would be much higher.

Possible limitations of the sampling and detection methods

In the Singapore experiments, an alternative possible explanation might be that the surface of the manikin's face may have been too smooth to capture these airborne droplets (unlike human facial skin and mucous membranes) and that even if the droplets were carrying significant numbers of viruses, the droplets simply 'bounced' off the manikin's face, without leaving any detectable influenza RNA. From the shadowgraph imaging, it is clear that exhalation flows certainly impact upon the manikin's face (this is especially obvious with the close-up coughing from about 0.1 m distance). For these Singapore experiments that used a thermal manikin (with a surface skin temperature similar to that of a human – around 33–35°C), the generated thermal plume may be an additional factor that could have reduce the amount of airborne virus actually settling on the manikin's skin surface. The human thermal plume has been described in various studies, and may act as a sort of natural, protective air curtain in this regard [38–40]. Perhaps both of these reasons may be relevant in these experiments, and further studies are required to resolve this issue.

In the Hong Kong experiments, a pump was used to extract air through filters, which will increase the evaporation rate of droplets deposited on the filter. Together with the accompanying shear stresses applied to the influenza virus (which is a relatively labile, lipid-enveloped RNA virus), this would also decrease the virus survival rate on the filter, though this should not significantly affect the PCR detection sensitivity of viral RNA. However, the SKC BioSampler also has limitations in that its collection efficiency decreases significantly with increasing particle diameter from about 100% with 4 μm particles to about 30% with 9μm particles [41]. This may underestimate the viral loads detected in larger particles. With the PTFE filter capture and detection methods, any loss of sensitivity was relatively limited, with the $\log_{10}$(inoculated) vs $\log_{10}$(detected) viral loads being mostly within 10% of each other, according to the baseline experiments.

Comparison with other similar studies

Two other studies by Bischoff and colleagues have estimated approximate viral concentrations at certain distances. A study on the potential transocular transmission of influenza suggested that exposure to aerosolised influenza at a distance of up to 1 foot, would be sufficient to inoculate (i.e. infect) most exposed human subjects via the ocular route [42]. However, this exposure may bear little resemblance to a natural exposure with wild-type seasonal influenza virus, as it consisted of a 20-minute exposure to a mechanical aerosol generator emitting a mono-dispersed aerosol (of approximately 4.9 mm diameter) of the live attenuated vaccine ('Flumist') strain of influenza. The virus concentrations of this artificially generated aerosol and the naturally generated aerosols are difficult to compare.

Bischoff et al. [43] subsequently attempted to define concentration contours around patients infected with influenza, using Andersen samplers to sample air at head level distances of ≤ 0.305 m (1 ft), 0.914 m (3 ft) and 1.829 m (6 ft) away the heads of influenza infected patients. The upper limits of the viral concentration measured at 0.305 m and 0.914 m were roughly similar at approximately 400–600 and 350–600 "influenza virus RNA copies per 10-L human respiratory minute volume". Although this unit is difficult to compare to the results of the Hong Kong and Singapore experiments exactly, it does seem to agree with the implications of Milton et al. [18] that the airborne viral load exhaled by infected patients/volunteers is not particularly high, and together with the dispersion calculations above, may well result in very little virus actually reaching and depositing within the breathing zone of a susceptible recipient up to 1 m away.

In summary, these two complementary sets of experiments from Hong Kong and Singapore, with naturally-infected human volunteers, exhaling in various respiratory modalities, directly onto manikin targets, resulted in no detectable transmission of influenza virus RNA. Taking into account other recent findings of the relatively low viral loads in aerosolised droplets [18], this suggests that influenza may not be particularly transmissible by the aerosol route in most circumstances. Further experiments are required to confirm these findings. However, this does not exclude the possible transmission of the virus in situations with longer exposure/contact periods, or in super-spreader individuals who may well shed higher levels of virus in aerosolised form.

Supporting Information

Video S1 A 21-year old male coughing onto the target thermal, breathing manikin from 0.1 m then 1 m distance. Images shot at 2000 frames-per-second (fps) on a Photron SA1.1 high-speed camera. Playback speed: 100 fps (about one quarter normal speed) for clarity.

Acknowledgments

We thank Mr Lee Hong Kai (Molecular Diagnosis Centre, Department of Laboratory Medicine, National University Hospital, Singapore) for useful discussions about the sensitivity of the in-house influenza PCR detection assay for the Singapore experiments.

Author Contributions

Conceived and designed the experiments: JWT CXG BJC GCK JSMP YL. Performed the experiments: JWT CXG GCK DC JP ADN CAK. Analyzed the data: JWT CXG GCK DC JP ADN CAK. Contributed reagents/materials/analysis tools: JWT CXG BJC GCK JP ADN CAK JSMP CS DKWC KWT ESCK YL. Contributed to the writing of the manuscript: JWT CXG BJC GCK DC. Recruited the influenza-infected volunteers for the Hong Kong study: AK KC WT. Assisted CXG in critically reviewing the manuscript for the Hong Kong study: BL CH.

References

1. Tellier R (2006) Review of aerosol transmission of influenza A virus. Emerg Infect Dis 12: 1657–1662.
2. Brankston G, Gitterman L, Hirji Z, Lemieux C, Gardam M (2007) Transmission of influenza A in human beings. Lancet Infect Dis 7: 257–265.
3. Moser MR, Bender TR, Margolis HS, Noble GR, Kendal AP, et al. (1979) An outbreak of influenza aboard a commercial airliner. Am J Epidemiol 110: 1–6.
4. Lowen AC, Mubareka S, Tumpey TM, Garcia-Sastre A, Palese P (2006) The guinea pig as a transmission model for human influenza viruses. Proc Natl Acad Sci U S A 103: 9988–9992.
5. Han K, Zhu X, He F, Liu L, Zhang L, et al. (2009) Lack of airborne transmission during outbreak of pandemic (H1N1) 2009 among tour group members, China, June 2009. Emerg Infect Dis 15: 1578–1581.
6. Wong BC, Lee N, Li Y, Chan PK, Qiu H, et al. (2010) Possible role of aerosol transmission in a hospital outbreak of influenza. Clin Infect Dis 51: 1176–1183.
7. Tang JW, Li Y, Eames I, Chan PK, Ridgway GL (2006) Factors involved in the aerosol transmission of infection and control of ventilation in healthcare premises. J Hosp Infect 64: 100–114.
8. Li YG (2011) The secret behind the mask. Indoor Air 21: 89–91.
9. Roy CJ, Milton DK (2004) Airborne transmission of communicable infection–the elusive pathway. N Engl J Med 350: 1710–1712.
10. Nicas M, Nazaroff WW, Hubbard A (2005) Toward Understanding the Risk of Secondary Airborne Infection: Emission of Respirable Pathogens. Journal of Occupational and Environmental Hygiene 2: 143–154.
11. Atkinson MP, Wein LM (2008) Quantifying the routes of transmission for pandemic influenza. Bull Math Biol 70: 820–867.
12. Weber TP, Stilianakis NI (2008) Inactivation of influenza A viruses in the environment and modes of transmission: A critical review. Journal of Infection 57: 361–373.
13. Chapin CV (1912) The Sources and Modes of Infection New York: John Wiley & Sons Inc.
14. Wells WF (1955) Airborne Contagion and Air Hygiene: an Ecological Study of Droplet Infection. Cambridge, MA: Harvard University Press. 423 p.
15. Fabian P, McDevitt JJ, DeHaan WH, Fung RO, Cowling BJ, et al. (2008) Influenza virus in human exhaled breath: an observational study. PLoS ONE 3: e2691.
16. Stelzer-Braid S, Oliver BG, Blazey AJ, Argent E, Newsome TP, et al. (2009) Exhalation of respiratory viruses by breathing, coughing, and talking. J Med Virol 81: 1674–1679.
17. Lindsley WG, Blachere FM, Thewlis RE, Vishnu A, Davis KA, et al. (2010) Measurements of airborne influenza virus in aerosol particles from human coughs. PLoS ONE 5: e15100.
18. Milton DK, Fabian MP, Cowling BJ, Grantham ML, McDevitt JJ (2013) Influenza virus aerosols in human exhaled breath: particle size, culturability, and effect of surgical masks. PLoS Pathog 9: e1003205.
19. Storey-Bishoff J, Noga M, Finlay WH (2008) Deposition of micrometer-sized aerosol particles in infant nasal airway replicas. J Aerosol Sci 39: 1055–1065.
20. Golshahi L, Noga ML, Vehring R, Finlay WH (2013) An In vitro Study on the Deposition of Micrometer-Sized Particles in the Extrathoracic Airways of Adults During Tidal Oral Breathing. Ann Biomed Eng 41: 979–989.
21. Fabian P, McDevitt JJ, Houseman EA, Milton DK (2009) Airborne influenza virus detection with four aerosol samplers using molecular and infectivity assays:

considerations for a new infectious virus aerosol sampler. Indoor Air 19: 433–441.
22. Cheng CKY, Cowling BJ, Chan KH, Fang VJ, Seto WH, et al. (2009) Factors affecting QuickVue Influenza A + B rapid test performance in the community setting. Diagnostic microbiology and infectious disease 65: 35–41.
23. Chan KH, Peiris JSM, Lim W, et al (2008) Comparison of nasopharyngeal flocked swabs and aspirates for rapid diagnosis of respiratory viruses in children. J Clin Virol 42: 65–69.
24. Tang JW, Nicolle A, Pantelic J, Koh GC, Wang LD, et al. (2012) Airflow dynamics of coughing in healthy human volunteers by shadowgraph imaging: an aid to aerosol infection control. PLoS One 7: e34818.
25. Tang JW, Nicolle AD, Klettner CA, Pantelic J, Wang L, et al. (2013) Airflow dynamics of human jets: sneezing and breathing - potential sources of infectious aerosols. PLoS One 8: e59970.
26. Lee HK, Loh TP, Lee CK, Tang JW, Chiu L, et al. (2012) A universal influenza A and B duplex real-time RT-PCR assay. J Med Virol 84: 1646–1651.
27. Lee CK, Lee HK, Loh TP, Lai FY, Tambyah PA, et al. (2011) Comparison of Pandemic (H1N1) 2009 and Seasonal Influenza Viral Loads, Singapore. Emerg Infect Dis 17: 287–291.
28. Lindsley WG, Pearce TA, Hudnall JB, Davis KA, Davis SM, et al. (2012a) Quantity and size distribution of cough-generated aerosol particles produced by influenza patients during and after illness. J Occup Environ Hyg 9: 443–449.
29. Lindsley WG, King WP, Thewlis RE, Reynolds JS, Panday K, et al. (2012b). Dispersion and exposure to a cough-generated aerosol in a simulated medical examination room. J Occup Environ Hyg 9: 681–690.
30. Lindsley WG, Noti JD, Blachere FM, Szalajda JV, Beezhold DH (2014) Efficacy of face shields against cough aerosol droplets from a cough simulator. J Occup Environ Hyg 11: 509–518.
31. Herfst S, Schrauwen EJ, Linster M, Chutinimitkul S, de Wit E, et al. (2012) Airborne transmission of influenza A/H5N1 virus between ferrets. Science 336: 1534–1541.
32. Kaminski MM, Ohnemus A, Staeheli P, Rubbenstroth D (2013) Pandemic 2009 H1N1 influenza A virus carrying a Q136K mutation in the neuraminidase gene is resistant to zanamivir but exhibits reduced fitness in the guinea pig transmission model. J Virol 87: 1912–1915.
33. Fábián TK, Hermann P, Beck A, Fejérdy P, Fábián G (2012) Salivary defense proteins: their network and role in innate and acquired oral immunity. Int J Mol Sci 13: 4295–4320.
34. Duguid JP (1946) Expulsion of pathogenic organisms from the respiratory tract. Br Med J 1: 265–268.
35. White MR, Helmerhorst EJ, Ligtenberg A, Karpel M, Tecle T, et al. (2009) Multiple components contribute to ability of saliva to inhibit influenza viruses. Oral Microbiol Immunol 24: 18–24.
36. Gupta JK, Lin CH, Chen Q (2009) Flow dynamics and characterization of a cough. Indoor Air 19: 517–525.
37. Gupta JK, Lin CH Chen QY (2010) Characterizing exhaled airflow from breathing and talking. Indoor Air 20: 31–39.
38. Tang JW, Liebner TJ, Craven BA, Settles GS (2009) A schlieren optical study of the human cough with and without wearing masks for aerosol infection control. J R Soc Interface 6(Suppl 6): S727–36. doi:10.1098/rsif.2009.0295.focus.
39. Licina D, Pantelic J, Melikov A, Sekhar C, Tham KW (2014) Experimental investigation of the human convective boundary layer in a quiescent indoor environment. Build Environ S0360-1323(14)00019-5. doi.org/10.1016/j.buildenv.2014.01.016 [Epub ahead of print].
40. Voelker C, Maempel S, Kornadt O (2014) Measuring the human body's micro-climate using a thermal manikin. Indoor Air doi:10.1111/ina.12112. [Epub ahead of print].
41. Kesavan J, Schepers D, McFarland AR (2010) Sampling and Retention Efficiencies of Batch-Type Liquid-Based Bioaerosol Samplers. Aerosol Sci Tech 44: 817–829.
42. Bischoff WE, Reid T, Russell GB, Peters TR (2011) Transocular entry of seasonal influenza-attenuated virus aerosols and the efficacy of n95 respirators, surgical masks, and eye protection in humans. J Infect Dis 204: 193–199.
43. Bischoff WE, Swett K, Leng I, Peters TR (2013) Exposure to influenza virus aerosols during routine patient care. J Infect Dis 207: 1037–1046.

Correlation of *Klebsiella pneumoniae* Comparative Genetic Analyses with Virulence Profiles in a Murine Respiratory Disease Model

Ramy A. Fodah[1☯], Jacob B. Scott[3,5☯], Hok-Hei Tam[4], Pearlly Yan[6,7], Tia L. Pfeffer[1], Ralf Bundschuh[6,7], Jonathan M. Warawa[1,2*]

1 Department of Microbiology and Immunology, University of Louisville, Louisville, Kentucky, United States of America, **2** Center for Predictive Medicine, University of Louisville, Louisville, Kentucky, United States of America, **3** Dental School, University of Louisville, Louisville, Kentucky, United States of America, **4** Department of Chemical Engineering, Massachusetts Institute of Technology, Cambridge, Massachusetts, United States of America, **5** College of Dentistry, Ohio State University, Columbus, Ohio, United States of America, **6** The Comprehensive Cancer Center and The James Cancer Hospital and Solove Research Institute, Division of Hematology, Department of Internal Medicine, Ohio State University, Columbus, Ohio, United States of America, **7** Departments of Physics and Chemistry & Biochemistry and Center for RNA Biology, Ohio State University, Columbus, Ohio, United States of America

Abstract

Klebsiella pneumoniae is a bacterial pathogen of worldwide importance and a significant contributor to multiple disease presentations associated with both nosocomial and community acquired disease. ATCC 43816 is a well-studied *K. pneumoniae* strain which is capable of causing an acute respiratory disease in surrogate animal models. In this study, we performed sequencing of the ATCC 43816 genome to support future efforts characterizing genetic elements required for disease. Furthermore, we performed comparative genetic analyses to the previously sequenced genomes from NTUH-K2044 and MGH 78578 to gain an understanding of the conservation of known virulence determinants amongst the three strains. We found that ATCC 43816 and NTUH-K2044 both possess the known virulence determinant for yersiniabactin, as well as a Type 4 secretion system (T4SS), CRISPR system, and an acetonin catabolism locus, all absent from MGH 78578. While both NTUH-K2044 and MGH 78578 are clinical isolates, little is known about the disease potential of these strains in cell culture and animal models. Thus, we also performed functional analyses in the murine macrophage cell lines RAW264.7 and J774A.1 and found that MGH 78578 (K52 serotype) was internalized at higher levels than ATCC 43816 (K2) and NTUH-K2044 (K1), consistent with previous characterization of the antiphagocytic properties of K1 and K2 serotype capsules. We also examined the three *K. pneumoniae* strains in a novel BALB/c respiratory disease model and found that ATCC 43816 and NTUH-K2044 are highly virulent (LD_{50}<100 CFU) while MGH 78578 is relatively avirulent.

Editor: José A. Bengoechea, Quuen's University Belfast, United Kingdom

Funding: This work was supported by internal funding at the University of Louisville. The funders had no role in study design, data collection and analysis, decision to publish, or preparation of the manuscript.

Competing Interests: The authors have declared that no competing interests exist.

* Email: jonathan.warawa@louisville.edu

☯ These authors contributed equally to this work.

Introduction

Klebsiella pneumoniae ssp. *pneumoniae* (*K. pneumoniae*) is responsible for emerging infectious disease and is a causative agent of both nosocomial and community acquired pneumonia (CAP) worldwide. The epidemiology of *K. pneumoniae* is complex, involving ecological persistence as well as carriage in both animal and human populations [1]. Carriage of *K. pneumoniae* is frequently associated with colonization of the upper respiratory tract or gastrointestinal (GI) tract, with the potential for GI tract amplification of antibiotic resistant strains of *K. pneumoniae* following antibiotic therapies [2]. *K. pneumoniae* opportunistically infects a variety of mucosal surfaces with the primary sites of infection including the urinary tract and the lower respiratory tract (LRT) [3].

K. pneumoniae pneumonia is a fatal disease with mortality rates of up to 22.7% [4,5]. The incidence of *K. pneumoniae* pneumonia in the United States is more commonly associated with nosocomial acquisition of disease rather than environmental sources [6,7], as *Klebsiella* is thought to contribute to only 1% of CAP in North America [8,9,10]. *K. pneumoniae* is the fifth most prevalent nosocomial bacterial pathogen in the United States for infections associated with UTIs, VAP and central line-associated bacteremia, and accounts for 6% of all nosocomial bacterial disease [11]. The emergence of *K. pneumoniae* as a nosocomial pathogen in the US and Europe may be due in part to the acquisition of antibiotic resistance markers providing a selective advantage in hospital settings, with particular concerns growing over an increasing prevalence of carbapenemase-expressing *K. pneumoniae* (KPC) strains [12]. Well characterized outbreaks of KPC dating back to 1988 have still not led to effective clinical diagnosis or control of these emerging pathogens in the US over 20 years later [13,14]. Recently instated surveillance programs have begun to characterize the increasing threat of *K. pneumoniae* in the US health care system, where it is understood that the threat of *K. pneumoniae*, and in particular KPC, may be underestimated, particularly in long-term acute care facilities [15].

Several virulence determinants are important in mediating the virulence of *K. pneumoniae* in the lung, including capsular polysaccharide, lipopolysaccharide, enterobacterial common antigen, OmpA, OmpK36, the AcrAB efflux pump, the regulator RamA, the biofilm related factor YciI, and yersiniabactin [16,17,18,19,20,21,22,23], however, additional undescribed systems may participate in *K. pneumoniae* virulence. To this end, numerous sequencing efforts have begun to characterize the genomes of *K. pneumoniae* strains including the first whole genome sequences of the clinical isolates MGH 78578 and NTUH-K2044 [24], and the more recent release of whole genome sequences of the strains HS11286 [25] and KCTC 2242 [26]. Comparative genetic analyses have successfully led to the identification and characterization of a novel allantoin metabolism locus required for GI tract disease which is present in the genome of NTUH-K2044, but absent from MGH 78578 [27].

The ATCC 43816 strain has been the focus of several studies characterizing the respiratory disease caused by *K. pneumoniae* [16,18,28], however this strain has not been sequenced, thus limiting investigations directed at identification of novel virulence determinants. To address this scientific gap, we have performed whole genome sequencing of ATCC 43816 to begin the characterization potential genomic differences relative to the sequenced *K. pneumoniae* strains.

We also decided to investigate host-pathogen interaction for the sequenced *K. pneumoniae* strains NTUH-K2044 and MGH 78578, for which little is known about their ability to cause respiratory disease or interact with professional phagocytes. We developed a novel pulmonary-specific delivery respiratory disease model in which to examine sequenced *K. pneumoniae* strains. Finally, we have characterized the ability of *K. pneumoniae* to modulate uptake and persist within multiple cultured murine macrophage cell lines.

Materials and Methods

Bacterial strains and media

K. pneumoniae strains were cultured routinely in Lennox Broth (LB) or LB agar plates at 37°C. *K. pneumoniae* was preconditioned for cell culture and animal studies by subculturing overnight broth cultures 1:25 into TSBDC [29] for an additional 3 hr of growth at 37°C. Briefly, TSBDC is formulated as a concentrate of a 30 g/L trypticase soy broth mixed with 5 g/L of Chelex 100 in a 1/10th volume, which is dialyzed from a 6–8 kDa dialysis tubing into a 1x volume of 1% glycerol, where the media consists of the small organic compounds which leave the dialysis tubing into the 1% glycerol solution. TSBDC is supplemented with 50 mM monosodium glutamate immediately prior to use. The bacterial cultures were washed into PBS and their concentration was estimated using OD_{600} measurements. The *K. pneumoniae* strains used in this study included ATCC 43816, MGH 78578 (kindly provided by Virginia Miller, UNC), NTUH-K2044 (kindly provided by Jin-Town Wang, NTUCM and Valley Stewart, UC Davis), and CIP 52.145 (Collection of Institut Pasteur). Where appropriate, antibiotics were used at the following concentrations unless otherwise stated: carbenicillin (100 µg/ml), kanamycin (25 µg/ml), zeocin (100 µg/ml), and gentamicin (20 µg/ml).

Sequencing of *K. pneumoniae* ATCC 43816

ATCC 43816 genomic DNA was isolated from ~5×10^9 bacteria grown in LB broth overnight. The DNA was isolated in TE buffer with 0.5% SDS extraction in the presence of proteinase K and RNase, followed by phenol:chloroform:isoamyl alcohol (25:24:1 v/v) purification, and alcohol precipitation. A 1.5 µg aliquot of chromosomal DNA was processed for Illumina Next Generation Sequencing based on the manufacturer's instructions. Briefly, fragmentase (NEB) was used to generate 100–300 bp DNA fragments which were end repaired, A-tailed, adaptor ligated, and PCR amplified using Phusion. Two lanes of 51 base reads were run to generate 22,422,915 reads of sequencing data, filtered to eliminate low quality reads, and assembled using Velvet [30]. We assembled 1763 contigs, of which 1550 contigs were > 200 bp and were deposited at DDBJ/EMBL/GenBank under the accession APWN00000000. The version described in this paper is the first version, APWN01000000. The contigs were aligned against the non-redundant nucleotide database using BLASTN [31] and hits to the full genomes of the NTUH-K2044 and MGH 78578 strains were retained separately. Manual sorting was conducted to identify contigs common to or unique from the NTUH-K2044 and MGH 78578 genomes, and unique sequence was aligned by BLASTN to identify homology to other bacterial species.

The capsular polysaccharide genetic cluster was manually sequenced to close contig gaps between five contigs, as described elsewhere [32], and the complete sequence for the ATCC 43816 capsular polysaccharide locus have been deposited with DDBJ/EMBL/GenBank with the accession number KJ541664.

Quantification of capsular polysaccharide production

Capsule production was quantified for *K. pneumoniae* from LB overnight cultures, as described elsewhere [33]. Briefly, PBS-washed bacteria were enumerated and subjected to hot phenol extraction before precipitating the chloroform-treated aqueous phase with 0.5 M sodium acetate and then 10 volumes of 95% ethanol. Polysaccharide was pelleted at 7200 g for 5 min after an overnight storage at −20°C. The pellet was resuspended in water, and uronic acid was measured from capsular polysaccharide preparations using a modified carbazole assay [34], with measurement calculated relative to a glucuronolactone standard.

Generation of capsular polysaccharide mutants

Capsular polysaccharide mutants were generated for *K. pneumoniae* strains ATCC 43816 and NTUH-K2044 by allelic exchange mutagenesis by initially PCR-amplifying upstream (5′) and downstream (3′) 1 kb fragments from a gene targeted for knock out (Table 1). The 1 kb homologous fragments were assembled in pSK (Stratagene) using a HindIII restriction site common to both the upstream and downstream fragments. A HindIII floxed zeocin cassette was inserted between the upstream and downstream fragments before the assembled construct was moved into an allelic exchange vector, pJMW106, which is a Km^R variant of pCVD442 [35]. Thus, an XbaI-KpnI fragment containing an in-frame 89.3% coding region deletion of the NTUH-K2044 *wzc* gene was cloned into pJMW106, and electroporated into *E. coli* strain S17-1 [36] to yield strain S17-1/pJMW106-NTUH Δ*wzc*::flox-zeo. Similarly, a XhoI-SpeI fragment containing an in-frame 90.4% coding region deletion of the ATCC 43816 *manC* gene was used to generate the strain S17-1/pJMW106-ATCC Δ*manC*::flox-zeo.

Allelic exchange was conducted over two stages, first by bacterial conjugation of the allelic exchange vectors from S17-1 to *K. pneumoniae* and selection of Cb^{R}Km^R merodiploid intermediates, and secondly by counter-selection of the suicide vector with 5% sucrose and zeocin. Confirmation of genome knock-out mutagenesis was confirmed on Km^S clones using PCR

Table 1. Primers used in this study.

5′ ATCC *manC* XbaI(+)	CTGCTCGAGATTACCAAAGATATCTTCACCAAGAAGGATGAAG
5′ ATCC *manC* HindIII(−)	GTAAAGCTTGCGAGACATCGGCCAGAGACGAC
3′ ATCC *manC* HindIII(+)	GAAAAGCTTGAGATCCAGTCGGGGTCGTACCTC
3′ ATCC *manC* KpnI(−)	GTGACTAGTTTTCGCTCCCGGCTGCTTCTGC
ATCC *manC* mut(+)	GTTATTCTACAATAAACTGACCAAGTCATCTTGTTTCCTCTCCTTCG
ATCC *manC* mut(−)	CTATCTTCCCGGGTTTCAGAAATTCGCCGTAGGC
5′ NTUH *wzc* XbaI(+)	CGTTCTAGAGCATAACGGTAAAGATACTAAGATCTCCTTATATGC
5′ NTUH *wzc* HindIII(−)	CAAAGCTTTATGATCAATAACTTCACCAATTAAACGACCTAGATCGATCC
3′ NTUH *wzc* HindIII(+)	CAAAGCTTTCGATGTTGCTAAAAATAGATTGGAACATAGCGGTGTTATAG
3′ NTUH *wzc* KpnI(−)	CTGGTACCTAATAATGAGGAGAACATTACCATAAAACGAGATGTATTTCG
NTUH *wzc* mut(+)	GGCAAAACTATGTTATTCGGACATTGGATAGGGCAACGAG
NTUH *wzc* mut(−)	CATTAATCGCAAGGCCAAATCCTTGTGATAATAGCATGCTTAGTATTC

analysis with 'mut' primers (Table 1) which flank the deletion site. The resulting strains were named ATCC Δ*manC* and NTUH Δ*wzc*.

Microscopic analysis of capsule mutants

Negative staining of *K. pneumoniae* capsule was conducted using nigrosin stain, as described elsewhere [37]. Briefly, LB overnight broth cultures of wild type and capsule mutant strains of ATCC 43816 and NTUH-K2044 were mixed 1:1 with 10% nigrosin and smeared onto 18×18 mm coverslips. The smear was air dried before mounting onto a glass slide. Samples were visualized with a 63x objective on a Zeiss Axio microscope, and images were analyzed with Zeiss Axiovision Vs40x64 and Imaris x64 (Bitplane).

Macrophage uptake assay

Both J774A.1 and RAW264.7 cell lines (ATCC) were cultured in DMEM (Invitrogen) supplemented with heat-inactivated 10% fetal bovine serum (FBS, HyClone) and seeded into 96 well microtiter plates at a density of 7.5×10^4 or 2×10^5 cells per well, respectively. Cells were challenged at an MOI of 10 with *K. pneumoniae* ATCC 43816, NTUH-K2044 or MGH 78578, or with capsule mutants ATCC Δ*manC* or NTUH Δ*wzc*. At one hour post infection, gentamicin was added to eliminate extracellular bacteria (20 µg/ml final, or 1000 µg/ml for the Gm^R MGH 78578 strain). Gentamicin concentrations were empirically determined to kill extracellular *K. pneumoniae* in DMEM/FBS at > 99.99% efficiency within a 1 hr window. At three hours post infection, monolayers were washed with PBS, lysed with 0.1% Triton X-100/PBS for 5 min, and serially diluted for bacterial enumeration on LB plates. Statistical analysis of data sets was conducted by One-way ANOVA with Tukey post-test of log-transformed data.

Macrophage survival assay

J774A.1 and RAW264.7 macrophages were cultured in 96 well microtiter plates as described above. Triplicate wells of macrophages were infected with *K. pneumoniae* in five replicate plates, and infections were conducted for 1 hr before the addition of gentamicin to kill extracellular bacteria, and antibiotic was maintained throughout the assay duration. At time points corresponding to 3, 4.5, 6, 9, and 12 hr post infection, a microtiter plate of samples was washed in PBS before releasing intracellular bacteria from macrophages using a 5 min treatment of 0.1% Triton X-100/PBS. Samples were serially diluted in PBS and plated onto LB plates to enumerate intracellular bacteria. Statistical analysis of growth between time point outgrowth was conducted by One-way ANOVA with Tukey post-test of log-transformed data.

Intratracheal infection of mice

Murine infection studies were approved by the University of Louisville Institutional Animal Care and Use Committee in accordance with National Institutes of Health guidelines (Protocol #10069). Groups of five 8 wk old female BALB/c mice (Charles River) were challenged using a non-surgical intratracheal infection procedure was developed to minimize trauma during pathogen delivery. Intubation-mediated intratracheal (IMIT) inoculations were conducted as demonstrated in detail elsewhere [38]. Briefly, isoflurane-anesthetized animals received 10 µl of 2% lidocaine anesthetic to the rear of the throat and were supported supine on a tilting platform raised to a 45° angle. Using a fine tipped cotton applicator, the tongue was retracted while an otoscope fitted with a cut-away specula was inserted into the oral cavity to visualize the glottis. An 18 G catheter, cast with a silicone rubber sleeve (10 mm of catheter exposed) was used to intubate mice, using a 20 mil guide wire to assist catheter placement. A 20 G blunt needle was used to instill a 50 µl PBS bacterial suspension directly into the lung via the catheter, followed by a 150 µl volume of air to aid distribution of the inoculum. Infected animals were monitored twice daily for indications of moribund disease, at which point they were humanely euthanized by isoflurane. Studies were concluded at 14 days. Statistical analysis of survival data was conducted using Log-rank (Mantel-Cox) and Gehan-Breslow-Wilcoxon Tests (GraphPad Prism 5). Probit analysis (StatPlus 2009 Professional) was used to calculate the LD_{50} (Lethal Dose 50%) and both the upper (UCL) and lower (LCL) reliable interval values.

Bacterial enumeration from key sites of infection

Groups of five BALB/c mice were infected using the IMIT model with $10^{2.2}$ CFU of either NTUH-K2044 or ATCC 43816. Moribund mice were euthanized at the presentation of lethargy, hunching, and labored breathing. Mice were euthanized by overdose of isoflurane, immediately followed by exsanguination by cardiac puncture with a 23 G needle, and the blood was collected to a Microtainer (K_2EDTA, BD Biosciences). Lung, liver and spleen were each collected into a sterile Whirl-Pak bag (Nasco) and homogenized in 1 ml of sterile PBS, by rolling the tissue with a 25 ml serological pipette. Blood and tissue homogenate were subjected to detergent lysis with 1% Triton X-100 for 5 min and subsequently serially diluted in a 96 well plate. LB plates were spot-plated with 10 µl aliquots of diluted bacterial suspensions, grown for 8 hrs at 37°C, and bacterial burdens were calculated based on dilution factor, tissue weight, and estimated tissue density. Neutral buoyancy testing in glycerol solutions revealed that the estimated tissue densities for lung, liver, and spleen were 1.03, 1.08, and 1.06 g/ml, respectively.

Results

Whole genome sequencing of strain ATCC 43816

K. pneumoniae ATCC 43816 is a well-studied strain, capable of causing a moribund respiratory disease in mouse models. However, limited genomic data is available to support future investigations of *K. pneumoniae* pathogenesis, thus we decided to perform whole genome sequencing. Next Generation Sequencing was used to sequence the ATCC 43816 genome, which was subsequently assembled into 1763 contigs consisting of 4.207 MB of sequence data (accession number APWN00000000). To investigate the genetic relatedness of sequenced *K. pneumoniae* strains, the ATCC 43816 genome was aligned to the complete genome sequences of the NTUH-K2044 and MGH 78578 strains (Figure 1A and B, respectively). A total of 1676 contigs (4.128 MB) aligned with the NTUH-K2044 chromosome representing 78.7% genome coverage. Similarly, 1668 contigs (4.098 MB) mapped to 77.1% of the MGH 78578 genome, which includes two contigs mapping to the toxin-antitoxin system of the pKPN4 plasmid. We identified no additional sequence homology to *K. pneumoniae* plasmids, and the homologous toxin-antitoxin system is maintained on the chromosome for the NTUH-K2044 strain, suggesting that *K. pneumoniae* strain ATCC 43816 does not possess plasmids.

A high degree of genetic conservation was observed between the three *K. pneumoniae* strains with 96.3% of ATCC 43816 sequence mapping to both MGH 78578 and NTUH-K2044. However, 69.71 kb of ATCC 43816 contigs uniquely map with the NTUH-K2044 genome and 44.67 kb with the MGH 78578 genome (1.66% and 1.06% total sequence data, respectively). While MGH 78578 shares primarily metabolic and hypothetical proteins with ATCC 43816, NTUH-K2044 shares the virulence-associated yersiniabactin biosynthetic operon, a Type IV secretion system, an iron transport system, a CRISPR locus, and an acetonin catabolism locus (Table 2). Given the conservation of known virulence determinants between ATCC 43816 and NTUH-K2044, the data suggests that NTUH-K2044 may share the same virulence potential as ATCC 43816 in disease models. Conversely, MGH 78578 lacks several of the virulence determinants previously identified as critical to the disease potential of ATCC 43816 in murine respiratory disease models, suggesting that MGH 78578 may have a reduced virulence in these models, though MGH 78578 is notably a clinical lung isolate from a presentation of pneumonia.

We also identified novel genetic sequences unique to ATCC 43816, and not present in either NTUH-K2044 or MGH 78578, notably including two bacteriophages, one of which is homologous to a bacteriophage found in the enteric *Escherichia coli* strain UMN026, and the other to the upper respiratory tract (URT) pathogen *Klebsiella rhinoscleromatis* strain ATCC 13884 (Table 2). Little has been reported regarding the clinical history of ATCC 43816, however the presence of both gastrointestinal (GI) and URT-related bacteriophages suggests that this *K. pneumoniae* strain may have previously been resident of both host niches.

Next Generation Sequencing provided an estimated 78% coverage of the ATCC 43816 genome, however sequencing of the capsular polysaccharide biosynthetic locus was under-represented at 22% coverage (determined retrospectively). Given the importance of capsule as a virulence determinant, we completed sequencing of a 34.6 kb region which includes the capsule locus as well as an adjacent region (*wzm* to *wbbO*) reported to be required for LPS biosynthesis (Fig. 2) [39]. The K2 capsular polysaccharide locus shares broad homology to sequenced capsule loci from the *galF* to *wzc* and *rfbP* to *uge* genes, but shares specific homology over the central *orf7* to *orf13* genes to a subset of sequenced *K. pneumoniae* strains of K2 serotype. Homology over the entire capsule locus is therefore highest (99% identity) to that of the recently fully sequenced strains CG43 (Accession CP006648), KCTC 2242 (CP002910), and Kp52.145 (FO834906), and also to the partially sequenced capsule biosynthetic loci of VGH525 (Accession AB371296) and Chedid (D21242). The central region of the capsule loci encodes for the antigenic diversity of capsules, which has previously supported the use of PCR as a methodology to identify capsule serotype [40,41].

Characterization of capsule production

K. pneumoniae capsular serotypes influence the virulence potential of strains, as could the regulated production of capsule. Thus, we investigated whether differences exist in the amount of capsule produced by the three clinical strains examined in this study. *K. pneumoniae* were examined for their ability to produce capsule from LB overnight cultures. We found that ATCC 43816, NTUH-K2044 and MGH 78578 strains produced 9.7, 13.5, and 6.1 fg/CFU of capsule, respectively. As a control, we also measured capsule production from previously characterized strain 52.145 which produced 21.7 fg/CFU of capsule in our studies, consistent with 52.145 being a significant producer of capsule [33]. Our measurement of NTUH-K2044 capsule production is consistent with previously reported levels of 17.3 fg/CFU of capsule from overnight LB cultures [42]. Thus, of the sequenced strains studied in this work, NTUH-K2044 produced the greatest amount of capsule at levels 1.4 and 2.2 fold greater than ATCC 43816 and MGH 78578. Similar amounts of capsule were measured from strains grown to mid-exponential phase in TSBDC (data not shown), suggesting that media and growth phase do not significantly impact capsule production.

Cell culture model

K. pneumoniae is internalized by a variety of host cell types both *in vivo* and in cell culture models, thus we investigated whether the three study strains exhibit differences in uptake rates in cultured murine macrophages. Given that capsular polysaccharide has been reported to mediate an antiphagocytic phenotype, we also generated capsular polysaccharide mutants of ATCC 43816 (Δ*manC*) and NTUH-K2044 (Δ*wzc*), and confirmed that the capsule mutants exhibited reduced exclusion of nigrosin staining (Figure 3). Both J774A.1 and RAW264.7 monolayers were challenged with *K. pneumoniae* strains at an MOI of 10, and internalized bacteria were detected using a gentamicin protection assay. In both J774A.1 and RAW264.7 cells, the MGH 78578 strain was phagocytosed more efficiently than the ATCC 43816 and NTUH-K2044 strains ($P<0.001$) (Figure 4). This suggests that the K52 serotype capsule of the MGH 78578 strain does not resist uptake by murine macrophages to the same degree as representative K1 and K2 serotype strains. In addition, ATCC 43816 was phagocytosed more efficiently than NTUH-K2044 in

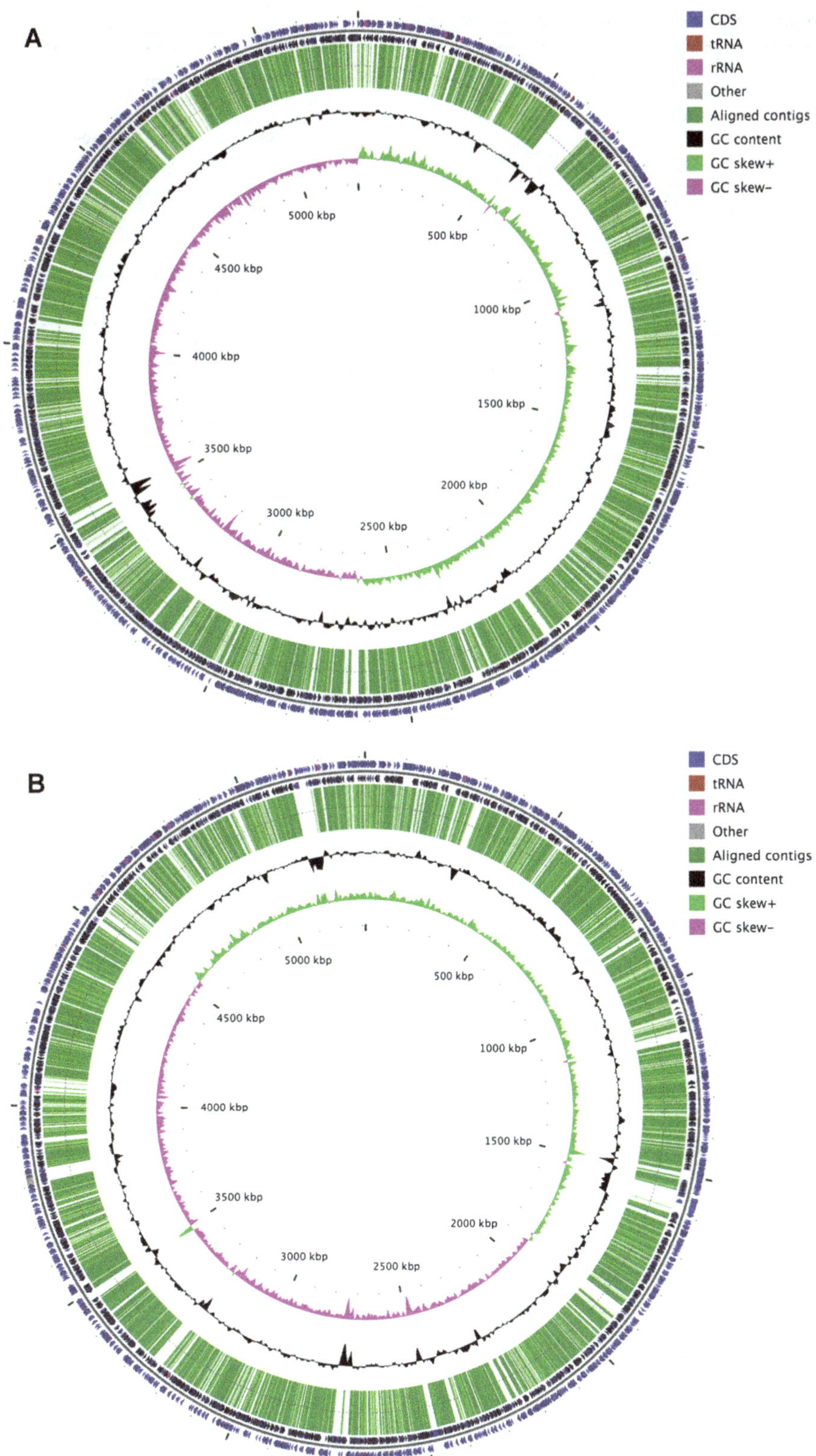

Figure 1. Alignment of the ATCC 43816 sequence to previously sequenced *K. pneumoniae* chromosomes. Next generation sequencing of ATCC 43816 produced 1763 contigs which were aligned to published NTUH-K2044 (Panel A) and MGH 78578 (Panel B) chromosomes. The locations of the contigs are shown as long green lines. The two outer tracks depict the annotated genes in the reference genomes (on both strands) while the two inner tracks show GC content and GC skew, respectively which strongly effects sequencing as can be seen from the coincidence of low GC content regions and gap in the contig alignments.

Table 2. Genetic elements common/unique to sequenced strains.

Genetic loci common to NTUH-K2044	Genes mapped (KP1_)
Yersiniabactin biosynthesis	3583–3586, 3588–3593, 3605–3609, 3611–3613
Type IV Secretion	3634, 3638–3641, 3643
Iron transport	1980–1989
CRISPR locus	3164–3166, 3171
Acetonin catabolism	1112–1121
Conserved and hypothetical genes	2362–2364, 2378–2385, 3239–3240, 3773
Genetic loci common to MGH 78578	**Genes mapped (KPN_)**
Metabolic	00033–00034, 00594–00598, 03359–03370, 03372, 04612–04613
Conserved and hypothetical genes	01146–01148, 01151–01164, 01432–01433, 01316–01317, 04518
ATCC 43816 genetic loci absent from NTUH-K2044 and MGH 78578	**Genes**
Escherichia coli UMN026-like bacteriophage	ECUMN_0964–0965, 0975, 0977–0986, 0994–0996
Klebsiella pneumoniae subsp. *rhinoscleromatis* ATCC 13884-like bacteriophage	HMPREF0484_4775, 4777–4779, 1182
Enterobacter radicincitans DSM 16656 acriflavine resistance	Y71_5381–5385
Klebsiella oxytoca 10-5243 fimbrial biosynthesis	HMPREF9687_02419–02420
Hypothetical protein *Salmonella enterica* subsp. *enterica* serovar Saintpaul str. SARA29	SeSPB_A4698
Hypothetical protein *Enterobacter hormaechei* ATCC 49162	HMPREF9086_3347
Hypothetical protein *Klebsiella* sp. 4_1_44FAA	HMPREF1024_04074
Hypothetical protein *Escherichia hermannii* NBRC 105704	EH105704_01_06400

both cell lines ($P<0.001$), suggesting that there may be differences in the antiphagocytic properties of K1 and K2 capsular polysaccharides or other surface exposed factors.

We therefore also investigated whether capsule alone mediates the antiphagocytic phenotype by comparing ATCC 43816 and NTUH-K2044 capsule mutants to relatively highly phagocytosed MGH 78578. Both ATCC Δ*manC* and NTUH Δ*wzc* capsule mutants were phagocytosed at significantly higher rates than their isogenic wild type parent strains in both cell lines (Figure 4), and furthermore, the NTUH Δ*wzc* was significantly less phagocytosed than the MGH 78578 strain. These data demonstrate that the NTUH Δ*wzc* capsule mutant retains antiphagocytic properties which are distinct from capsular polysaccharide, suggesting that additional factors additionally mediate the antiphagocytic phenotype of *K. pneumoniae*. The ATCC Δ*manC* was phagocytosed at levels similar to the MGH 78578 K52 strain, and it is therefore not possible to conclude whether ATCC 43816 possesses non-capsule antiphagocytic determinants using the K52 MGH 78578 strain which may itself be antiphagocytic. Due to the intrinsic antibiotic resistance of the MGH 78578 strain to common antibiotic markers used for molecular biology, we were unable to generate an acapsular MGH 78578 strain for these studies.

We decided to investigate whether *K. pneumoniae* is replication-competent within cultured macrophages after internalization. Both RAW264.7 and J774A.1 murine macrophages were infected at an MOI of 10 with subsequent evaluation of bacterial colonization at time points 3, 4.5, 6, 9 and 12 hr post infection. As observed previously, MGH 78578 was internalized at the highest levels in both cell lines, while NTUH-K2044 had the lowest level of internalization at the 3 hr time point (Figure 5). Proliferation of *K. pneumoniae* was observed for all bacterial strains, however during 9 hr of observation between the 3 and 12 hr time points the average fold increase in bacterial number was just 3.0–4.6 fold in J774A.1 cells. Higher rates of proliferation were observed for ATCC 43816 and MGH 78578 in RAW264.7 cells, however NTUH-K2044 saw only a 2.9 fold increase in bacterial numbers from 3 hr to 12 hr. These data indicate that the K1 (NTUH-K2044) and K2 (ATCC 43816) strains of *K. pneumoniae* are internalized at relatively low rates but are replication competent in cultured macrophages. However, the K52 strain, MGH 78578, was phagocytosed at relatively high levels in both cell lines, and proliferated significantly in RAW264.7 cells. Importantly, intracellular ATCC 43816 and MGH 78578 exhibited significant outgrowth in cultured macrophages between the 3 and 12 hr time

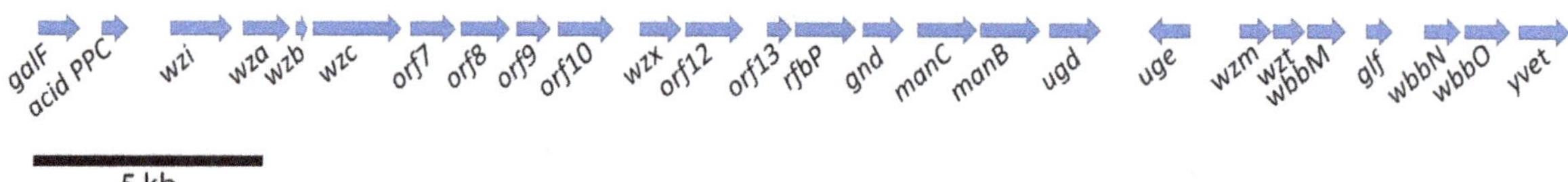

Figure 2. Genetic organization of the ATCC 43816 K2 capsule locus. Scale representation of the capsular polysaccharide biosynthetic locus (*galF-uge*) and LPS locus (*wzm-yvet*). The central domain of the capsule locus (*orf7-orf13*) represents the antigenic diversity region unique to K2 serotype capsules, while the remainder of the locus is well conserved with other *K. pneumoniae* capsule loci.

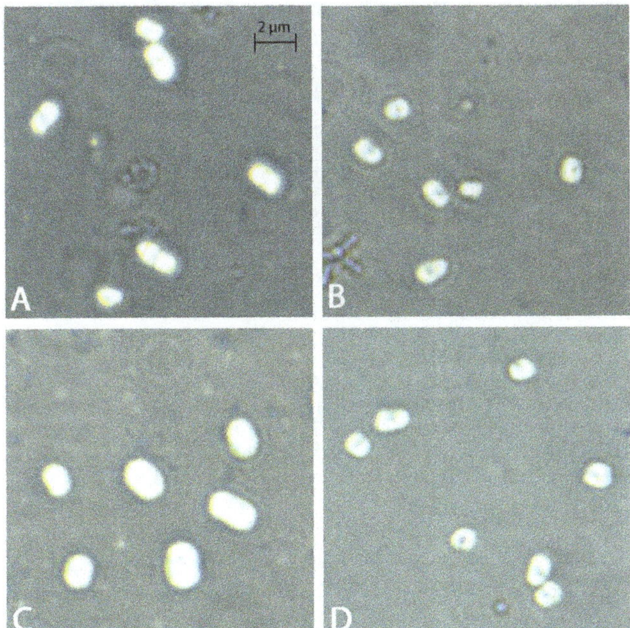

Figure 3. Negative staining of capsular polysaccharide from ATCC 43816 and NTUH-K2044 strains. Overnight bacterial suspensions of ATCC 43816 (A), ATCC Δ*manC* (B), NTUH-K2044 (C) and NTUH Δ*wzc* (D) were mixed in 1:1 ratio with 10% nigrosin. The loss of the capsular polysaccharide from the mutant strains were illustrated by the decrease exclusion of the nigrosin dye which was visualized with Zeiss Axio microscope (63x magnification). Imaris analysis identified that the cross-sectional areas of ATCC Δ*manC*, and NTUH Δ*wzc* mutants were reduced by 36.21%, and 28.59%, relative to their isogenic parents.

points (both J774A. 1 and RAW264.7, P<0.001), indicating that *K. pneumoniae* possesses replicative viability within macrophages, in spite of its classification as an extracellular pathogen. These data suggest that differences between *K. pneumoniae* serotype, and potentially other genetic determinants, could impact the preferred host niche during disease, including the propensity to persist within macrophages.

Respiratory murine model of *K. pneumoniae* infection

We decided to investigate the virulence potential of the three sequenced *K. pneumoniae* strains in a murine respiratory disease model. Because *K. pneumoniae* is known to colonize the upper respiratory tract (URT) in mammals, we developed a novel infection model to deliver *K. pneumoniae* non-surgically into the lung of mice using intubation-mediated intratracheal (IMIT) instillation, specifically modeling lower respiratory tract (LRT) disease. Female BALB/c mice were challenged with one of the three *K. pneumoniae* study strains using the IMIT infection method using multiple challenge doses to estimate the 50% lethal dose (LD_{50}). Both ATCC 43816 and NTUH-K2044 were found to be highly virulent strains of *K. pneumoniae* (LD_{50}<100) while the MGH 78578 strain is significantly less virulent, with an LD_{50}> $10^{5.4}$ fold higher than the virulent strains (Table 3). *K. pneumoniae* respiratory disease in the IMIT mouse model is associated with an acute course of disease with minimally lethal doses resulting in moribund disease within 3–4 days (Figure 6).

Groups of mice infected with minimally lethal doses of ATCC 43816 and NTUH-K2044 ($10^{2.2}$ CFU) were necropsied to investigate bacterial burdens in host tissues. Bacteria were enumerated by plate count from blood, and homogenates of lung, liver, and spleen. Moribund mice were found to have the highest levels of host colonization in both blood and lung, followed by liver and spleen (Figure 7). One-way ANOVA with Tukey Post Test revealed no significant difference between ATCC 43816 and NTUH-K2044 bacterial burdens in any of the host samples examined. These data reveal that both ATCC 43816 and NTUH-K2044 *K. pneumoniae* pneumonia is associated with development of a significant bacteremia and systemic spread to multiple organs.

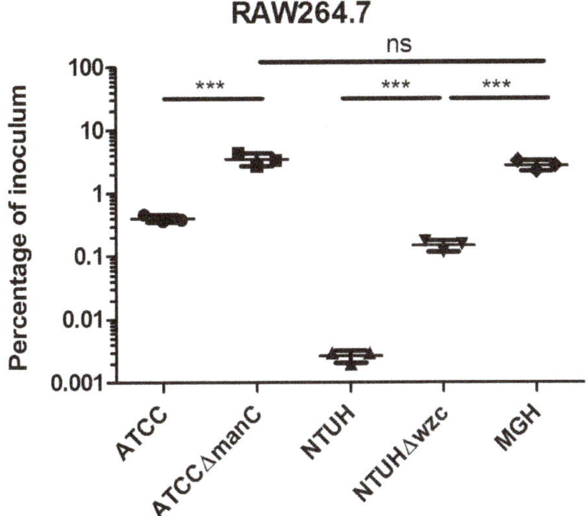

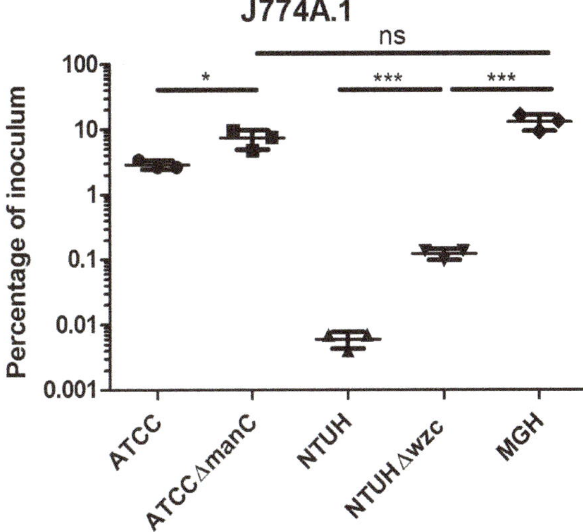

Figure 4. Uptake of *K. pneumoniae* wild type and capsular polysaccharide mutants strains into cultured murine macrophages. *K. pneumoniae* strains ATCC 43816 (K2), NTUH-K2044 (K1) and MGH 78578 (K52) or capsule mutants ATCC Δ*manC*, and NTUH Δ*wzc* were incubated in the presence of cultured murine macrophage cell lines J774A.1 or RAW264.7 at an MOI of 10 in 96 well plates. At one hour post-infection, gentamicin was introduced to eradicate extracellular bacteria, and uptake of *K. pneumoniae* strains into macrophages was assessed at 3 hr post-infection by plate counting. Triplicate samples were enumerated and data analyzed as a percentage of the inoculum, with the results representative of at least two independent trials.

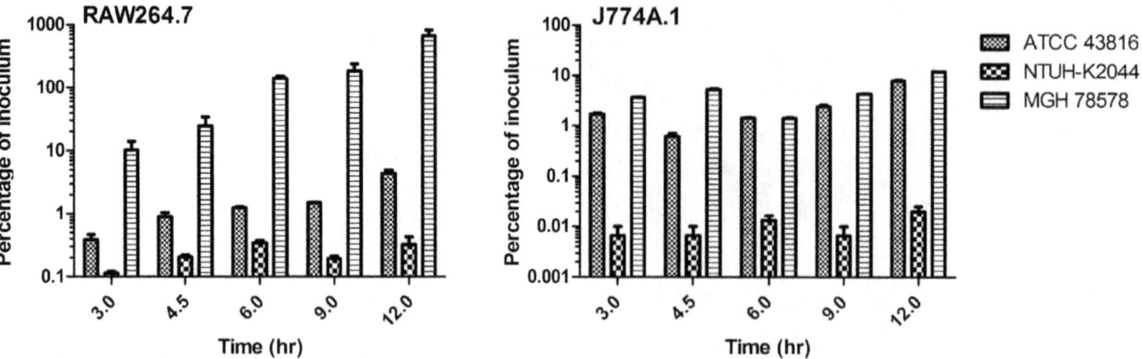

Figure 5. Growth potential of *K. pneumoniae* strains in cultured murine macrophages. *K. pneumoniae* strains ATCC 43816 (K2), NTUH-K2044 (K1) and MGH 78578 (K52) were incubated in the presence of cultured murine macrophage cell lines J774A.1 or RAW264.7 at an MOI of 10 in 96 well plates. At one hour post-infection, gentamicin was introduced to eradicate extracellular bacteria. At 3, 4.5, 6, 9, and 12 hr post-infection, a triplicate set of samples was processed for enumeration of intracellular bacteria. The data is representative of at least three independent trials.

Discussion

K. pneumoniae respiratory infections may result from several mechanisms of pathogen introduction into susceptible hosts including inhalation of environmental sources of bacteria, as it relates to community acquired pneumonia (CAP), or nosocomial foreign body introduction of *K. pneumoniae* into the respiratory system, as in ventilator associated pneumonia (VAP). Thus, respiratory infections with *K. pneumoniae* are clinically important both to nosocomial pneumonia in hospital settings as well as CAP in developing areas of the world. The primary focus of this work was to gain insight into the molecular mechanisms which contribute to the respiratory disease caused by virulent *K. pneumoniae*. We therefore sequenced one of the commonly researched strains, capable of causing pneumonia in surrogate animal models. The ATCC 43816 strain was successfully sequenced by Next Generation approaches at approximately 80% coverage, based on estimated total sequence data relative to the NTUH-K2044 genome size. The majority of ATCC 43816 sequence (>96%) was well conserved to both the highly virulent NTUH-K2044 and the minimally virulent MGH78578 strains suggesting that *K. pneumoniae* strains may have large core genomes, and that key differences in virulence potential may be related to a small number of pathogenicity islands.

Based on the data from our murine respiratory disease model, we identified NTUH-K2044 and ATCC 43816 as highly virulent *K. pneumoniae* strains, and MGH 78578 as a low virulence strain. These findings are consistent with clinical evidence that K1 and K2 serotypes of *K. pneumoniae* are most commonly associated with severe disease presentations, including CAP, invasive presentations, as well as lethality in a mouse intravenous challenge model [7,43]. To the best of our knowledge, this current study provides the first experimental evidence demonstrating that a representative K52 clinical isolate is relatively avirulent in a murine respiratory disease model. Thus, phenotypic evidence links the newly sequenced ATCC 43816 strain to the fully sequenced NTUH-K2044 rather than MGH 78578 strain. The genetic systems found to be shared between NTUH-K2044 and ATCC 43816, but absent from MGH 78578 included iron acquisition genes (yersiniabactin biosynthesis and iron transport), a Type 4 secretion system (T4SS), a CRISPR locus, and an acetonin catabolism locus. Yersiniabactin biosynthetic operon has been previously demonstrated to be important to the function of ATCC 43816 in a murine intranasal respiratory disease model [16,17], where yersiniabactin is thought to contribute to evasion of the activity of lipocalin2 in the lung – a host factor which neutralizes enterobactin-based iron acquisition [44]. The T4SS present in the virulent ATCC 43816 and NTUH-K2044 strains has been proposed to potentially represent a DNA conjugation system, and is also present in the related *K. variicola* environmental isolate strain 342 [45,46], thus future studies will be required to investigate the virulence potential of this secretion system in *K. pneumoniae*. This study supports previous findings that the capsular serotype and the presence of the yersiniabactin iron acquisition systems contribute significantly to the disease potential of highly virulent *K. pneumoniae* strains, with the additional possibility that T4SS or acetonin catabolism may be important for *K. pneumoniae* disease.

In this study, we investigated whether there were any significant differences in the ability of *K. pneumoniae* strains to persist within cultured macrophages. *K. pneumoniae* is considered to be primarily an extracellular pathogen, although there is evidence that this organism may be internalized in human epithelial cell lines [47,48]. Furthermore, *K. pneumoniae* can be taken up into cultured murine peritoneal macrophages, and are also internalized *in vivo* in alveolar macrophages [49]. However, capsular polysac-

Table 3. Probit analysis of IMIT-infections of BALB/c mouse using *K. pneumoniae* strains.

Strain	LD_{50} (95% CI.*)
ATCC 43816	4.71×10^{1} ($1.36\times10^{1}-1.63\times10^{2}$)
NTUH-K2044	2.33×10^{1} ($5.4\times10^{0}-1.01\times10^{2}$)
MGH 78578	1.37×10^{7} ($9.50\times10^{6}-1.97\times10^{7}$)

*95% confidence interval.

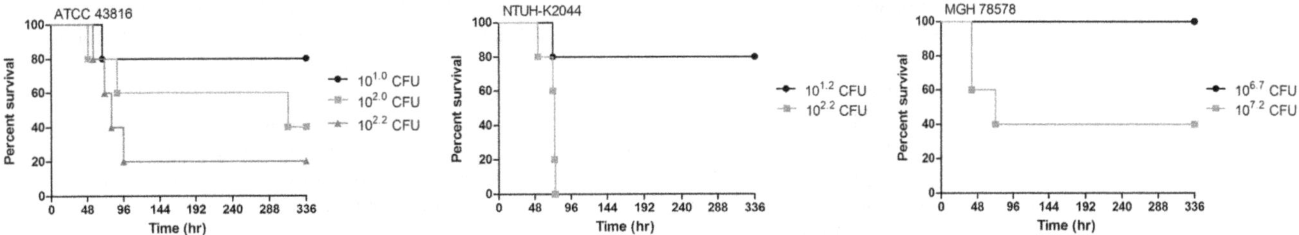

Figure 6. Survival analysis of *K. pneumoniae* respiratory challenge. Groups of five female BALB/c mice were challenged with *K. pneumoniae* strains ATCC 43816 (K2), NTUH-K2044 (K1) or MGH 78578 (K52) by IMIT respiratory infection. Mice were monitored for 14 days, and moribund mice were euthanized. The challenge dose for each survival curve group is indicated.

charide may mediate blocking the initial attachment of bacteria to cells, reducing internalization [50]. Given the importance of capsule in mediating the uptake of *K. pneumoniae* into phagocytic cells, we anticipated that the representative K2 strain in our study, ATCC 43816, may resist uptake into cultured macrophages given the previous discovery that the K2 serotype is associated with an absence of mannose residues in the capsular polysaccharide [51]. Similarly, the *gmd* and *wcaG* genes, present in K1 serotype capsular loci, are required for the modification of mannose to fucose, and a corresponding low level of mannose/high level fucose in *K. pneumoniae* isolates which possess these genes [52]. We had observed that the K1 strain NTUH-K2044 exhibited particularly low uptake into cultured murine macrophages in our studies, and that the K2 strain ATCC 43816 also had a lower level of uptake than the K52 strain MGH78578. Similarly, capsule has been demonstrated to mediate anti-phagocytosis in both amoeba and alveolar macrophages, suggesting that this role for capsule is ubiquitously important across a range of host-pathogen interactions with professional phagocytes [21,53]. Given the potential role of the mannose receptor in facilitating phagocytosis, and the reduced level of mannose residues in K1 and K2 serotype capsules, it is possible that modulation of the polysaccharide surface of *K. pneumoniae* may represent an important strategy for evading host defense.

Consistent with prior studies, we found that acapsular *K. pneumoniae* mutants also exhibited increased uptake into macrophages, however, we also observed that the increase in uptake of the NTUH-K2044 capsule mutant did not achieve the level of uptake of the representative K52 serotype strain. This finding suggests that the NTUH-K2044 strain possesses additional non-capsule antiphagocytic factors, or that the MGH78578 strain actively promotes its uptake into macrophages. Given that *K. pneumoniae* capsule does possess antiphagocytic properties as a strategy to act primarily as an extracellular pathogen, we hypothesize that the K52 MGH 78578 strain does not promote its own uptake, and instead, we hypothesize that the function of

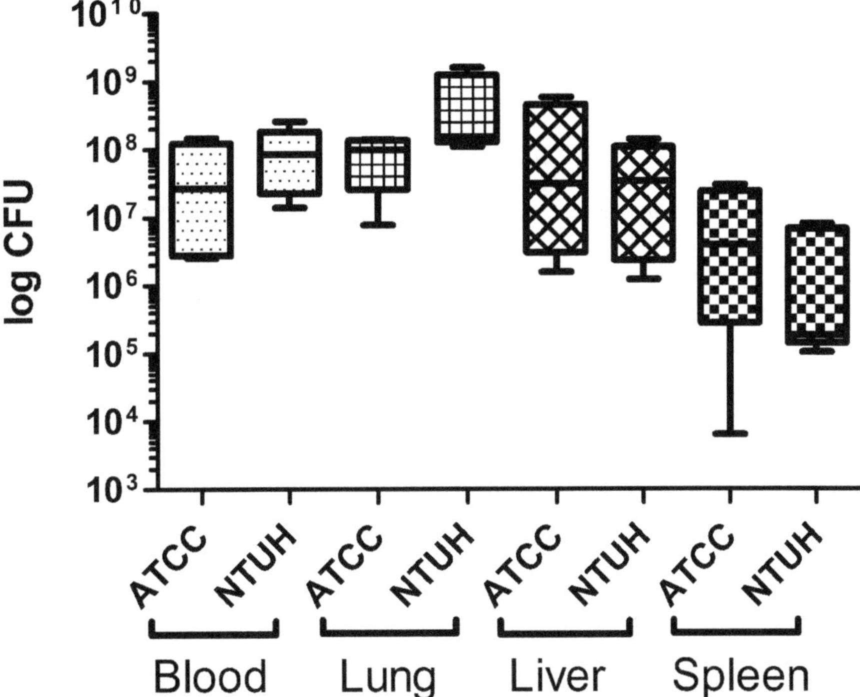

Figure 7. Bacterial burden of *K. pneumoniae*-infected mice. Groups of five female BALB/c mice were infected with *K. pneumoniae* strains ATCC 43816 or NTUH-K2044 and tissues were harvested at the onset of moribund disease, and homogenized in 1 ml of PBS Bacteria were enumerated from blood and from homogenates of lung, liver, and spleen. The results present a min/max box and whisker plot for each infected tissue (n = 5). Statistical analysis was carried out by one way ANOVA and Tukey post test.

K52 capsules would be as an antiphagocytic determinant consistent with other serotype capsules. Thus, we interpret that the NTUH-K2044 strain possesses multiple mechanisms to resist phagocytosis, which is consistent with previous findings that capsule, LPS, carnitine metabolism, and the ClpX protease are all required to resist entry into amoeba and human neutrophils [53]. We conclude that *K. pneumoniae* antiphagocytosis is mediated by a multifactorial process and that capsule alone is insufficient to account for this phenotype. This conclusion is consistent with prior published findings that additional genetic loci participate in mediating *K. pneumoniae* antiphagocytosis, including genes for LPS, the ClpX protease, and carnitine metabolism [53].

In our respiratory challenge studies, the K1 and K2 serotype strains possessed a significantly higher virulence in mice than the K52 serotype strain, supporting the possibility that evasion of phagocytosis is a strategy employed by *K. pneumoniae* to enhance virulence in mammalian hosts. Thus, these finding support the characterization of *K. pneumoniae* as an extracellular pathogen, whereby the most virulent strains are also the most antiphagocytic. These results are consistent with previous reports which have demonstrated that antiphagocytic properties of *K. pneumoniae* capsule are associated with highly virulent K1 and K2 serotypes in panels of Asian strain isolates [54,55]. It is however noteworthy that several additional virulence-associated genetic determinants are common to the K1 and K2 representative strains investigated in this study, including mechanisms of iron acquisition, highlighting that *K. pneumoniae* serotype is not the sole distinguishing factor for predicting disease potential in mammalian hosts.

Our data supports a link between evasion of phagocytosis and virulence potential as an interpretation that *K. pneumoniae* is primarily an extracellular pathogen. However, we interestingly demonstrate that *K. pneumoniae* strains are fit to replicate within macrophages once internalized. This is an intriguing finding that may suggest that a subpopulation of *K. pneumoniae* may use an intracellular lifestyle as part of the disease process. Future studies will be required to characterize to what extent *K. pneumoniae* has adapted to intracellular host-pathogen interaction, and what role the intracellular lifestyle might play *in vivo*.

We developed a novel respiratory disease model to study *K. pneumoniae* pneumonia which facilitated an investigation of the lower respiratory tract (LRT) colonization in the absence of the involvement of other primary sites of infection. Our motivation to develop this model system was in part shaped by our observations that bacterial pathogens may opportunistically infect the upper respiratory tract (URT) in a process which is unique from that observed during human disease [56]. Direct non-surgical instillation directly into the LRT also directly mimics a normal route of nosocomial acquisition of *K. pneumoniae* associated with VAP. Our novel intubation-mediated intratracheal (IMIT) delivery of bacteria facilitates: i) the use of a flow meter to validate the placement of a catheter into the trachea, ii) the ability to instill bacteria directly into the lung via a blunt needle inserted through the catheter lumen, iii) delivery of bacteria into the lower lobes of the lung under positive pressure, and iv) minimal trauma to the host owing to the non-surgical nature of the procedure.

We found that our novel IMIT infection model lowered previously reported LD_{50} values for both i.n. and surgical i.t. infection models, suggesting that targeted delivery of a reduced number of bacteria to the lungs enhances the disease potential of *K. pneumoniae*. The LD_{50} for the ATCC 43816 strain in the IMIT model is $10^{1.8}$–$10^{2.8}$ fold less than previously published LD_{50} values using intranasal models [16,57,58], suggesting that the IMIT model provides a lower LD_{50} due to the ability of the intubation tubing to briefly occlude the air space, allowing for positive pressure delivery of organisms deep into the lung, rather than passive delivery into the lung in shallowly breathing anesthetized animals. Thus, our IMIT model improves the disease potential of *K. pneumoniae* in lung-specific disease, and may be an excellent instillation method for therapeutic and diagnostic reagents in studies requiring LRT delivery.

In summary, our study has provided a first draft sequence of the ATCC 43816 genome which will support future investigations of *K. pneumoniae* function. We also have provided the first description of the growth potential of *K. pneumoniae* in cultured murine macrophages, supporting a growing body of evidence that *K. pneumoniae* may not be exclusively an extracellular pathogen. Finally, we have developed and employed a novel non-surgical, lung-specific infection model which allows for targeted low dose inoculation of *K. pneumoniae* giving rise to a lethal pneumonia in mice, and revealing a significant difference in the disease potential of clinical isolates.

Acknowledgments

We would like to thank Dr. Matthew Lawrenz for critical review of this manuscript.

Author Contributions

Conceived and designed the experiments: JMW. Performed the experiments: JBS RAF HT PY TLP JMW. Analyzed the data: JBS RAF HT PY RB JMW. Contributed reagents/materials/analysis tools: PY RB JMW. Wrote the paper: RB JMW.

References

1. Bagley ST (1985) Habitat association of *Klebsiella* species. Infect Control 6: 52–58.
2. Kesteman AS, Perrin-Guyomard A, Laurentie M, Sanders P, Toutain PL, et al. (2010) Emergence of resistant *Klebsiella pneumoniae* in the intestinal tract during successful treatment of *Klebsiella pneumoniae* lung infection in rats. Antimicrobial agents and chemotherapy 54: 2960–2964.
3. Highsmith AK, Jarvis WR (1985) *Klebsiella pneumoniae*: selected virulence factors that contribute to pathogenicity. Infect Control 6: 75–77.
4. Chung DR, Song JH, Kim SH, Thamlikitkul V, Huang SG, et al. (2011) High prevalence of multidrug-resistant nonfermenters in hospital-acquired pneumonia in Asia. American journal of respiratory and critical care medicine 184: 1409–1417.
5. Paganin F, Lilienthal F, Bourdin A, Lugagne N, Tixier F, et al. (2004) Severe community-acquired pneumonia: assessment of microbial aetiology as mortality factor. The European respiratory journal: official journal of the European Society for Clinical Respiratory Physiology 24: 779–785.
6. Podschun R, Ullmann U (1998) *Klebsiella* spp. as nosocomial pathogens: epidemiology, taxonomy, typing methods, and pathogenicity factors. Clinical microbiology reviews 11: 589–603.
7. Yu VL, Hansen DS, Ko WC, Sagnimeni A, Klugman KP, et al. (2007) Virulence characteristics of *Klebsiella* and clinical manifestations of *K. pneumoniae* bloodstream infections. Emerging infectious diseases 13: 986–993.
8. Marrie TJ, Durant H, Yates L (1989) Community-acquired pneumonia requiring hospitalization: 5-year prospective study. Reviews of infectious diseases 11: 586–599.
9. Fang GD, Fine M, Orloff J, Arisumi D, Yu VL, et al. (1990) New and emerging etiologies for community-acquired pneumonia with implications for therapy. A prospective multicenter study of 359 cases. Medicine 69: 307–316.
10. Marston BJ, Plouffe JF, File TM Jr, Hackman BA, Salstrom SJ, et al. (1997) Incidence of community-acquired pneumonia requiring hospitalization. Results of a population-based active surveillance Study in Ohio. The Community-Based Pneumonia Incidence Study Group. Archives of internal medicine 157: 1709–1718.
11. Hidron AI, Edwards JR, Patel J, Horan TC, Sievert DM, et al. (2008) NHSN annual update: antimicrobial-resistant pathogens associated with healthcare-associated infections: annual summary of data reported to the National Healthcare Safety Network at the Centers for Disease Control and Prevention, 2006–2007. Infection control and hospital epidemiology: the official journal of the Society of Hospital Epidemiologists of America 29: 996–1011.

12. CDC (2009) Guidance for control of infections with carbapenem-resistant or carbapenemase-producing *Enterobacteriaceae* in acute care facilities. MMWR Morbidity and mortality weekly report 58: 256–260.
13. Meyer KS, Urban C, Eagan JA, Berger BJ, Rahal JJ (1993) Nosocomial outbreak of *Klebsiella* infection resistant to late-generation cephalosporins. Annals of internal medicine 119: 353–358.
14. Doyle T, Sanderson R (2008) Survey of hospital microbiology laboratories regarding *Klebsiella pneumoniae* carbapenemase (KPC)-producing organisms. Epi Update: Florida Department of Health: 9–12.
15. Marquez P, Terashita D (2010) Carbapenem-resistant Klebsiella pneumoniae (CRKP) surveillance Los Angeles County, June-December 2010. Special Studies Report: LA County Public Health: 25–26.
16. Lawlor MS, Hsu J, Rick PD, Miller VL (2005) Identification of *Klebsiella pneumoniae* virulence determinants using an intranasal infection model. Mol Microbiol 58: 1054–1073.
17. Lawlor MS, O'Connor C, Miller VL (2007) Yersiniabactin is a virulence factor for *Klebsiella pneumoniae* during pulmonary infection. Infect Immun 75: 1463–1472.
18. Lavender HF, Jagnow JR, Clegg S (2004) Biofilm formation *in vitro* and virulence *in vivo* of mutants of *Klebsiella pneumoniae*. Infection and immunity 72: 4888–4890.
19. Padilla E, Llobet E, Domenech-Sanchez A, Martinez-Martinez L, Bengoechea JA, et al. (2010) *Klebsiella pneumoniae* AcrAB efflux pump contributes to antimicrobial resistance and virulence. Antimicrobial agents and chemotherapy 54: 177–183.
20. March C, Moranta D, Regueiro V, Llobet E, Tomas A, et al. (2011) *Klebsiella pneumoniae* outer membrane protein A is required to prevent the activation of airway epithelial cells. The Journal of biological chemistry 286: 9956–9967.
21. March C, Cano V, Moranta D, Llobet E, Perez-Gutierrez C, et al. (2013) Role of bacterial surface structures on the interaction of *Klebsiella pneumoniae* with phagocytes. PLoS ONE 8: e56847.
22. Insua JL, Llobet E, Moranta D, Perez-Gutierrez C, Tomas A, et al. (2013) Modeling *Klebsiella pneumoniae* pathogenesis by infection of the wax moth *Galleria mellonella*. Infection and immunity 81: 3552–3565.
23. Izquierdo L, Coderch N, Pique N, Bedini E, Corsaro MM, et al. (2003) The *Klebsiella pneumoniae wabG* gene: role in biosynthesis of the core lipopolysaccharide and virulence. Journal of bacteriology 185: 7213–7221.
24. Wu KM, Li LH, Yan JJ, Tsao N, Liao TL, et al. (2009) Genome sequencing and comparative analysis of *Klebsiella pneumoniae* NTUH-K2044, a strain causing liver abscess and meningitis. J Bacteriol 191: 4492–4501.
25. Liu P, Li P, Jiang X, Bi D, Xie Y, et al. (2012) Complete genome sequence of *Klebsiella pneumoniae* subsp. *pneumoniae* HS11286, a multidrug-resistant strain isolated from human sputum. Journal of bacteriology 194: 1841–1842.
26. Shin SH, Kim S, Kim JY, Lee S, Um Y, et al. (2012) Complete genome sequence of the 2,3-butanediol-producing *Klebsiella pneumoniae* strain KCTC 2242. Journal of bacteriology 194: 2736–2737.
27. Chou HC, Lee CZ, Ma LC, Fang CT, Chang SC, et al. (2004) Isolation of a chromosomal region of *Klebsiella pneumoniae* associated with allantoin metabolism and liver infection. Infect Immun 72: 3783–3792.
28. Cano V, Moranta D, Llobet-Brossa E, Bengoechea JA, Garmendia J (2009) *Klebsiella pneumoniae* triggers a cytotoxic effect on airway epithelial cells. BMC Microbiol 9: 156.
29. Brett PJ, Deshazer D, Woods DE (1997) Characterization of *Burkholderia pseudomallei* and *Burkholderia pseudomallei*-like strains. Epidemiol Infect 118: 137–148.
30. Zerbino DR, Birney E (2008) Velvet: algorithms for de novo short read assembly using de Bruijn graphs. Genome research 18: 821–829.
31. Altschul SF, Madden TL, Schaffer AA, Zhang J, Zhang Z, et al. (1997) Gapped BLAST and PSI-BLAST: a new generation of protein database search programs. Nucleic acids research 25: 3389–3402.
32. Scott JB (2013) Genetic characterization of the K2 serotype capsule of Klebsiella pneumoniae ATCC 43816 and the development of a bioluminescent strain. Louisville: University of Louisville.
33. Campos MA, Vargas MA, Regueiro V, Llompart CM, Alberti S, et al. (2004) Capsule polysaccharide mediates bacterial resistance to antimicrobial peptides. Infect Immun 72: 7107–7114.
34. Bitter T, Muir HM (1962) A modified uronic acid carbazole reaction. Analytical biochemistry 4: 330–334.
35. Donnenberg MS, Kaper JB (1991) Construction of an eae deletion mutant of enteropathogenic Escherichia coli by using a positive-selection suicide vector. Infect Immun 59: 4310–4317.
36. Simon R, Priefer U, Pühler A (1983) A broad range mobilization system for in vivo genetic engineering: transposon mutagenesis in gram-negative bacteria. Bio/Technology 1: 784–791.
37. Struve C, Krogfelt KA (2003) Role of capsule in *Klebsiella pneumoniae* virulence: lack of correlation between *in vitro* and *in vivo* studies. FEMS microbiology letters 218: 149–154.
38. Lawrenz MB, Fodah RA, Gutierrez M, Warawa J (2014) Intubation-mediated intratracheal (IMIT) instillation: A non-invasive, lung-specific delivery system JoVE in press.
39. Hsieh PF, Lin TL, Yang FL, Wu MC, Pan YJ, et al. (2012) Lipopolysaccharide O1 antigen contributes to the virulence in *Klebsiella pneumoniae* causing pyogenic liver abscess. PLoS ONE 7: e33155.
40. Liao CH, Huang YT, Lai CC, Chang CY, Chu FY, et al. (2011) *Klebsiella pneumoniae* bacteremia and capsular serotypes, Taiwan. Emerging infectious diseases 17: 1113–1115.
41. Pan YJ, Fang HC, Yang HC, Lin TL, Hsieh PF, et al. (2008) Capsular polysaccharide synthesis regions in *Klebsiella pneumoniae* serotype K57 and a new capsular serotype. J Clin Microbiol 46: 2231–2240.
42. Srinivasan VB, Vaidyanathan V, Mondal A, Rajamohan G (2012) Role of the two component signal transduction system CpxAR in conferring cefepime and chloramphenicol resistance in *Klebsiella pneumoniae* NTUH-K2044. PLoS ONE 7: e33777.
43. Keynan Y, Rubinstein E (2007) The changing face of *Klebsiella pneumoniae* infections in the community. Int J Antimicrob Agents 30: 385–389.
44. Bachman MA, Oyler JE, Burns SH, Caza M, Lepine F, et al. (2011) *Klebsiella pneumoniae* yersiniabactin promotes respiratory tract infection through evasion of lipocalin 2. Infection and immunity 79: 3309–3316.
45. Brisse S, Fevre C, Passet V, Issenhuth-Jeanjean S, Tournebize R, et al. (2009) Virulent clones of *Klebsiella pneumoniae*: identification and evolutionary scenario based on genomic and phenotypic characterization. PLoS One 4: e4982.
46. Fouts DE, Tyler HL, DeBoy RT, Daugherty S, Ren Q, et al. (2008) Complete genome sequence of the N2-fixing broad host range endophyte *Klebsiella pneumoniae* 342 and virulence predictions verified in mice. PLoS Genet 4: e1000141.
47. Fumagalli O, Tall BD, Schipper C, Oelschlaeger TA (1997) N-glycosylated proteins are involved in efficient internalization of *Klebsiella pneumoniae* by cultured human epithelial cells. Infection and immunity 65: 4445–4451.
48. Oelschlaeger TA, Tall BD (1997) Invasion of cultured human epithelial cells by *Klebsiella pneumoniae* isolated from the urinary tract. Infection and immunity 65: 2950–2958.
49. Lau HY, Clegg S, Moore TA (2007) Identification of *Klebsiella pneumoniae* genes uniquely expressed in a strain virulent using a murine model of bacterial pneumonia. Microb Pathog 42: 148–155.
50. Sahly H, Podschun R, Oelschlaeger TA, Greiwe M, Parolis H, et al. (2000) Capsule impedes adhesion to and invasion of epithelial cells by *Klebsiella pneumoniae*. Infection and immunity 68: 6744–6749.
51. Kabha K, Nissimov L, Athamna A, Keisari Y, Parolis H, et al. (1995) Relationships among capsular structure, phagocytosis, and mouse virulence in *Klebsiella pneumoniae*. Infection and immunity 63: 847–852.
52. Pan PC, Chen HW, Wu PK, Wu YY, Lin CH, et al. (2011) Mutation in fucose synthesis gene of *Klebsiella pneumoniae* affects capsule composition and virulence in mice. Experimental biology and medicine 236: 219–226.
53. Pan YJ, Lin TL, Hsu CR, Wang JT (2011) Use of a *Dictyostelium* model for isolation of genetic loci associated with phagocytosis and virulence in *Klebsiella pneumoniae*. Infection and immunity 79: 997–1006.
54. Yeh KM, Kurup A, Siu LK, Koh YL, Fung CP, et al. (2007) Capsular serotype K1 or K2, rather than *magA* and *rmpA*, is a major virulence determinant for *Klebsiella pneumoniae* liver abscess in Singapore and Taiwan. Journal of clinical microbiology 45: 466–471.
55. Lin JC, Chang FY, Fung CP, Xu JZ, Cheng HP, et al. (2004) High prevalence of phagocytic-resistant capsular serotypes of *Klebsiella pneumoniae* in liver abscess. Microbes and infection/Institut Pasteur 6: 1191–1198.
56. Warawa JM, Long D, Rosenke R, Gardner D, Gherardini FC (2011) Bioluminescent diagnostic imaging to characterize altered respiratory tract colonization by the *Burkholderia pseudomallei* capsule mutant. Frontiers in microbiology 2: 133.
57. Yadav V, Sharma S, Harjai K, Mohan H, Chhibber S (2003) Induction & resolution of lobar pneumonia following intranasal instillation with *Klebsiella pneumoniae* in mice. The Indian journal of medical research 118: 47–52.
58. Ye P, Rodriguez FH, Kanaly S, Stocking KL, Schurr J, et al. (2001) Requirement of interleukin 17 receptor signaling for lung CXC chemokine and granulocyte colony-stimulating factor expression, neutrophil recruitment, and host defense. The Journal of experimental medicine 194: 519–527.

8

GBA2-Encoded β-Glucosidase Activity is Involved in the Inflammatory Response to *Pseudomonas aeruginosa*

Nicoletta Loberto[2]⁹, Maela Tebon[1]⁹, Ilaria Lampronti[3], Nicola Marchetti[4], Massimo Aureli[2], Rosaria Bassi[2], Maria Grazia Giri[5], Valentino Bezzerri[1], Valentina Lovato[1], Cinzia Cantù[1], Silvia Munari[1], Seng H. Cheng[6], Alberto Cavazzini[4], Roberto Gambari[3], Sandro Sonnino[2], Giulio Cabrini[1], Maria Cristina Dechecchi[1]*

1 Laboratory of Molecular Pathology, Department of Pathology and Diagnostics, University Hospital of Verona, Verona, Italy, **2** Department of Medical Biotechnology and Translational Medicine, University of Milano, Milano, Italy, **3** Department of Life Sciences and Biotechnology, Section of Biochemistry and Molecular Biology, University of Ferrara, Ferrara, Italy, **4** Department of Chemistry and Pharmaceutical Sciences, University of Ferrara, Ferrara, Italy, **5** Medical Physics Unit, Department of Pathology and Diagnostics, University Hospital of Verona, Verona, Italy, **6** Genzyme, a Sanofi Company, Framingham, Massachusetts, United States of America

Abstract

Current anti-inflammatory strategies for the treatment of pulmonary disease in cystic fibrosis (CF) are limited; thus, there is continued interest in identifying additional molecular targets for therapeutic intervention. Given the emerging role of sphingolipids (SLs) in various respiratory disorders, including CF, drugs that selectively target the enzymes associated with SL metabolism are under development. Miglustat, a well-characterized iminosugar-based inhibitor of β-glucosidase 2 (GBA2), has shown promise in CF treatment because it reduces the inflammatory response to infection by *P. aeruginosa* and restores F508del-CFTR chloride channel activity. This study aimed to probe the molecular basis for the anti-inflammatory activity of miglustat by examining specifically the role of GBA2 following the infection of CF bronchial epithelial cells by *P. aeruginosa*. We also report the anti-inflammatory activity of another potent inhibitor of GBA2 activity, namely *N*-(5-adamantane-1-yl-methoxy)pentyl)-deoxynojirimycin (Genz-529648). In CF bronchial cells, inhibition of GBA2 by miglustat or Genz-529648 significantly reduced the induction of IL-8 mRNA levels and protein release following infection by *P. aeruginosa*. Hence, the present data demonstrate that the anti-inflammatory effects of miglustat and Genz-529648 are likely exerted through inhibition of GBA2.

Editor: Dominik Hartl, University of Tübingen, Germany

Funding: This research was supported by Italian Cystic Fibrosis Research Foundation (grant FFC # 14/2012) with the contribution of "Picasso. Capolavori dal Museo Nazionale Picasso di Parigi", Festa d'Estate Villa Sigurtà Verona, Delegazione FFC Lago di Garda e Arezzo. The funders had no role in study design, data collection and analysis, decision to publish, or preparation of the manuscript.

Competing Interests: Seng H. Cheng is an employee and shareholder of Genzyme, a Sanofi Company, when the work was performed. This work is also part of a patent application titled "Amorphous and a crystalline form of Genz 112638 hemitartrate as inhibitor of glucosylceramide synthase" (International Application No: PCT/US20130137743A1).

* Email: cristina.dechecchi@ospedaleuniverona.it

⁹ These authors contributed equally to this work.

Introduction

Cystic fibrosis (CF) lung disease is characterized by progressive chronic infection and inflammation of the airways. The prolonged airway inflammation is an important aspect of the obstructive lung disease noted in CF patients. Resultant progressive remodeling leads to irreversible damage and fibrosis, which is a major cause of mortality in patients [1]. Significant efforts have been invested into developing therapies that address the underlying basis of CF. For example, recent efforts to identify small-molecule drugs that target a mutant CF transmembrane conductance regulator (CFTR) led to the successful development of a potentiator (Kalydeco) for patients who harbor the mutant G551D-CFTR [2]. Moreover, phase 3 clinical trials of Kalydeco in combination with the corrector lumacaftor for people with two copies of the F508del-CFTR mutation showed significant improvements in lung function and other key measures of the disease (http://www.cff.org/about CFFoundation/NewsEvents/2014NEWSArchive/6-24-Vertex Phase-3-Results_Lumacaftor_Ibvacaftor.cfm). However, despite these very encouranging results, adjuvant therapies that abate the decline in pulmonary function in other patients are still needed. Examples include the potential deployment of new antibiotics, anti-mucolytic and anti-inflammatory drugs [3]. To date, the only non-steroidal anti-inflammatory agent that has been shown to be beneficial in CF patients is ibuprofen; however, its use can be associated with severe adverse effects, such as gastrointestinal bleeding [4]. Hence, the identification and development of novel and more potent anti-inflammatory drugs for CF airway disease remains a priority. The chemokine IL-8 is abundantly expressed at sites of chronic inflammation and appears to play a major role in driving the formation of neutrophil (PMN)-rich exudates in the lungs of CF patients [5–8]; thus its reduction is a key therapeutic goal in CF.

Sphingolipids (SLs) are a large group of lipids that are thought to modulate the pathophysiology of several respiratory disorders, including CF [9–11]. Ceramide, the central hub of SL metabolism, is generated by *de novo* synthesis or hydrolysis of complex SLs, such as sphingomyelin (SM) by acid sphingomyelinase (ASM) and glucosylceramide (GlcCer) by glucocerebrosidases [12]. Ceramide plays an important role in the infection by *P. aeruginosa* by reorganizing lipid rafts on cellular membranes into larger signaling platforms, which is a feature conducive to internalizing bacteria, inducing apoptosis and regulating the cytokine response [13]. Controversial findings on the association between abnormalities in SL metabolism and inflammation in CF have been reported. For example, ceramide has been identified as a key regulator of inflammation in CF airways in different CFTR-/- mouse models [14]. In contrast, decreased ceramide levels have been demonstrated in CFTR KO mice [15], and no significant difference has been found in basal ceramide levels in CFTR KO lung homogenates compared to wild type mice [16]. The possible explanation for this discrepancy appears to be the special diet required for the survival of CFTR KO mice, which severely affects the concentration of SLs [14]. Interestingly, an accumulation of ceramide, which has been directly correlated with neutrophilic lung inflammation, has been demonstrated in the lower airway of CF patients [17]. These findings suggest that the CF pathophysiology associated with infection by *P. aeruginosa* can be corrected, in part, by modulating ceramide levels to their normal physiological range, independent of the conflicting results obtained in different CF models. To date, there is some evidence that supports pharmacological interventions in SL metabolism as therapeutic agents for CF lung disease [14–21].

Given the emerging importance of SLs in respiratory disorders, novel drugs that selectively target different enzymes involved in SL metabolism are under development. Recently developed iminosugar-based inhibitors of GBA2 are of particular interest because of their good oral bioavailability and specific immune modulatory and chaperoning activities [22]. A well-characterized inhibitor is miglustat (*N*-butyldeoxynojirimycin, NB-DNJ), which is FDA-approved and EMA-designated for use in Europe and the USA for the treatment of type I Gaucher and other SL storage diseases. We previously demonstrated that miglustat exhibits an anti-inflammatory effect *in vitro* and *in vivo* by reducing *P. aeruginosa* induced immunoreactive ceramide levels [20,23]. Moreover, miglustat can restore F508del-CFTR chloride channel activity in respiratory and pancreatic cells *in vitro* [24,25] and in CF mice [26]. However, a recent clinical trial in CF patients did not provide evidence of efficacy, which may be related to the intra-individual variability of nasal potential difference (NPD) measurements or the short duration of exposure [27]. Nevertheless, a drug that is able to correct both the CF channel defect and reduce the inflammatory response is of interest and warrants further attention. Miglustat inhibits the enzyme ceramide glucosyl-transferase (GlcCerT), which catalyzes the first step in the glycosphingolipid biosynthetic pathway [28] with IC50 values in the low micromolar range. It also inhibits the activities of two different GlcCer degrading enzymes, glucocerebrosidase (GBA1) and the non-lysosomal β-glucosidase 2 (GBA2), with IC50 values in the high micromolar and nanomolar range, respectively [29,30]. In addition, it is also a potent inhibitor of α-glucosidase [31]. Therefore, miglustat could affect the host response to *P. aeruginosa* through one or more of these SL metabolism pathways. The galactose analog of miglustat, *N*-butyldeoxygalactonojirimycin (NB-DGJ), also inhibits GlcCerT and GBA2, whereas its effect on GBA1 is less clear [30,32,33]. Similar to miglustat, NB-DGJ produces an anti-inflammatory effect in bronchial epithelial cells [25], which suggests a potential involvement of GlcCerT and/or GBA2 in the response of bronchial cells to *P. aeruginosa*. The non-lysosomal β-glucosidase GBA2, which is extremely sensitive to deoxynojirimycin-type inhibitors [34], is a membrane-associated enzyme located in the plasma membrane and ER of cells [29,35]. GBA2 has been described as a single pass transmembrane protein with its catalytic domain facing the extracellular environment [29]. Because this enzyme can hydrolyze GlcCer directly at the cell surface, it might be involved in affecting transient local changes in bioactive SL concentrations.

To gain greater insights into the molecular basis of the anti-inflammatory activity of miglustat, we explored the potential involvement of GBA2 in the ceramide-mediated signaling processes following *P. aeruginosa* infection of CF bronchial epithelial cells. The effects of a potent inhibitor of GBA2, *N*-(5-adamantane-1-yl-methoxy)pentyl)- deoxynojirimycin or Genz-529648 as it is referred to in this report [4,36], on the inflammatory response to *P. aeruginosa* were investigated and compared to miglustat and NB-DGJ. We also examined the impact of lowering the expression of GBA2 in human CF bronchial epithelial cells exposed to *P. aeruginosa* using siRNA oligonucleotides. The results obtained here demonstrate that GBA2 is a target of the anti-inflammatory effects of miglustat and Genz-529648. Thus, these compounds provide novel insights into the role of GBA2 in the signaling cascade activated by *P. aeruginosa* in CF bronchial epithelial cells.

Methods

Cell models

IB3-1 (LGC Promochem GmbH, Teddington, Middlesex, United Kingdom)[37] and CuFi-1 (a generous gift of A. Klingelhutz, P. Karp and J. Zabner, University of Iowa, Iowa City)[38] are human bronchial epithelial cells grown as previously described [24]. Primary airway epithelial cells, i.e., mainstem human bronchi, derived from CF individuals were obtained from "Servizio Colture Primarie" of the Italian Cystic Fibrosis Research Foundation and cultured as previously described [39].

Bacterial strains

The reference *P. aeruginosa* strain, PAO1, was kindly provided by A. Prince (Columbia University, New York) and grown in trypticase soy broth (TSB) or agar (TSA) (Difco) as previously described [25]. Some experiments were conducted with organisms killed by heating to 65°C for 30 minutes.

Inhibitors of SL metabolism

Miglustat and NB-DGJ were obtained from Toronto Research Chemicals, North York, ON, Canada. Genz-529648 was obtained from Genzyme, a Sanofi Company; amitriptyline was obtained from Sigma.

Inflammatory response *in vitro*

Cells were treated with different inhibitors or solvent alone and then infected with PAO1 for 4 hours at 37°C as previously described [25]. The inflammatory response to PAO1 infection was studied at the transcriptional level by measuring IL-8 chemokine expression as previously described [20]. An enzyme-linked immunosorbent assay for the quantitative measurement of IL-8 protein release was performed using the Human IL-8 Instant ELISA kit (Bender MedSystems, Vienna, Austria).

Cell toxicity

The effects of Genz-529648 on cell proliferation, viability and apoptosis were studied to evaluate the potential toxicity as detailed in the Supplement S3.

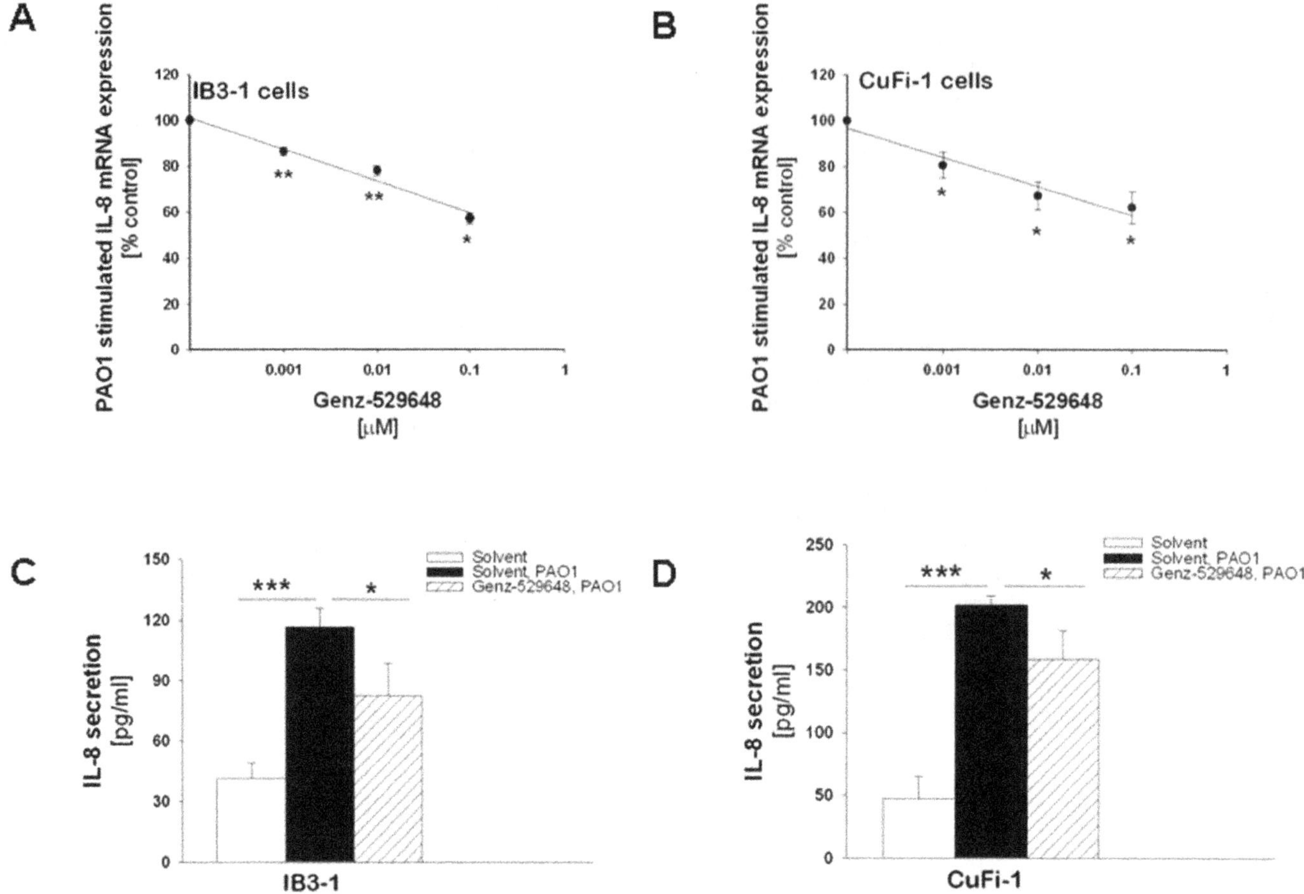

Figure 1. Genz-529648 reduces *P. aeruginosa* stimulated IL-8 mRNA expression and protein release. *Panels A and B. Genz-529648 reduces P. aeruginosa stimulated IL-8 mRNA expression.* IB3-1 (A) and CuFi-1 (B) cells were treated with a range of doses of Genz-529648 (1–100 nM) or solvent alone for 1 hour and then infected with PAO1 for 4 hours at 37°C. The inflammatory response was evaluated by studying the expression of IL-8 mRNA, which was measured by Real-time qPCR and obtained by comparing the ratio IL-8 and the housekeeping gene GAPDH between non-infected and infected cells. The results are expressed as the % of untreated cells and represent the mean ± standard error of the mean of 4 independent experiments in duplicate. Comparisons between groups were made by using Student's *t* tests. *Panels C and D. Genz-529648 reduces the P. aeruginosa induced IL-8 secretion.* IB3-1 (C) and CuFi-1(D) cells were treated with Genz-529648 (100 nM) for 1 hour prior to infection with heat killed PAO1 for 24 hours. Data reported are the mean ± standard error of the mean of 4 independent experiments in duplicate. Comparisons between groups were made by using Student's *t* tests.

GBA2 silencing

To perform silencing experiments of the GBA2 gene, a TriFECTa RNAi Kit (Integrated DNA technologies, Coralville, Iowa, IA) was used. Cells were transiently transfected with specific siRNA for GBA2 (sequence GGAUCAUGUUUGGAGCUA) or scrambled (CGUUAAUCGCGUAUAAUACGCGUAT) duplexes complexed with cationic liposomes Lipofectamine 2000 (Invitrogen, Carlsbad, CA) diluted in 1 ml serum-free cell culture medium. GBA2 siRNA or scrambled duplexes (10 nM) were added and incubated for 10 minutes. Liposome:duplex complexes (500 μL) were added to the cells grown in 2 cm^2 wells and incubated at 37°C for 6 hours. The cells were washed twice with culture medium and maintained at 37°C for an additional 18 or 42 hours.

Analysis of cell ceramide content

The analysis of cell ceramide content was performed via two different approaches: by the LC-MS and LC-MS/MS method [40] and by the metabolic labeling of cell SLs using (^{3}H)sphingosine as a precursor. Both methods are detailed in the Supplement S1 and S2.

Enzymatic activity

IB3-1 or CuFi-1 cells were treated with 2 μM miglustat, 10 nM Genz-529648 or solvent alone for 1 hour and the infected with heat-killed PAO1 for 4 hours. The cells were then scraped and centrifuged; the cellular pellets were resuspended in water containing protease inhibitors and sonicated. After protein determination, the β-glucosidase activities were assayed in the total cell lysates using the fluorigenic substrate 4-methylumbelliferyl-β-D-glucopyranoside (MUB-Glc) as previously described [41]. To discriminate between GBA1 and GBA2 β-glucosidase activity, the enzymatic assays were performed in the presence of 5 nM of Genz-529648 or 500 μM of Conduritol B Epoxide (CBE), respectively.

Statistics

Results are expressed as the mean ± standard error of the mean. Comparisons between groups were made using Student's t

Table 1. Inhibition of *P. aeruginosa* stimulated IL-8 mRNA expression by alkylated iminosugars in IB3-1 and CuFi-1 cells.

IB3-1 cells					CuFi-1 cells			
Inhibitor	*IC_{50}*	*CI*	*Maximal Inhibition*	*CI*	*IC_{50}*	*CI*	*Maximal Inhibition*	*CI*
	(µM)	*(µM)*	*(%)*	*(%)*	*(µM)*	*(µM)*	*(%)*	*(%)*
Miglustat	2.2	1.4–3.4	51.6	51.1–53.3	1.98	1.4–2.7	51.5	51.0–57.3
NB-DGJ	0.27	0.16–0.44	45.0	39.0-52-0	0.39	0.004–3.8	53.0	41.0–55.0
Genz-529648	0.009	0.004–0.018	51.4	46.0–57.0	0.002	0.002–0.003	46.0	38.0–53.0

IB3-1 and CuFi-1 cells were treated with a range of doses of the alkylated iminosugars miglustat or NB-DGJ (0.5–100 µM) or Genz-529648 (1–100 nM) for 1 hour prior to infection with PAO1 (10–50 CFU/cell) for 4 hrs, and IL-8 mRNA expression was measured. IC_{50} values were calculated by fitting with a non-linear regression experimental data obtained in 4 different independent experiments performed in each cell line treated with each inhibitor. IC_{50} values (*i.e.*, inhibitor concentration that results in 50% inhibition) were calculated by fitting experimental data with a non-linear regression according to the following formula: -log(*I*) = *pKi* + log (V−v)/v.
I = inhibitor concentration; v = % inhibition; *pKi* = IC_{50}; V = maximal inhibition; CI = confidence interval 95%.

tests. Statistical significance was defined by $p<0.05$. In order to calculate the IC_{50} values, experimental data were fitted by nonlinear regression using the software "R Core Team, 2013, "R: A language and environment for statistical Computing", R Foundation for Statistical Computing, Vienna, Austria, URL http://www.R-project.org.

Results

Genz-529648 reduces the expression of IL-8 in CF bronchial epithelial cells

Several hydrophobic deoxynojirimycin derivatives have been generated that can be used as research tools to probe the physiological relevance of GBA2. Complete inhibition of GBA2 can be realized in cells treated with low nanomolar concentrations of *N*-(5-adamantane-1-yl-methoxy)pentyl)- deoxynojirimycin (Genz-529648). GlcCerT and oligosaccharide chain-trimming glucosidases, which are sensitive to other hydrophobic deoxynojirimycin derivatives, are unaffected by Genz-529648 [34]. To determine a possible involvement of GBA2 in the inflammatory response to *P. aeruginosa* in bronchial epithelial cells, the effect of Genz-529648 was investigated and compared to miglustat and NB-DGJ. IB3-1 and CuFi-1 cells were treated with increasing amounts (1–100 nM) of the inhibitors for 1 hour prior to infection with *P. aeruginosa* (strain PAO1), and the IL-8 expression was then analyzed 4 hours post-infection. As shown in panels A and B in figure 1, Genz-529648 reduced the PAO1 induced increase in IL-8 mRNA levels by approximately 40% in both cell lines. These experiments were extended by measuring IL-8 chemokine secretion in the supernatants of IB3-1 and CuFi-1 cells. Thus, the cells were treated with Genz-529648 (100 nM) for 1 hour prior to infection with heat killed PAO1, and the supernatants were collected 24 hours later. Heat killed organisms were used to prevent bronchial cell death during the 24 hours of bacterial challenge. Figure 1, panels C and D, shows that Genz-529648 significantly decreased the amount of IL-8 released from the CF bronchial cells infected by PAO1 by approximately 30%, which is consistent with the results obtained at the transcriptional level (figure 1, panels A and B).

The effects of Genz-529648 in bronchial cells were then compared to miglustat and NB-DGJ, which also exhibit anti-inflammatory effects [25]. IB3-1 and CuFi-1 cells were treated with different concentrations of miglustat, NB-DGJ or Genz-529648 and infected with PAO1 as previously described; the IL-8 mRNA levels were then measured. As summarized in table 1, a similar maximal inhibition of approximately 50% was observed in both cell lines treated with miglustat, NB-DGJ or Genz-529648. However, the IC_{50} values of Genz-529648 in IB3-1 and CuFi-1 cells were considerably lower compared to miglustat or NB-DGJ, which indicated that it is a more potent inhibitor of the inflammatory response in CF bronchial cells. Moreover, the IC_{50} values of Genz-529648 at inhibiting IL-8 expression were of the same order of magnitude compared to that reported at inhibiting GBA2 [35], which suggests that the reduction in the inflammatory response to *P. aeruginosa* may have been mediated through its action on GBA2.

Although Genz-529648 is active at nanomolar concentrations, its potential toxicity on bronchial epithelial cells was investigated. To determine the impact on cell proliferation, IB3-1 cells were treated with increasing concentrations of Genz-529648 (from 0.001 to 1 µM), and the cell number/ml was analyzed after 4, 24, 48 and 72 hours. The results, which were derived from three independent experiments, indicate that the IC_{50} values calculated at these time points were always greater than 1 µM, which

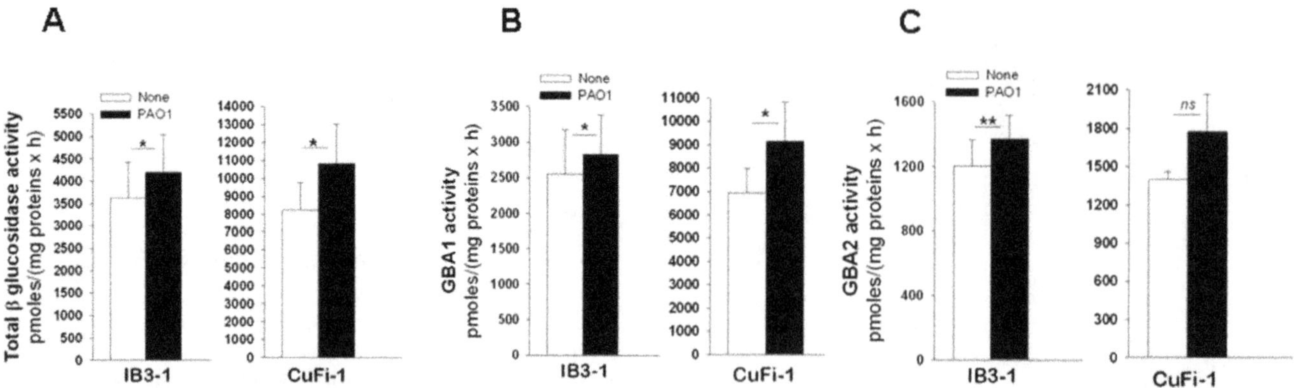

Figure 2. Infection with PAO1 increases β-glucosidase activity in IB3-1 and CuFi-1 cells. IB3-1 and CuFi-1 cells were infected with heat-killed PAO1 for 4 hours. The cells were then scraped and centrifuged; the cellular pellets were resuspended in water containing protease inhibitors and sonicated. Similar amounts of cellular proteins were used to perform the enzymatic assays to detect the activities of total β-glucosidase (A), GBA1 (B) and GBA2 (C), as reported in the Methods section. The data reported are the mean ± standard error of the mean of 4 (IB3-1) or 3 (CuFi-1) independent experiments in triplicate. Comparisons between groups were made by using Student's *t* tests.

supports the concept that this compound is not cytotoxic at nanomolar concentrations and does not display inhibitory activity on CF bronchial cells. Cell viability, which was measured after 4 and 24 hours of treatment (figure S1), was always similar to the untreated cells and between 91.3 and 97.6%. At the same time points, treatment with Genz-529648 did not cause apoptotic effects, even when used at the 1 μM concentration (figures S2 and S3).

Miglustat and Genz-529648 inhibit GBA2 activity in *P. aeruginosa* infected CF bronchial epithelial cells

To ascertain the possible involvement of GBA2 in the signaling processes associated with *P. aeruginosa* infection, total β-glucosidase, GBA1 and GBA2 activities in the lysates of both IB3-1 and CuFi-1 cells infected by heat killed PAO1 were measured. To prevent potential interference because of bacterial glucosidase activities, the infected cells were subjected to washes with PBS that removed most bacteria; moreover, heat killed instead of living organisms were used. In addition, the residual GBA1 and GBA2 activities associated with heat killed bacteria were measured by enzymatic assays on the amounts of heat killed PAO1 from 20 to 30-fold higher compared to those used for the cell infection. The fluorescence associated with the PAO1 samples, which was the result of hydrolysis of the artificial substrate MUB-Glc, was less or the same extent of that identified in the negative controls, which indicates that heat killed PAO1 does not have detectable β-glucosidase activity. As shown in figure 2, a significant increase in total β-glucosidase (figure 2, panel A), GBA1 (figure 2, panel B) and GBA2 (figure 2, panel C) activities were observed in response to infection. The effects of pre-treatment with miglustat or Genz-529648 on β-glucosidase activity were then studied in both IB3-1 and CuFi-1 cells infected with PAO1. Total β-glucosidase was slightly reduced in both cell lines treated with the two inhibitors (figure 3, panel A), whereas GBA1 activity remained unchanged (figure 3, panel B). Importantly, both miglustat and Genz-529648 significantly decreased GBA2 activity in bronchial cells infected with *P. aeruginosa* (figure 3, panel C). These results demonstrate that miglustat and Genz-529648 inhibited the activity of GBA2 and support the hypothesis that GBA2 could be a target of the anti-inflammatory effects of deoxynojirimycin-type inhibitors.

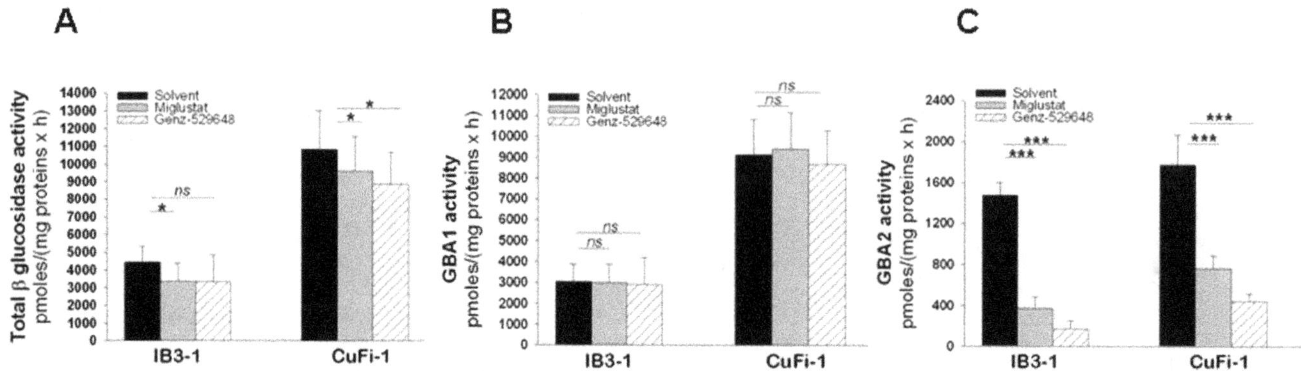

Figure 3. Miglustat and Genz-529648 inhibit GBA2 activity in IB3-1 and CuFi-1 cells infected by *P. aeruginosa*. IB3-1 and CuFi-1 cells were treated with [2 μM] miglustat, [10 nM] Genz-529648 or solvent alone for 1 hour prior to infection with heat-killed PAO1 for 4 hours. Total β-glucosidase (A), GBA1 (B) and GBA2 (C) activities were measured as indicated in figure 2. The data reported are the mean ± standard error of the mean of 3 (IB3-1) or 2 (CuFi-1) independent experiments in triplicate. Comparisons between groups were made by using Student's *t* tests.

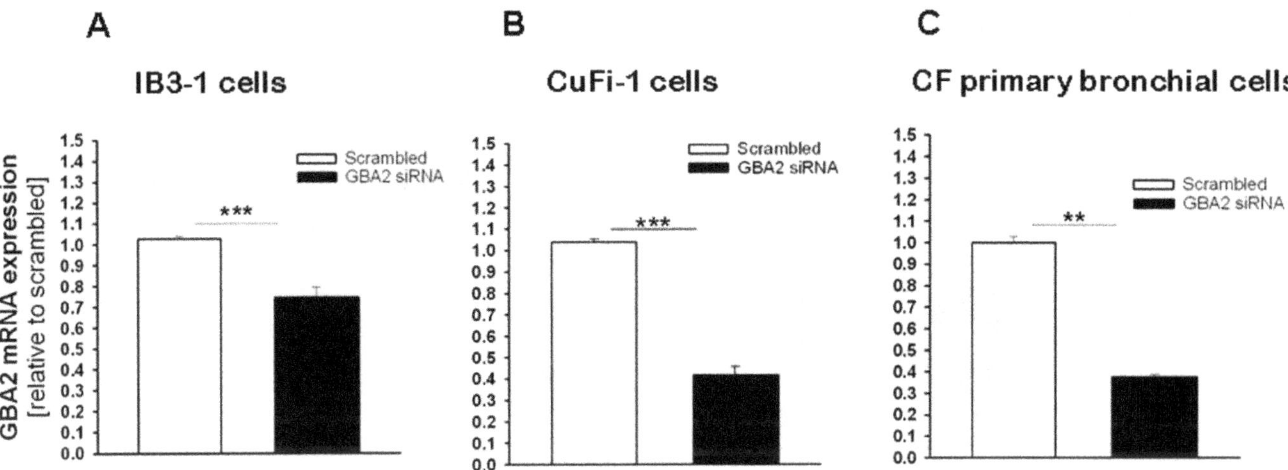

Figure 4. Transfection with GBA2 siRNA reduces the expression of GBA2 in CF bronchial cells. IB3-1 (A), CuFi-1 (B) or CF primary bronchial cells (C) were transfected with GBA2 siRNA or scrambled oligonucleotides for 24 h. GBA2 mRNA expression was measured by Real-time qPCR and obtained by comparing the ratio GBA2 and the housekeeping gene GAPDH between scrambled or siRNA treated cells. The data reported on the y-axis are relative to scrambled-treated cells and represent the mean ± SE of five (IB3-1, panel A), eight (CuFi-1, panel B) and four (CF primary bronchial, panel C) independent experiments performed in duplicate. Comparisons between groups were made by using Student's *t* tests.

siRNA-mediated silencing of GBA2 in CF bronchial cells decreases IL-8 expression

To confirm if GBA2 is involved in the signaling cascade activated by *P. aeruginosa* infection of CF bronchial cells, the levels of IL-8 were measured following GBA2 silencing with siRNA oligonucleotides. The cells were transiently transfected with a siRNA that specifically targeted the degradation of human GBA2 mRNA or a control duplex scrambled siRNA. As shown in figure 4, panel A, transfection of IB3-1 cells with the GBA2-specific siRNA significantly reduced (30%) the level of expression of GBA2 mRNA. Transfection of CuFi-1 cells with the GBA2 siRNA produced a greater decrease (60%) in GBA2 mRNA levels (figure 4, panel B). The experiments were then repeated in primary CF bronchial cells, a cell model that closely resembles the native epithelium, where a decrease of GBA2 expression (~60%) was also identified after transfection with the GBA2 specific siRNA (figure 4, panel C). As shown in figure 5, the silencing of GBA2 expression decreased IL-8 transcription in both uninfected cells (figure 5, panels A, B and C) and cells infected by *P. aeruginosa* (figure 5, panels D, E and F); however, in IB3-1 cells, the IL-8 reduction was not significant (figure 5, panels A and D). These findings were confirmed by measuring IL-8 protein levels in the supernatants of CuFi-1 cells at 4 hours post-infection with PAO1. As expected, the decrease in IL-8 mRNA expression was accompanied by a significant reduction in the secretion of IL-8 into the supernatant (figure 6). To provide evidence that the reduction of IL-8 levels is related to a decrease in GBA2 function, GBA2 activity was measured in GBA2 silenced CuFi-1 cells. Therefore, the cells were transiently transfected as previously described, and the total β-glucosidase and GBA2 activities in cell lysates were measured 18 and 42 hours after transfection. As shown in figure 7, panel A, GBA2 activity was significantly decreased at 18 hours after transfection. A further reduction of GBA2 activity resulted from measurements performed 42 hours after silencing. In these experimental conditions, transfection with siRNA that targeted GBA2 had an impact only on GBA2 activity, as demonstrated by the slight decrease of total β-glucosidase activity identified in GBA2 silenced cells (figure 7, panel B). These data, which demonstrate that lowering the expression and activity of GBA2 leads to a concomitant reduction in IL-8 levels, suggest a role for GBA2 in the inflammatory response induced by *P. aeruginosa* infection of CF bronchial cells.

Increase of cell ceramide content induced by *P. aeruginosa* in CF bronchial cells

Inhibiting the catabolism of GlcCer by GBA2 could also lower ceramide levels and thereby reduce pulmonary inflammation in CF patients. We have previously shown that miglustat reduced the expression of immunoreactive ceramides (measured by immunofluorescence) induced by *P. aeruginosa* [20]. To assess the effect of *P. aeruginosa* infection on the total cell ceramide content, LC-MS and LC-MS/MS analyses were performed as detailed in the Supplement S1. In the PAO1 infected IB3-1 and CuFi-1 cells, a significant increase in ceramides was identified (figure 8, panels A and B), which indicated that the infection up-modulated whole cell ceramide levels. Treatment with miglustat or Genz-529648 significantly reduced whole cell ceramide in IB3-1 cells by approximately 50% (figure 8, panel A), whereas in CuFi-1 cells, a small, albeit not significant decrease in ceramide levels was identified (figure 8, panel B).

To better evaluate the contribution of GSL catabolism to the ceramide increase following PAO1 infection, cell SL metabolic labeling was performed with the radioactive precursor sphingosine, which enables labeling of SLs at the steady-state. Thus, the effects of drug treatment on the radioactive ceramide content are only because of the modulation of the SL catabolism, thereby excluding the *de novo* pathway. To discriminate between the ceramide derived from SM catabolism and GSLs, we treated cells with amitriptyline alone, which is an inhibitor of ASM activity, or in combination with Genz-529648. IB3-1 and CuFi-1 cells were also subjected to the SL metabolic labeling with (1-^{3}H) sphingosine and were then differently treated with 10 μM amitriptyline alone or in combination with 10 nM Genz-529648 and infected with PAO1 as detailed in the Supplement S2. The total lipid extracts (ELT) obtained from cells were subjected to HPTLC separation to distinguish ceramide from the other SLs. The radioactive ceramide was quantified by digital autoradiography (figure 9, panel A). In the CuFi-1 cells, the ceramide levels were under the

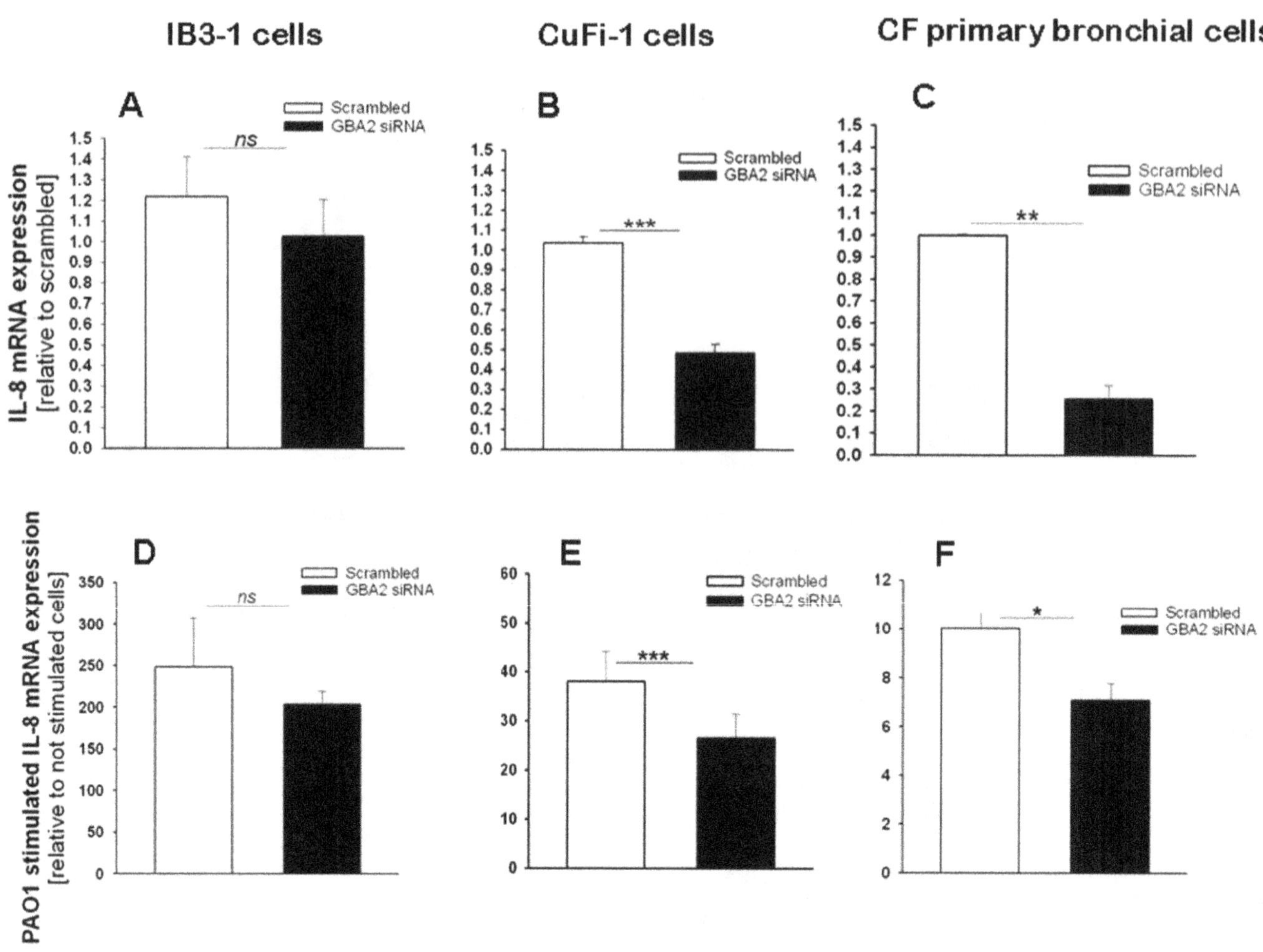

Figure 5. Reduction of IL-8 is associated with a relevant decrease of GBA2 expression in CF bronchial cells. IB3-1 (A), CuFi-1 (B) or CF primary bronchial cells (C) were transfected with GBA2 siRNA or scrambled oligonucleotides for 24 h and then infected with PAO1 (10–50 CFU/cell). IL-8 mRNA expression was measured as indicated in figure 1. The data reported on the y-axis are relative to scrambled-treated cells (A, B and C) or scrambled-treated uninfected cells (D, E and F) and represent the mean ± SE of five (IB3-1, panels A and D), eight (CuFi-1, panels B and E) and four (CF primary bronchial, panels C and F) independent experiments performed in duplicate. Comparisons between groups were made by using Student's *t* tests.

sensitivity threshold of the digital autoradiograph used. By contrast, a significant increase in the ceramide content after PAO1 infection was observed in the IB3-1 cells. The treatment of cells with amitriptyline caused a slight reduction of ceramide, whereas a significant decrease of the ceramide content was observed when infected cells were treated with both amitriptyline and Genz-529648; these findings support a direct involvement of GBA2 in ceramide production (figure 9, panel B).

Discussion

Recent advances in glycobiology have encouraged a search for novel drug molecules that address new biochemical targets. Iminosugars, which are carbohydrate-mimetics with a nitrogen atom replacing oxygen, have many attributes that make them suitable as small-molecule drug candidates. Pharmaceutical interest in these compounds is related to their ability to modulate carbohydrate processing, control cancer cell glycosylation, reduce viral and bacterial infectivity, alter immune responses and bind carbohydrate receptors [22]. The iminosugar miglustat, which was approved to treat type I Gaucher disease and Niemann-Pick type C disease, exerts an anti-inflammatory effect in CF human bronchial epithelial cells infected by *P. aeruginosa* and down modulates the neutrophil chemotaxis in murine lungs *in vivo* [20,23]. Here, we report that the non-lysosomal β-glucosidase 2, is a target of the anti-inflammatory effects of miglustat and other deoxynojirimycin-type inhibitors used in this study. This contention is supported by the findings that: *i)* treatment of *P. aeruginosa* infected CF bronchial cells with Genz-529648, a potent inhibitor of GBA2, reduced the extent of inflammation; *ii)* the IC_{50} value of the anti-inflammatory effect of Genz-529648 was similar compared to the effect reported toward inhibiting GBA2 activity (33); *iii)* treatment of CF bronchial cells with miglustat or Genz-529648 inhibited GBA2; and *iv)* inhibition of GBA2 by siRNA lowered the expression of IL-8.

The alkylated iminosugars miglustat, NB-DGJ and Genz-529648 employed in this study inhibit GlcCerT, GBA1 and GBA2. However, the impact of these compounds on GlcCerT and GBA activities depends greatly on their dosage [30]. Lower concentrations of iminosugars primarily affect GBA2, whereas higher doses inhibit all enzymes. Notably, we obtained a reduction of *P. aeruginosa* stimulated IL-8 mRNA expression in CF bronchial cells treated with Genz-529648 at very low nanomolar

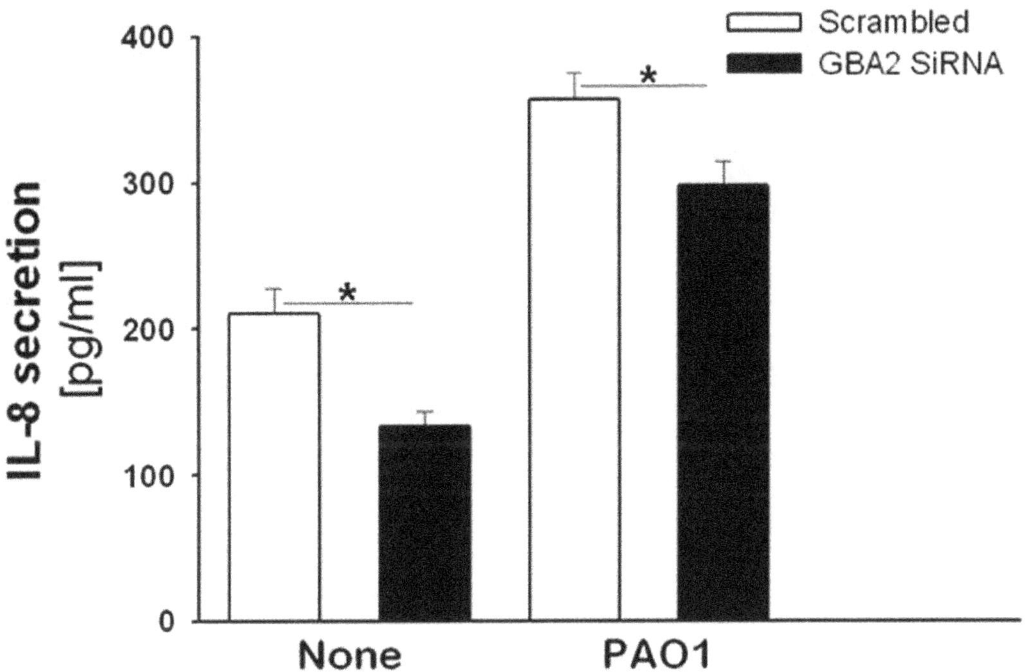

Figure 6. GBA2 silencing reduces the IL-8 protein release in CuFi-1 cells. CuFi-1 cells were transfected with GBA2 siRNA or scrambled oligonucleotides and then infected with PAO1 as indicated in figure 5. The supernatants were collected at the end of infection, and IL-8 protein release was measured as detailed in the "Methods" section. The data reported are the mean ± SE of eight independent experiments performed in duplicate. Comparisons between groups were made by using Student's *t* tests.

concentrations, which completely inhibited GBA2 activity, but not GBA1 or GlcCerT [34]. Measurements of the sensitivity of GlcCerT, GBA1 and GBA2 to the inhibition by miglustat in different mammalian cells/tissues revealed IC_{50} values in the low µM, high µM and nM range, respectively. This finding indicates that GBA2 is more sensitive to miglustat compared to GlcCerT and GBA1 [30]. Although the IC_{50} values of miglustat at inhibiting *P. aeruginosa* stimulated IL-8 mRNA expression in CF bronchial cells (table 1) are higher compared to the IC_{50} values for inhibiting GBA2, they are substantially lower compared to GlcCerT and GBA1. Hence, GlcCerT and GBA1 are unlikely to have been the targets of the anti-inflammatory effects of miglustat. Furthermore, we previously reported that miglustat down modulates neutrophil chemotaxis *in vivo* at doses that are lower (100 mg/Kg) [20] compared to the doses necessary to affect GlcCerT (1800–2400 mg/Kg) [42], which further supports the notion that the primary effect of miglustat is on GBA2 activity.

GBA2 plays a role in extra-lysosomal GlcCer catabolism, producing ceramide that can then be rapidly converted into sphingomyelin [29]. Although the mechanism and function of extra-lysosomal GlcCer degradation are not well understood, GBA2 has recently been implicated in various pathologic conditions, such as neuronal diseases [43] or cancer [44], which supports a role of GlcCer in cell growth, proliferation and immunity. The present novel findings suggest that GBA2 may also be involved in modulating the inflammatory response to *P. aeruginosa* infection in CF bronchial epithelial cells. Indeed, total β-glucosidase, GBA1 and GBA2 activities were elevated in CF bronchial cells infected by *P. aeruginosa* (figure 2). As for the effects of infection on SLs, it should be noted that infection of host epithelial cells with *P. aeruginosa* activates host ASM levels, which leads to the generation of plasma membrane ceramide-enriched platforms that promote the internalization of bacteria, induce apoptosis and regulate the cytokine storm [13]. Based on the observations noted in our studies, it is possible that in addition to ASM, an overall activation of β-glucosidase activity may also be involved in the host cell response to infection. However, additional studies are needed to validate this assumption. Importantly, miglustat or Genz-529648, at the concentrations used in this study, strongly inhibited only GBA2 activity (figure 3); in parallel, we demonstrated a reduction of *P. aeruginosa* stimulated IL-8 mRNA expression and protein release in CF bronchial cells when GBA2 expression (figure 5) and function (figures 1 and 7) were decreased. These findings support the contention that GBA2 is involved in the inflammatory response to *P. aeruginosa*. GBA2 is typically associated with plasma- and/or ER-membranes in close proximity to the sites of GlcCer synthesis and ceramide conversion to SM [45]. Therefore, as GBA2 is in a key position for GlcCer-mediated signaling, it could be activated following interactions between *P. aeruginosa* and the host cell. It has been shown that GBA2 activation causes the phosphorylation of eukaryotic initiation factor 2α (eIF2α), and this event is associated with an increased expression of the ATF4 family of transcription factors [44]. Interestingly, phosphorylation of eIF2α has been observed in models of acute infection with *Clostridium difficile*, as part of the mucosal inflammatory response [46]. It can be speculated that GBA2 activation by *P. aeruginosa* leads to increased expression of the transcription factors that regulate the pro-inflammatory genes in CF bronchial cells.

The airway epithelium is known to play a key role in the initiation and regulation of inflammatory processes in response to pathogens. In addition to the classical cytokines and chemokines that are released by the respiratory epithelium, ceramide is another important factor in pulmonary host defense [11]. Here, we report an increase in whole cell ceramides in response to infection by *P. aeruginosa* (figures 8 and 9) in CF bronchial

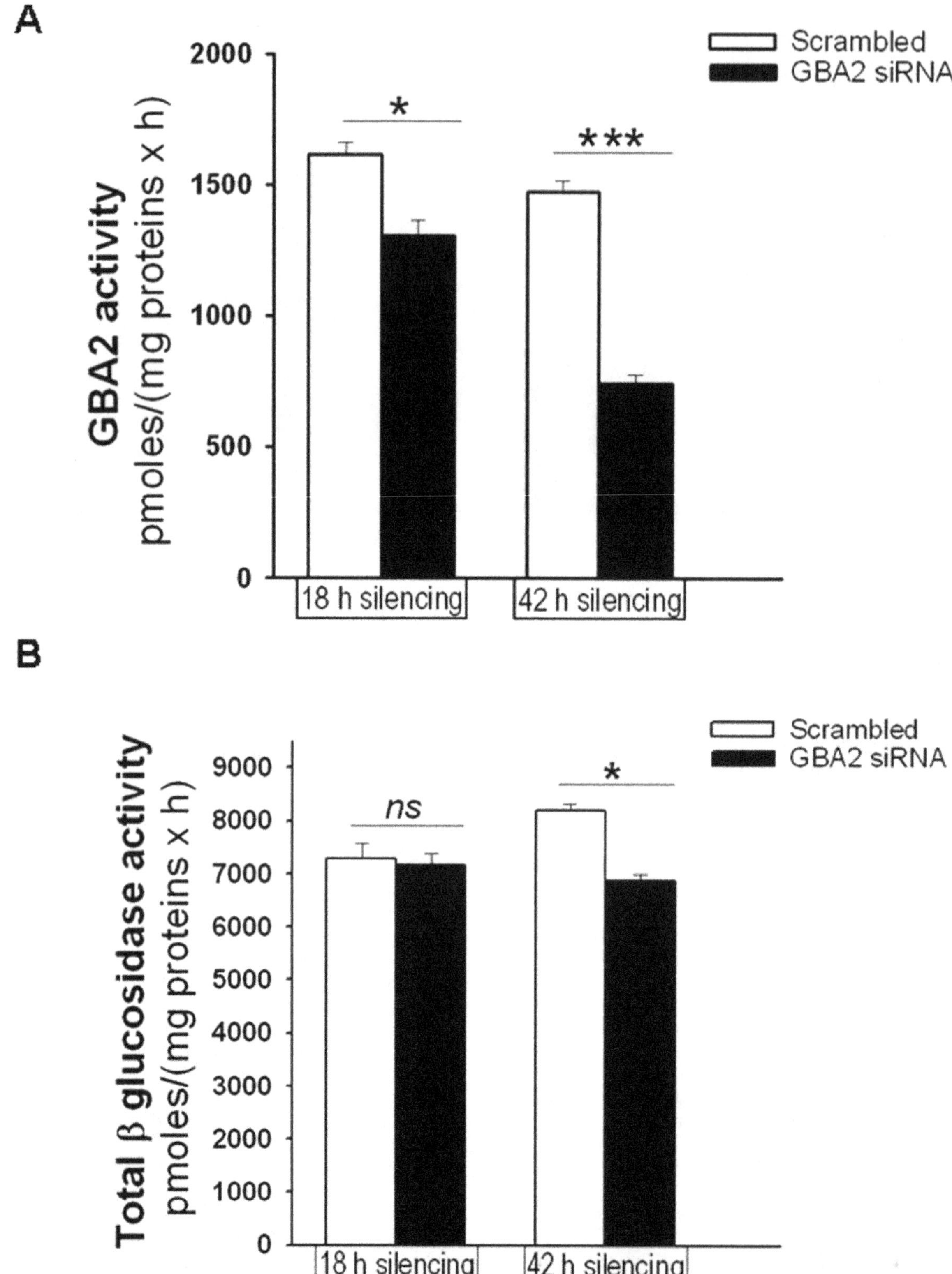

Figure 7. GBA2 silencing reduces GBA2 activity in CuFi-1 cells. CuFi-1 cells were transfected with GBA2 siRNA or scrambled oligonucleotides as indicated in figure 5. Eighteen or 42 hours after transfection, the cells were scraped and treated as indicated in figure 2. Total β-glucosidase (B) and GBA2 (A) activities were measured as reported in the Methods section. The data reported are the mean ± standard error of the mean of 2 independent experiments in triplicate. Comparisons between groups were made by using Student's *t* tests.

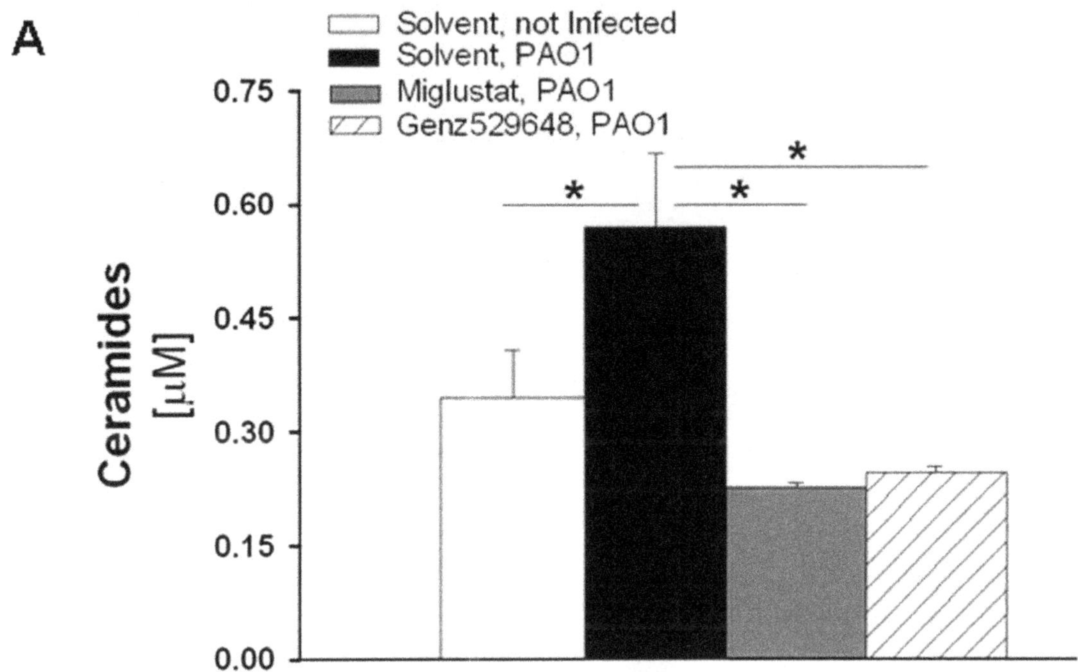

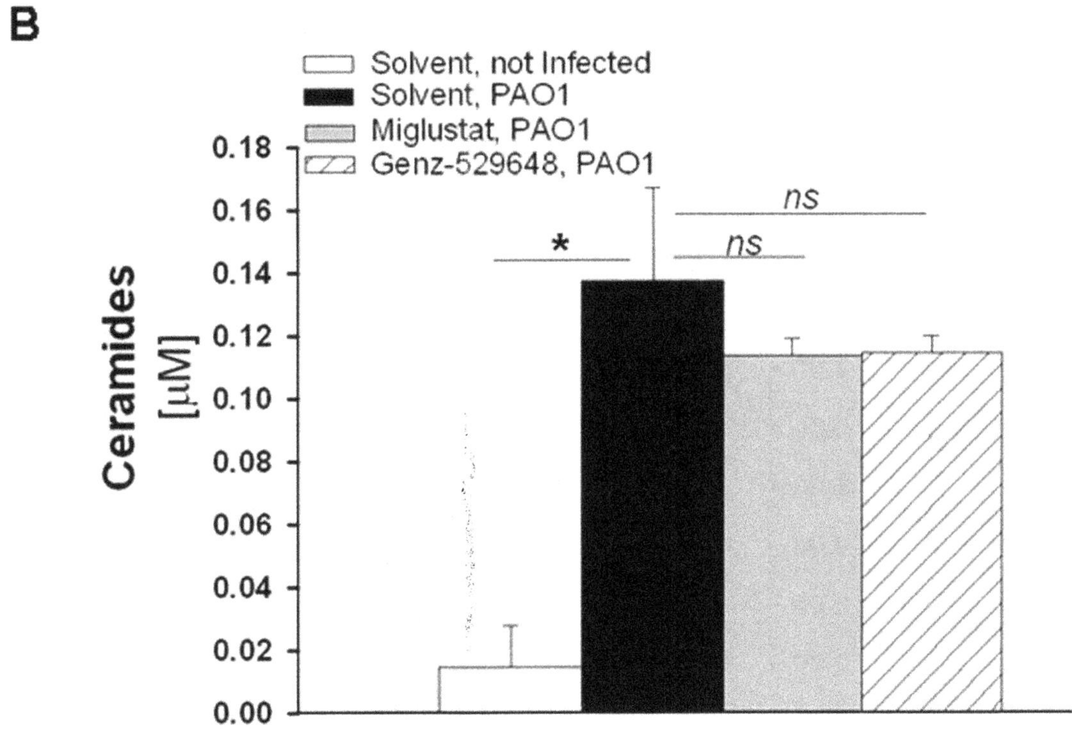

Figure 8. Infection with PAO1 increases whole cell ceramides in CF bronchial epithelial cells. IB3-1 (A) and CuFi-1 (B) cells were treated with [2 μM] miglustat, [10 nM] Genz-529648 or solvent alone and infected with PAO1 as indicated in figure 3. After infection, whole cell ceramides were analyzed by LC-MS and LC-MS/MS methods as described in the online supplement. The data reported are the mean ± SE of three independent experiments performed with both cell lines. Comparisons between groups were made by using Student's *t* tests.

epithelial cells, which is consistent with the rise of ceramide levels at the plasma membrane previously described [20]. In CuFi-1 cells, which have a lower ceramide content compared to IB3-1 cells, we observed a slight decrease in ceramide levels by miglustat or Genz-529648 (figure 8, panel B). By contrast, IB3-1 cells infected with PAO1 and treated with both miglustat and Genz-

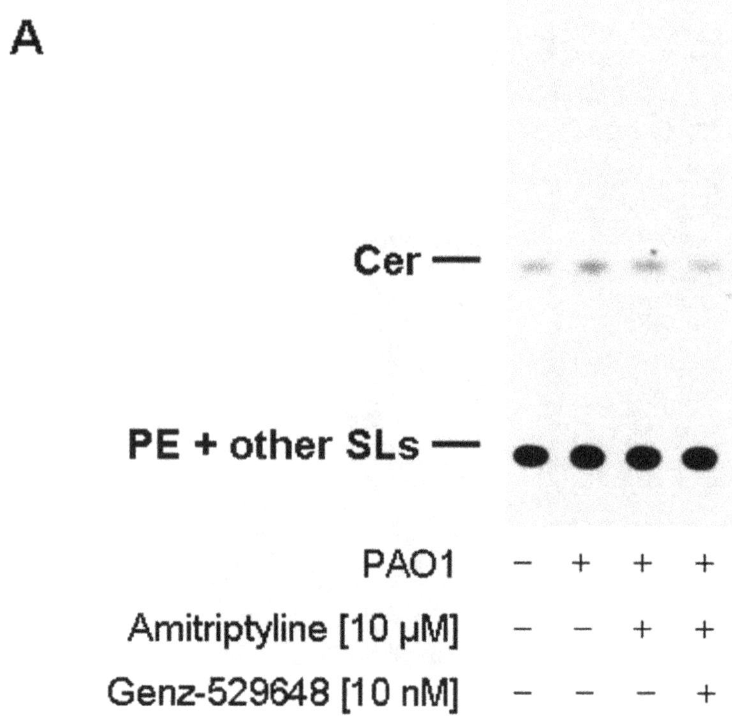

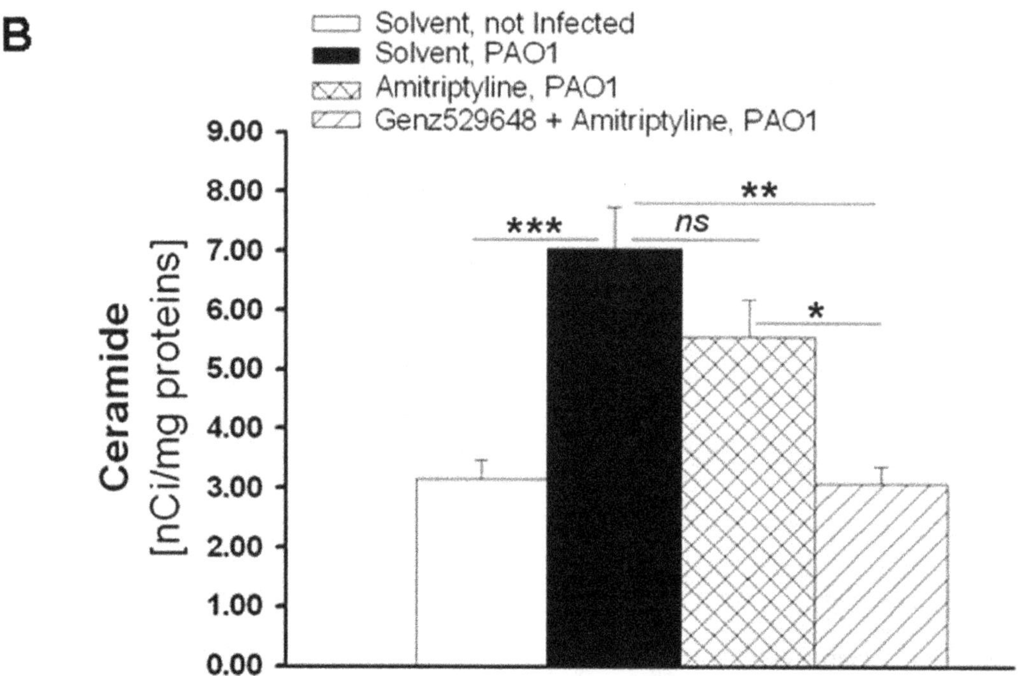

Figure 9. Treatment with Genz-529648 reduces the ceramide content in IB3-1 cells infected with PAO1. IB3-1 cells subjected to the SL metabolic labeling with (1-^{3}H)sphingosine were treated with [10 μM] amitriptyline alone, in combination with [10 nM] Genz-529648, or with solvent alone and infected with PAO1 as indicated in figure 3. After lipid extraction, (^{3}H)ceramide was separated from the other radioactive SLs by HPTLC, as detailed in the online supplement, and detected by digital autoradiography (total lipid extracts amounts corresponding to 4 μg of cellular proteins were applied on a 4-mm line. Time of acquisition: 48 hours). The digital autoradiography represents data obtained in three different experiments (A). The ceramide content was quantified by specific β-Vision software, and the data reported are the mean ± SE of three independent experiments. Comparisons between groups were made by using Student's *t* tests (B).

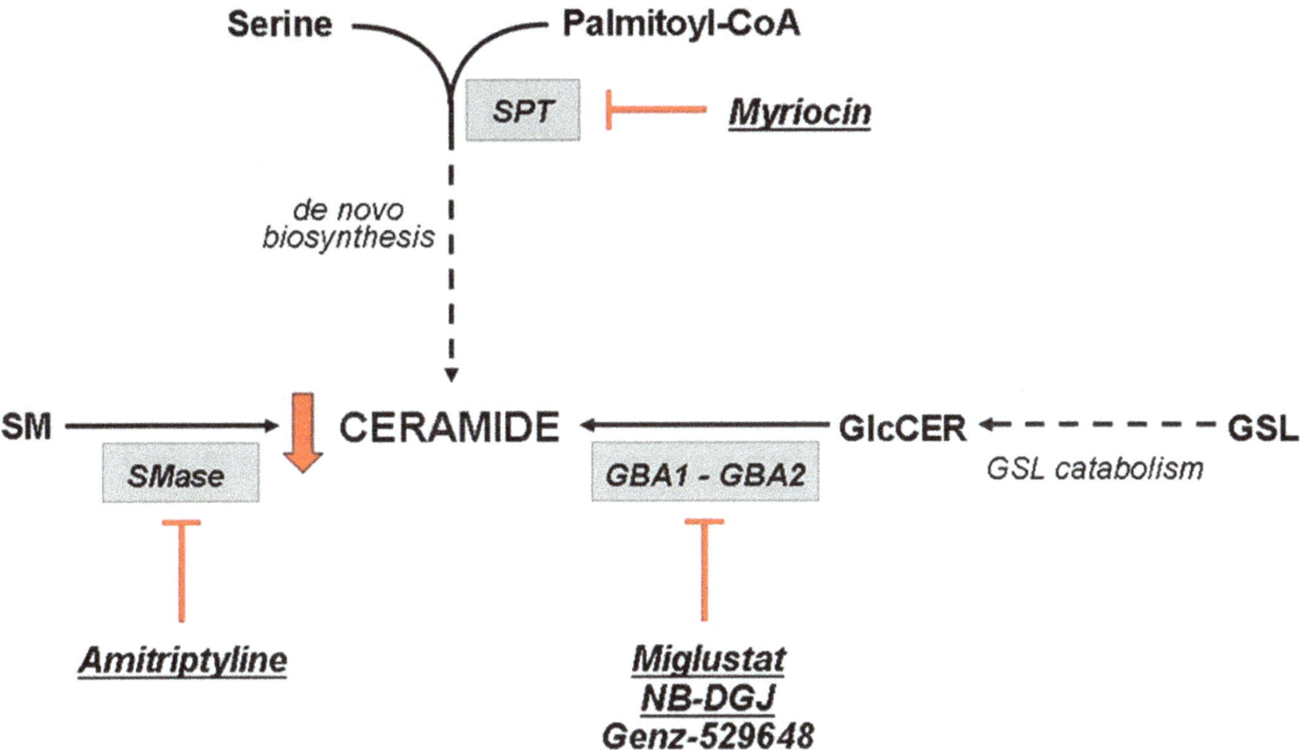

Figure 10. Metabolic pathways involved in ceramide formation. Schematic representation of the primary metabolic pathways involved in ceramide production. Ceramide can be produced by the *de novo* biosynthesis, the hydrolysis of sphingomyelin (SM) by the action of sphingomyelinases and the catabolism of glycosphingolipids (GSL). In particular, it has been observed that in CF bronchial epithelial cells, the use of inhibitors of these pathways resulted in a reduction of ceramide. Myriocin acts on the first step of the *de novo* biosynthesis through the inhibition of the Serine-palmitoyl transferase (SPT); amitriptyline inhibits the acid SMase (ASM) responsible for SM catabolism; and miglustat, NB-DGJ and Genz-529648 are inhibitors of the β-glucosidases GBA1 and GBA2, which are involved in the hydrolysis of the glucosylceramide (GlcCer).

529648 showed a marked decrease of ceramide content (figure 8, panel A). The increase in ceramide content following infection by PAO1 could be a result of different pathways, including the *de novo* biosynthesis [21], SM catabolism [13] and GSL degradation. When we evaluated the effects of drug treatment on the radioactive ceramide content that resulted only because of the modulation of SL catabolism, thus excluding the *de novo* pathway, we identified a marked increase in the cell ceramide content after PAO1 infection (figure 9). After ASM inhibition, we observed a slight decrease and a further, more significant ceramide reduction after the addition of the specific inhibitor of GBA2, Genz-529648 (figure 9), which strongly supports the direct involvement of GBA2 in the ceramide production after PAO1 infection of human bronchial epithelial cells. Thus, the information derived from the literature and the data presented here provide evidence that different inhibitors, such as miglustat and Genz-529648, amitriptyline [14] and myriocin [21], that target GBA2, ASM and ceramide *de novo* synthesis, respectively, could represent therapeutic tools to reduce ceramide levels and limit excessive lung inflammation in CF patients (figure 10). Nevertheless, drugs that target SL metabolism must be carefully titrated to normalize ceramide levels in CF airways, but not reduce ceramide concentrations below a critical level that would impair normal biological functions. Notably, systemic inhibition of ASM could negatively affect the host defense, which has been demonstrated by studies in mice that completely lack ASM and are unable to control infections [13]. Interestingly, no increased susceptibility to bacterial infections has been identified in patients affected by Gaucher disease, treated with miglustat [47] or in a mouse model of Sandhoff disease treated with Genz-529648 [48].

In summary, our study proposes GBA2 as a novel target to reduce the inflammatory response to *P. aeruginosa* in CF bronchial cells. These results further support the use of modulators of SL metabolism for CF lung inflammation. In addition, as GBA2 is sensitive to very low doses of miglustat, other alkylated iminosugars (NB-DGJ) and Genz-529648, our findings provide evidence to develop therapeutic options for CF lung inflammation using iminosugars, which can be effective at even low doses, thus limiting potential adverse effects.

Supporting Information

Figure S1 Viability profile of IB3-1 cells treated for 24 hours with the indicated concentrations of Genz-529648.

Figure S2 Apoptosis profile of IB3-1 cells treated for 24 hours with the indicated concentration of Genz-529648.

Figure S3 Apoptotic IB3-1 cells after 4 and 24 hours of treatment with the indicated concentrations of Genz-529648.

Supplement S1 Analysis of cell ceramide levels using LC-MS and LC-MS/MS.

Supplement S2 Analysis of cell ceramide levels by cell SLs labeling with (^{3}H)sphingosine.

Supplement S3 Cellular toxicity of Genz-529648.

Acknowledgments

We are grateful to: A. Tamanini for helpful discussions, A. Prince for the *P. aeruginosa* laboratory strain PAO1, "In Vitro Model and Cell Culture Care" of the University of Iowa, Iowa, U.S.A. for providing CuFi-1 cells and to "Servizio Colture Primarie" of the Italian Cystic Fibrosis Research Foundation at the Laboratory of Molecular Genetics, G. Gaslini Institute, Genova, Italy, for CF primary cells. This research was supported by the Italian Cystic Fibrosis Research Foundation (grant FFC # 14/2012) with the contribution of *"Picasso. Capolavori dal Museo Nazionale Picasso di Parigi", Festa d'Estate Villa Sigurtà Verona, Delegazione FFC Lago di Garda e Arezzo.*

Author Contributions

Conceived and designed the experiments: MCD MA SS GC. Performed the experiments: NL MT IL NM RB VB VL CC SM. Analyzed the data: MCD MA NL NM MGG AC RG. Contributed reagents/materials/ analysis tools: SHC MGG. Wrote the paper: MCD SHC MA RB NL .

References

1. Welsh JM, Ramsey BW, Accurso F, Cutting GR (2001) Cystic Fibrosis in Scriver CR, Beaudet AL, Sly WS, Valle D (Eds). *The Metabolic and Molecular Bases of Inherited Diseases*. McGraw-Hill, New York.
2. Ramsey BW, Davies J, McElvaney NG, Tullis E, Bell SC, et al. (2011) VX08-770-102 Study Group A CFTR Potentiator in Patients with Cystic Fibrosis and the *G551D* Mutation. New England J of Medicine 365: 1663–1672.
3. Hoffman LR, Ramsey BW (2013) Cystic Fibrosis Therapeutics. The road ahead. Chest 143(1): 207–213.
4. Konstan MW, Schluchter MD, Xue W, Davis PB (2007) Clinical use of Ibuprofen is associated with slower Fev1 decline in children with cystic fibrosis. Am J Respir Crit Care Med 176 (11): 1084–1089.
5. Khan TZ, Wagener JS, Bost T, Martinez J, Accurso FJ, et al. (1995) Early pulmonary inflammation in infants with cystic fibrosis. Am J Respir Crit Care Med 151: 1075–1082.
6. Noah TL, Black HR, Cheng PW, Wood RE, Leigh MW (1997) Nasal and bronchoalveolar lavage fluid cytokines in early cystic fibrosis. J Infect Dis 175: 638–647.
7. Tirouvanziam R, de Bentzmann S, Hubeau C, Hinnrasky J, Jacquot J, et al. (2000) Inflammation and infection in naive human cystic fibrosis airway grafts. Am J Respir Cell Mol Biol 23(2): 121–127.
8. Chmiel JF, Berger M, Konstan MW (2002) The role of inflammation in the pathophysiology of CF lung disease. Clin Rev Allergy Immunol 23: 5–27.
9. Lahiri S, Futerman AH (2007) The metabolism and function of shingolipids and glycoshingolipids. Cell Mol Life Sci 64: 2270–2284.
10. Uhlig S, Gulbins E (2008) Sphingolipids in the lungs. Am J Respir Crit Care Med 178(11): 1100–1114.
11. Yang Y, Uhlig S (2001) The role of sphingolipids in respiratory disease. Ther Adv Respir Dis 5: 325–344.
12. Hannun YA, Obeid LM (2008) Principles of bioactive lipid signalling: lessons from sphingolipids. Nat Rew Mol Cell Biol 9: 139–150.
13. Grassme' H, Jendrossek V, Riehle A, von Kürthy G, Berger J, et al. (2003) Host defense against *Pseudomonas aeruginosa* requires ceramide-rich membrane rafts. Nature Medicine 9: 322–330.
14. Teichgraber V, Ulrich M, Endlich N, Riethmüller J, Wilker B, et al. (2008) Ceramide accumulation mediates inflammation, cell death and infection susceptibility in cystic fibrosis. Nature Med 14: 382–391.
15. Guilbault C, De Sanctis JB, Wojewodka G, Saeed Z, Lachance C, et al. (2008) Fenretinide corrects newly found ceramide deficiency in cystic fibrosis. Am J Respir Cell Mol Biol 38(1): 47–56.
16. Yu H, Zeidan YH, Wu BX, Jenkins RW, Flotte TR, et al. (2009) Defective acid sphingomyelinase pathway with *Pseudomonas aeruginosa* infection in cystic fibrosis. American Journal of Respiratory Cell and Molecular Biology 41: 367–375.
17. Brodlie M, McKean MC, Johnson GE, Gray J, Fisher AJ, et al. (2010) Ceramide is Increased in the Lower Airway Epithelium of People with Advanced Cystic Fibrosis Lung Disease. Am J Respir Crit Care Med 182 (3): 369–375.
18. Bodas M, Min T, Mazur S, Vij N (2011) Critical modifier role of membrane-cystic fibrosis transmembrane conductance regulator-dependent ceramide signaling in lung injury and emphysema. J Immunol 186: 602–613.
19. Nährlich L, Mainz JG, Adams C, Engel C, Herrmann G, et al. (2013) Therapy of CF-patients with amitriptyline and placebo-a randomised, double-blind, placebo-controlled phase IIb multicenter, cohort-study. Cell Physiol Biochem 31(4–5): 505–312.
20. Dechecchi MC, Nicolis E, Mazzi P, Cioffi F, Bezzerri V, et al. (2011) Modulators of sphingolipid metabolism reduce lung inflammation. Am J Respir Cell Mol Biol 45(4): 825–833.
21. Caretti A, Bragonzi A, Facchini M, De Fino I, Riva C, et al. (2014) Anti-inflammatory action of lipid nanocarrier-delivered myriocin: therapeutic potential in cystic fibrosis. Biochim Biophys Acta 1840(1): 586–594.
22. Nash RJ, Kato A, Yu C-Y, Fleet GWJ (2011) Iminosugars as therapeuthic agents:recent advances and promising trends. Future Med Chem 3(12): 1–9.
23. Dechecchi MC, Nicolis E, Mazzi P, Paroni M, Cioffi F, et al. (2012) Pharmacological modulators of sphingolipid metabolism for the treatment of cystic fibrosis lung inflammation. In Dinesh D and Sriramulu D editors. Cystic Fibrosis - the Human Agony, ISBN 979-953-307-059-8, Germany.
24. Norez C, Noel S, Wilke M, Bijvelds M, Jorna H, et al. (2006) Rescue of functional delF508-CFTR channels in cystic fibrosis epithelial cells by the α-glucosidase inhibitor miglustat. FEBS Lett 580: 2081–2086.
25. Dechecchi MC, Nicolis E, Norez C, Bezzerri V, Borgatti M, et al. (2008) Anti-inflammatory effect of miglustat in bronchial epithelial cells. J Cyst Fibros 7(6): 555–565.
26. Lubamba B, Lebacq J, Lebecque P, Vanbever R, Leonard A (2009) Airway delivery of low-dose miglustat normalizes nasal potential difference in F508del cystic fibrosis mice. Am J Respir Crit Care Med 179: 1022–1028.
27. Leonard A, Lebecque P, Dingemanse J, Leal T (2012) A randomized placebo-controlled trial of miglustat in cystic fibrosi based on nasal potential difference. J Cystic Fibrosis 11(3): 231–236.
28. Inokuchi J, Mason I, Radin NS (1987) Antitumor activity via inhibition of glycosphingolipid biosynthesis. Cancer Lett 38: 23–30.
29. Boot RG, Verhoek M, Donker-Koopman W, Strijland A, van Marle J, et al. (2007) Identification of the non-lysosomal glucosylceramidase as beta-glucosidase 2. J Biol Chem 282: 1305–1312.
30. Ridley CM, Thur KE, Shanahan J, Thillaiappan NB, Shen A, et al. (2013) β-Glucosidase 2 (GBA2) activity and imino sugar pharmacology. J Biol Chem 288(36): 26052–26066.
31. Dwek RA, Butters TD, Platt FM, Zitzmann N (2002) Targeting glycosylation as a therapeutic approach. Nat Rev Drug Discov 1: 65–75.
32. Platt FM, Neises GR, Karlsson GB, Dwek RA, Butters TD (1994) N-butyldeoxygalactonojirimycin inhibits glycolipid biosynthesis but does not affect N-linked oligosaccharide processing. J Biol Chem 269 (43): 27108–27114.
33. Weenekes T, Meijer AJ, Groen AK, Boot RG, Groener JE, et al. (2010) Large-Scale synthesis of the glucosylceramide synthase inhibitor N-[5-(Adamantan-1-yl-methoxy)-pentyl]-1-deoxynojirimycin. J Med Chem 53: 689–698.
34. Overkleeft HS, Renkema Hg, Neele J, Vianello P, Hung IO, et al. (1998) Generation of specific deoxynojirimycin-type inhibitors of the non-lysosomal glucosylceramidase. J Biol Chem 273 (41): 26522–26527.
35. Yildiz Y, Matern H, Thompson B, Allergood JC, Warren RL, et al. (2006) Mutation of beta-glucosidase 2 causes glycolipid storage disease and impaired male fertility. J Clin Invest 116: 2985–2994.
36. Aerts JM, Ottenhoff R, Powlson AS, Grefhorst A, van Eijk M, et al. (2007) Pharmacological inhibition of glucosylceramide synthase enhances insulin sensitivity. Diabetes 56(5): 1341–1349.
37. Zeitlin PL, Lu L, Rhim J, Cutting G, Stetten G, et al. (1991) A cystic fibrosis bronchial epithelial cell line: immortalization by adeno-12-SV40 infection. Am J Respir Cell Mol Biol 4: 313–319.
38. Zabner J, Karp P, Seiler M, Phillips Sl, Mitchell CJ, et al. (2003) Development of cystic fibrosis and non cystic fibrosis airway cell lines. Am J Physiol Lung Cell Mol Physiol 284: L844–L854.
39. Scudieri P, Caci E, Bruno S, Ferrera L, Schiavon M, et al. (2012) Association of TMEM16A chloride channel overexpression with airway goblet cell metaplasia. J Physiol 590 (23): 6141–6155.
40. Sullards MC, Allegood JC, Kelly S, Wang E, Haynes CA, et al. (2007) Structure-specific, quantitative methods for analysis of sphingolipids by LC-tandem MS: "inside-out" sphingolipids. Methods in Enzymology 432: 83–115.
41. Aureli M, Loberto N, Bassi R, Ferraretto A, Perego S, et al. (2012) Plasma membrane-associated glycohydrolases activation by extracellular acidification due to proton exchangers. Neurochem Res 37(6): 1296–1307.
42. Platt FM, Reinkensmeier G, Dwek RA, Butters TD (1996) Extensive glycosphingolipid depletion in the liver and lymphoid organs of mice treated with *N*- butyldeoxynojirimycin. J Biol Chem 272: 19365–19372.
43. Martin E, Schüle R, Smets K, Rastetter A, Boukhris A, et al. (2013) Loss of function of glucocerebrosidase GBA2 is responsible for motor neuron defects in hereditary spastic paraplegia. Am J Hum Genet 92(2): 238–244.
44. Sorli SC, Colié S, Albinet V, Dubrac A, Touriol C, et al. (2013) The nonlysosomal β-glucosidase GBA2 promotes endoplasmic reticulum stress and impairs tumorigenicity of human melanoma cells. FASEB J 27(2): 489–498.
45. Körschen HG, Yildiz Y, Raju DN, Schonauer S, Bönigk W, et al. (2013) The non-lysosomal β-glucosidase GBA2 is a non-integral membrane-associated protein at the endoplasmic reticulum (ER) and Golgi. J Biol Chem 288(5): 3381–3393.

9

Transcription Analysis of the Porcine Alveolar Macrophage Response to *Mycoplasma hyopneumoniae*

Li Bin[1,2]*, Du Luping[1], Sun Bing[1], Yu Zhengyu[1,2], Liu Maojun[1,2], Feng Zhixin[1,2], Wei Yanna[1,2], Wang Haiyan[1,2], Shao Guoqing[1,2], He Kongwang[1,2]*

1 Institute of Veterinary Medicine, Jiangsu Academy of Agricultural Sciences, Key Laboratory of Veterinary Biological Engineering and Technology, Ministry of Agriculture, Nanjing, Jiangsu Province, China, **2** Jiangsu Co-innovation Center for Prevention and Control of Important Animal Infectious Diseases and Zoonoses, Yangzhou, China

Abstract

Mycoplasma hyopneumoniae is considered the major causative agent of porcine respiratory disease complex, occurs worldwide and causes major economic losses to the pig industry. To gain more insights into the pathogenesis of this organism, the high throughput cDNA microarray assays were employed to evaluate host responses of porcine alveolar macrophages to *M. hyopneumoniae* infection. A total of 1033 and 1235 differentially expressed genes were identified in porcine alveolar macrophages in responses to exposure to *M. hyopneumoniae* at 6 and 15 hours post infection, respectively. The differentially expressed genes were involved in many vital functional classes, including inflammatory response, immune response, apoptosis, cell adhesion, defense response, signal transduction, protein folding, protein ubiquitination and so on. The pathway analysis demonstrated that the most significant pathways were the chemokine signaling pathway, Toll-like receptor signaling pathway, RIG-I-like receptor signaling pathway, nucleotide-binding oligomerization domains (Nod)-like receptor signaling pathway and apoptosis signaling pathway. The reliability of the data obtained from the microarray was verified by performing quantitative real-time PCR. The expression kinetics of chemokines was further analyzed. The present study is the first to document the response of porcine alveolar macrophages to *M. hyopneumoniae* infection. The data further developed our understanding of the molecular pathogenesis of *M. hyopneumoniae*.

Editor: Yung-Fu Chang, Cornell University, United States of America

Funding: This work was supported by the National Natural Sciences Foundation of China (31001066 and 31370208) and the Jiangsu province Natural Sciences Foundation (BK20131330). The funders had no role in study design, data collection and analysis, decision to publish, or preparation of the manuscript.

Competing Interests: The authors have declared that no competing interests exist.

* Email: libinana@126.com (LB); Kongwanghe@126.com (HK)

Introduction

Mycoplasma hyopneumoniae is the etiological agent of swine enzootic pneumonia, a chronic nonfatal disease affecting pigs of all ages. It is characterised by high morbidity and low mortality, resulting in significant economic losses due to decreased performance of pigs and the cost of medication [1]. *M. hyopneumoniae* predisposes animals to concurrent infections with other respiratory pathogens including bacteria, parasites and viruses. *M. hyopneumoniae* is also considered to be one of the primary agents involved in the porcine respiratory disease complex (PRDC) [2].

M. hyopneumoniae has been found to attach to the cilia of epithelial cells in the lungs of swine. They cause cilia to stop beating (ciliostasis), clumping and loss of cilia, eventually leading to epithelial cell death, which is the source of the lesions found in the lungs of pigs with porcine enzootic pneumonia [3]. On a cellular level, mononuclear cell infiltration of peribronchiolar and perivascular areas occurs. Then, *M. hyopneumoniae* actively suppresses immune systems of the host during early stages of pneumonia by inhibiting macrophage-mediated phagocytosis. The response of the host immune system causes the lesions seen in the lung tissue of infected swine by increasing phagocytic and cytotoxic activities of macrophages and initiating the chronic inflammatory response [4]. Increased production of proinflammatory cytokines, including interleukin (IL)-1β, tumor necrosis factor (TNF)-α, IL-6, IL-8 and IL-18 in the *M. hyopneumoniae* infected host also leads to a greater recruitment of neutrophils [4–9]. However, the factors involved in promoting protective immunity and/or the inflammatory responses against *M. hyopneumoniae* are not fully understood, and the cellular sensors and signaling pathway involved in these process has not yet been elucidated.

Innate immunity is the first line of defense for host protection against invading pathogens. Pattern recognition receptors (PRRs) are expressed in cells of the innate immune system, it include Toll-like receptors (TLR), RIG-I-like receptors (RLR) and NOD-like receptors (NLR). Pathogen-associated molecular patterns (PAMPs), derived from different pathogens, are recognized by PRRs, resulting in the release of inflammatory cytokines and interferons, and the boosting of host defenses. As a major component of the host innate immunity, macrophages have essential roles in host defense to infection [10,11]. Host-pathogen interactions during *M. hyopneumoniae* infection are complicated, the interactions between *M. hyopneumoniae* with porcine alveolar macrophages have been less studied [7,8], but the detailed mechanisms of how porcine alveolar macrophages response to *M. hyopneumoniae* infection are not well elucidated. To study the molecular mechanisms underlying the host response to pathogenic microorganisms in macrophages, microarrays have been widely used in recent years [12–15]. In the current study, we applied this high throughput cDNA microarray assay to improve our understanding of the innate immune response of macrophages to *M. hyopneumoniae* infection.

Results

Gene expression analysis during *M. hyopneumoniae* infection

To investigate the pathogenesis of *M. hyopneumoniae*, the differential gene (DE) expression profile of PAM, after infection with *M. hyopneumoniae* was determined. Genes whose relative transcription levels showed a fold change (FC)≥2 ($p \leq 0.05$) were considered to be up-regulated, and those with a FC≤0.5 ($p \leq 0.05$) were considered to be down-regulated. Genes whose relative transcription levels had a FC greater than 0.5 or less than 2 were considered to have no notable change in expression levels. In this study, 1033 and 1235 DE genes were detected for active infection with *M. hyopneumoniae* compared with the control group at 6 and 15 hpi, respectively, $p \leq 0.05$ (Figure 1A and 1C). At 6 hpi, 747 genes were up-regulated and 286 down-regulated, whilst at 15 hpi 706 genes were up-regulated and 529 down-regulated.

qRT-PCR validated DE genes

Microarray experiments yield a large amount of data, therefore it is important to validate differential expression by independent methods. To confirm the statistical significance of our findings, we performed quantitative real-time PCR (qRT-PCR) analysis on the relevant genes from our original samples used in the microarray study. Five up-regulated and five down-regulated genes, were selected for qRT-PCR analysis. Table 1 compares the results obtained from the microarray analysis with those of qRT-PCR. The results demonstrated that changes in expression levels of the ten selected genes as detected by qRT-PCR, were consistent with the changes (up-regulation or down-regulation) predicted by microarray analysis. However, the FCs differed markedly between microarray and qRT-PCR. This discrepancy may be attributable to technical differences encountered in the methods of analysis and

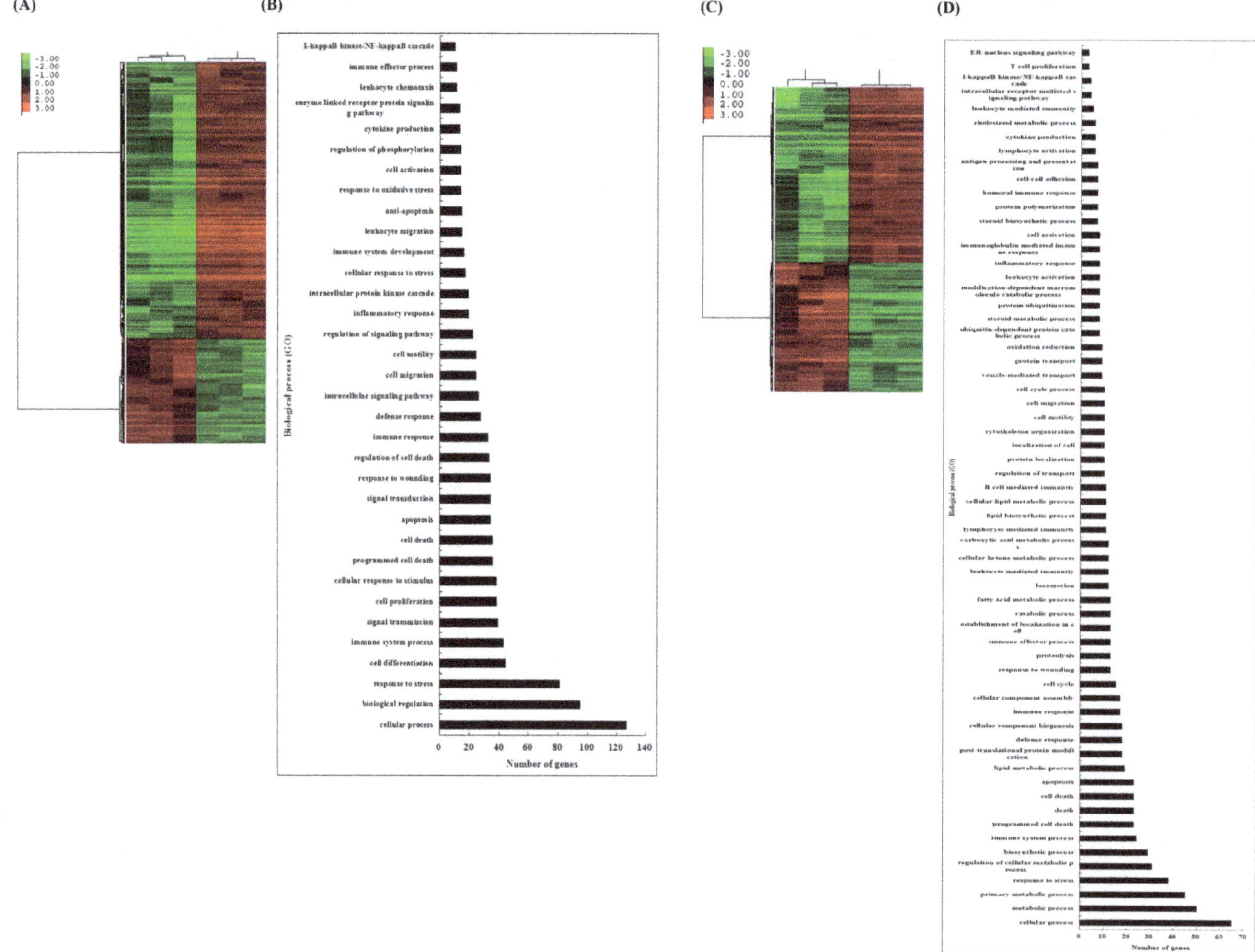

Figure 1. Clustering and characterization of the differential expression of genes. (A) The DE genes showing clear functional annotation at 6 HPI have been selected for cluster analysis which is described in methods. Each row represents a separate gene, and each column represents a experiment sample. Color legend is on the left, the color scale ranges from saturated green for log ratios −3.0 and above to saturated red for log ratios 3.0 and above. Red indicates increased gene expression levels; green indicates decreased levels compared with normal samples. (B) Categories of annotated genes based on biological process GO term at 6 HPI. (C) The genes showing clear functional annotation at 15 HPI have been selected for cluster analysis. (D) Categories of annotated genes based on biological process GO term at 15 HPI.

Table 1. Validation of microarray results by qRT-PCR.

GenBank ID	Gene symbol	Primers sequence (5′-3′)	Regulation	Microarray FC*	Real-time PCR FC
NM_214055	IL1β	F:GTGATGCCAACGTGCAGTCT	up	41.07	56.25
		R:TGGGCCAGCCAGCACTAG			
NM_213867	IL8	F:AGTTTTCCTGCTTTCTGCAGCT	up	4.16	8.26
		R:TGGCATCGAAGTTCTGCACT			
NM_214194	CD40	F:AGAACCACCCACTTCATGCAA	up	2.08	4.23
		R:TGGCGGGCACAAATTACA			
NM_001164511	BCL2A1	F:TTTGCATTTGAAGGTATTCTCATGA	up	4.15	8.95
		R:AATCTCCTTGTACGTGTCCACATC			
NM_214022	TNF-α	F:CGTTGTAGCCAATGTCAAAGCC	up	6.88	10.79
		R:TGCCCAGATTCAGCAAAGTCCA			
NM_001110425	CD302	F:TGGTTTCACCACAGTTTTCTCAA	down	2.48	3.25
		R:CCTCTGCAACTACCAAAACACAAT			
NM_001206441	TAP2	F:GGACTCTTCGGCTTCATGCT	up	2.16	2.03
		R:CGCTATCGTGAGAGGCATCTG			
NM_001113707	SLA	F:CACACACACCCAACCCTTCTG	down	3.01	2.85
		R:TGGTTTTGGCCACTTGCA			
NM_214162	CASP1	F:GCCAAGAGGGAGCCTCAAG	down	2.1	6.71
		R:CTCTGCTGACTTTTCTTTCCATAGC			
NM_001204769	NLRX1	F:TCTGCTGCGCAAATACATGTT	down	2.11	5.32
		R: CCATAGCGGCCCACATACTT			
NM_213779	CCL4	F: GCAAGACCATGAAGCTCTGC			
		R: AAGCTTCCGCACGGTGTATG			
NM_001164515	CCL8	F:AAGACCAAAGCCGACAAGGA			
		R: TCATGGAATTCTGGACCCACT			
NM_001001861	CXCL2	F: CCGTGCAAGGAATTCACCTC			
		R: TGCGGGGTTGAGACAAACTT			
NM_001008691	CXCL10	F: CCCACATGTTGAGATCATTGC			
		R CATCCTTATCAGTAGTGCCG			
	GAPDH	F:ACATGGCCTCCAAGGAGTAAGA			
		R:GATCGAGTTGGGGCTGTGACT			

*Fold change.

normalization. Alternatively, the data could indicate that results from the microarray analysis are good indicators of overall changes in gene expression.

Analysis of DE genes by gene ontology (GO)

All DE genes were annotated on the basis of the gene ontology (GO) database using Visualization and Integrated Discovery (DAVID). At 6 hpi, the DE genes mainly clustered into functional groups: inflammatory response (e.g. IL-1β, CCL4, CXCL10, CD14, TNF-α), immune response (e.g. TLR2, NFKBIA, IL7R, IL-8), apoptosis and anti-apoptosis (e.g. CASP10, BCL2A1, PIK3R1, NFKBIA, BTG2, PSEN1), programmed cell death (e.g. CXCR4, SOD2, NFKB1, PRK), defense response (e.g. TLR2, S100A8, CCL3L1, CD40), signal transmission, signal transduction cytokine production, I-kappaB kinase/NF-κB cascade and so on (Figure 1B).

Of interest, was the over-expression of up-regulated genes associated with immune responses and inflammatory responses, suggesting an important role for these genes in *M. hyopneumoniae* infections (Table 2). Of these genes, 20 genes were up-regulated more than five-fold, and 8 genes (CCL4, IL1β, IL1α, CCL2, ISG15, CCL8, LOC780407, CXCL2) up-regulated more than 10-fold.

In addition to the functional groups observed at 6 hpi (namely inflammatory response, immune response, apoptosis, programmed cell death, signal transduction and so forth), the following functional groups of DE genes were observed at 15 hpi: cell-cell adhesion (e.g. CD274, CCN2, CLDN7, CD2), protein ubiquitination (e.g. MAPK9, PSMB8, PSMD10, PSMA5, ISG15), T cell proliferation, protein transport and so forth (Figure 1D). Similarly, a greater number of genes associated with immune and inflammatory responses were found at 15 hpi (Table S1).

Pathway analysis

To gain insights into the different biological processes associated with *M. hyopneumoniae* infections at different times post-infection,

Table 2. The DE genes associated with immune and inflammatory responses at 6 hpi.

SEQ_ID	p-value	FC Change	GeneName	description
NM_213779	0.000298	52.12223	CCL4	Sus scrofa chemokine (C-C motif) ligand 4 (CCL4), mRNA.
NM_214055	0.000173	41.07524	IL1B	Sus scrofa interleukin 1, beta (IL1B), mRNA.
NM_214029	0.001527	20.72427	IL1A	Sus scrofa interleukin 1, alpha (IL1A), mRNA.
NM_214214	0.000228	13.97029	CCL2	Sus scrofa chemokine (C-C motif) ligand 2 (CCL2), mRNA.
NM_001128469	0.0000129	13.800437	ISG15	Sus scrofa ISG15 ubiquitin-like modifier (ISG15), mRNA.
NM_001164515	0.000172	12.3193	CCL8	Sus scrofa chemokine (C-C motif) ligand 8 (CCL8), mRNA.
NM_001161434	7.71E-05	10.32473	LOC780407	Sus scrofa chemokine ligand 24-like protein (LOC780407), mRNA.
NM_001001861	0.000775	10.01722	CXCL2	Sus scrofa chemokine (C-X-C motif) ligand 2 (CXCL2), mRNA.
NM_001146128	0.008214	8.429539	IL7R	Sus scrofa interleukin 7 receptor (IL7R), mRNA.
ENSSSCT0000 0013077	0.000562	7.193156	NFKBIZ	Sus scrofa chromosome 13 Sscrofa10.2 partial sequence 165990981..166988044 reannotated via EnsEMBL
NM_214084	0.003889	7.036763	VEGFA	Sus scrofa vascular endothelial growth factor A (VEGFA), mRNA.
NM_214022	0.00066	6.881882	TNF	Sus scrofa tumor necrosis factor (TNF), mRNA.
XM_001929223	6.41E-05	6.076357	PNP	PREDICTED: Sus scrofa purine nucleoside phosphorylase (PNP), mRNA.
NM_214061	0.000237	5.901434	MX1	Sus scrofa myxovirus (influenza virus) resistance 1, interferon-inducible protein p78 (mouse) (MX1), mRNA.
NM_001008691	0.007205	5.879376	CXCL10	Sus scrofa chemokine (C-X-C motif) ligand 10 (CXCL10), mRNA.
NM_001100194	0.011522	5.642215	IFIH1	Sus scrofa interferon induced with helicase C domain 1 (IFIH1), mRNA.
NM_001160271	1.18E-05	5.595223	S100A8	Sus scrofa S100 calcium binding protein A8 (S100A8), mRNA.
XM_001925952	0.002127	4.301922	IFIT5	PREDICTED: Sus scrofa interferon-induced protein with tetratricopeptide repeats 5 (IFIT5), mRNA.
NM_213867	0.000619	4.162192	IL8	Sus scrofa interleukin 8 (IL8), mRNA.
NM_001164511	0.000316	4.145637	BCL2A1	Sus scrofa BCL2-related protein A1 (BCL2A1), mRNA.
NM_001048232	0.000114	4.033666	NFKB1	Sus scrofa nuclear factor of kappa light polypeptide gene enhancer in B-cells 1 (NFKB1), mRNA.
NM_001044552	5.65E-05	3.686546	LOC733 603	Sus scrofa serum amyloid A2 (LOC733603), mRNA.
NM_214303	4.32E-06	3.381383	OAS1	Sus scrofa 2'-5'-oligoadenylate synthetase 1, 40/46kDa (OAS1), mRNA.
XM_003127915	0.009899	3.04153	IFI44	PREDICTED: Sus scrofa interferon-induced protein 44 (IFI44), mRNA.
NM_001031796	0.000513	2.980078	OAS2	Sus scrofa 2'-5'-oligoadenylate synthetase 2, 69/71kDa (OAS2), mRNA.
XM_001924787	0.00041	2.957249	LOC1001 57000	PREDICTED: Sus scrofa chromosome 6 open reading frame 4, transcript variant 1 (LOC100157000), mRNA.
NM_001097416	0.012537	2.864776	MX2	Sus scrofa myxovirus (influenza virus) resistance 2 (mouse) (MX2), mRNA.
NM_001097445	0.000273	2.848918	CD14	Sus scrofa CD14 molecule (CD14), mRNA.
NM_001005150	2.73E-05	2.829609	NFKBIA	Sus scrofa nuclear factor of kappa light polypeptide gene enhancer in B-cells inhibitor, alpha (NFKBIA), mRNA.
NM_001177906	0.001647	2.748172	S100A9	Sus scrofa S100 calcium binding protein A9 (S100A9), mRNA.
NM_214379	0.006056	2.74367	PPARG	Sus scrofa peroxisome proliferator-activated receptor gamma (PPARG), mRNA.
NM_001244354	0.026452	2.451839	SEC61A1	Sus scrofa Sec61 alpha 1 subunit (S. cerevisiae) (SEC61A1), mRNA.
NM_001033011	0.008059	2.327992	FCGR1A	Sus scrofa Fc fragment of IgG, high affinity Ia, receptor (CD64) (FCGR1A), mRNA.
NM_001243435	0.025967	2.307106	ADORA3	Sus scrofa adenosine A3 receptor (ADORA3), transcript variant 1, mRNA.
NM_213761	0.016065	2.221215	TLR2	Sus scrofa toll-like receptor 2 (TLR2), mRNA.

Table 2. Cont.

SEQ_ID	p-value	FC Change	GeneName	description
AM177151	0.03376	2.168304	LOC1001 25542	Sus scrofa partial VDJ heavy chain gene for immunoglobulin heavy chain variable region, clone Pig3 CD5+ C13.
NM_214194	0.004432	2.082431	CD40	Sus scrofa CD40 molecule, TNF receptor superfamily member 5 (CD40), mRNA.
XM_003122031	0.001052	2.061163	TRIM14	PREDICTED: Sus scrofa tripartite motif containing 14 (TRIM14), mRNA.
NM_001078667	0.01484	2.051649	PSEN1	Sus scrofa presenilin 1 (PSEN1), mRNA.
AM177169	0.034076	2.033368	LOC100 125541	Sus scrofa partial VDJ heavy chain gene for immunoglobulin heavy chain variable region, clone Pig3 CD5- F12.
NM_001160272	6.64E-05	2.027732	S100A12	Sus scrofa S100 calcium binding protein A12 (S100A12), mRNA.
AF248289	0.048925	2.001558	LOC100 037926	Sus scrofa clone 3 immunoglobulin heavy chain mRNA, partial cds.

pathway mapping of DE genes according to the Kyoto Encyclopedia of Genes and Genomes (KEGG) pathway database was performed. At 6 hpi, the predominant pathways included the cytokine-cytokine receptor interaction, chemokine signaling pathway, RIG-I-like receptor signaling pathway, Toll-like receptor signaling pathway, nucleotide-binding oligomerization domains (Nod)-like receptor (NLR) signaling pathway, proteasome, apoptosis signaling pathway, Cell adhesion molecules, Jak-STAT signaling pathway and PPAR signaling pathway. These results suggest that at an early stage of infection, the host initiated different strategies to activate immune and inflammatory responses to prevent infection (Table 3).

At 15 hpi, the phagosome, antigen processing and presentation, protein processing in endoplasmic reticulum became the most significant pathways. Other dominant pathways at late stages of infection included phagosome, RIG-I-like receptor signaling pathway, PPAR signaling pathway gap junction and tight junction (Table S2).

STRING analysis of the relationships between DE genes

DE genes were analyzed using STRING for predicting network of proteins encoded by DE genes [16,17]. Predictions of functional association networks for all DE genes encoded proteins at 6 hpi are presented in Figure 2. The results indicated that genes MAP3KB, NFKB1, TNF, IL-1β, IL-8, TLR2, IKBA, BCL2L1, CD14, CXCR4, CXCL10 and IL-1R2 are associated according to experimental evidence, with involvement in many signaling pathways and other immune responses. The IL-1β, TLR2, PLK2, TNF-α, IKBA, IL-18 and TANK genes are involved in the NF-kappa-B pathway and in other immune responses. According to the STRING analysis a number of proteins (e.g. IL-1β, NFKB1, TLR2, IRF3, IL-7R, S100A8, BCL2A1, and ISG15) are integral molecules, linking to other proteins. However, many proteins failed to link to other proteins, and as such their functions were unrelated or unknown.

Based on database evidence, inflammatory cytokines IL-1β, IL-8 and TNF-α are the central genes of these protein interaction networks. According to text mining data, more than 60 DE genes were associated with inflammatory cytokines, including MYD88,

Table 3. DE genes analysis base on KEGG at 6 hpi.

Pathway Name	Number	Gene
Cytokine-cytokine receptor interaction	15	CCL2, CCL3L1, CCL4, CD40, CXCL10, CXCR4, IFNAR2, IL10RB, IL18, IL1A, IL1B, IL1R2, IL7R, IL8, TNF
Chemokine signaling pathway	13	CCL2, CCL3L1, CCL4, CCL8, CRK, CXCL10, CXCL2, CXCL2, CXCR4, IL8, NFKB1, NFKBIA, SRC
RIG-I-like receptor signaling pathway	11	CASP10, CXCL10, DHX58, IFIH1, IL8, IRF3, ISG15, NFKB1, NFKBIA, TANK, TNF
Toll-like receptor signaling pathway	11	CD14, CD40, CXCL10, IFNAR2, IL1B, IL8, IRF3, NFKB1, NFKBIA, TLR2, TNF
NOD-like receptor signaling pathway	8	CCL2, IL18, IL1B, IL8, NFKB1, NFKBIA, TNF, TNFAIP3
Phagosome	8	ATP6V1B2, C1R, CALR, CD14, FCGR1A, OLR1, SEC61A1, TLR2
Apoptosis	7	BIRC3, CASP10, IL1A, IL1B, NFKB1, NFKBIA, TNF
Cell adhesion molecules	7	CD274, CD40, CLDN4, CLDN7, ITGB8, SDC4, VCAM1
Jak-STAT signaling pathway	7	IFNAR2, IL10RB,IL7R, MYC, PIAS2, SOCS1, SOCS7
PPAR signaling pathway	6	ACSL1, ACSL4, ACSL5, GK, OLR1, PPARG

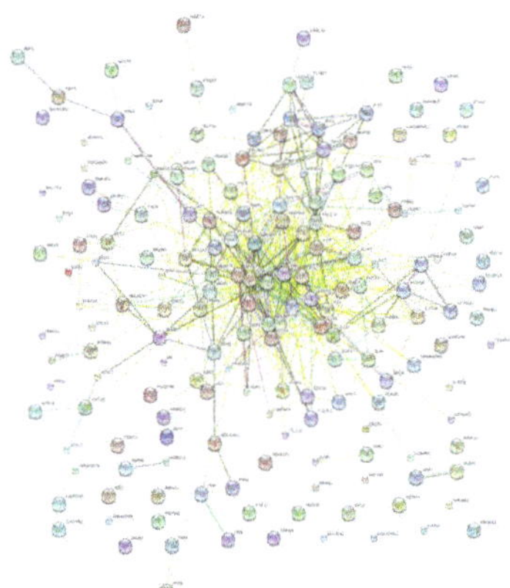

Figure 2. STRING analysis of the relationship between DE genes. The DE genes in PAM cells infected *M. hyopneumoniae* were analyzed using the STRING database. The network nodes represent the proteins encoded by the DE genes. Seven different colored lines link a number of nodes and represent seven types of evidence used in predicting associations. A red line indicates the presence of fusion evidence; a green line represents neighborhood evidence; a blue line represents coocurrence evidence; a purple line represents experimental evidence; a yellow line represents textmining evidence; a light blue line represents database evidence and a black line represents co-expression evidence.

CD14, AKT1, IRF7, IRF3, CCL4, CCL8, CCL2, CXCL2, CXCL10, BCL2A1, PPARG, CD40, ADORA3 and so on.

Expression analyses of chemokines

When compared with the mock-inoculated PAMs, *M. hyopneumoniae*-infected PAMs inducted significantly higher levels of the chemokines from the transcription analysis data (Table 2). To understand the pattern of some chemokines expression in PAMs infected with *M. hyopneumoniae*, RNAs were extracted at different times post inoculation from the infected group and controls, and subjected to qRT-PCR analysis. The results showed that PAMs infected with *M. hyopneumoniae* exhibited significantly increased expression of CCL4, CXCL2 and CXCL10 mRNA at 6 h post-infection, and decreased at a steady-state level, with maximal production at 6 h post-infection. The CCL8 exhibited significantly increased expression at 6–24 h post-infection, and the maximal production was at 12 h post-infection (Figure 3).

(A)

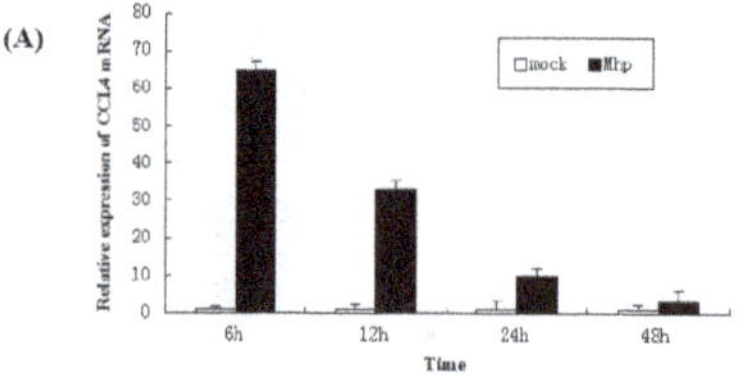

(B)

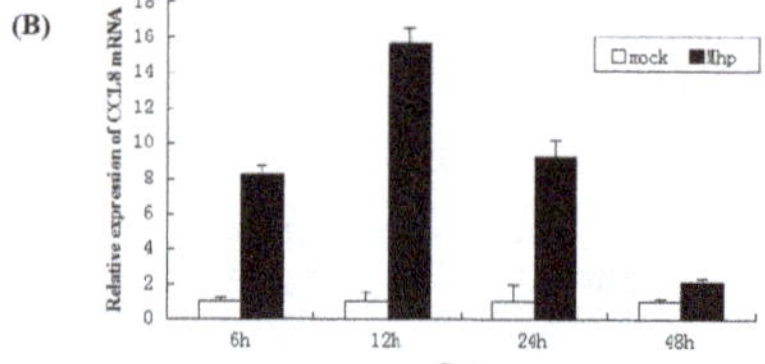

(C)

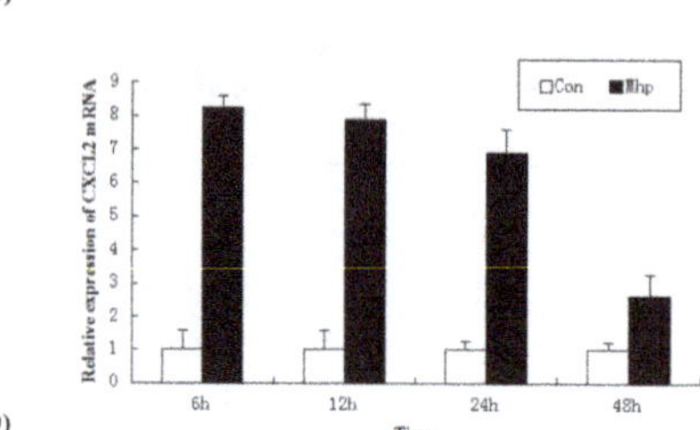

(D)

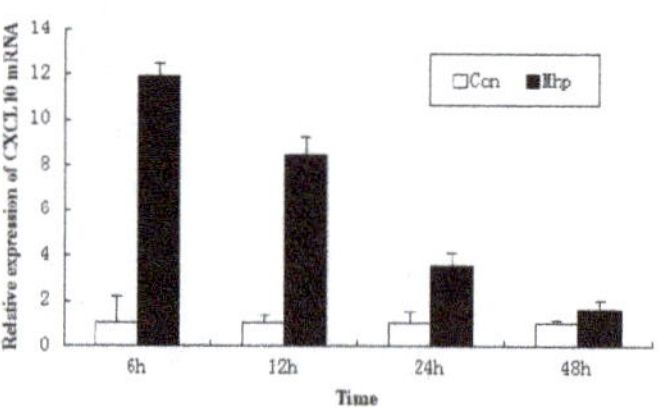

Figure 3. Expression kinetics of chemokines in PAM. PAMs were mock-infected, infected with *M. hyopneumoniae*. Cells were collected at the indicated time points, and subjected to real-time PCR to analyze the expression of CCL4 (A), CCL8 (B), CXCL2 (C) and CXCL10 (D).

Discussion

M. hyopneumoniae is the primary cause of a chronic respiratory disease in pigs. And Mycoplasma infection correlates with the infection of other secondary respiratory pathogens by inducing the immunomodulation of host animals [18–21]. However, the mechanisms of immunomodulation are elusive. The previous study reported that the lung tissue injury about *M. hyopneumoniae* infections appear to be mainly caused by the host response [22]. And it indicated that the expression of proinflammatory cytokines were increased in the lung of *M. hyopneumoniae*-infected pigs [4–9]. These studies also suggested that the activation of host immune system played an important role in the pathogenesis and immune mechanisms for *M. hyopneumoniae* infection. Despite the fact that the current vaccine strategy can efficiently control *M. hyopneumoniae* infection, immunization failures exist in the field, and the molecular mechanisms underlying PRDC caused by *M. hyopneumoniae* remain largely unknown [23]. The present study aimed to identify genes involved in the immune response against *M. hyopneumoniae* in primary alveolar macrophages. Furthermore, by generating a comprehensive transcriptomic profile of the temporal *M. hyopneumoniae* pathogenic process in the host cells, we hoped to gain insights into the underlying molecular interactions and signaling pathways in the *M. hyopneumoniae* infection process.

This study is the first to report the use of GeneChip Porcine Genome Array for the investigation of transcriptional responses to *M. hyopneumoniae* infection. We found that more than 2000 transcripts with significant differential expression were produced in response to *M. hyopneumoniae* infections of PAM (Figure 1). Results from Gene Ontology, KEGG pathway and STRING analysis suggested that these DE genes belonged to a variety of functional categories and signal pathways.

Analysis of the expression of porcine genes after infection with *M. hyopneumoniae* showed that a large set of DE genes were involved in the immune response. TLR signaling plays an essential role in the innate immune response. TLR2 (up-regulated 2.22-fold) belongs to the TLR family and is expressed most abundantly in PAM (Table 2). TLR2 mediates the host response to mycoplasmal lipoproteins and has a fundamental role in pathogen recognition and activation of innate immunity. NF-κB (up-regulated 7.19 fold) is a family of inducible transcription factors involving pathogen- or cytokine-induced immune and inflammatory responses as well as cell proliferation and survival [24,25]. The previously study indicated that *M. hyopneumoniae* infection could induce pro-inflammatory cytokines by the activation of the NF-κB [26]. These studies implied that *M. hyopneumoniae* might have developed sophisticated strategies for activation or inhibition of NF-κB pathway in order to survive in host cells. Further investigation to evaluate the exact mechanisms of *M. hyopneumoniae* in modulating NF-κB pathway will be required. Another receptor for bacteria, CD14 (up-regulated 2.85-fold) cooperates with TLR4 (which also recognizes lipopolysaccharides) via MYD88, leading to inflammatory responses in mycoplasmal infections [27,28]. The signal transducer MYD88 (up-regulated 2.1 fold) is an adapter for almost all TLR signaling pathways, and acts via interferon regulatory factor 7 (IRF7), leading to activation of NF-κB, cytokine secretion and the inflammatory response. It was similar to the reports, which suggested that the interaction of *M. arthritidis* mitogen with TLR2 and TLR4 might play an important role in disease outcomes by *M. arthritidis* [29].

Many DE genes in this study are involved in the inflammatory response, including CCL4, IL-1β, IL-1α, CCL2, CCL8, CXCL2, TNF-α, CXCL10, IL-8, S100A8, PPARG; (peroxisome proliferator-activated receptor gamma), CD40 and so on. Furthermore, eleven genes involved with the TLR signaling pathway, eleven with the RLR signaling pathway, eight with the NLR signaling pathway, and thirteen with the chemokine signaling pathway, were found to be regulated (Table 3). These results reflect the up-stream signal cascades that could lead to secretion of inflammatory cytokines and chemokines.

Cytokines and chemokines are central mediators during host-pathogen interactions, including the clearance of invading microorganisms, as well as the initiation, progression, and resolution of inflammation in response to various microbes. In this study, chemokines CCL4, CCL2, CCL8, CXCL2 and CXCL10 was up-regulated more than 5-fold. CCL4, also known as macrophage inflammatory protein-1β (MIP-1β) is a CC chemokine with specificity for CCR5 receptors. It is a chemoattractant for natural killer cells, monocytes and a variety of other immune cells [30]. Cytokine CCL2 (chemokine (C-C motif) ligand 2, up-regulated 26.14-fold) is thought to bind to chemokine receptors CCR2 and CCR4. Studies demonstrating the contribution of T cells to disease pathogenesis, suggest the recruitment of T cells by chemokines (CCL4 and CCL8) elicited at the site of infection would most likely contribute to the pathogenesis of mycoplasma disease [31]. CXCL2 and CXCL10 are chemokines of the CXC subfamily, and CXC chemokines are particularly significant for leukocyte infiltration in inflammatory diseases. The expression kinetics of some chemokines showed that PAMs infected with *M. hyopneumoniae* exhibited significantly increased expression of these chemokines mRNA at 6 h post-infection, and decreased at a steady-state level, with maximal production at 6 h post-infection (Fig. 3A, 3C and 3D). It suggested that *M. hyopneumoniae* induced an inflammatory response at the early time point (6 HPI) of infection.

IL-1β, IL-8 and TNF-α are acute-phase proinflammatory mediators that promote inflammation and induce fever, tissue destruction, and, in some cases, shock and death [32], they play an integral role in shaping the inflammatory response against pathogens. Our study showed that *M. hyopneumoniae* could induce IL-1β, IL-8 and TNF-α expression (Table 2) in PAMs at 6 hpi. These results are in good agreement with previous study [4–9]. These results suggested that *M. hyopneumoniae* infection modulates the immune response of pigs by inducing several cytokines, and promotes the inflammatory response. Then it maybe cause immunosuppression to infected pigs.

Cell adhesion molecules (CAMs) perform various functions in fundamental cellular processes, including polarization, movement, proliferation and survival [33]. We discovered several DE genes that were related to cell adhesion during *M. hyopneumoniae* infection, including CD274, CLDN4, CLDN7, ITGB8, SDC4 and VCAM1. CD274 (up-regulated 4.11-fold) also known as programmed cell death 1 ligand 1 (PD-L1), which has been speculated to play a major role in suppressing the immune system during particular events such as pregnancy, tissue allografts, autoimmune disease and other disease states [34]. The VCAM-1(up-regulated 2.68-fold) also known as vascular cell adhesion molecule 1 or cluster of differentiation 106 (CD106), mediates the adhesion of lymphocytes, monocytes, eosinophils, and basophils to vascularendothelium. It also functions in leukocyte-endothelial cell signal transduction [35]. These cell adhesion molecules maybe play a important role in pathogenicity of *M. hyopneumoniae.*

Apoptosis plays an essential role in the development and maintenance of homeostasis in multicellular organisms. Moreover, apoptosis plays a crucial role in the pathogenesis of a number of infections [36]. Apoptosis is often considered as an innate defense mechanism that limits pathogen infection by eliminating infected cells. Bai et al indicated that the LAMP derived from *M. hyopneumoniae* induced apoptosis in porcine alveolar macrophage cell line through enhancing the production of NO, superoxide burst, and activation of caspase-3 [37]. In this study, 34 of the DE genes identified were known to be involved in apoptosis after *M. hyopneumoniae* infection. Such as, the caspase-10, TIMP1 (tissue inhibitor of metalloproteinases 1), BCL2-related protein A1, and PMAIP1 (Phorbol-12-myristate-13-acetate-induced protein 1) were up-regulated at 6 hpi to various degrees. Furthermore, seven genes were involved in the apoptosis signaling pathway (Table 3). BCL2-related protein A1 belongs to the Bcl-2 protein family, and is considered a pivotal player in apoptosis, especially for mitochondria-mediated apoptosis. Expression of PMAIP1 is regulated by the tumor suppressor p53, and PMAIP1 has been shown to be involved in p53-mediated apoptosis [38]. The glycoprotein TIMP1 is expressed from several tissues of biological organisms, is able to promote cell proliferation in a wide range of cell types, and may also possess an anti-apoptotic function [39]. Not surprisingly, pathogens target these proteins to induce or inhibit apoptosis. These findings were beneficial to research the mechanisms about *M. hyopneumoniae* infection induces apoptosis, and will contribute to a greater understanding of pathogenesis.

In summary, this is the first study to evaluate the gene expression profile of *M. hyopneumoniae* infected PAMs *in vitro*. Microarray analysis showed that the expressions of more than 2000 genes were altered after *M. hyopneumoniae* infection. These DE genes were involved in the inflammatory response, innate immune response, apoptosis, defense response, signal transduction, cell adhesion and so on. The data generated from the analysis of the overall pattern of innate immune signaling and proinflammatory, apoptotic and cell adhesion pathways activated by *M. hyopneumoniae* infection, could be used to screen potential host agents for reducing prevalence of *M. hyopneumoniae* infection, and to develop a greater understanding of the pathogenesis of *M. hyopneumoniae*.

Materials and Methods

Ethics

All pigs were purchased from the farm of Jiangsu Center of Disease Control, Nanjing, China. The healthy pigs (serologically negative for PRRSV, *M. hyopneumoniae* and porcine circovirus type 2) were sacrificed by the bloodletting after anesthesia under ethical approval granted by the Jiangsu Academy of Agricultural Sciences. The protocol was approved by the Science and Technology Agency of Jiangsu Province. The approval ID is NKYVET 2012-0035, granted by the Jiangsu Academy of Agricultural Sciences Experimental Animal ethics committee. All efforts were made to minimize animal's suffering. The PAMs were obtained from the sacrificed pigs under ethical approval for the purposes of research. The diseased piglets were not sacrificed.

M. hyopneumoniae and cells

M. hyopneumoniae field strain XLW-1 was isolated from diseased pigs in Jiangsu Province, China. Porcine alveolar macrophages (PAMs) obtained from three 4–5-week-old *M. hyopneumoniae*-negative piglets, and serologically negative for PRRSV and porcine circovirus type 2 (PCV2), were prepared as described previously [14,15]. Prior to infection, PAMs were mixed and confirmed negative for *M. hyopneumoniae*, PRRSV, PCV2, pseudorabies virus, and classical swine fever virus by PCR and RT-PCR. RPMI 1640 medium and fetal bovine serum (FBS) were obtained from GIBCO (Invitrogen). The isolated cells were grown and maintained in RPMI 1640 medium containing 10% (v/v) FBS at 37°C with 5% CO_2.

In order to simulate natural conditions of *M. hyopneumoniae* infection, the tracheal ring were infected first. Tracheas were collected as previously described [40]. Briefly, the tracheas were excised aseptically from pigs and submerged in chilled PBS. Tracheas were washed with PBS, and transverse sections (approximately 0.5 cm thick) were prepared by making an incision between the tracheal rings. Each tracheal ring was placed in a 30-mm culture plate insert (Millipore, Bedford, Mass.) containing 3 ml of complete medium.

Experimental design

The controls included uninfected PAMs and tracheas. *M. hyopneumoniae* (10^8 CCU/ml) was inoculated onto the tracheal rings 10 h prior to their addition to PAMs (approximately 10^7 cells). The *M. hyopneumoniae* group included the *M. hyopneumoniae*-infected tracheal ring, and the corresponding supernatant was transferred to culture PAMs. The mixture incubated at 37°C with 5% CO_2. PAMs were harvested from the vessels' surface with a cell scraper at 6 and 15 hpi, and stored at −80°C until use.

RNA preparation

Total RNA were extracted from PAM of each groups with Trizol (Invitrogen) then quantified using the Nano-Drop 1000 Spectrophotometer (Thermo Fisher Scientific Inc., USA). The quality of the RNA was checked by formaldehyde denaturing gel electrophoresis in 1.2% agarose gels, which showed dispersed bands (28S and 18S) without any obvious smearing patterns that would indicate degradation.

Microarray hybridization

The RNA samples were sent to KangChen Bio-tech, China, for microarray hybridization. Each RNA sample from different PAM treatments was hybridized to one Roche NimbleGen Porcine Genome Expression Array (Roche). Briefly, double-stranded cDNA was synthesized from 6 mg of total RNA using a T7-oligo (dT) primer. The cDNA was further purified and converted into cRNA using an in vitro transcription reaction. Five *mg* cRNA was reverse transcribed to cDNA, fragmented, and then labeled with Cy3-dCTP (GE Healthcare) using Klenow. These labeled cDNA fragments were hybridized to NimbleGen Porcine Genome Expression Arrays for 16 h at 42°C using the Roche NimbleGen Hybridization System. Afterwards, the GeneChips were washed, stained, and then scanned with a Roche-NimbleGen MS200. The Roche NimbleGen Porcine Genome Expression Array contains over 135,000 probe sets, representing 45,023 transcripts and variants of pig from the database of RefSeq, Unigene and TIGR.

Microarray data analysis

Raw data and statistical analyses were performed with Feature Extraction software. Normalization was performed per chip (normalized to 50th percentile) and per gene (normalized to the median) respectively. A statistical analysis of variance (ANOVA) model was applied to the data and the significance was showed by accepting a false discovery rate (FDR) of 0.05. A further cut-off threshold was applied based on a fold change of 2.0 between infected and control cells. Then all the DE genes were performed for hierarchical cluster (Ver.3.0) and TreeView (Ver.1.1.1) analyses. Genes with significant similarities to the transcripts in nr database based on BLASTX searches were selected for GO analysis, performed by MAS 3.0 software which was based on DAVID database (CapitalBio, Beijing, China). Annotation results were obtained by inputting the list of gene symbol as identifier. The pathway analysis was done by using the MAS 3.0 software which was based on the Kyoto Encyclopedia of Genes and Genomes (KEGG) database (http://www.genome.jp/kegg/pathway.html). Differentially expressed (DE) genes in porcine PAM infected with WD or KO were analyzed using STRING (http://string-db.org/), a database of known and predicted protein interactions. The raw and processed data discussed in this publication have been deposited in NCBI's Gene Expression Omnibus and are accessible through GEO series accession number GPL17577.

Quantitative RT-PCR analysis

Quantitative RT-PCR (qRT-PCR) was used to validate selected data from the microarray experiments, and to follow the expression of a subset of genes over time. For each group, total RNA was extracted from PAMs using Trizol (Invitrogen), and 5 μg included as template for first strand cDNA synthesis using the Superscript II cDNA amplification System (Invitrogen), according to the manufacturer's instructions. GAPDH was included as an endogenous control. The specific primers used in the qRT-PCR assays are listed in Table 1. qRT-PCR was performed in triplicate for all reactions using the SYBR green detection system and an ABI 7500 real-time PCR system (Applied Biosystems, Warrington, UK). Relative standard curves for target and endogenous control primer pairs were performed to verify comparable PCR efficiencies, and once established the comparative (2-delta-delta) Ct method was applied.

Expression analyses of chemokines

Total RNA was extracted from PAMs harvested at different times post-inoculation from each infection groups. CCL4, CCL8, CXCL2, CXCL10 expression were measured using specific primers (Table 1) and qRT-PCR, as described above. GAPDH was used as the endogenous control.

Statistical analysis of qRT-PCR data

Statistical analyses were carried out using Microsoft Excel 2007 (Microsoft Co., USA). Differences between groups were assessed by one-way repeated measures ANOVA, followed by Tukey's multiple comparison tests. *P*-values less than 0.05 were considered to be statistically significant.

Author Contributions

Conceived and designed the experiments: LB HK SG. Performed the experiments: LB. Analyzed the data: LB. Contributed reagents/materials/analysis tools: DL SB YZ LM FZ WY WH. Wrote the paper: LB.

References

1. Maes D, Verdonck M, Deluyker H, Kruif A (1996) Enzootic pneumonia in pigs. Vet Q 18: 104–9.
2. Thacker E (2006) Mycoplasmal diseases. The Iowa State University Press, Ames, IA, pp. 701–717.
3. Blanchard B, Vena M, Cavalier A, Lannic J, Gouranton J, et al. (1992) Electron microscopic observation of the respiratory tract of SPF piglets inoculated with *Mycoplasma hyopneumoniae*. Vet Microbiol 30: 329–341.
4. Sarradell J, Andrada M, Ramairez AS, Fernandez A, Gaomez JC, et al. (2003) A morphologic and immunohistochemical study of the bronchus-associated lymphoid tissue of pigs naturally infected with *Mycoplasma hyopneumoniae*. Vet Pathol 40: 395–404.
5. Baskerville A (1972) Development of the early lesions in experimental enzootic pneumonia of pig: an ultrastructural and histological study. Res Vet Sci 13: 570–578.
6. Muneta Y, Minagawa Y, Shimoji Y, Ogawa Y, Hikono H, et al. (2008) Immune response of gnotobiotic piglets against *Mycoplasma hyopneumoniae*. J. Vet. Med. Sci 70: 1065–1070.
7. Lorenzo H, Quesada O, Assunçao P, Castro A, Rodríguez F (2006) Cytokine expression in porcine lungs experimentally infected with *Mycoplasma hyopneumoniae*. Vet Immunol Immunopathol 109: 199–207.
8. Rodriguez F, Ramirez GA, Sarradell J, Andrada M, Lorenzo H (2004) Immunohistochemical labelling of cytokines in lung lesions of pigs naturally infected with *Mycoplasma hyopneumoniae*. J Comp Pathol 130: 306–12.
9. Meyns T, Maes D, Calus D, Ribbens S, Dewulf J, et al. (2007) Interactions of highly and low virulent *Mycoplasma hyopneumoniae* isolates with the respiratory tract of pigs. Vet Microbiol 120: 87–95.
10. McGuire K, Glass EJ (2005) The expanding role of microarrays in the investigation of macrophage responses to pathogens. Vet Immunol Immunop 105:259–275.
11. Nau GJ, Richomond JF, Schlesinger A, Jennings EG, Lander ES, et al. (2002) Human macrophage activation programs induced by bacterial pathogens. P Natl Acad Sci USA 99:1503–1508.
12. Liu ML, Fang LR, Tan C, Long TS, Chen HC, et al. (2011) Understanding Streptococcus suis serotype 2 infection in pigs through a transcriptional Approach. BMC Genomics 12: 253
13. Ma Z, Zhang H, Yi L, Fan H, Lu C (2012) Microarray analysis of the effect of Streptococcus equi subsp zooepidemicus M-like protein in infecting porcine pulmonary alveolar macrophage. PLoS One 7: e36452.
14. Li W, Liu S, Wang Y, Deng F, Yan W, et al. (2013) Transcription analysis of the porcine alveolar macrophage response to porcine circovirus type 2. BMC Genomics 14: 353.
15. Wang Y, Liu C, Fang Y, Li W, Liu S, et al. (2012) Transcription analysis on response of porcine alveolar macrophages to Haemophilus parasuis. BMC Genomics 13:68.
16. Bonetta L (2010) Protein-protein interactions: Interactome under construction. Nature 468: 851–854.
17. Von MC, Jensen LJ, Snel B, Hooper SD, Krupp M, et al. (2005) STRING: known and predicted protein-protein associations, integrated and transferred across organisms. Nucleic Acids Res 33: 433–437.
18. Kyriakis SC, Saoulidis K, Lekkas S, Miliotis CC, Papoutsis PA, et al. (2002) The effects of immunomodulation on the clinical and pathological expression of postweaning multisystemic wasting syndrome. J. Comp. Pathol 126: 38–46.
19. Thacker EL, Halbur PG, Ross RF, Thanawongnuwech R, Thacker BJ (1999). *Mycoplasma hyopneumoniae* potentiation of porcine reproductive and respiratory syndrome virus-induced pneumonia. J. Clin. Microbiol 37: 620–627.
20. Yazawa S, Okada M, Ono M, Fujii S, Okuda Y, et al. (2004) Experimental dual infection of pigs with an H1N1 swine influenza virus (A/Sw/Hok/2/81) and *Mycoplasma hyopneumoniae*. Vet Microbiol 98: 221–8.
21. Opriessnig T, Thacker EL, Yu S, Fenaux M, Meng XJ, et al. (2004) Experimental reproduction of postweaning multisystemic wasting syndrome in pigs by dual infection with *Mycoplasma hyopneumoniae* and porcine circovirus type 2. Vet Pathol 41: 624–40.
22. Thacker E, Nilubol D, Halbur P (2006) Efficacy of Aureomycin1 chlortetracycline (CTC) granulated premix in decreasing the potentiation of PRRSV pneumonia by *Mycoplasma hyopneumoniae*. In: Proceedings of the 37th Annual Meeting, Am. Assoc. Swine Vet., Kansas City, Missouri, pp. 153–155.
23. Maes D, Segales J, Meyns T, Sibila M, Pieters M, et al. (2008) Control of *Mycoplasma hyopneumoniae* infections in pigs. Vet Microbiol 126: 297–309.
24. Caamano J, Hunter CA (2002) NF-kappaB family of transcription factors: central regulators of innate and adaptive immune functions. Clin microbiol rev 15:414–429.
25. Li Q, Verma IM (2002) NF-kappaB regulation in the immune system. Nat Rev Immunol 2:725–734.
26. Damte D, Lee SJ, Hwang MH, Gebru E, Choi MJ, et al. (2011) Inflammatory responses to *Mycoplasma hyopneumoniae* in murine alveolar macrophage cell lines. N Z Vet J. 59: 185–90.
27. He J, You X, Zeng Y, Yu M, Zuo L, et al. (2009) Mycoplasma genitalium-derived lipid-associated membrane proteins activate NF-kappaB through toll-like receptors 1, 2, and 6 and CD14 in a MyD88-dependent pathway. Clin Vaccine Immunol 16: 1750–7.
28. He J, Wang S, Zeng Y, You X, Ma X, et al. (2013) Binding of CD14 to mycoplasma genitalium-Derived lipid-Associated membrane proteins upregulates TNF-α. Inflammation 9: 26.
29. Mu HH, Hasebe A, Van Schelt A, Cole BC (2011) Novel interactions of a microbial superantigen with TLR2 and TLR4 differentially regulate IL-17 and Th17-associated cytokines. Cell Microbiol, 13: 374–87.
30. Bystry RS, Aluvihare V, Welch KA, Kallikourdis M, Betz AG (2001) B cells and professional APCs recruit regulatory T cells via CCL4. Nat Immunol 2: 1126–32.
31. Sun X, Jones HP, Hodge LM, Simecka JW (2006) Cytokine and chemokine transcription profile during *Mycoplasma pulmonis* infection in susceptible and resistant strains of mice: macrophage inflammatory protein 1beta (CCL4) and monocyte chemoattractant protein 2 (CCL8) and accumulation of CCR5+ Th cells. Infect Immun 74: 5943–54.
32. Dinarello CA (2000) Proinflammatory cytokines. Chest 118:503–508.
33. Rikitake Y, Takai Y (2008) Interactions of the cell adhesion molecule nectin with transmembrane and peripheral membrane proteins for pleiotropic functions. Cell Mol Life Sci 65: 253–263.
34. Chemnitz JM, Parry RV, Nichols KE, June CH, Riley JL (2004) SHP-1 and SHP-2 associate with immunoreceptor tyrosine-based switch motif of programmed death 1 upon primary human T cell stimulation, but only receptor ligation prevents T cell activation. J Immunol 173: 945–54.
35. Wu TC (2007) The role of vascular cell adhesion molecule-1 in tumor immune evasion. Cancer Res 67: 6003–6.
36. Rudin CM, Thompson CB (1997) Apoptosis and disease: regulation and clinical relevance of programmed cell death. Annu Rev Med 48: 267–281.
37. Bai FF, Ni B, Liu MJ, Feng ZX, Xiong QY, et al. (2013) *Mycoplasma hyopneumoniae*-derived lipid-associated membrane proteins induce apoptosis in porcine alveolar macrophage via increasing nitric oxide production, oxidative stress, and caspase-3 activation. Vet Immunol Immunopathol 155: 155–161.
38. Hijikata M, Kato N, Sato T, Kagami Y, Shimotohno K (1990) Molecular cloning and characterization of a cDNA for a novel phorbol-12-myristate-13-acetate-responsive gene that is highly expressed in an adult T-cell leukemia cell line. J Virol 64: 4632–9.
39. Reichenstein M, Reich R, LeHoux JG, Hanukoglu I (2004) ACTH induces TIMP-1 expression and inhibits collagenase in adrenal cortex cells. Mol Cell Endocrinol 215: 109–14.
40. Thanawongnuwech R, Thacker B, Halbur P, Thacker EL (2004) Increased production of proinflammatory cytokines following infection with porcine reproductive and respiratory syndrome virus and *Mycoplasma hyopneumoniae*. Clin Diagn Lab Immunol 11: 901–908.

10

Integrative Model of the Immune Response to a Pulmonary Macrophage Infection: What Determines the Infection Duration?

Natacha Go[1,2]*, Caroline Bidot[1], Catherine Belloc[2], Suzanne Touzeau[3,4]

1 UR341 MIA, INRA, Jouy-en-Josas, France, **2** LUNAM Université, Oniris, INRA UMR 1300 BioEpAR, Nantes, France, **3** UMR1355 ISA, INRA, Université Nice Sophia Antipolis, CNRS, Sophia Antipolis, France, **4** BIOCORE, Inria, Sophia Antipolis, France

Abstract

The immune mechanisms which determine the infection duration induced by pathogens targeting pulmonary macrophages are poorly known. To explore the impact of such pathogens, it is indispensable to integrate the various immune mechanisms and to take into account the variability in pathogen virulence and host susceptibility. In this context, mathematical models complement experimentation and are powerful tools to represent and explore the complex mechanisms involved in the infection and immune dynamics. We developed an original mathematical model in which we detailed the interactions between the macrophages and the pathogen, the orientation of the adaptive response and the cytokine regulations. We applied our model to the Porcine Respiratory and Reproductive Syndrome virus (PRRSv), a major concern for the swine industry. We extracted value ranges for the model parameters from modelling and experimental studies on respiratory pathogens. We identified the most influential parameters through a sensitivity analysis. We defined a parameter set, the reference scenario, resulting in a realistic and representative immune response to PRRSv infection. We then defined scenarios corresponding to graduated levels of strain virulence and host susceptibility around the reference scenario. We observed that high levels of antiviral cytokines and a dominant cellular response were associated with either short, the usual assumption, or long infection durations, depending on the immune mechanisms involved. To identify these mechanisms, we need to combine the levels of antiviral cytokines, including IFN_{γ}, and IL_{10}. The latter is a good indicator of the infected macrophage level, both combined provide the adaptive response orientation. Available PRRSv vaccines lack efficiency. By integrating the main interactions between the complex immune mechanisms, this modelling framework could be used to help designing more efficient vaccination strategies.

Editor: Francesco Pappalardo, University of Catania, Italy

Funding: Financial support for this research was provided by ABIES (AgroParisTech) INRA, and the French Research Agency (ANR), program Investments for the future, project ANR-10-BINF-07 (MIHMES). The funders had no role in study design, data collection and analysis, decision to publish, or preparation of the manuscript.

Competing Interests: The authors have declared that no competing interests exist.

* Email: Natacha.Go@jouy.inra.fr

Introduction

Respiratory pathogens, which enter the body through the mucosal surfaces of the respiratory tract, are responsible for local inflammation and tissue damages [1,2]. They initiate the infection and the immune response. The first interaction between the pathogen and the immune system involves the innate immune system. This first line of defence, which includes epithelial surfaces, inflammation process, complement system and innate cells, provides an immediate but non-specific response. The innate cells mainly consist of the pulmonary macrophages, the dendritic cells and the natural killers. Macrophages and dendritic cells phagocyte the pathogens, whereas the natural killers destroy the host infected cells. If pathogens successfully evade the innate response, a second layer of protection is provided by the adaptive immune system, which is activated by the innate response and confers specific long-lasting protective immunity to the host. The adaptive immune system mainly involves the cellular, the humoral and the regulatory responses. The cellular effectors destroy the infected cells, whereas the humoral effectors release antibodies, which are responsible for the neutralisation of free viral particles. The regulatory response mainly inhibits the adaptive response. Innate and adaptive immune cells synthesise cytokines, small proteins which regulate the immune mechanisms in complex ways.

The best strategy to control the severity of respiratory pathogens is to limit the inflammation while maintaining an efficient immune response. Some pathogens, such as influenza viruses, *Mycobacterium tuberculosis* or the Porcine Reproductive and Respiratory Syndrome virus, replicate in the cells of the respiratory tract, including pulmonary macrophages. They hinder the immune functions of the macrophages and consequently reduce the efficacy of the immune response. With these pathogens, activated macrophages (i) either phagocyte and destroy the pathogen, or are infected and excrete the pathogen; (ii) produce cytokines that promote the migration of immune cells to the infection site; (iii) synthesise cytokines that regulate the adaptive immunity; (iv) express antigen proteins on their cell surface that activate the adaptive response. In turn, the adaptive cell effectors and cytokines regulate the immune functions of macrophages. However, the influence of macrophage–pathogen interactions on the immune response has been poorly studied and needs more insight [1–4]. The two major reasons are that the innate mechanisms are very difficult to explore by experimentation *in vivo* and that they have been considered as having little impact compared to the adaptive response.

Here, we were interested in identifying the immune mechanisms which determine the infection duration induced by pathogens targeting pulmonary macrophages. The immune response is a highly complex system involving numerous interactions between cells and cytokines. An additional level of complexity is due to the between-host and between-pathogen variability. Pathogens use multiple strategies, that vary among pathogens but also among strains, resulting in various virulence levels. The host response depends on the host genotype or housing conditions, resulting in various susceptibility levels to a given pathogen. Consequently, to explore the impact of pathogens targeting pulmonary macrophages, it is indispensable to integrate the various immune mechanisms and to take into account the variability in pathogen virulence and host susceptibility.

In this context, mathematical models are powerful tools to represent and explore the complex mechanisms involved in the infection and immune dynamics [3,5]. They complement experimentation. On the one hand, they are based on experimental data. On the other hand, they can be used to test biological hypotheses or assess the impact of control strategies, which would not be feasible or would be too expensive by experimentation. They can also guide experimentation by identifying key parameters or mechanisms that need further exploration. Mathematical models have been developed to explore the immune and infection dynamics for various human and animal diseases. However, very few models represent the innate mechanisms explicitly and macrophage–pathogen interactions need to be better represented in models [6]. Several models describe pathogens targeting macrophages, such as influenza viruses [5–7], *Mycobacterium tuberculosis* [8,9], or Porcine Respiratory and Reproductive Syndrome virus [10]. These models focused more on the adaptive than on the innate response, which was fairly simplified or even missing. In particular, none of these models included the macrophage and natural killer immune functions explicitly and innate the cytokine regulations were simplified. Moreover, none took into account the regulatory adaptive response.

So we proposed an original model of the immune response to a virus infecting pulmonary macrophages in the lung. We considered with particular attention the macrophage–virus interactions. We highly detailed the mechanisms of the innate response and the cytokine regulations. We included the cellular, the humoral and the regulatory orientation of the adaptive response, as well as their main functions. We represented the interactions between innate and adaptive components. We applied our model to the Porcine Respiratory and Reproductive Syndrome virus (PRRSv). PRRSv is a major concern for the swine industry, as it is responsible for significant economic losses worldwide [11,12]. This pathogen is of particular interest because: (i) it exhibits a strong tropism for the pulmonary macrophages [11–14]; (ii) it induces a prolonged viremia thanks to its ability to hamper the immune response [11,12,15]; and (iii) the infection and immune dynamics are highly variable between hosts and viral strains. Depending on the studies, various components of the immune response have been highlighted as having an impact on PRRSv infection duration: (i) the macrophage permissiveness and excretion rate; (ii) the levels of antiviral and immuno-modulatory cytokines; and (iii) the balance between the cellular, humoral and regulatory responses [16]. We used our integrative model to identify the immune mechanisms determining the infection duration and to explore the relevance of these three assumptions, taking into account the variability in pathogen virulence and host susceptibility.

First, we built our model by synthesising knowledge on the immune mechanisms from published studies on PRRSv. Experimental studies on PRRSv are numerous, but cannot provide all our model parameter values. So we compiled data from the literature by reviewing experimental and modelling studies on pathogens targeting pulmonary macrophages and obtained large value ranges for our model parameters. We explored the influence of these parameters on the viral and macrophage dynamics by a sensitivity analysis. We then identified a parameter set resulting in realistic infection and immune dynamics. Finally, we explored the influence of host susceptibility and viral virulence on the infection outcome and we identified the associated immune mechanisms.

Methods

In this section, we first present the dynamic model and its calibration, based on literature data. We then describe the sensitivity analysis method used to quantify the influence of model parameters on outputs of interest, among which the viral titer. Finally, we define scenarios which represent the variability in host susceptibility and strain virulence, in order to assess the impact of this variability on the model outputs.

Model description

We built a deterministic dynamic model of ordinary differential equations to simulate the infection and immune dynamics induced by a pathogen targeting pulmonary macrophages in the lung. The functional diagram of the model appears in Figure 1. We selected the immune components and their interactions from current knowledge on the immune mechanisms induced by pathogens targeting pulmonary macrophages. Our modelling assumptions are detailed and justified in the complete model description given in Appendix S1. In particular, the cytokine regulations and syntheses represented in our model, as well as the related literature references, are summarised in Table S1 and Table S2 respectively.

The model is characterised by 18 state variables: the free viral particles (V); five effectors of the innate response: four macrophage states and the natural killers (NK); three effectors of the adaptive response and nine cytokines. A macrophage can either be susceptible (M_S), phagocyting (M_P), or infected; in this latter case, it is either latent (M_L) or excreting the virus (M_E). For the adaptive response, the effectors represent the regulatory (R_r), humoral (R_h) and cellular (R_c) responses. The nine cytokines included are the major pro-inflammatory ($IL_{1\beta}$, IL_6, IL_8), the innate antiviral (TNF_α, IFN_α) and the immuno-regulatory (IFN_γ, IL_{10}, TGF_β, IL_{12}) cytokines. IFN_γ also exhibits an antiviral function. TNF_α is generally considered as a pro-inflammatory cytokine, but we were here more interested is its antiviral function. The model describes the evolution over time of the state variable concentrations in the lung.

The main processes that drive the evolution of these state variables and that are integrated in the model are: the phagocytosis of the viral particles by the macrophages (rate η); the macrophage infection by the virus (rate β); the excretion of free viral particles by the infected macrophages (rate e); the recruitment (rate A_m) and decay/migration of the macrophages (rates μ_M); the activation (rates α) and decay/migration of the other effectors (rates μ); the cytokine productions by the immune cells (rates ρ) and their decay (rates μ_C); the cytokine regulations (functions κ). Figure 2 gives a schematic representation of the model (without regulations). Parameter descriptions and values are synthesised in

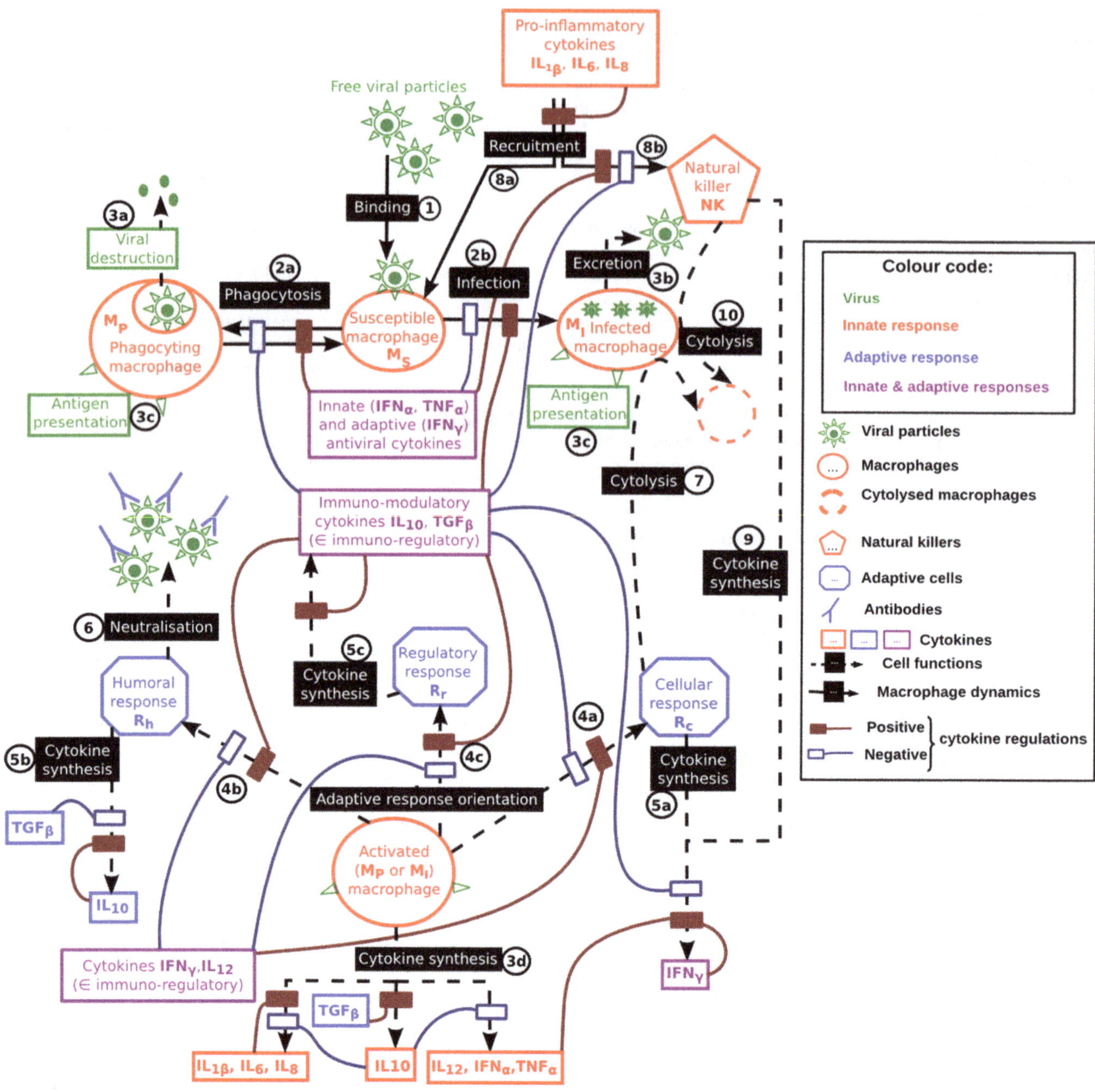

Figure 1. Functional diagram of the immune response to a virus targeting macrophages. Interactions between macrophages and virus (1) result in macrophage activation by either phagocytosis (2a, amplified by antiviral cytokines and inhibited by immuno-modulatory cytokines) or macrophage infection (2b, amplified by immuno-modulatory cytokines and inhibited by antiviral cytokines) releasing viral particles (3b). The activated macrophages initiate the adaptive response (4a–c). IFN_γ and IL_{12} orient the adaptive response towards the cellular response (4a), whereas immuno-modulatory cytokines orient the response towards the humoral and regulatory responses (4b–c). The cellular response and the natural killers are responsible for the destruction of infected cells by cytolysis (7 & 10, respectively). The humoral response is responsible for the viral neutralisation through antibodies (6). The recruitment of susceptible macrophages and natural killers is amplified by the pro-inflammatory cytokines (8a & 8b, respectively). Cytokines are produced by activated macrophages (3d), natural killers (9) and adaptive cells (4a–c). These syntheses are regulated by various cytokines.

Table 1. A complete description of the model and the corresponding equations is given in Appendix S1. Here we describe the main components of the model, illustrated by a few representative equations.

When a free viral particle encounters a susceptible macrophage (1 in Figure 1), it can either be phagocyted (rate η, 2a in Figure 1), resulting in viral destruction (3a in Figure 1), or it can infect the cell (rate β, 2b in Figure 1), resulting in viral replication (3b in Figure 1). The phagocytosis is amplified by antiviral cytokines (TNF_α, IFN_α and IFN_γ) and inhibited by immuno-modulatory cytokines (IL_{10} and TGF_β, 2a in Figure 1). The infection (linked to the macrophage permissiveness) is amplified by IL_{10} and inhibited by innate antiviral cytokines (IFN_α,TNF_α) and TGF_β (2b in 1). Phagocyting macrophages revert to a susceptible status after viral destruction (rate γ); it is amplified by the antiviral

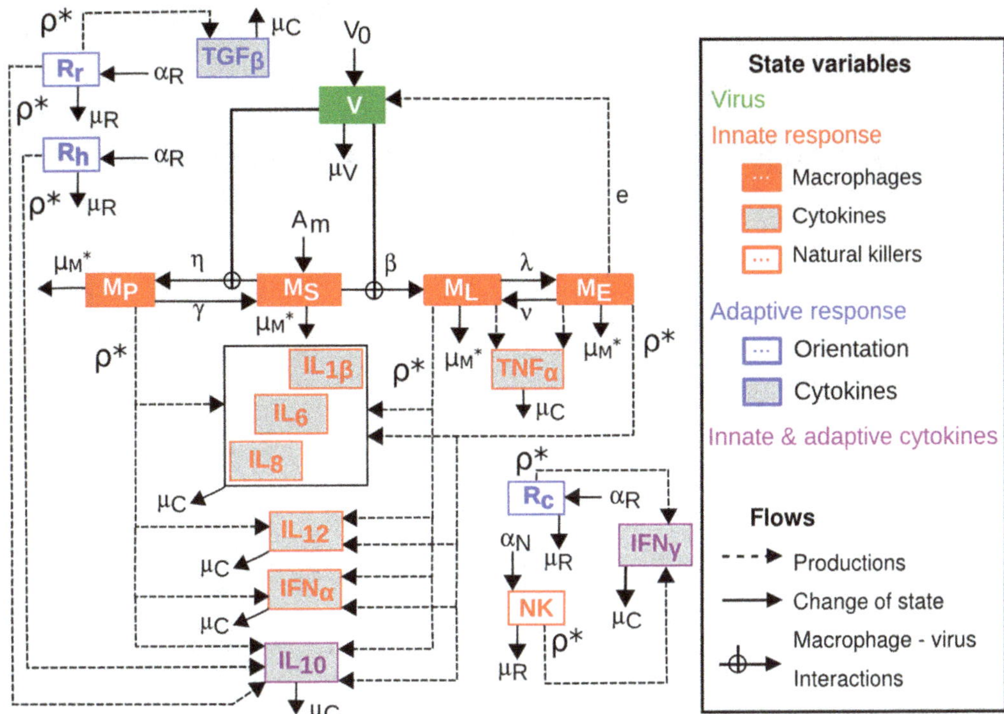

Figure 2. Conceptual model: state variables and flows without regulations. The state variables consist of: the free viral particles (V); the susceptible (M_S), phagocyting (M_P), latent (M_L) and excreting (M_E) macrophages; the natural killers (NK); the cellular (R_c), humoral (R_h) and regulatory (R_r) adaptive cells; the pro-inflammatory cytokines ($IL_{1\beta}$, IL_6 & IL_8; grouped in the box), the innate antiviral cytokines (IFN_α & TNF_α) and the immuno-regulatory cytokines (IL_{12}, IFN_γ, IL_{10} & TGF_β). The flows represented are: the inoculation of free viral particles (V_0); the recruitment of susceptible macrophages (A_m); the activation of natural killers (α_N) and cells of the adaptive response (α_R); the decay of the free viral particles (μ_v), the macrophages (μ_M*), the natural killers (μ_N), the adaptive cells (μ_R) and the cytokines (μ_C); the macrophage state changes, *i.e.* phagocytosis (η and γ), infection (β) and transient excretion (λ and ν); the excretion of free viral particles by infected macrophages (e) and the cytokine syntheses by activated immune cells (ρ*). For the sake of readability, the cytokine and cell regulations and not drawn and some parameter notations (marked with *) are simplified.

cytokines and inhibited by IL_{10} (2a in Figure 1). Activated macrophages (infected or phagocyting macrophages) produce pro-inflammatory cytokines (3d in Figure 1), which amplify the recruitment of susceptible macrophages (inflow A_m, 8a in Figure 1) [4,17–19]. Finally, susceptible macrophages undergo natural decay (rate μ_M^{nat}) and TNF_α-induced apoptosis (rate $\mu_M^{\inf}$) [20]. The resulting susceptible macrophage dynamics is shown in Equation (1) and Figure 3.

$$\begin{aligned}\dot{M}_S = \;& A_m\,[1+\kappa(IL_{12},IL_6)]\,[1+\kappa(IL_8)] && \leftarrow \text{recruitment}\\ & -\eta\, M_S\, V\,\frac{[1+\kappa(TNF_\alpha)]\,[1+\kappa(IFN_\alpha)]\,[1+\kappa(IFN_\gamma)]}{[1+\kappa(IL_{10})]\,[1+\kappa(TGF_\beta)]} && \leftarrow \text{phagocytosis}\\ & +\gamma\, M_P\,\frac{[1+\kappa(TNF_\alpha)]\,[1+\kappa(IFN_\alpha)]\,[1+\kappa(IFN_\gamma)]}{1+\kappa(IL_{10})} && \leftarrow \text{phagocytosis ending}\\ & -\beta\, M_S\, V\,\frac{1+\kappa(IL_{10})}{[1+\kappa(TNF_\alpha)]\,[1+\kappa(IFN_\alpha)]\,[1+\kappa(TGF_\beta)]} && \leftarrow \text{infection}\\ & -M_S\,(\mu_M^{nat}+\mu_M^{\inf}\,TNF_\alpha) && \leftarrow \text{decay}\end{aligned} \tag{1}$$

The cytokine environment is not static in our model, as we explicitely represented the evolution of the cytokine concentrations over time. Cytokines are produced by activated immune cells. In turn, they modulate the cellular functions through their recognition by specific receptors, inducing cascaded reactions within the cells. The higher the cytokine concentration, the stronger the effect. However, there is a limited number of cytokine receptors on the cell surface, so the effect saturates above a given cytokine concentration. We formalised the cytokine effects by a Michaelis–Menten function (κ) of the cytokine concentration (C_i) [8,21,22] as follows:

$$\kappa(C_i)=\frac{K\,C_i}{C_i+k},$$

where K represents the saturation factor and k the half-saturation concentration. A cytokine can have three possible effects listed below on a given flow (R).

- Activation: $R\,\kappa(C_i)$. The flow is only possible in the presence of the cytokine and it increases with the cytokine concentration.

Table 1. Model parameters.

Parameter	Description	Tested values			Reference value	Unit	References
Macrophage dynamics							
A_m	recruitment rate of M_S	$5\ 10^4$	10^5	$1.5\ 10^5$	$5\ 10^4$	$(\mathrm{ml.d})^{-1}$	[21,62]
η	phagocytosis rate	10^{-10}	10^{-8}	10^{-6}	$5\ 10^{-7}$	ml/d*	[68]
β	infection rate	10^{-10}	10^{-8}	10^{-6}	10^{-6}	ml/d*	[14]
γ	1/phagocytosis duration	24	48	96	96	d^{-1}	[23]
λ	1/duration of M_L state	6	12	24	6	d^{-1}	[14]
ν	1/duration of M_E state	6	12	24	6	d^{-1}	–
μ_M^{nat}	natural death rate	0.1	0.2	0.3	0.2	d^{-1}	[22]
δ_μ	over-mortality rate of M_I	0.9	1	1.1	1.1	no unit	–
μ_M^{ap}	apoptosis rate by TNF_α	10^{-7}	$10^{-4.5}$	10^{-2}	10^{-2}	ml/(pg.d)	[69]
μ_M^{inn}	cytolysis rate of M_I by NK	10^{-8}	$10^{-5.5}$	10^{-3}	10^{-3}	ml/d	[69]
μ_M^{ad}	R_c cytolysis rate of M_I by	10^{-8}	$10^{-5.5}$	10^{-3}	10^{-3}	ml/d	[69]
Virus dynamics							
V_0	initial viral inoculation	10^4	10^5	10^7	$2\ 10^6$	$\mathrm{TCID_{50}/ml}$	[38,39]
e	excretion rate	0.1	1	10	0.2	$\mathrm{TCID_{50}/d}$	–
μ_V^{nat}	natural death rate	0.1	0.2	0.3	0.2	d^{-1}	–
μ_V^{ad}	neutralisation rate by R_h	10^{-4}	10^{-3}	10^{-2}	10^{-4}	ml/d	–
Adaptive cell (R) and natural killer (NK) dynamics							
α_R	M_a activation rate of R by	10^{-6}	10^{-5}	10^{-4}	10^{-5}	d^{-1}	[21]
α_N	activation rate of NK	0.1	1	10	10	$(\mathrm{ml.d})^{-1}$	[21]
p_R	proliferation rate of R	0.05			0.05	d^{-1}	–
δ_{R_c}	death rate of R by AICD	10^{-3}	10^{-2}	10^{-1}	10^{-1}	ml/d	–
μ_R	natural death rate	0.01	0.03	0.05	0.05	d^{-1}	–
Cytokine dynamics							
ρ_{P_i}	M_a synthesis rate of P_i by	10^{-2}	10	10^2	10^{-2}	pg/d	–
$\rho_{\mathrm{IL}_{12}}$	synthesis rate of IL_{12} by M_a	10^{-2}	10	10^2	10^{-2}	pg/d	–
ρ_{A_i}	synthesis rate of A_i by M_a	10^{-2}	10	10^2	$5\ 10^{-2}$	pg/d	–
$\rho_{\mathrm{IL}_{10}}^{inn}$	synthesis rate of IL_{10} by M_a	10^{-2}	10	10^2	$2\ 10^{-2}$	pg/d	–
$\rho_{\mathrm{IL}_{10}}^{ad}$	R synthesis rate of IL_{10} by	10^{-2}	10	10^2	2	pg/d	–
$\rho_{\mathrm{IFN}_\gamma}^{inn}$	synthesis rate of IFN_γ by NK	10^{-2}	10	10^2	10	pg/d	–
$\rho_{\mathrm{IFN}_\gamma}^{ad}$	synthesis rate of IFN_γ by R	10^{-2}	10	10^2	10	pg/d	–
$\rho_{\mathrm{TGF}_\beta}$	synthesis rate of TGF_β by R	10^{-2}	10	10^2	10	pg/d	–
μ_C	natural death rate	10	20	40	20	d^{-1}	[22]

Table 1. Cont.

Parameter	Description	Tested values			Reference value	Unit	References
k	half-saturation concentration	5	10^2	$1.5\ 10^3$	30	pg/ml	[22]
K	saturation factor	0.5	1	1.5	1.5	no unit	-

The minimal and maximal values tested were issued from the literature when we found some information, otherwise they were assumed (-). Macrophages: susceptible (M_S), latent (M_L), excreting (M_E), infected ($M_I = M_L + M_E$), phagocyting (M_P), activated ($M_a = M_L + M_E + M_P$). Adaptive cells R: cellular (R_c), humoral (R_h) and regulatory (R_r) effectors.
* The unit of η and β is given for the macrophage equation and is different in the virus equation (ml/(d.TCID$_{50}$)); nevertheless, the parameter values are the same since we considered that the phagocytosis and macrophage infection consume one TCID$_{50}$ of virus per macrophage.

- Amplification: $R\,[1+\kappa(C_i)]$. The flow increases with the cytokine concentration.
- Inhibition: $R/[1+\kappa(C_i)]$. The flow decreases with the cytokine concentration.

Regulations often involve several cytokines (C_i and C_j), which can act

- either independently: $R\,[\kappa(C_i)+\kappa(C_i)]$ for an activation, $R\,[1+\kappa(C_i)]\,[1+\kappa(C_j)]$ for an amplification, or $R/([1+\kappa(C_i)]\,[1+\kappa(C_j)])$ for an inhibition;
- or in synergy: $R\,\kappa(C_i,C_j)=R\,\kappa(C_i)\,\kappa(C_j)$ for an activation, $R\,[1+\kappa(C_i,C_j)]$ for an amplification, or $R[1+\kappa(C_i,C_j)]$ for an inhibition.

For example, the recruitment of susceptible macrophages (8a in Figure 1) is amplified by three cytokines, as shown in Equation (1): two act in synergy (IL_{12} and IL_6) and the third one acts independently (IL_8).

The dynamics of natural killers, given by Equation (2), offers a more complex example of cytokines acting independently and in synergy. We represented the dynamics of activated natural killers and only included the regulations by the most influential cytokines [4,19,23,24]. The recruitment of natural killers from the bloodstream (rate α_N, 8b in Figure 1) is activated by pro-inflammatory cytokines: IL_{12} and IL_6 co-activate the recruitment, whereas IL_8 acts independently. Natural killers are then activated by IFN_γ and IL_{12}, whereas IL_{10} inhibits the activation. They are submitted to natural death or/and migration (rate μ_R). Activated natural killers destroy infected cells (10 in Figure 1) and synthesise IFN_γ (9 in Figure 1) [4,19,23,24].

$$\begin{aligned}\dot{NK} = {} & \alpha_N \frac{[\kappa(IL_{12},IL_6)+\kappa(IL_8)]\ [\kappa(IFN_\gamma)+\kappa(IL_{12})]}{[1+\kappa(IL_{10})]} && \leftarrow \text{recruitment \& activation} \\ & -\mu_R\,NK && \leftarrow \text{decay} \qquad (2)\end{aligned}$$

Activated macrophages present the viral antigens to the adaptive cells (3c in Figure 1). The subsequent orientation of the adaptive response depends on the immuno-regulatory cytokines (4a – c in Figure 1). We represented the adaptive response by three effectors corresponding to the three main orientations: cellular, humoral and regulatory responses [1,4,13,25–31]. As for the natural killers, we only represented the dynamics of the activated effectors. Based on the model proposed by Yates *et al.* for the regulation of T helper cell populations [31], we synthesised the dynamics of each adaptive effector by three steps: activation by activated macrophages (rate α_R), proliferation (rate p_R) and decay. We represented the regulations of the activation and proliferation steps by the most influential cytokines: IFN_γ, IL_{12}, IL_{10} and TGF_β (assumptions and references detailed in Appendix S1). The decay includes the natural decay (rate μ_R) and the Activation Induced Cell Death (AICD) induced by the interaction with a type 1 T helper cell from the R_c compartment (basic rate δ_{R_c}) [31].

- Cellular response: R_c represents the type 1 T helper cells and the cytotoxic lymphocytes. Its dynamics is described in Equation (3). Activation is amplified by IFN_γ and IL_{12} and inhibited by IL_{10}; proliferation is activated by IFN_γ and IL_{12} and inhibited by IL_{10} and TGF_β (4a in Figure 1). R_c synthesises IFN_γ (5a in Figure 1) and destroys infected macrophages (7 in Figure 1).

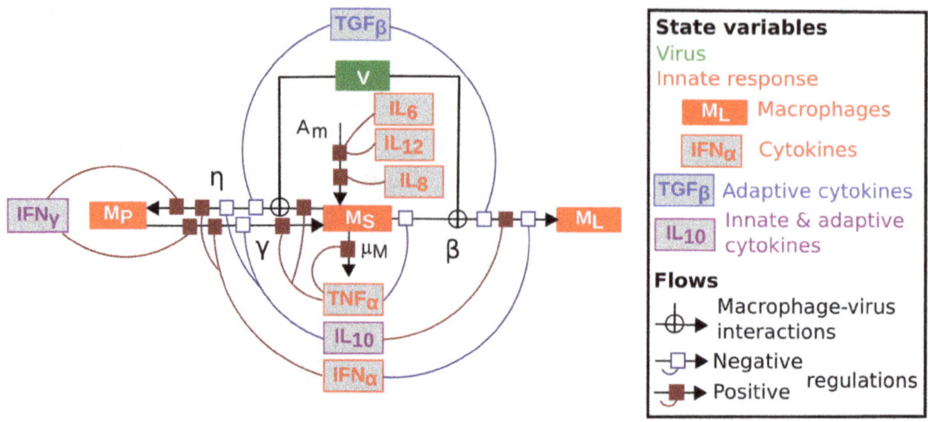

Figure 3. Susceptible macrophage dynamics with cytokine regulations. The state variables represented are: the free viral particles (V); the susceptible (M_S), phagocyting (M_P) and latent (M_L) macrophages; the pro-inflammatory cytokines (IL_6 & IL_8), the innate antiviral cytokines (IFN_α & TNF_α) and the immuno-regulatory cytokines (IL_{12}, IFN_γ, IL_{10} & TGF_β). All processes that impact the susceptible macrophages are included: recruitment (A_m), decay (μ_M, simplified notation), phagocytosis (η and γ) and infection (β); their positive and negative regulations by cytokines are also drawn.

$$\begin{aligned}\dot{R}_c = \quad & \alpha_R\,[M_P+M_L+M_E]\,\frac{[1+\kappa(\mathrm{IFN}_\gamma)]\,[1+\kappa(\mathrm{IL}_{12})]}{1+\kappa(\mathrm{IL}_{10})} && \leftarrow \text{ activation}\\ & +p_R\,R_c\,\frac{[\kappa(\mathrm{IFN}_\gamma)+\kappa(\mathrm{IL}_{12})]}{[1+\kappa(\mathrm{IL}_{10})]\,[1+\kappa(\mathrm{TGF}_\beta)]} && \leftarrow \text{ proliferation}\\ & -\mu_R\,R_c-\delta_{R_c}\,R_c^{\,2} && \leftarrow \text{ decay}\end{aligned} \tag{3}$$

- Humoral response: R_h represents the type 2 T helper cells, the B lymphocytes and the antibodies. Activation is amplified by IL_{10} and inhibited by IFN_γ and IL_{12}; proliferation is activated by IL_{10} and inhibited by IFN_γ, IL_{12} and TGF_β (4b in Figure 1). R_h synthesises IL_{10} (5b in Figure 1) and neutralises free viral particles through antibodies (6 in Figure 1).
- Regulatory response: R_r represents the regulatory T cells. Activation is amplified by IL_{10} and TGF_β and inhibited by IFN_γ and IL_{12}; proliferation is activated by TGF_β and inhibited by IL_{10}, IFN_γ and IL_{12} (4c in Figure 1). R_r synthesises IL_{10} and TGF_β (5c in Figure 1).

Simulations. The model was implemented in Scilab 5.3.3 (http://www.scilab.org/). For all simulations, the initial conditions were set to represent an initial viral inoculation in a PRRSv-naive host and were chosen as follows: $V(0)=V_0\in[10^4,10^7]\mathrm{TCID}_{50}/\mathrm{ml}$ for the viral titer; $M_S(0)=5\ 10^5\mathrm{cells/ml}$ for the susceptible macrophages; all remaining variables were set to zero. The model parameters are summarised in Table 1.

Model calibration

Published experimental data on PRRSv infection (reviewed in [11,12,16,32–37]) are highly heterogeneous and differ on: (i) the monitoring duration, (ii) the measured immune components, (iii) the viral strain, (iv) the pig genotype. Moreover, among the variables included in our model, only a few were monitored in each experimental study and there were few measures over time. Consequently, based on these data, classical parameter estimation methods were not suitable to calibrate our model and we had to design an *ad hoc* procedure.

The first step of the calibration procedure was to synthesise data from experimental infections to identify the variation ranges of our model parameters. When PRRSv studies could not provide parameter values, we reviewed models applied to tuberculosis and influenza. The value ranges obtained for the model parameters and the corresponding references are given in Table 1 (ranges defined by the minimum and maximum tested values). The second step was to explore the parameter space defined by these value ranges. We used a design of experiments which is described in the Sensitivity analysis section below. The simulations resulting from this exploration exhibited very contrasted outputs (Figures S2–S4). So the third step was to define the characteristics of the infection and immune dynamics corresponding to a realistic response to PRRSv infection. We chose to represent an average response as our reference scenario (S0). This step is detailed below. Finally, the fourth step was to select a parameter set corresponding to this reference scenario. We used the sensitivity analyses presented below to focus first on the most sensitive parameters, *i.e.* parameters which had the greatest impact on the model outputs.

For the reference scenario, we chose to represent the infection of a weaned pig by a single PRRSv inoculation. Weaned pigs are supposed to be naive to PRRSv and to have lost their maternal immunity. In experimental PRRSv infection studies, the inoculation dose ranged between 4 and 7 $\log_{10}(\mathrm{TCID}_{50}/\mathrm{ml})$ [38,39]; we chose an inoculation dose of 6.3 $\log_{10}(\mathrm{TCID}_{50}/\mathrm{ml})$. PRRSv infection usually lasts between 28 to 42 days in the blood [12,16,40] and around 56 days in the lung [12]. However, the infection duration is highly variable between pigs and viral strains and can be higher than 200 days [16,41]. So we chose an infection duration in the lung of around 70 days. Few quantitative data are available for the immune dynamics. The cytokine levels are highly variable between studies [11,13] and poorly documented in the lung. Their magnitude ranges between 10^{-1} and 10^3 pg/ml. IL_{10} levels in response to PRRSv infection and other respiratory pathogens are similar. They are higher than the levels of pro-inflammatory, antiviral (innate and adaptive) and other immuno-regulatory (IL_{12}, IFN_γ and TGF_β) cytokines. Without infection, macrophage concentrations in the lung were observed around 10^5 cells/ml. To our knowledge, only one experimental study tracked infected macrophages, which peaked during the first days of PRRSv infection at around 40% among all macrophages [39]. Little is known about the phagocyting macrophages, except that the phagocyting state is transient and that PRRSv promotes macrophage infection over phagocytosis [42,43]. Reported levels of natural killers during PRRSv infection were low compared to other respiratory pathogens [15,33]. The humoral response to PRRSv infection is similar to other respiratory pathogens, whereas the cell-mediated immunity is delayed and weak. The regulatory response has been poorly studied and results are controversial [13,44–46]. Moreover, the orientation of the adaptive response varied considerably between studies. Consequently, we chose a balanced adaptive response orientation for our reference scenario.

Sensitivity analysis

We were interested in identifying the most influential parameters on the infection dynamics thanks to a global sensitivity analysis. Consequently, the first two outputs selected were the viral titer (V) and the percentage of infected macrophages among the total concentration of macrophages ($\%M_I = \%(M_L + M_E)$). We were also interested in characterising the phagocytosis activity, which directly limits the macrophage infection. The phagocytosis is a transient macrophage state, which explains why, whatever the parameter combination selected in the parameter ranges, the percentage of phagocyting macrophages ($\%M_P$) was low compared to the percentage of infected macrophages ($\%M_I$) at any time during the course of infection (Figure **S1**). However, it does not mean that the phagocytosis activity was necessarily low. We compared the phagocytosis flow (susceptible macrophages becoming phagocyting macrophages per unit of time) and the infection flow (susceptible macrophages becoming infected macrophages per unit of time) during the course of infection. Depending on the parameter values, the phagocytosis inflow was higher or lower than the infection inflow (Figure **S1**). Consequently, the cumulative number of phagocyting macrophages (cM_P), which corresponds to the phagocytosis flow integrated over time, is a good representation of the phagocytosis activity. So we selected this variable as the third output of interest. We used a design of experiments to define which simulations to run. The resulting outputs were analysed to produce the sensitivity indices, which quantify the influence of the parameters on the model outputs. We used the R software, version 3.0.2, (http://www.r-project.org/) for these analyses.

We selected 30 among the 31 model parameters for the sensitivity analysis. We did not include the proliferation rate of the adaptive effectors (p_R), because the combination of high p_R and high IL_{10} synthesis rates led to the explosion of the R_h and R_r dynamics, which resulted in a numerical integration failure of the model. For each of the 30 parameters, we chose to test three values among the value range identified in the calibration procedure: the lower and upper bounds of the range, as well as an intermediate value (Table 1). Testing all parameter combinations, *i.e.* a complete factorial design, would have required 3^{30} simulations, which was not feasible. Consequently, fractional factorial designs were used instead. A preliminary analysis was conducted to estimate the main effects of the 30 parameters on the model outputs, without taking into account the interactions between parameters. A fractional design of size 243, determined as the minimum size to correctly estimate the main effects, was implemented: 243 parameter combinations were defined and the corresponding simulations were performed and analysed. From this preliminary analysis, the ten most influential parameters on each of the three outputs were identified. We then performed a sensitivity analysis on each output, aiming at estimating the main effects and two-parameter interactions of the corresponding ten most influential parameters, to which we potentially added extra parameters assumed to have an impact on the corresponding output. For instance, we added the macrophage mortality rates for the $\%M_I$ output. We selected 17 parameters for the viral titer, 10 parameters for the cumulative M_P and 21 parameters for the percentage of infected macrophages (Figure 4). The smallest design that correctly estimates the main effects and two-parameter interactions for 21 parameters ($\%M_I$ output) requires $3^8 = 6561$ parameter combinations. We chose to use the same design size for all outputs, so 6561 simulations were performed and analysed for each of the three outputs. The Planor R package (http://cran.r-project.org/web/packages/planor/index.html) was used to construct the fractional designs.

Sensitivity indices were calculated for each parameter on each output in the preliminary analysis (30 parameters $\times$ 3 outputs) and the subsequent analyses taking into account two-factor interactions. Sensitivity indices quantify the fraction of output variance among simulations explained by the variation of each parameter within its value range [47]. Our model outputs being time-dependent variables, we used a method adapted to multivariate outputs, which is based on a decomposition of the variable using a principal component analysis (PCA) [48]. As a result of the PCA, an inertia proportion is attributed to each component. It represents the variability among simulations carried by the component. Moreover, each simulation is given a "score" on each component, a scalar which represents the projection of the simulation on the component. Then, for each component, an ANOVA is performed on these scores to estimate the influence of each parameter on the output. The sensitivity index associated with each term, main effect of a parameter or interaction between parameters, is defined as the ratio between the sum of squares corresponding to that term and the total sum of squares. Finally, a generalised sensitivity index (GSI) is calculated for each term (main effect or interaction) as the the sum of the sensitivity indices corresponding to that term on each PCA component, weighted by the inertia of the component. The total generalised sensitivity index (tGSI) of a parameter is defined as the sum of the sensitivity indices corresponding to this parameter (main effect mGSI plus sum of interactions involving the parameter iGSI). We used the Multisensi R package (http://cran.r-project.org/web/packages/multisensi/index.html) for this analysis.

GSI results are presented below. For each output, key parameters are defined as the most influential parameters for which the cumulative total GSI is higher than 75%.

Variability in host susceptibility and strain virulence

PRRSv exhibits an important genotypic diversity associated with various virulence levels [13]. The European genotype is less virulent than the American genotype [35], but the virulence also differs among strains within a genotype [49]. The highly virulent strains are associated with a prolonged viremia, a high viral replication rate and a high humoral response [50]. Moreover, the genetic component of the host susceptibility to PRRSv has been demonstrated [51,52]. Pig susceptibility can also depend on other factors such as herd management. The more susceptible pigs

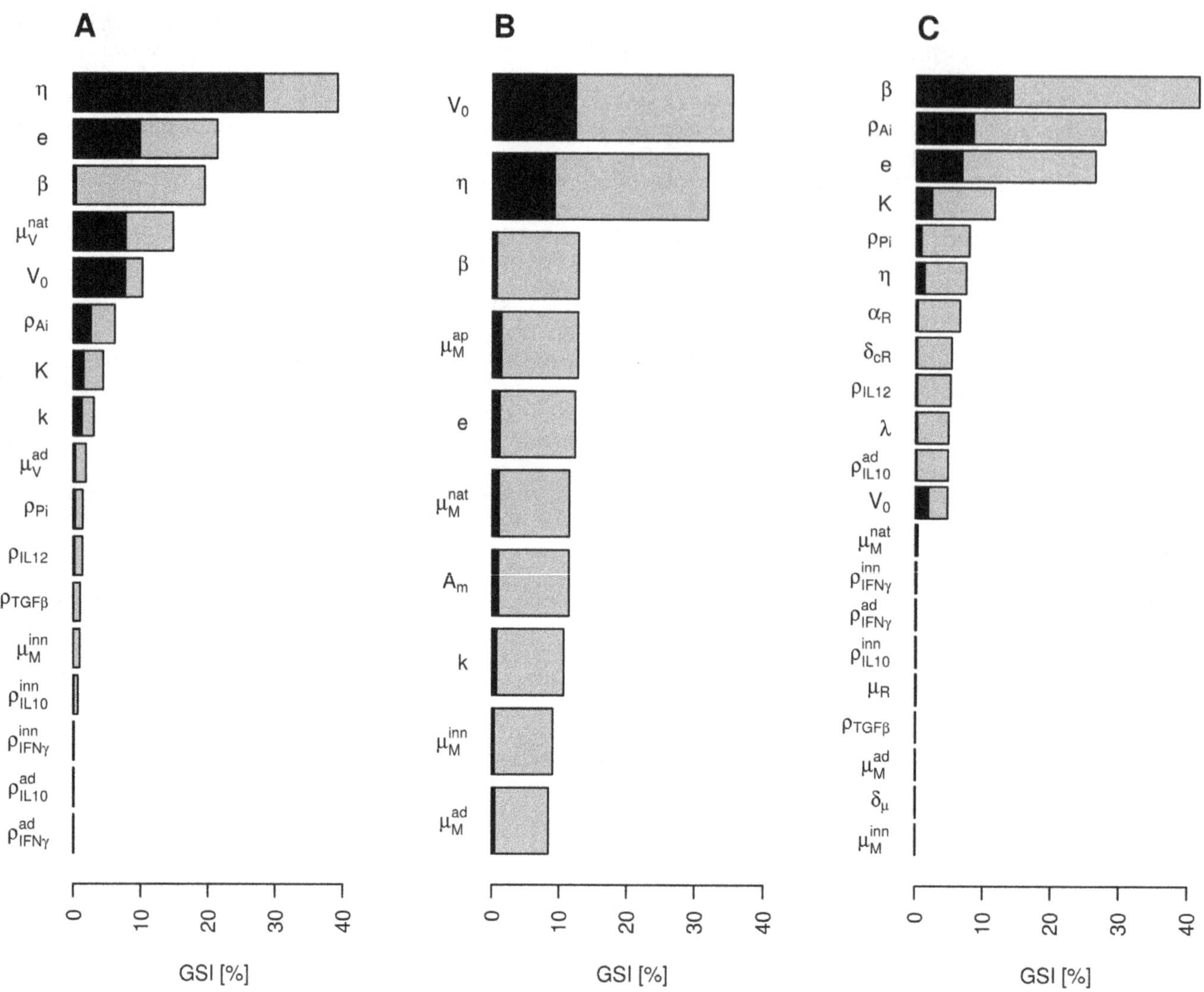

Figure 4. Generalised sensitivity indices (GSI) for the three outputs of interest. **A**: Viral titer V ($R^2=0.93$). **B**: Cumulative number of phagocyting macrophages cM_P ($R^2=0.92$). **C**: Percentage of infected macrophages among all macrophages $\%M_I$ ($R^2=0.96$). Total GSI (bars) are represented for an output-dependent selection of influential parameters. For each parameter, the total GSI is split into main parameter effect (black bar) and the sum of two-parameter interactions involving the parameter (grey bar). R^2 corresponds to the fraction of output variance explained by the parameters. NB: As the two-parameter interactions are counted for both parameters, the sum of the total GSI is higher than 100%.

develop prolonged viremia, with low titers of neutralising antibodies [10,52], probably linked to a high macrophage permissiveness and/or specific cytokine profiles [51].

Both viral virulence and pig susceptibility seem linked to: (i) the virus capacity to infect the cell and replicate, (ii) the host capacity to synthesise antiviral *vs* immuno-modulatory cytokines in response to PRRSv infection, and (iii) the activation and orientation of the adaptive response. Recent studies hypothesise that these variations of the immune dynamics are due to cascaded reactions initiated by the macrophage–virus interactions [33,34,49,51]. Consequently, we focused on the macrophage infection and cytokine synthesis capacities. Both macrophage permissiveness and viral replication impact the cytokine synthesis, which in turn regulates them. Discriminating the respective influence of the macrophage permissiveness and the cytokine synthesis rate is very difficult experimentally, but it can be achieved by a modelling approach. To explore the influence of both mechanisms, scenarios were defined by varying a selection of parameters chosen according to the sensitivity analysis results and to the hypotheses presented above. We tested 19 graduated values of: (i) the macrophage permissiveness, promoting either the phagocytosis (scenarios S0 to S1: S0→S1), or the macrophage infection and viral excretion (scenarios S0→S2); and (ii) the cytokine synthesis rates, promoting either the antiviral cytokine synthesis (scenarios S0→SB), or the immuno-modulatory cytokine synthesis (scenarios S0→SA). Scenarios are defined in Table 2. Compared to the reference scenario (S0), scenarios S0→S1 and S0→SB correspond to low host susceptibility and strain virulence, whereas scenarios S0→S2 and S0→SA correspond to high susceptibility and virulence. The parameter ranges were set to cover the variation range of the viral titer reported in the literature.

We used the area under the curve (AUC) to synthesise our model outputs. As the shapes of the immune and viral output curves were similar across the scenarios, characterising each curve by a well-chosen number was appropriate and facilitated the comparisons between scenarios. Choosing the AUC was relevant,

Table 2. Definition of the host susceptibility and strain virulence scenarios.

	Macrophage permissiveness			Cytokine synthesis capacities					
Scenarios	e	β	η	ρ_{A_i}	$\rho^{inn}_{IFN_\gamma}$	$\rho^{ad}_{IFN_\gamma}$	$\rho^{inn}_{IL_{10}}$	$\rho^{ad}_{IL_{10}}$	ρ_{TGF_β}
S1	0.15	5 10^{-7}	10^{-6}	**0.05**	**10**	**10**	**0.02**	**2**	**10**
SB	**0.2**	**10^{-6}**	**5 10^{-7}**	0.5	100	100	0.005	0.5	2.5
S0	**0.2**	**10^{-6}**	**5 10^{-7}**	**0.05**	**10**	**10**	**0.02**	**2**	**10**
SA	**0.2**	**10^{-6}**	**5 10^{-7}**	0.005	0.1	0.1	0.08	8	40
S2	0.25	2 10^{-6}	2.5 10^{-7}	**0.05**	**10**	**10**	**0.02**	**2**	**10**

Scenarios S1 and S2 differ from the reference scenario S0 by their respectively low and high macrophage permissiveness. Scenarios S1→S2 correspond to 19 intermediate scenarios (including S0) obtained by gradually varying the following parameter values: excretion rate (e), macrophage infection rate (β) and phagocytosis rate (η). Scenarios SB and SA differ from the reference scenario S0 by their cytokine synthesis capacities: scenario SB promotes antiviral over immuno-modulatory cytokine synthesis, and *vice versa* for scenario SA. Scenarios SB→SA correspond to 19 intermediate scenarios (including S0) obtained by varying gradually the synthesis rates of the following cytokines: the innate antiviral cytokines IFN_α and TNF_α (both ρ_{A_i}); the immuno-regulatory cytokines IFN_γ ($\rho^{inn}_{IFN_\gamma}$ & $\rho^{ad}_{IFN_\gamma}$), IL_{10} ($\rho^{inn}_{IL_{10}}$ & $\rho^{ad}_{IL_{10}}$) and TGF_β (ρ_{TGF_β}). Low/high susceptibility and virulence levels correspond to scenarios with low/high macrophage permissiveness (S1/S2) and scenarios which promote the antiviral/immuno-modulatory cytokine synthesis (SB/SA). The parameter values corresponding to the reference scenario are in boldface.

as it reflects the entire curve [53]. Relative AUC were defined as percentages of output AUC among a group of outputs.

Several linear regressions were performed to extract trends from our results and facilitate the interpretations. In particular, to highlight the links between immuno-regulatory cytokines and the orientation of the adaptive response, we performed linear regressions between (i) the relative AUC of relevant cytokines and (ii) the relative AUC of the adaptive response effectors (R_c, R_h & R_r). To highlight the immune mechanisms determining the infection duration, we performed linear regressions between (i) the AUC of relevant immune components, which are assumed to have a strong influence on the infection duration in the literature and (ii) the infection duration. We used the R software, version 3.0.2, for these analyses.

The infection duration is defined as the time elapsed between the initial viral inoculation and the virus clearance. In our model, we assumed that there was no more infection when the virus titer was below 0.01 $TCID_{50}$/ml.

Results

Model calibration and sensitivity analysis

The reference scenario (S0) was characterised by a 72-day infection duration, an infected macrophage peak at 40% of the total macrophage concentration, a balanced adaptive response orientation and high IL_{10} levels compared to antiviral and pro-inflammatory cytokine levels. Its parameter values are given in Table 1 and it is represented in Figue 5 (black curves).

In the preliminary sensitivity analysis, with all 30 parameters but no interactions between parameters, the variance explained by the parameters retained for the main sensitivity analysis on each output was 89% for the viral titer, 89% for the cumulative number of phagocyting macrophages and 70% for the percentage of infected macrophages. The results of the main sensitivity analyses with two-parameters interactions are shown in Figure 4; for each output, the total global sensitivity index defined for each parameter is split into the parameter main effect and its interactions. At least 92% of the total output variance was explained by the parameters and two-parameter interactions for all three outputs. Three key parameters (explaining together more than 75% of the variance) were identified for each output. Their impact is detailed in Table 3. Most of them were involved in macrophage–virus interactions. The infection rate β was a key parameter for the three outputs of interest. The excretion rate e was a key parameter for the viral titer and the percentage of infected macrophages. The phagocytosis rate η was a key parameter for the viral titer and the cumulative number of phagocyting macrophages. The remaining key parameters were the inoculation dose V_0 for the cumulative number of phagocyting macrophages and the synthesis rate of innate antiviral cytokines ρ_{A_i} for the percentage of infected macrophages. The main effects of the key parameters ranged between 0.4% (β on the viral titer) and 28% (η on the viral titer). Key parameters also exhibited high interactions (*e.g.* 27% for interactions involving β on the percentage of infected macrophages), in particular between two key parameters (results not shown).

The initial inoculation dose V_0 was a key parameter for the cumulative number of phagocyting macrophages (tGSI = 35%), but neither for the viral titer (tGSI = 11%), nor for the percentage of infected macrophages (tGSI = 5%). This result can be explained by the fact that the phagocytosis activity mostly occurs during the first days of the infection, whereas the viral titer and infected macrophages are impacted all along the infection course (Figures S2–S4).

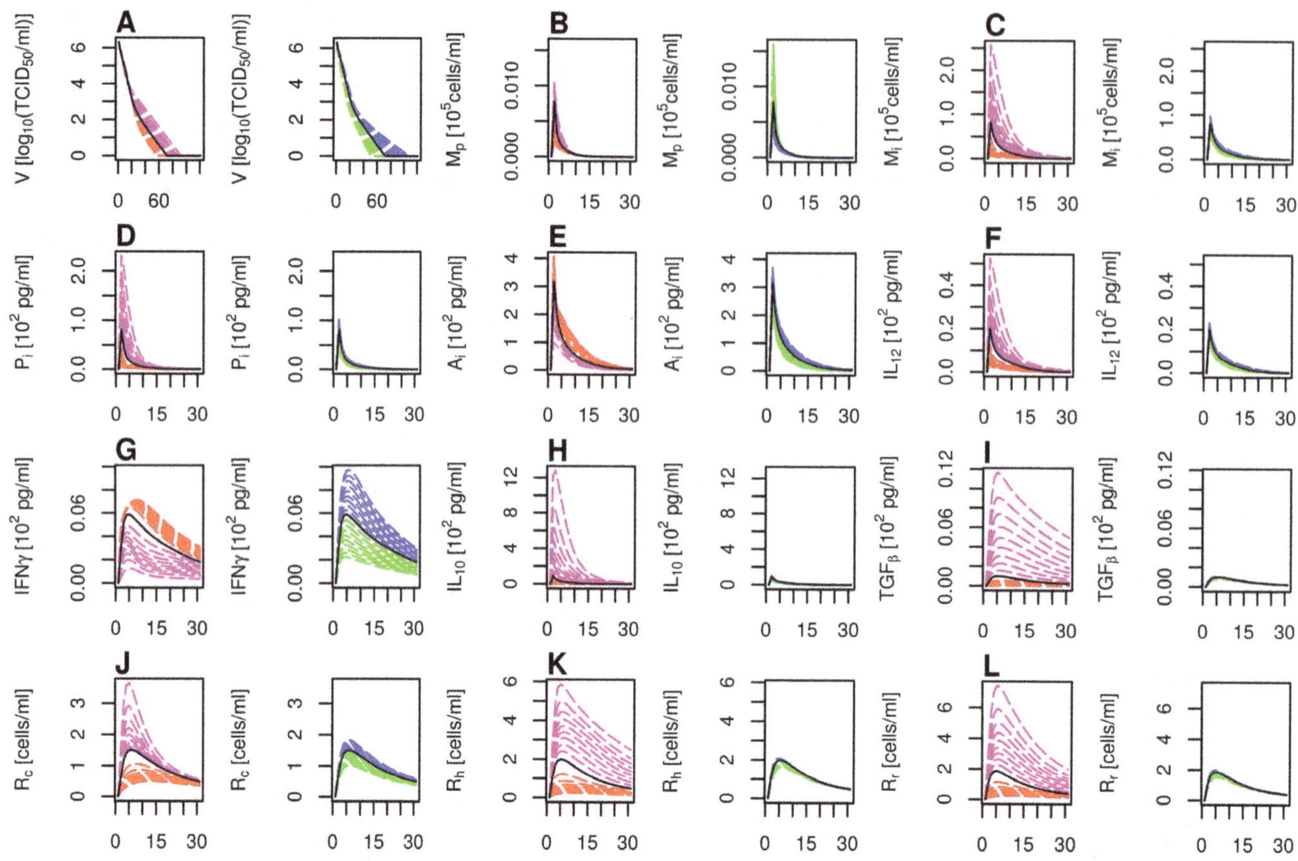

Figure 5. Immune and infection dynamics for variable host susceptibility and strain virulence. Evolution of twelve variables (panels **A** to **L**) during the first 30 days of infection (unless specified). **A**: Viral titer (V, during 120 days). **B**: Phagocyting macrophages (M_P). **C**: Infected macrophages ($M_I = M_L + M_E$). **D**: Pro-inflammatory cytokines ($P_i = \mathrm{IL}_{1\beta} + \mathrm{IL}_6 + \mathrm{IL}_8$). **E**: Innate antiviral cytokines ($A_i = \mathrm{TNF}_\alpha + \mathrm{IFN}_\alpha$). **F–I**: Immuno-regulatory cytokines (**F**: IL_{12}, **G**: IFN_γ, **H**: IL_{10} and **I**: TGF_β). **J**: Adaptive cellular effectors (R_c). **K**: Adaptive humoral effectors (R_h). **L**: Adaptive regulatory effectors (R_r). For each variable, the left plot corresponds to scenarios SB→SA, in which the antiviral cytokine synthesis is higher (S0→SB, red) or lower (S0→SA, magenta) than in the reference scenario (S0, black). The right plot corresponds to scenarios S1→S2, in which the macrophage permissiveness is lower (S0→S1, green) or higher (S0→S2, blue) than in the reference scenario (S0, black). Low susceptibility and virulence levels correspond to scenarios which promote the antiviral cytokine synthesis (red) and scenarios with low macrophage permissiveness (green). High susceptibility and virulence levels correspond to scenarios which promote the immuno-modulatory cytokine synthesis (magenta) and scenarios with high macrophage permissiveness (blue) Scenarios are defined in Table 2.

The infection rate β had less impact on the viral titer variability (tGSI = 19.4%, mGSI = 0.4%) than the phagocytosis rate η (tGSI = 39%, mGSI = 28%) and the excretion rate e (tGSI = 22%, mGSI = 10%). Macrophage infection results in viral excretion and has a positive impact on the free viral particles, but it is attenuated by the virus mobilisation by infected macrophages.

The infection rate β and the excretion rate e exhibited a strong interaction on the viral titer and the percentage of infected macrophages (GSI around 8%). Indeed, the viral replication needs macrophages to be infected and conversely, macrophage infection is induced by free viral particles which are released through viral excretion.

Impact of host susceptibility and strain virulence on the infection resolution and associated immune mechanisms

The 37 scenarios corresponding to graduated levels of host susceptibility and strain virulence were simulated. The results are illustrated in Figure 5 and summarised in Table 4. The infection durations (52–118 days according to the scenario) were consistent with literature data [12,16,40,41]. All scenarios had a notable impact on the infection duration. The scenarios related to macrophage permissiveness (S1→S2) induced higher differences in infection duration than the scenarios related to the cytokine synthesis (SB→SA), even if the parameter variations were lower for scenarios S1→S2 than for scenarios SB→SA (Table 2). Consequently, the infection duration seems more sensitive to the parameters involved in the macrophage permissiveness than the antiviral cytokine synthesis rate.

The dynamics of immune components were similarly bell-shaped but differed quantitatively. More severe and longer infections were overall associated with higher levels of immune responses (Figure 5), but the relative proportions of the immune components varied (Table 4).

Concerning the innate response, we found a significant and positive correlation ($R^2 = 0.97$) between the levels of infected macrophages and IL_{10}, a cytokine which amplifies macrophage permissiveness and viral replication (results not shown).

There was no evidence of a link between the proportions of IL_{12} and TGF_β and the orientation of the adaptive response. The proportions of IL_{10} and IFN_γ, however, were linked to the adaptive response orientation (Table 4 & Figure 5). The proportion of IL_{10} among IL_{10} and IFN_γ was negatively correlated with

Table 3. Generalised sensitivity indices and influence of the key parameters on the three outputs of interest.

	V			cM_P			$\%M_I$		
Key parameters	**mGSI**	**iGSI**	**Influence**	**mGSI**	**iGSI**	**Influence**	**mGSI**	**iGSI**	**Influence**
Initial inoculation V_0	8	3	↑	**12**	**23**	↑	2	3	↑
Excretion rate e	**10**	**12**	↑	1	11	↑	**7**	**20**	↑
Infection rate β	**0.4**	**19**	↑	**0.6**	**12**	↓	**14**	**27**	↑
Phagocytosis rate η	**28**	**11**	↓	**9**	**23**	↑	1	6	↓
A_i synthesis rate ρ_{Ai}	3	4	↑	-	-	↑	**8**	**19**	↓

The outputs are the viral titer (V), the cumulative number of phagocyting macrophages (cM_P), and the percentage of infected macrophages among all macrophages ($\%M_I$). Three key parameters were identified for each output (corresponding GSI in bold). For each parameter and each output, the generalised sensitivity index of the parameter main effect (mGSI, in %) and of the sum of two-parameter interactions involving the parameter (iGSI, in %) are given. Increasing the parameter value can induce an increase (↑) or decrease (↓) of the output.

the percentage of cellular response ($R^2=0.91$) and positively correlated with both the humoral ($R^2=0.94$) and regulatory responses ($R^2=0.84$).

Scenarios S1→S2 resulted in immune dynamics rather close to the reference scenario, except for IFN_γ levels (Figure 5). On the one hand, high infection capacities (S0→S2) resulted in long infection durations despite high levels of IFN_γ (Figure 5) and the adaptive response was oriented towards the cellular response ($\%R_c=40\%$, Table 4). However, IFN_γ percentages were similar to the reference scenario. On the other hand, low infection capacities (S1→S0) resulted in short infection durations despite high percentages of IL_{10} and the adaptive response was oriented towards the humoral response ($\%R_h=41\%$,Table 4). IL_{10} levels were similar to the reference scenario (Figure 5).

Scenarios SB→SA resulted in more contrasted immune dynamics (Figure 5) and influenced the adaptive response orientation more than scenarios S1→S2 (Table 4). Low antiviral capacities (S0→SA) resulted in long infection durations associated with high levels (Figure 5) and percentages of IL_{10}, and co-dominant humoral and regulatory responses (Table 4). High antiviral capacities (SB→S0) resulted in short infection durations associated with high levels (Figue 5) and percentages of IFN_γ, and an orientation towards the cellular response (Table 4).

To extract trends more easily from these results, we investigated the correlations between the infection duration and the levels of seven key immune components of interest: infected and phagocyting macrophages, innate antiviral and pro-inflammatory cytokines and percentages of IL_{10} and IFN_γ (Figure 6). Considering all scenarios together, no significant correlations could be extracted. Consequently, we split the scenarios in two groups: those with varying macrophage capacities (S1→S2) and those with varying cytokine synthesis capacities (SB→SA). All correlations were significant. The AUC of infected macrophages and pro-inflammatory cytokines were positively correlated with the infection duration for both groups. Otherwise, both groups exhibited opposite correlations.

In summary, low virulence and susceptibility scenarios induced short infection durations by promoting the phagocytosis or the synthesis of antiviral cytokines. On the contrary, high virulence and susceptibility scenarios resulted in long infection durations by promoting the infection and viral excretion or the synthesis of immuno-modulatory cytokines. Infection durations were always positively correlated with the levels of infected macrophages and pro-inflammatory cytokines. We observed that longer durations were associated with higher percentages of infected macrophages among activated macrophages. However, high levels of antiviral cytokines compared to immuno-regulatory cytokines, inducing a dominant cellular response, can be associated with either (i) long (scenarios related to macrophage permissiveness) or (ii) short infection durations (scenarios related to cytokine synthesis capacities).

Discussion

Modelling approach

In this paper, we presented an integrative dynamic model of the immune response in the lung to a virus targeting pulmonary macrophages: the PRRSv. The complexity level of the model is a good compromise between detailed intra-cellular models which focus on specific immune mechanisms and global models which give general trends [8]. Our model offers a comprehensive representation of the interactions between the virus and the immune response, which is necessary to explore the influence of the immune mechanisms on the infection duration. It is an original

Table 4. Summary of the virus and immune dynamics for variable host susceptibility and strain virulence.

	Susceptibility and virulence:				
	low		reference	high	
	S1	SB	S0	SA	S2
Virus - Infection duration [d]	**52**	**57**	**72**	**93**	**118**
Innate response - AUC					
$M_P/(M_I+M_P)$ [%]	1.4	1.6	0.5	0.2	0.2
M_P	0.030	0.008	0.009	0.030	0.008
M_I	2.1	0.48	3.5	18	5.1
NK	71	15	225	866	559
$P_i = IL_{1\beta} + IL_6 + IL_8$	1.2	0.28	2.4	10.8	3.6
$A_i = IFN_\alpha + TNF_\alpha$	9	26	16	7	23
Adaptive response - AUC					
$IL_{12} + IFN_\gamma + IL_{10} + TGF_\beta$	3.2	2.5	6.6	107	10.3
$R_c + R_h + R_r$	108	36	124	455	146
Cytokines - relative AUC [%]*					
IL_{12}	21	9	16	2.8	14
IFN_γ	1	85	22	0.2	30
IL_{10}	71	4.5	59	93	54
TGF_β	7	0.5	3	4	2
Orientation - relative AUC [%]*					
R_c	23	54	32	14	40
R_h	41	23	36	43	32
R_r	36	23	32	43	28

Scenarios S1: low macrophage permissiveness; SB: high antiviral and low immuno-modulatory cytokine synthesis; S0: reference; SA: high macrophage permissiveness; S2: low antiviral and high immuno-modulatory cytokine synthesis. AUC (area under the curve) units: macrophages [10^5 d/ml], other cells [d/ml], cytokines [10^2 pg.d/ml]. Macrophages: infected (M_I), phagocyting (M_P). Adaptive effectors: cellular (R_c), humoral (R_h) and regulatory (R_r) orientations.
*Relative AUC are defined within a group of outputs (*e.g.* the four cytokines IL_{12}, IFN_γ, IL_{10} and TGF_β) as the AUC of the outputs expressed as percentages of the sum of the AUC within the group.

approach that takes into account the innate mechanisms, the adaptive response orientation and their complex interactions and regulations involving cytokines. We chose to represent the activation and orientation of the adaptive response, even if they occur outside the lung, because they interact with the immune and infection dynamics. Therefore, we did not detail the intermediate differentiation and proliferation steps of the adaptive response, but we represented its main immune functions and regulations. We hence obtained a realistic qualitative dynamic of the adaptive response. We did not represent the dendritic cells, major antigen presenting cells which influence the adaptive response activation and orientation. These cells maturate during their migration from the infection site to the lymph nodes, where they synthesise cytokines. They influence the infection dynamics through the cytokines they synthesise, which is consequently negligible in the lung. Moreover, dendritic cells and macrophages drive the adaptive response orientation in a similar way. As our model does intend to represent the orientation of the adaptive response between the different types and not the quantitative levels of adaptive cells, we trust that our simplification did not distort the results. This simplification is even more appropriate when dealing with PRRSv, as the virus also infects dendritic cells. Dendritic cells and macrophages hence have very similar dynamics and impacts during PRRSv infection [54,55].

The model was built to describe a single infection by a stable pathogen at the within-host scale. We used it to study the impact of PRRSv strains, which exhibit various virulence levels. Our model could be easily adapted to other pathogens targeting pulmonary macrophages, such as influenza viruses. As influenza also infects epithelial cells, these target cells would have to be included in the model. As for other pathogens, the immune dynamic part of our model constitutes a good basis to study the innate response, given the fact that it is strongly simplify in most of the published models.

Model calibration and scenario definition

The variation range of our model parameters were based on literature data. To complement these data and deal with the high variability on the parameter values and output levels, we developed an *ad hoc* method based on large parameter space exploration and sensitivity analysis. We defined a reference scenario, which corresponds to an average dynamics within the observed immune and infection dynamics. To study the impact of host and strain variability, we also defined parameter sets based on published assumptions and resulting in infection durations which were consistent with the literature [12,16,40,41]. However, a quantitative calibration based on the viral dynamics and immune response data was not feasible. The levels of strain virulence and susceptibility of pigs are not quantified, the viral strains and pig breeds are not always informed and only few combinations of breeds and strains have been tested, so the comparisons between

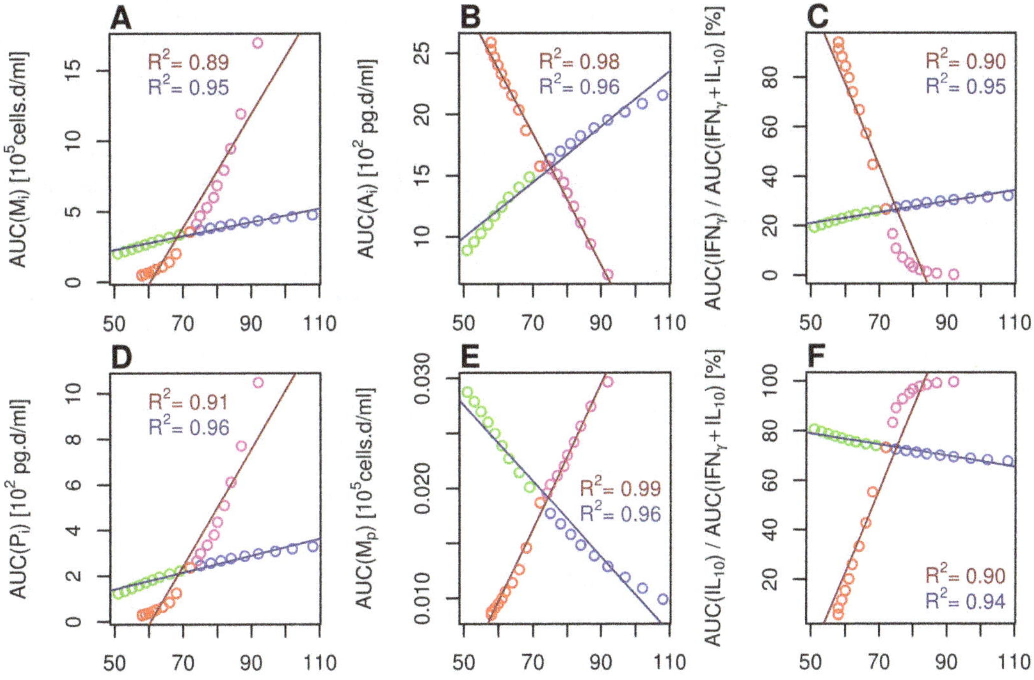

Figure 6. Linear regressions between the infection duration and immune components of interest. The immune components selected are the area under the curve (AUC) of **A:** infected macrophages ($M_I = M_L + M_E$), **B:** innate antiviral cytokines ($A_i = \mathrm{TNF}_\alpha + \mathrm{IFN}_\alpha$), **D:** pro-inflammatory cytokines ($P_i = \mathrm{IL}_{1\beta} + \mathrm{IL}_6 + \mathrm{IL}_8$), and **E:** phagocyting macrophages (M_P); and the relative AUC of **C:** IFN_γ and **F:** IL_{10}. Two regressions were performed for each component: (i) for scenarios SB→SA (dark red), in which the antiviral cytokine synthesis is higher (S0→SB, red dots) or lower (S0→SA, magenta dots) than in the reference scenario; (ii) for scenarios S1→S2 (dark blue), in which the macrophage permissiveness is lower (S0→S1, green dots) or higher (S0→S2, blue dots) than in the reference scenario. Scenarios are defined in Table 2.

our scenarios and the literature are limited, especially for the immune response.

The sensitivity analysis highlighted five key parameters with a strong influence on the macrophage and virus dynamics: the viral inoculation dose V_0, the viral excretion rate e, the macrophage infection rate β, the phagocytosis rate η and the antiviral cytokine synthesis rate ρ_{A_i}. The inoculation dose is measured in experimental studies but is difficult to assess in field conditions. The other three key parameters are not easy to inform. Distinguishing between infected and phagocyting macrophages is an experimental challenge, so their dynamics are rarely observed and the related parameter values are not measured in the literature. Further experimentation would be needed to track the dynamics of our outputs of interest, especially viral titer and ideally both infected and phagocyting macrophages, or at least activated macrophages. The sensitivity analysis also exhibited high interactions between parameters, which partly explain the difficulties encountered to calibrate the model.

In terms of viral dynamics, the simulated infection durations ranged between 52 and 118 days according to the scenarios. Experimental studies show that the resolution generally occurs in the serum between 28 and 42 days after a PRRSv infection [12,16,40] and in the lung after 56 days on average [12,56–59]. Infections longer than 240 days have been observed [16]. Consequently, the variation range of the simulated infection durations is realistic. Few studies measure the infection duration in the sera and in the lung simultaneously [40,60,61]. Combining these studies, we estimated that the infection duration in the lung is around 1.6 times longer than in the sera. This approximation allowed us to compare the infection duration in the lung from our simulation results to the infection duration in the blood (viremia) from experimental results. Few experimental studies focus on the response variability due to the viral strain or pig breed susceptibility. In a resistant pig breed, the viral load was around 35 days in the sera (estimated around 56 days in the lung) [52] and around 52 days in the lung with a low virulent strain [62]. Conversely, a more susceptible pig breed showed a 72-day viremia (estimated around 115 days in the lung) [52]. Infections by a highly virulent strain resulted in a viremia of 36 days (estimated around 58 days in the lung) [59] or the presence of viral particles in the lung for more than 67 days [63]. Our results were consistent with these data, but exhibited a larger range of infection durations.

In terms of immune response, the main trends found in the literature are the following: high virulence and susceptibility are associated with (i) a high activation of the immune response [64]; (ii) a dominant humoral response [38] with high levels of IL_{10}; (iii) a lower cellular response with low levels antiviral cytokines [33,34,50,64,65]. However, trends (ii) and (iii) do not always hold. Some reviews point out that levels of antiviral and IL_{10} cytokines are highly variable between hosts and viral strains [11,13]. An infection by a highly virulent strain can result in high levels of IFN_γ [59]. A strong cellular response is not necessarily correlated with a short infection duration [57]. Our results are qualitatively consistent with these data: high virulence and susceptibility scenarios were associated with high levels of the immune response and various orientations of the adaptive response. A common trend detected throughout all scenarios was the correlation between IL_{10} and the infected macrophages. Unlike the infected macrophages, IL_{10} can be easily be measured. However, this result should be confirmed by experimentation before using IL_{10} as a proxy for infected macrophages. We also found that high levels of pro-inflammatory cytokines were associated with longer infections.

It has been suggested that inflammatory responses in the lung are an indicator of the severity and duration of the PRRSv infection rather than an indicator of the immune response efficacy [17].

Assessing the impact of variability in host susceptibility and strain virulence

The strain virulence and pig susceptibility variability impact the infection duration, but the underlying mechanisms are still incompletely understood. Several hypotheses are formulated to explain PRRSv infection duration. Early immunological findings link prolonged viremia with (i) a weak innate antiviral response, (ii) high levels of immuno-modulatory cytokines (IL_{10} and TGF_{β}) and (iii) low levels of IFN_{γ}, resulting in the orientation towards an inefficient humoral response; in contrast the cellular response could be protective. These results are challenged in more recent studies. All this knowledge is synthesised and discussed in terms of between-host and between-strain variability in recent reviews [16,33,34,37]. In the following discussion sections, we confront our simulation results to the above-mentioned hypotheses.

Innate response. PRRSv has been reported to have various negative effects on innate immune functions, which probably contribute to the long survival of the virus in infected pigs. It suppresses the phagocyting activity, it fails to elicit any significant innate antiviral cytokines and it alters of the innate cytokine patterns compared to other respiratory pathogens [33,37]. Consequently, we could expect negative correlations between the infection duration and both innate antiviral cytokines (A_i) and phagocyting macrophages (M_P). However, we found that long PRRSv infections were correlated as follows: either positively with A_i and negatively with M_P, or positively with M_P and negatively A_i. To explain these questioning results, we need to consider the levels of the other immune components and the parameter values used.

For scenarios S1→S2, we gradually promoted the infection and excretion while limiting the phagocytosis. It resulted in longer infection durations, a high increase of A_i, a decrease of M_P and a moderate increase of infected macrophages (M_I). As A_i are mainly synthesised by M_I, promoting infection results in increasing A_i. In turn, A_i inhibits the infection and should reduce M_I. However, promoting the excretion and limiting the phagocytosis increase the free viral particles (V) and M_I. This last mechanism was dominant in these scenarios and countered the effect of A_i.

For scenarios SB→SA, we gradually promoted the synthesis of immuno-modulatory cytokines (IL_{10} and TGF_{β}) and limited the synthesis of A_i and IFN_{γ}. It resulted in longer infection durations, an increase of M_P and a high increase of M_I and IL_{10}. Promoting IL_{10} and TGF_{β} should increase the infection and reduce the phagocytosis, both contributing to an increase of V. In turn, V activates the phagocytosis and infection. This last mechanism was dominant in these scenarios and countered the cytokine effect. As a net result, M_P increased.

Our results suggest that despite high correlations between components of the innate response and the infection duration, measuring the innate response alone is insufficient to explain and predict the infection duration.

Adaptive response. The orientation towards the cellular, humoral or regulatory responses is supposed to have a high influence on the infection duration, but the mechanisms governing the orientation still need more insight. In experimental studies, the orientation towards the humoral and cellular responses is usually approximated by the levels of IL_{10} and IFN_{γ} respectively. However, few studies consider the cellular and humoral responses simultaneously, as well as the associated cytokines, and most studies neglect the regulatory response. Reviews on PRRSv infection suggest that high levels of IL_{10} are capable of shifting the immune response towards a humoral response and that in the absence of IFN_{γ}, there is no cellular response [16,33]. As the neutralisation of IL_{10} inhibits the regulatory response [37], levels of IL_{10} and regulatory response are assumed to be linked. In our model, the three orientations were represented, as well as their regulations and interactions. We found that the orientation of the adaptive response did not depend on specific cytokine levels, but on the proportions of IFN_{γ} and IL_{10}. This result is consistent with the literature, as it points out the crucial role of IFN_{γ} and IL_{10} on the adaptive response orientation. However, it also points out the limits of the usual approximation of the adaptive response orientation by IFN_{γ} or IL_{10} levels.

The cellular response is considered as protective against a wide variety of viral infections but its influence is controversial in the case of PRRSv infections [16,33]. Reviews suggest that the suppression of IFN_{γ} may have little influence on the *in vivo* disease progression [16,66]. Moreover, long-term persistence of the virus in the host associated with a strong cellular response has been observed [33]. Both findings suggest that the cellular response alone cannot curtail the infection. Correlations between the strength of the cellular response and the PRRSv infection duration are highly variable between hosts and strains [34]. We also found that a dominant cellular response and high percentages of IFN_{γ} can be associated with either long or short infection durations. Scenarios SB→SA are consistent with the usual assumption that confers a protective role to the cellular response. However, in scenarios S1→S2, long infection durations were associated with a dominant cellular response. To explain this result, we need to consider simultaneously the levels of the other immune components and the parameter values used. Long infection durations were associated with high levels of IFN_{γ} and A_i, moderate levels of IL_{10} and infected macrophages, as well as an orientation towards the cellular response. We previously explained the high increase of A_i and the moderate increase of M_I (see Innate response above). Being produced by M_I, IL_{10} also increases, but less than A_i (lower production rate). As M_I increases, the activation of the immune response also increases. In particular, the natural killers increase. They synthesise IFN_{γ}, which promotes the cellular response, whose effectors synthesise IFN_{γ}, resulting in the orientation towards the cellular response. IL_{10} does not increase enough to prevent this orientation. As A_i, the cellular response and IFN_{γ} inhibit the infection, but not enough to compensate the high excretion and infection rates.

The high influence of the excretion rate on the infection duration is consistent with the results of the sensitivity analysis. The scenarios explored could correspond to real conditions. Indeed, an experimental study showed that pig genotypes can influence the alveolar macrophage abilityto suppress the viral replication [67]. Moreover, virulent strains vary in their ability to induce the synthesis of antiviral [16] and IL_{10} [37] cytokines. So scenarios S0→S2 could correspond to a pig that is not able to inhibit the viral replication and that is infected by a highly virulent type 2 PRRSv field strain, inducing a strong antiviral response and a moderate IL_{10} production.

Neutralising antibodies play a key role in the immunological control of a wide variety of viral infections [16,33]. Consequently, a strong humoral response, should result in a short infection duration. PRRSv infections induce high levels of IL_{10} compared to the other cytokines and the humoral response levels are similar to the levels encountered in other viral infection. However, the levels of neutralising antibodies remain low. The combination of high levels of IL_{10} and a strong but inefficient humoral response is often proposed to explain the long infection duration [11]. Indeed, IL_{10}

is a major regulator of the immune response and its inhibitory effects on numerous immune functions could explain several immunological phenomena observed in PRRSv infection [33,34,37]. However, the variability in host susceptibility and viral virulence challenges this hypothesis. PRRSv infections by virulent or attenuated strains showed no correlation between the IL_{10} levels and the infection duration [16]. In a variety of studies, PRRSv infection resolution was observed without the development of neutralising antibodies [16]. We found that a dominant humoral response and high percentages of IL_{10} can be associated with either long or short infection durations. Scenarios SB→SA are consistent with the usual assumption of the ineffective humoral response. However, scenarios S1→S0 associated short infection durations with a dominant humoral response. This result is due to the low excretion and macrophage infection rates, despite the low levels of innate and adaptive antiviral cytokines.

Concerning TGF_{β} and the regulatory response, few studies explored their influences on the immune dynamics and the subsequent infection resolution. The induction of regulatory T lymphocytes (T_{reg}) during the early stages of infection is considered as one of the mechanisms that establish chronic or persistent viral infections [16,33]. According to this hypothesis, our results showed that a strong regulatory response was associated with very high levels of IL_{10} and that it resulted in a prolonged infection (scenarios S0→SA). Further experimentation considering the T_{reg} cells and TGF_{β} cytokines are needed to validate our model results.

Conclusion

We built an original and integrative model of the immune response in the lung to a pathogen targeting pulmonary macrophages, applied here to PRRSv. This model provides an interesting framework to explore the macrophage–pathogen interactions while representing the adaptive response. We used the model to explore the influence of macrophage permissiveness and cytokine synthesis capacities on the infection duration and immune dynamics. A recent review suggests that the concepts proposed to explain prolonged PRRSv infection have not been experimentally proved; in particular, the roles of the cytokines and the orientation of the adaptive response need to be more clearly elucidated [16]. Our integrative model allowed to simulate contrasted dynamics in terms of immune response and infection duration, suggesting hypotheses to explain the apparent contradictions between published results.

In addition, we extracted some synthetic and original elements from our work.

1. Among the immune variables that can be easily measured, some were found to characterise immune mechanisms: (a) the proportions of IL_{10} and IFN_{γ} were good indicators of the adaptive response orientation; and (b) the level of IL_{10} was a good indicator of the level of infected macrophages.
2. Whatever the strain virulence and host susceptibility, the infection duration was linked to some immune variables: (a) the level of pro-inflammatory cytokines was a good indicator of the infection duration; and (b) a dominant regulatory response was associated with a prolonged infection.

However, to identify and understand the immune mechanisms responsible for the infection duration, the entire immune response had to be considered. At least (i) the levels of innate antiviral cytokines, (ii) the level of IL_{10}, and (iii) the relative levels of IL_{10} and IFN_{γ} were needed.

We found that the macrophage permissiveness and the cytokine synthesis capacities both influence the infection duration through various immune mechanisms. Promoting antiviral cytokines or limiting the macrophage permissiveness and viral replication in order to reduce the infection duration has only been suggested [33,34,57]. Classically, two main approaches are associated to limit the infection: (i) appropriate housing conditions to reduce the pig susceptibility and (ii) vaccination to improve the immune response efficiency. Moreover, it has been shown that pig genotypes can influence the alveolar macrophage ability to suppress viral replication [51]. Our results suggest that the viral replication rate is highly influential on the infection duration. So selecting resistant pigs should be efficient to prevent severe infections. Concerning the vaccination strategies, vaccines capable of promoting the synthesis of antiviral cytokines or minimising IL_{10} production have been considered in the literature and numerous experimentation have been carried out, but the current results are not convincing (reviewed in [16,37]). Obviously, vaccination strategies need more insight. Our integrative model provides a powerful framework to go beyond experimental constraints. In particular, such an approach could be used to help designing efficient vaccination strategies.

Supporting Information

Figure S1 Preliminary sensitivity analysis: comparison of the phagocytosis and infection activities. This figure results from the 243 simulations performed for the preliminary sensitivity analysis. **A**: Percentage of phagocyting macrophages among all macrophages over time (maximum 14%). **B**: Percentage of infected macrophages over time (maximum 100%). **C**: Phagocytosis activity as a percentage of the phagocytosis and infection flows, *i.e.* the ratio between the concentration of susceptible macrophages becoming phagocyting macrophages per unit of time and the concentration of susceptible macrophages becoming phagocyting or latent infected macrophages per unit of time × 100. At a given time, if a simulation is above the 50% red line, its phagocytosis flow is higher than its infection flow. These figures show that, even if there are few phagocyting macrophages at all times, the phagocytosis activity can be dominant over the infection activity at given times for susceptible macrophages.

Figure S2 Parameter space exploration: viral titer. This figure results from the 6561 simulations performed for the sensitivity analysis. **A**: Viral titer over time (red curve: reference scenario S0). **B**: Distribution of the viral titer at day 200. Some simulations resulted in infection persistence, others in infection resolution occurring at various dates. The viral titer at day 200 was heterogeneously distributed: 56% of the simulations had a viral titer lower than $2\log_{10}(TCID_{50}/ml)$, which is usually considered as the infection resolution; the remaining simulations had viral titers ranging between 2 and $8.96\log_{10}(TCID_{50}/ml)$. More precisely: (i) 3.7% of the simulations had a viral titer higher than the maximal initial inoculation titer ($7\log_{10}(TCID_{50}/ml)$) and (ii) 90% of the simulations had a viral titer lower than its corresponding inoculation titer (4, 5 or $7\log_{10}(TCID_{50}/ml)$). In the lung, PRRSv infection lasts 56 days on average [12] and can be longer than 200 days [16,41].

Figure S3 Parameter space exploration: cumulative number of phagocyting macrophages. This figure results from the 6561 simulations performed for the sensitivity analysis. **A**: Cumulative number of phagocyting macrophages (cM_P) over time (red curve: reference scenario S0). **B**: Distribution of cM_P at day 1. **C**: Distribution of cM_P at day 200. cM_P was highly variable between simulations: between 0.5 and $10^{6.7}$ macrophages/ml on the first day, and between 1.4 and $10^{8.4}$ macrophages/ml at day 200. Most simulations rapidly increased during the first days and then tended to a threshold. This means that the phagocytosis activity was maximal at the beginning of the infection, which is consistent with the literature. Simulations that did not saturate corresponded to persistent infection. To our knowledge, there are no experimental studies that measure the concentration of phagocyting macrophages during a PRRSv infection.

Figure S4 Parameter space exploration: percentage of infected macrophages. This figure results from the 6561 simulations performed for the sensitivity analysis. **A**: Percentage of infected macrophages among all macrophages ($\%M_I$) over time (red curve: reference scenario S0). **B**: Distribution of the $\%M_I$ peak value. **C**: Distribution of the $\%M_I$ peak date. The peak is defined as the maximum value of $\%M_I$ over the course of infection. The $\%M_I$ dynamics was highly variable among simulations but tended to decrease after the first weeks of infection. At day 200, $\%M_I$ was higher than 60% for only 4% of the simulations and lower than 1% for 84% of the simulations. 55% of the simulations peaked during the first week. For 80% of the simulations, the $\%M_I$ peak was lower than 20%. Some experimental studies showed a peak of infected macrophages of around 40% during the first week of a PRRSv infection [39]. During the first week, only 5% of the simulations had $\%M_I$ peaking between 20 and 60%, which is consistent with the experimental results.

File S1.

Author Contributions

Analyzed the data: NG ST C. Bidot. Contributed reagents/materials/analysis tools: C. Bidot. Wrote the paper: NG ST C. Belloc. Biological expertise: NG C. Belloc. Modelling & analysis expertise: NG ST C. Bidot. Model implementation & simulations: NG.

References

1. Braciale TJ, Sun J, Kim TS (2012) Regulating the adaptive immune response to respiratory virus infection. Nature Reviews Immunology 12: 295–305.
2. Kohlmeier JE, Woodland DL (2009) Immunity to respiratory viruses. Annual Review of Immunology 27: 61–82.
3. Heffernan JM (2011) Mathematical immunology of infectious diseases. Mathematical Population Studies 18: 47–54.
4. Rouse BT, Sehrawat S (2010) Immunity and immunopathology to viruses: what decides the outcome? Nature Review Immunology 10: 514–526.
5. Beauchemin C, Handel A (2011) A review of mathematical models of influenza A infections within a host or cell culture: lessons learned and challenges ahead. BMC Public Health 11.
6. Smith AM, Perelson AS (2011) Influenza A virus infection kinetics: quantitative data and models. Wiley Interdisciplinary Reviews: Systems Biology and Medicine 3: 429–445.
7. Dobrovolny HM, Reddy MB, Kamal MA, Rayner CR, Beauchemin CAA (2013) Assessing mathematical models of influenza infections using features of the immune response. PLoS ONE 8: e57088.
8. Gammack D, Ganguli S, Marino S, Segovia-Juarez J, Kirschner D (2005) Understanding the immune response in tuberculosis using different mathematical models and biological scales. Multiscale Modeling & Simulation 3: 312–345.
9. Marino S, Linderman JJ, Kirschner DE (2011) A multifaceted approach to modeling the immune response in tuberculosis. Wiley Interdisciplinary Reviews: Systems Biology and Medicine 3: 479–489.
10. Doeschl-Wilson AB, Kyriazakis I, Vincent A, Rothschild MF, Thacker E, et al. (2009) Clinical and pathological responses of pigs from two genetically diverse commercial lines to porcine reproductive and respiratory syndrome virus infection. Journal of Animal Science: 1638–1647.
11. Darwich L, Díaz I, Mateu E (2010) Certainties, doubts and hypotheses in porcine reproductive and respiratory syndrome virus immunobiology. Virus Research 154: 123–132.
12. Zimmerman J, Benfield DA, Murtaugh MP, Osorio F, Stevenson GW, et al. (2006) Porcine reproductive and respiratory syndrome virus (porcine arterivirus). In: Straw BE, Zimmerman JJ, D'Allaire S, Taylor DL, editors, Diseases of swine, Blackwell, chapter 24. Ninth edition, pp. 387–418.
13. Gómez-Laguna J, Salguero FJ, Pallarés FJ, Carrasco L (2013) Immunopathogenesis of porcine reproductive and respiratory syndrome in the respiratory tract of pigs. The Veterinary Journal 195: 148–155.
14. Murtaugh MP (2005) PRRSV/host interaction. In: PRRS fatti vs speculazioni. Parma, Italy: Università degli Studi di Parma, Dipartimento di Salute Animale, pp.73–80.
15. Murtaugh MP, Xiao Z, Zuckermann F (2002) Immunological responses of swine to porcine reproductive and respiratory syndrome virus infection. Viral immunology 15: 533–547.
16. Murtaugh MP, Genzow M (2011) Immunological solutions for treatment and prevention of porcine reproductive and respiratory syndrome (PRRS). Vaccine 29: 8192–8204.
17. Van Reeth K, Van Gucht S, Pensaert M (2002) In vivo studies on cytokine involvement during acute viral respiratory disease of swine: troublesome but rewarding. Veterinary Immunology and Immunopathology 87: 161–168.
18. Roth AJ, Thacker EL (2009) Immune sytem. In: Straw BE, Zimmerman JJ, D'Allaire S, Taylor DL, editors, Diseases of swine, Blackwell, chapter 2. Ninth edition, pp.15–36.
19. Tosi MF (2005) Innate immune responses to infection. Journal of Allergy and Clinical Immunology 116: 241–249.
20. Choi C, Chae C (2002) Expression of tumour necrosis factor alpha is associated with apoptosis in lungs of pigs experimentally infected with porcine reproductive and respiratory syndrome virus. Research in Veterinary Science 72: 45–49.
21. Marino S, Myers A, Flynn JL, Kirschner DE (2010) TNF and IL-10 are major factors in modulation of the phagocytic cell environment in lung and lymph node in tuberculosis: A next-generation two-compartmental model. Journal of Theoretical Biology 265: 586–598.
22. Wigginton JE, Kirschner D (2001) A model to predict cell-mediated immune regulatory mechanisms during human infection with Mycobacterium tuberculosis. The Journal of Immunology 166: 1951–1967.
23. DeFranco AL, Locksley RM, Robertson M, Cunin R (2009) Immunité: la réponse immunitaire dans les maladies infectieuses et inflammatoires. DeBoeck, Bruxelles, 2nd edition.
24. Vidal SM, Khakoo SI, Biron CA (2011) Natural killer cell responses during viral infections: flexibility and conditioning of innate immunity by experience. Current Opinion in Virology 1: 497–512.
25. Bosch AATM, Biesbroek G, Trzcinski K, Sanders EAM, Bogaert D (2013) Viral and bacterial interactions in the upper respiratory tract. PLoS Pathogens 9: e1003057.
26. Borghetti P (2005) Cell-mediated immunity and viral infection in pig. In: PRRS fatti vs speculazioni. Parma, Italy: Università degli Studi di Parma, Dipartimento di Salute Animale, pp.27–46.
27. Coquerelle C, Moser M (2010) DC subsets in positive and negative regulation of immunity. Immunological Reviews 234: 317–334.
28. Kidd P (2003) Th1/Th2 balance: the hypothesis, its limitations, and implications for health and disease. Alternative Medicine Review 8: 223–246.
29. LeRoith T, Ahmed SA (2012) Regulatory T cells and viral disease. In: Khatami M, editor, Inflammation, Chronic Diseases and Cancer: Cell and Molecular Biology, Immunology and Clinical Bases, InTech, chapter 6. pp.121–144. doi:10.5772/28502.
30. Knosp CA, Johnston JA (2012) Regulation of CD4+ T-cell polarization by suppressor of cytokine signalling proteins. Immunology 135: 101–111.
31. Yates A, Bergmann C, Van Hemmen JL, Stark J, Callard R (2000) Cytokine-modulated regulation of helper T cell populations. Journal of Theoretical Biology 206: 539–560.
32. Darwich L, Gimeno M, Sibila M, Díaz I, de la Torre E, et al. (2011) Genetic and immunobiological diversities of porcine reproductive and respiratory syndrome genotype I strains. Veterinary Microbiology 150: 49–62.
33. Kimman TG, Cornelissen LA, Moormann RJ, Rebel JMJ, Stockhofe-Zurwieden N (2009) Challenges for porcine reproductive and respiratory syndrome virus (PRRSV) vaccinology. Vaccine 27: 3704–3718.
34. Lunney JK, Chen H (2010) Genetic control of host resistance to porcine reproductive and respiratory syndrome virus (PRRSV) infection. Virus Research 154: 161–169.
35. Mateu E, Díaz I (2008) The challenge of PRRS immunology. The Veterinary Journal 177: 345–351.
36. Nauwynck HJ, Van Gorp H, Vanhee M, Karniychuk U, Geldhof M, et al. (2012) Micro-dissecting the pathogenesis and immune response of PRRSV infection paves the way for more efficient PRRSV vaccines. Transboundary and Emerging Diseases 59: 50–54.

37. Thanawongnuwech R, Suradhat S (2010) Taming PRRSV: Revisiting the control strategies and vaccine design. Virus Research 154: 133–140.
38. Johnson W, Roof M, Vaughn E, Christopher-Hennings J, Johnson CR, et al. (2004) Pathogenic and humoral immune responses to porcine reproductive and respiratory syndrome virus (PRRSV) are related to viral load in acute infection. Veterinary Immunology and Immunopathology 102: 233–247.
39. Labarque G, van Gucht S, Nauwynck H, van Reeth K, Pensaert M (2003) Apoptosis in the lungs of pigs infected with porcine reproductive and respiratory syndrome virus and associations with the production of apoptogenic cytokines. Veterinary Research 34: 249–260.
40. Duan X, Nauwynck HJ, Pensaert MB (1997) Virus quantification and identification of cellular targets in the lungs and lymphoid tissues of pigs at different time intervals after inoculation with porcine reproductive and respiratory syndrome virus (PRRSV). Veterinary Microbiology 56: 9–19.
41. Albina E, Pirou L, Hutet E, Cariolet R, L'Hospitalier R (1998) Immune response in pigs infected with porcine reproductive and respiratory sydrome virus (PRRSV). Veterinary immunology and immunopathology 61: 49–66.
42. Costers S, Delputte PL, Nauwynck HJ (2006) Porcine reproductive and respiratory syndrome virus-infected alveolar macrophages contain no detectable levels of viral proteins in their plasma membrane and are protected against antibody-dependent, complement-mediated cell lysis. Journal of General Virology 87: 2341–2351.
43. Gaudreault N, Rowland R, Wyatt C (2009) Factors affecting the permissiveness of porcine alveolar macrophages for porcine reproductive and respiratory syndrome virus. Archives of Virology 154: 133–136.
44. Gómez-Laguna J, Rodríguez-Gomez IM, Barranco I, Pallarés FJ, Salguero FJ, et al. (2012) Enhanced expression of TGF_{β} protein in lymphoid organs and lung, but not in serum, of pigs infected with a European field isolate of porcine reproductive and respiratory syndrome virus. Veterinary Microbiology 158: 187–193.
45. Silva-Campa E, Flores-Mendoza L, Reséndiz M, Pinelli-Saavedra A, Mata-Haro V, et al. (2009) Induction of T helper 3 regulatory cells by dendritic cells infected with porcine reproductive and respiratory syndrome virus. Virology 387: 373–379.
46. Wongyanin P, Buranapraditkun S, Chokeshai-usaha K, Thanawonguwech R, Suradhat S (2010) Induction of inducible CD4+CD25+Foxp3+ regulatory T lymphocytes by porcine reproductive and respiratory syndrome virus (PRRSV). Veterinary Immunology and Immunopathology 133: 170–182.
47. Saltelli A, Chan K, Scott EM, editors (2000) Sensitivity analysis. Wiley Series in Probability and Statistics. Wiley.
48. Lamboni M, Monod H, Makowski D (2011) Multivariate sensitivity analysis to measure global contribution of input factors in dynamic models. Reliability Engineering & System Safety 96: 450–459.
49. Gimeno M, Darwich L, Díaz I, de la Torre E, Pujols J, et al. (2011) Cytokine profiles and phenotype regulation of antigen presenting cells by genotype-I porcine reproductive and respiratory syndrome virus isolates. Veterinary Research 42.
50. Díaz I, Gimeno M, Darwich L, Navarro N, Kuzemtseva L, et al. (2012) Characterization of homologous and heterologous adaptive immune responses in porcine reproductive and respiratory syndrome virus infection. Veterinary Research 43.
51. Ait-Ali T, Wilson AD, Carré W, Westcott DG, Frossard JP, et al. (2011) Host inhibits replication of European porcine Reproductive and respiratory syndrome virus in macrophages by altering differential regulation of type-I interferon transcriptional responses. Immunogenetics 63: 437–448.
52. Reiner G, Willems H, Pesch S, Ohlinger V (2010) Variation in resistance to the porcine reproductive and respiratory syndrome virus (PRRSV) in Pietrain and Miniature pigs. Journal of Animal Breeding and Genetics 127: 100–106.
53. Duan F, Simeone S, Wu R, Grady J, Mandoiu I, et al. (2012) Area under the curve as a tool to measure kinetics of tumor growth in experimental animals. Journal of Immunological Methods 382: 224–228.
54. Flores-Mendoza L, Silva-Campa E, Reséndiz M, Osorio FA, Hernndez J (2008) Porcine reproductive and respiratory syndrome virus infects mature porcine dendritic cells and up-regulates interleukin-10 production. Clinical and Vaccine Immunology 15: 720–725.
55. Park JY, Kim HS, Seo SH (2008) Characterization of interaction between porcine reproductive and respiratory syndrome virus and porcine dendritic cells. Journal of Microbiology and Biotechnology 18: 1709–1716.
56. Molina RM, Cha SH, Chittick W, Lawson S, Murtaugh MP, et al. (2008) Immune response against porcine reproductive and respiratory syndrome virus during acute and chronic infection. Veterinary immunology and immunopathology 126: 283–292.
57. Murtaugh MP (2004) PRRS immunology: what are we missing? In: 35th Annual Meeting of the American Association of Swine Veterinarians. Des Moines (Iowa), USA, pp.359–367.
58. Petry DB, Holl JW, Weber JS, Doster AR, Osorio FA, et al. (2005) Biological responses to porcine respiratory and reproductive syndrome virus in pigs of two genetic populations. Journal of Animal Science 83: 1494–1502.
59. Wesley DR, Lager KM, Kehrli ME (2006) Infection with porcin reproductive and respiratory syndrome virus stimulates an early gamma interferon response in the serum of pig. Canadian Journal Veterinary Research 70: 176–182.
60. Beyer J, Fichtner D, Schirrmeir H, Polster U, Weiland E, et al. (2000) Porcine reproductive and respiratory syndrome virus (PRRSV): Kinetics of infection in lymphatic organs and lung. Journal of Veterinary Medicine, Series B 47: 9–25.
61. Karniychuk U, Geldhof M, Vanhee M, Van Doorsselaere J, Saveleva T, et al. (2010) Pathogenesis and antigenic characterization of a new East European subtype 3 porcine reproductive and respiratory syndrome virus isolate. BMC veterinary research 6.
62. Labarque GG, Nauwynck HJ, Van Reeth K, Pensaert MB (2000) Effect of cellular changes and onset of humoral immunity on the replication of porcine reproductive and respiratory syndrome virus in the lungs of pigs. Journal of General Virology 81: 1327–1334.
63. Xiao Z, Batista L, Dee S, Halbur P, Murtaugh MP (2004) the level of virus-specific T-cell and macrophage recruitment in porcine reproductive and respiratory syndrome virus infection in pigs is independent of virus load. Journal of Virology 78: 5923–5933.
64. Petry DB, Lunney J, Boyd P, Kuhar D, Blankenshi E, et al. (2007) Differential immunity in pigs with high and low responses to porcine reproductive and respiratory syndrome virus infection. Journal of Animal Science 85: 2075–2092.
65. Weesendorp E, Morgan S, Stockhofe-Zurwieden N, Graaf DJ, Graham SP, et al. (2013) Comparative analysis of immune responses following experimental infection of pigs with european porcine reproductive and respiratory syndrome virus strains of differing virulence. Veterinary Microbiology 163: 1–12.
66. Mogler M (2012) Evaluation of replicon particle vaccines for porcine reproductive and respiratory syndrome virus. Ph.D. thesis, Iowa State University. URL http://lib.dr.iastate.edu/etd/12841.
67. Ait-Ali T, Wilson AD, Westcott DG, Clapperton M, Waterfall M, et al. (2007) Innate immune responses to replication of porcine Reproductive and respiratory syndrome virus in isolated swine alveolar macrophages. Viral immunology 20: 105–118.
68. Gammack D, Doering CR, Kirschner DE (2004) Macrophage response to Mycobacterium tuberculosis infection. Journal of Mathematical Biology 48: 218–242.
69. Marino S, Kirschner DE (2004) The human immune response to Mycobacterium tuberculosis in lung and lymphe node. Journal of Theoretical Biology 227: 463–486.

Modeling the Dynamics and Migratory Pathways of Virus-Specific Antibody-Secreting Cell Populations in Primary Influenza Infection

Hongyu Miao[1,9], Mark Y. Sangster[2,9], Alexandra M. Livingstone[2], Shannon P. Hilchey[3], Le Zhang[1], David J. Topham[2], Tim R. Mosmann[2], Jeanne Holden-Wiltse[1], Alan S. Perelson[4], Hulin Wu[1¶], Martin S. Zand[3*¶]

1 Department of Biostatistics and Computational Biology, University of Rochester Medical Center, Rochester, New York, United States of America, 2 David H. Smith Center for Vaccine Biology & Immunology, Department of Microbiology and Immunology, University of Rochester Medical Center, Rochester, New York, United States of America, 3 Department of Medicine, University of Rochester Medical Center, Rochester, New York, United States of America, 4 Theoretical Biology and Biophysics, Los Alamos National Laboratory, Los Alamos, New Mexico, United States of America

Abstract

The B cell response to influenza infection of the respiratory tract contributes to viral clearance and establishes profound resistance to reinfection by related viruses. Numerous studies have measured virus-specific antibody-secreting cell (ASC) frequencies in different anatomical compartments after influenza infection and provided a general picture of the kinetics of ASC formation and dispersion. However, the dynamics of ASC populations are difficult to determine experimentally and have received little attention. Here, we applied mathematical modeling to investigate the dynamics of ASC growth, death, and migration over the 2-week period following primary influenza infection in mice. Experimental data for model fitting came from high frequency measurements of virus-specific IgM, IgG, and IgA ASCs in the mediastinal lymph node (MLN), spleen, and lung. Model construction was based on a set of assumptions about ASC gain and loss from the sampled sites, and also on the directionality of ASC trafficking pathways. Most notably, modeling results suggest that differences in ASC fate and trafficking patterns reflect the site of formation and the expressed antibody class. Essentially all early IgA ASCs in the MLN migrated to spleen or lung, whereas cell death was likely the major reason for IgM and IgG ASC loss from the MLN. In contrast, the spleen contributed most of the IgM and IgG ASCs that migrated to the lung, but essentially none of the IgA ASCs. This finding points to a critical role for regional lymph nodes such as the MLN in the rapid generation of IgA ASCs that seed the lung. Results for the MLN also suggest that ASC death is a significant early feature of the B cell response. Overall, our analysis is consistent with accepted concepts in many regards, but it also indicates novel features of the B cell response to influenza that warrant further investigation.

Editor: James M. McCaw, University of Melbourne, Australia

Funding: This work was funded by the National Institute of Allergy and Infectious Diseases contract HHSN272201000055C and R01 AI069351 (MZ). The funders had no role in study design, data collection and analysis, decision to publish, or preparation of the manuscript.

Competing Interests: The authors have declared that no competing interests exist.

* Email: martin_zand@urmc.rochester.edu

9 These authors contributed equally to this work.

¶ These authors are joint senior authors on this work.

Introduction

The antibody (Ab) response against influenza infection involves activation and progressive differentiation of virus-specific B cells into Ab-secreting cells (ASCs). A similar process occurs during intramuscular influenza vaccination. In both cases, Ab-mediated immunity develops after influenza-specific B cells produce high affinity Abs, most importantly against the haemagglutinin (HA) protein responsible for viral binding to target respiratory epithelial cells. B cells activated by influenza infection or vaccination may develop into ASCs secreting the IgM Ab class, or may undergo class switching during the differentiation process and form IgG or IgA ASCs. The Ab class reflects functional capabilities of the immunoglobulin molecule, such as complement activation, Fc receptor binding, and transcytosis of epithelial cells at mucosal surfaces.

Studies by several groups have characterized ASC formation during primary influenza A virus infection using murine models [1–5]. Influenza-specific ASCs first develop in lymph nodes that drain the respiratory tract and a day or so later in the spleen. In sites of ASC formation, a peak of IgM ASCs typically precedes increasing numbers of IgG and IgA ASCs. Influenza-specific ASC numbers in the regional lymph nodes and spleen gradually wane after clearance of infectious virus, but in the course of the response ASCs traffic to the respiratory tract and bone marrow and establish long-lasting populations. A rapid increase in serum levels of influenza-specific IgM and IgG beginning approximately 7 days after infection closely follows initial ASC formation. Serum IgM levels peak at 8–10 days and then gradually decline, reflecting the

IgM ASC numbers in lymphoid tissues. However, high serum levels of IgG are maintained long-term, primarily by ASCs in the bone marrow [6,7]. Although much has been learned, B cell dynamics in the context of primary influenza infection have not been well characterized in a quantitative manner. Specifically, we know little about the dynamics of ASC division, death and migration, the routes taken by ASCs after they migrate from sites of formation, the rates of ASC trafficking from site-to-site, and the number and source of ASCs that migrate to the site of infection in the lung.

The key dynamic parameters mentioned above are very difficult to measure experimentally. For example, direct measurement of the rate at which activated B cells transit from regional lymph nodes to bone marrow requires real-time measurement and direct tracking of labeled cells over a period of 12–24 hours in a live mouse. However, such kinetic parameters can be estimated using quantitative mathematical models. This approach has been used by other groups to estimate the survival time of free virus and virus-infected cells at particular stages of infection, the relative contributions of different Ab classes to viral clearance, and the relative importance of host lymphoid tissues in generating antiviral effector T cells that migrate to sites of infection [6,8–13]. In the current study, we applied mathematical modeling to investigate the dynamics of virus-specific ASCs over the 2-week period immediately following primary influenza infection in mice. High frequency time-course measurements of IgM, IgG, and IgA ASC frequencies in a regional lymph node, the spleen, and the lung provided the basis for the development of mathematical models to describe ASC appearance, disappearance, and migration. To refine parameter estimates, semi-mechanistic models were also considered and best models were selected based on model comparison criteria. Our combination of experimental data and mathematical modeling provides a precise depiction of early ASC dynamics in the context of influenza infection.

Materials and Methods

Mouse Infection and Sampling

All animal experiments were performed under a protocol approved and monitored by the University Committee on Animal Research (UCAR) at the University of Rochester Medical Center, and in compliance with the United States Public Health Service (PHS) Policy on Humane Care and Use of Laboratory Animals.

C57BL/6NCr mice at 8 to 10 weeks of age were anesthetized using 2,2,2-tribromoethanol (Avertin) and then infected intranasally with 10^5 EID_{50} H3N2 A/Hong Kong/X31 (X31) influenza virus [13]. On the day of organ harvest, mice ($n = 9$/day) were euthanized. The mediastinal lymph node (MLN) and spleen were collected and disrupted to generate single-cell suspensions. Lungs were disrupted and strained through a nylon mesh. Red blood cells were lysed using buffered ammonium chloride solution (Gey's solution). Pelleted lung cells were resuspended in 5 ml of complete minimum essential medium (cMEM), layered over 5 ml of Histopaque 1083 (Sigma, St. Louis, MO), and centrifuged for 18 min at 1,800×g. After centrifugation, cells at the interface were removed, washed, and resuspended in cMEM.

ELISpot Assay

Influenza-specific ASCs were enumerated by ELISpot assay. Plates were coated with purified X31 and single cell suspensions were plated and incubated as previously described [14]. Plates were washed and alkaline phosphatase-conjugated goat anti-mouse Abs specific for IgM, IgG, or IgA (KPL, Gaithersburg, MD) were added to the appropriate wells. After overnight incubation at 4°C, plates were washed thoroughly and incubated with alkaline phosphatase substrate kit III (Vector Laboratories, Burlingame, CA) for 30 min at room temperature. Plates were washed and dried after optimal spot development and spots were counted using a CTL ImmunoSpot plate reader (Cellular Technology Limited, Cleveland, OH).

Mathematical Models

We first developed a mechanistic ordinary differential equation (ODE) model to describe the dynamics of virus-specific ASC populations in the blood, MLN, spleen, and lung compartments following primary influenza infection. Model construction was based on a set of assumptions derived from our current understanding of the processes of ASC formation and dispersion (reviewed in [15]). To briefly outline these processes, as influenza virus replicates in the respiratory tract, B cell responses are initiated by the delivery of viral antigens to draining lymph nodes and to the spleen. Virus-specific ASC formation is largely a T cell-dependent process that involves the proliferation and differentiation of activated B cells and Ab class switching. Activated B cells can progress along an extrafollicular differentiation pathway to form short-lived ASCs, or can enter germinal center reactions where affinity maturation of expressed Abs takes place and long-lived ASCs are produced. ASCs induced by influenza infection exit the draining lymph nodes (initially via efferent lymphatics) and the spleen (directly into the blood) and are transported in the blood to establish long-lasting populations in the respiratory tract and bone marrow. Some trafficking of ASCs from responding lymph nodes to spleen is predicted because of the phase of blood-borne migration. Specific assumptions for model construction (illustrated in Fig. 1) are as follows: (i) ASC numbers in the MLN are affected by differentiation and proliferation within the lymph node, migration to spleen, migration to lung, migration to other compartments that were not experimentally measured (e.g., bone marrow), and cell death (a term used to encompass all mechanisms of cell death as well as processes resulting in loss of Ab secretion by living cells); (ii) ASC numbers in the spleen reflect differentiation and proliferation, influx from MLN, migration to lung, migration to other compartments, and loss through cell death; and (iii) ASC numbers in the lung reflect influx from both MLN and spleen, with loss due to cell death. ASC transition from a cell secreting a particular Ab class into a cell secreting a different Ab class (for example, transition from an IgM ASC to an IgG ASC) was not incorporated into our model. This is an unlikely event, since transcriptional programming for ASC formation is associated with down-regulation of Ab class switching [16]. We denote ASC numbers by B (for B cell-derived); superscripted letters denote the anatomical compartment (N for MLN, S for spleen, and L for lung) and subscripted letters denote the secreted Ab class (M for IgM, G for IgG, and A for IgA). For example, B_M^N denotes the number of IgM ASCs in the MLN.

The virus-specific B cell response to influenza infection in the MLN and spleen is largely dependent on cognate help delivered by CD4 T cells. For simplicity, we do not explicitly represent the effect of T cell help, but instead parameterize the model with a general term representing the strength of B cell activation. This formulation allows the magnitude and timing of the activation strength to take any reasonable value and is thus flexible enough to allow for both cognate and non-cognate B cell help (see the stimulation strength coefficient and the time delay parameters in Model 1 below).

ASC loss from a compartment results from emigration and cell death. The rate of ASC migration via pathways involving the MLN, the spleen, or the lung is denoted by the symbol γ, together

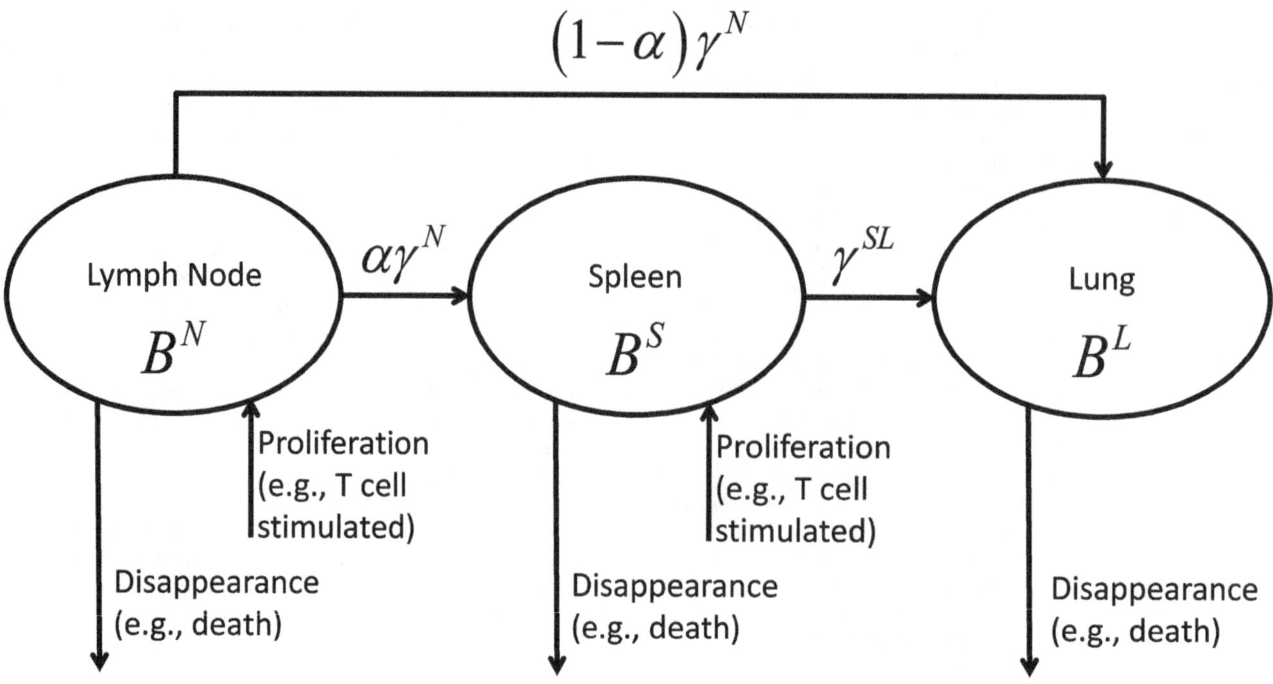

Figure 1. Schematic diagram of ASC migration pathways involving MLN, spleen, and lung following influenza infection.

with a one- or two-letter superscript to identify aspects of cell migration (see Table 1). We use the symbol δ to denote the rate of ASC disappearance, with disappearance specifically defined as ASC loss resulting from migration to sites not explicitly included in our model (e.g., bone marrow and liver) or from cell death. The mechanistic model has exactly the same structure for IgM, IgG, and IgA ASCs, so we only show the model structure for IgM ASCs

$$\begin{cases} \dfrac{dB_M^N}{dt} = \left[\rho_M^N S^N(t-\tau_1) - \delta_M^N\right] B_M^N - \gamma_M^N B_M^N \\ \dfrac{dB_M^S}{dt} = \left[\rho_M^S S^S(t-\tau_2) - \delta_M^S\right] B_M^S + \alpha\gamma_M^N B_M^N - \gamma_M^{SL} B_M^S, \\ \dfrac{dB_M^L}{dt} = (1-\alpha)\gamma_M^N B_M^N + \gamma_M^{SL} B_M^S - \delta_M^L B_M^L \end{cases} \quad (1)$$

where S^N and S^S represent the temporal patterns of the synergistic effects on B cell activation in lymph node and spleen, respectively, and their parametric forms are derived from the antigen-presenting cell data [17–19] (Supplementary Material S1). Also, we introduce the stimulation strength coefficient (denoted by ρ) to allow the estimation of the actual magnitude of the stimulation strength [13]. Furthermore, τ_1 and τ_2 denote the time delay between infection and ASC growth in MLN and spleen, respectively.

A concern about the mechanistic model (Model 1) described above is that it may not fully accommodate the complexity of factors that modulate ASC formation and trafficking following influenza infection, and may therefore not sufficiently describe experimental observations. For example, the effects of innate mechanisms such as type I interferon production and complement activation on B cell activation are not explicitly taken into account. In addition, dendritic cell and T cell effects may have different temporal patterns that are not accommodated in Model 1. We therefore considered an alternative semi-mechanistic model (Model 2) in which the terms S^N and S^S in Model 1 are replaced by the nonparametric time-varying parameter $S(t)$ (Supplementary Material S2). Since no explicit assumption is made about the temporal pattern of $S(t)$, this term can represent the different temporal patterns of innate and adaptive immune mechanisms that drive ASC formation. Model 2 for IgM ASCs is written as

$$\begin{cases} \dfrac{dB_M^N}{dt} = \rho_M^N S(t-\tau_1) B_M^N - \gamma_M^N B_M^N \\ \dfrac{dB_M^S}{dt} = \rho_M^S S(t-\tau_2) B_M^S + \alpha\gamma_M^N B_M^N - \gamma_M^{SL} B_M^S. \\ \dfrac{dB_M^L}{dt} = (1-\alpha)\gamma_M^N B_M^N + \gamma_M^{SL} B_M^S - \delta_M^L B_M^L \end{cases} \quad (2)$$

Using the implicit function theorem method [20], one of the standard structural identifiability analysis techniques [21], we verified that the parameters δ^N (for MLN) and δ^S (for spleen) in Model 1 cannot be explicitly included in Model 2. However, δ^N and δ^S are implicitly included in the terms $\rho_M^N S(t-\tau_1)$ and $\rho_M^S S(t-\tau_2)$, which represent the net rates of increase of ASC populations in MLN and spleen, respectively.

Assumptions and model structures were tested using our experimental data and the statistical methods described below. Mathematical notations and parameter definitions are summarized in Table 1.

Statistical Methods

We first performed structural identifiability analysis for the ODE models and verified that all parameters were theoretically identifiable [21,22]. Outliers in the time-course data set of virus-specific ASC numbers for model fitting were automatically identified and removed using the median absolute deviation (MAD) method [23]. Absolute ASC counts represented the difference between counts from virus-coated wells and control wells. Variability resulted in negative ASC counts at some time points and these were assigned a value of zero for analysis since

Table 1. Parameter and variable definitions in Models 1–2 (subscripts for antibody isotypes are not shown).

Variable/Parameter	Definition	Units	Assay	Description
B^N	antigen-specific ASC in MLN	cells per MLN	ELISpot	in all models
B^S	antigen-specific ASC in spleen	cells per spleen	ELISpot	in all models
B^L	antigen-specific ASC in lung	cells per lung	ELISpot	in all models
S^N	B cell activation stimulus (e.g. antigen presenting cells)	cells per MLN	parametric form adapted from literatures [17–19]	in Model 1 only
S^S	B cell activation stimulus (e.g. antigen presenting cells)	cells per spleen	parametric form adapted from literatures [17–19]	in Model 1 only
ρ^N	stimulation strength coefficent in MLN	day^{-1} per cell per MLN	estimated	in all models
ρ^S	stimulation strength coefficent in spleen	day^{-1} per cell per spleen	estimated	in all models
δ^N	disappearance rate of plasma cells in MLN	day^{-1}	estimated	in Model 1 only
δ^S	disappearance rate of plasma cells in spleen	day^{-1}	estimated	in Model 1 only
δ^L	disappearance rate of plasma cells in lung	day^{-1}	estimated	in all models
α	percentage of plasma cells from MLN to spleen	dimensionless	estimated	in all models
γ^N	migration rate of plasma cells out of MLN	day^{-1}	estimated	in all models
γ^{SL}	migration rate of plasma cells from spleen to lung	day^{-1}	estimated	in all models
τ_1	lag time for B cell activation in MLN	day	estimated	in all models
τ_2	lag time for B cell activation in spleen	day	estimated	in all models
$S_{(t)}$	temporal pattern of B cell activation stimulus	cells per organ	nonparametric, estimated	in Model 2 only, time-varing

cell counts must be non-negative. Models were fitted to $\log_{10}$-transformed data using the robust nonlinear least squares (RNLS) method [24], which is less senstive to data noise (e.g., outliers) than the ordinary NLS. More specifically, instead of the normal distribution assumption, we assumed that the log-transformed data follow a Lorentzian (or Cauchy) distribution and its probability density function is given as

$$f(\varepsilon;\varepsilon_0,\gamma)=\frac{1}{\pi}\cdot\frac{\gamma}{\gamma^2+(\varepsilon-\varepsilon_0)^2},$$

where ε denotes the measurement error, ε_0 is the location parameter and γ is the scale parameter. In our implementation, the location parameter was fixed as zero and the scale parameter was chosen as the data standard deviation. The Lorentzian distribution has heavier tails so more frequent occurrence of outliers is allowed; therefore, the mean estimation is more robust against outliers than that obtained under the normal distribution assumption. Parameter estimates were obtained using the hybrid optimization algorithm DESQP, which has a superior performance over many alternative methods [25] and has been used in sevearl previous studeis [6,13,26,27]. The 95% confidence intervals for all parameter estimates were calculated using the bootstrap method [28] since the asymptotic confidence intervals calculated using Fisher information matrix (FIM) turned out to be numerically sensitive and unstable. Alternative models were evaluated based on the AICc score, which has a sample size correction and is thus recommended over AIC [29]

$$\text{AICc}=n\ln\left(\frac{RSS}{n}\right)+\frac{2nk}{n-k-1},$$

where RSS denotes the residual sum of squares, n is the number of observations, and k is the number of unknown parameters. A smaller AICc score indicates a better model. Finally, all the computing methods have been implemented and performed in C++ based on the MathStat Library (https://cbim.urmc.rochester.edu/software/mathstat/).

Results

Model fitting and evaluation

Experimental data for model fitting was obtained by high frequency sampling during the primary response to intranasal influenza infection. Cell suspensions prepared from MLN, spleen, and lung on days 0 to 14 after infection were analyzed by ELISpot assay to determine virus-specific ASC numbers. ASC counts for samples collected prior to day 4 were generally close to zero in virus-coated and control wells. Because of occasional inconsistencies (deemed as outliers) at early time-points, only data from days 4 to 14 were used for model fitting.

Models 1 and 2 (called the full models, see Table 1 and Fig. 1), together with sub-models derived by setting some parameter values in the full model to zero, were fitted to the experimental data and evaluated based on AICc score [29]. Model 1 outperformed Model 2 for each of the IgM, IgG, and IgA ASC populations, indicating that the increase in ASC populations can be well estimated without introducing the non-parametric form of the synergistic stimulation effects as in Model 2. Point estimates and 95% confidence intervals from Model 1 are presented in Table 2. The 95% confidence intervals were estimated for all model parameters. Curves predicted by Model 1 fitted well with the experimental data (Fig. 2), evidenced by the fact that the p-values from the χ^2 test against the saturated model [30] are greater than 0.3.

ASC population dynamics in MLN and spleen

The ASC time delay estimates the time from initiation of infection to the initial increase in size of virus-specific ASC populations (Table 3), essentially when the first derivative becomes non-zero. The initial rise in ASC population sizes can be due to either proliferation or differentiation. ASC populations began to increase approximately 1–2 days earlier in MLN than in spleen, consistent with a more rapid delivery of antigen to the MLN via direct lymphatic drainage from the lung.

Parameter values shown in Table 2 were used to calculate measures of ASC population dynamics (Table 3). The results are expressed as *population* doubling times, which are distinct from mitotic duration times of individual cells. Population doubling times were generally shorter for IgM ASCs, consistent with the differentiation and appearance of most of these cells during the early ASC response. Interestingly, the doubling time for the isotype-switched IgA ASC population was substantially shorter in MLN than in spleen, but this was not the case for IgG ASCs. This observation fits with evidence for rapid, T cell-dependent IgA ASC formation in the MLN after influenza infection [2]. As calculated ($\ln 2/\delta$), the half-life more precisely represents the half-disappearance time and encompasses ASC population loss from death or functional inactivation and from migration to sites not sampled in this study such as the bone marrow. The half-disappearance time of IgG and IgA ASC populations were shorter in spleen than in MLN, perhaps reflecting rapid ASC exit from the spleen. The relatively short half-disappearance time times of IgG and IgA ASC populations in the lung suggest that many of the

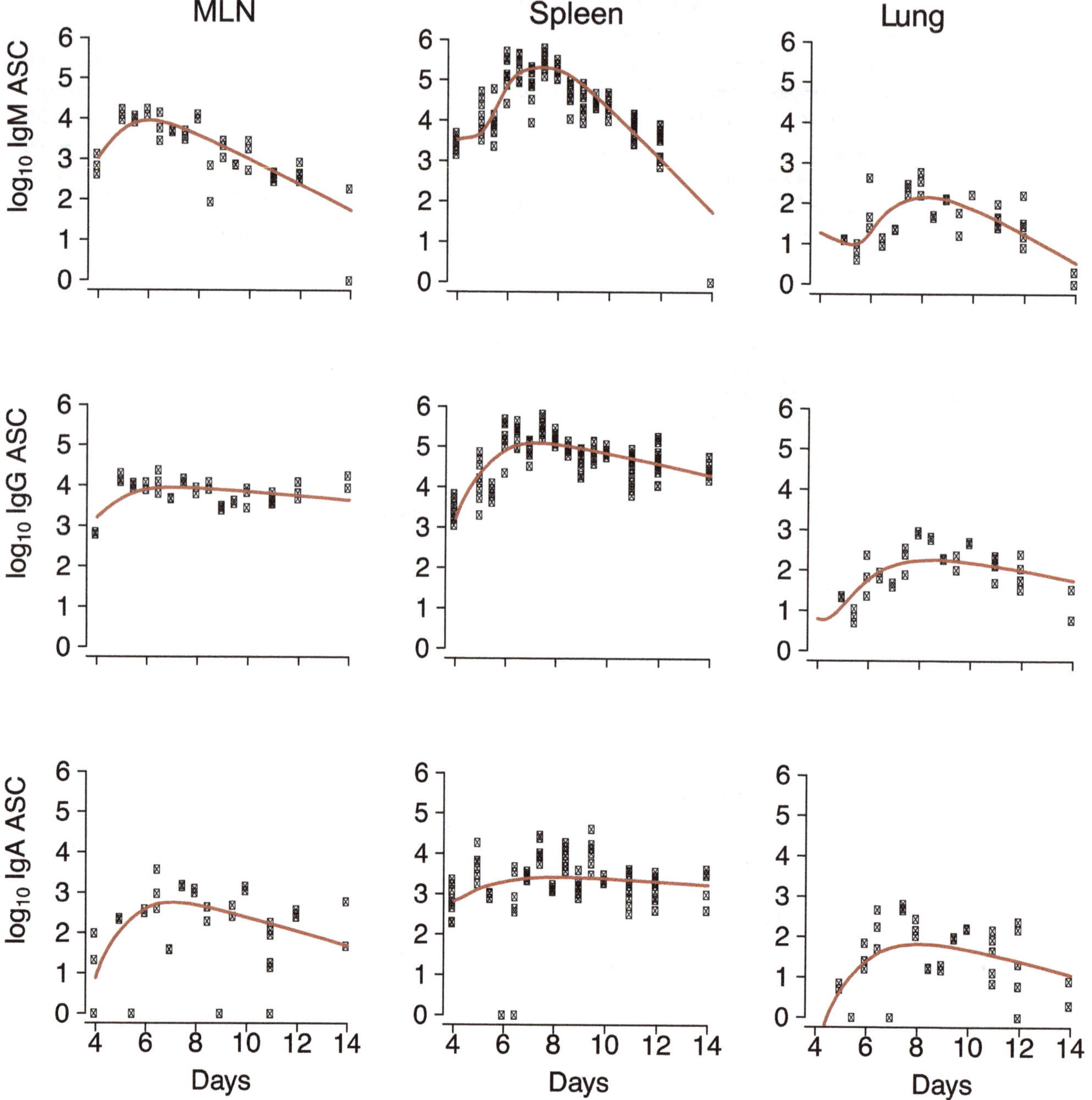

Figure 2. Model fitting results using parameter estimates shown in Table 2 (derived from Model 1), together with experimental data (individual symbols) plotted against days after infection. Outliers have been removed.

Table 2. Point estimates based on the best sub-models (derived from Model 1) selected using AICc and the 95% confidence intervals (insignificant parameter estimates selected by AICc are labelled as dropped).

Parameters (unit)	IgM-secreting B cells	IgG-secreting B cells	IgA-secreting B cells
initial B^N cells per MLN	1.1E+3 (2.0E+1, 9.4E+4)	1.6E+3 (7.7E+1, 4.8E+4)	7.6E+0 (1.6E−1, 9.8E+1)
initial B^S cells per spleen	3.4E+3 (3.0E+1, 9.7E+4)	1.6E+3 (5.0E+1, 4.8E+4)	6.5E+2 (2.5E+0, 9.8E+2)
initial B^L cells per lung	1.8E+1 (1.7E+0, 9.4E+3)	6.2E+0 (2.9E−1, 9.8E+2)	0 dropped
ρ^N day^{-1} per cell per MLN	1.3E−4 (4.3E−6, 9.4E−1)	6.6E−5 (2.2E−5, 9.5E−1)	1.0E−4 (NA, 9.6E−1)
ρ^S day^{-1} per cell per spleen	9.6E−5 (2.1E−5, 9.7E−1)	1.1E−4 (3.3E−5, 9.7E−1)	1.9E−5 (NA, 9.5E−1)
δ^N day^{-1}	7.3E−1 (1.2E−3, 9.6E+0)	1.2E−1 (3.9E−3, 2.9E+0)	0 dropped
δ^S day^{-1}	1.5E+0 (3.4E−3, 9.6E+0)	3.2E−1 (2.2E−3, 2.9E+0)	1.1E−1 (3.0E−2, 4.9E+0)
δ^L day^{-1}	8.3E−1 (5.1E−3, 9.8E+0)	7.8E−1 (8.4E−3, 4.8E+0)	9.5E−1 (5.4E−2, 9.4E+0)
α (%)	0 dropped	0 dropped	6.8E−1 (2.7E−3, 9.7E−1)
γ^N day^{-1}	0 dropped	0 dropped	4.2E−1 (2.4E−2, 9.8E+0)
γ^{SL} day^{-1}	7.6E−4 (5.6E−4, 9.7E−1)	1.4E−3 (4.7E−4, 9.7E−1)	0 dropped
τ_1 day	0 dropped	0 dropped	7.4E−1 (2.6E−2, 5.8E+0)
τ_2 day	2.5E+0 (1.1E−3, 5.7E+0)	6.2E−1 (3.8E−3, 5.8E+0)	1.4E+0 (2.6E−2, 5.8E+0)
$S_{(t)}$ cells per organ	-	-	-
RSS	6.0E+1	3.2E+1	2.0E+2
AICc	−8.9E+2	−1.2E+3	−3.4E+2

The lower bound for some highly-skewed parameters are not available and labeled as NA.

early ASC immigrants are short-lived, even though long-lasting resident ASC populations are established in the lung [3,4,31].

ASC migration from MLN and spleen

To assess the characteristics of ASC loss from MLN and spleen, estimated migration rates and disappearance rates of ASC populations were plotted against sampling time (Fig. 3). Our assumptions related to migration pathways from MLN and spleen were described in the previous section (see Fig. 1). Disappearance essentially accounted for all IgM and IgG ASC loss from the MLN, with negligible loss occurring through migration to spleen or lung. In contrast, IgA ASC loss from the MLN primarily resulted from migration to spleen or lung and not from disappearance. Disappearance accounted for most of the IgM, IgG, and IgA ASC loss from the spleen, although there was some IgM and IgG ASC migration from spleen to lung. These observations fit with the estimated half-migration times for ASC populations exiting the MLN and for ASC populations migrating from spleen to lung (Table 3). The half-migration time for the IgA ASC population in the MLN was only 1.7 days, but was substantially longer for IgM and IgG ASC populations. Half-migration times for trafficking to the lung were relatively long for all ASC populations in the spleen. This was particularly the case

Table 3. Summary of doubling time, half life and half migration time (∞denotes a large value greater than 10^4, and insignificant parameter estimates selected by AICc are labelled as dropped).

Parameters (unit)	IgM-secreting B cells	IgG-secreting B cells	IgA-secreting B cells
doubling time in MLN (days) $\ln 2 \Big/ \left[\frac{1}{(t_1-t_0)}\int_{t_0}^{t_1} \rho^N S^N dt\right]$	1.6 (2.2E−4, 4.7E+1)	3.1 (2.1E−4, 9.2E+0)	1.1 (6.8E−5, NA)
doubling time in spleen (days) $\ln 2 \Big/ \left[\frac{1}{(t_1-t_0)}\int_{t_0}^{t_1} \rho^S S^S dt\right]$	0.64 (6.3E−5, 6.4E+1)	1.2 (7.4E−5, 3.2E+0)	4.1 (6.3E−5, NA)
half-life in MLN (days) $\ln 2/\delta^N$	0.94 (1.4E−1, 5.8E+2)	5.7 (2.4E−1, 1.8E+2)	∞
half-life in spleen (days) $\ln 2/\delta^S$	0.46 (7.2E−2, 2.1E+2)	2.2 (2.4E−1, 3.2+2)	6.5 (1.4E−1, 2.3E+1)
half-life in lung (days) $\ln 2/\delta^L$	0.84 (7.1E−2, 1.4E+2)	0.89 (1.4E−1, 8.3E+1)	0.73 (7.4E−2, 1.3E+1)
percentage of cells from MLN to spleen (%) α	0 dropped	0 dropped	0.68 (2.7E−3, 9.7E−1)
half egress time from MLN (days) $\ln 2/\gamma^N$	∞	∞	1.7 (7.1E−2, 2.9E+1)
half migration time from spleen to lung (days) $\ln 2/\delta^{SL}$	910 (7.1E−1, 1.2E+3)	502 (7.2E−1, 1.5E+3)	∞
stimulation delay in MLN (days) τ_1	0 dropped	0 dropped	0.74 (2.6E−2, 5.8E+0)
stimulation delay in spleen (days) τ_2	2.5 (1.1E−3, 5.7E+0)	0.62 (3.8E−3, 5.8E+0)	1.4 (2.6E−2, 5.8E+0)

The uppper bound for some highly-skewed parameters are not available and labeled as NA.

for the IgA ASC population, consistent with minimal IgA ASC migration from spleen to lung.

The difference between MLN and spleen in their contribution to ASC populations in the lung is also shown in Fig. 3. Interestingly, the MLN contributed most of the lung IgA ASCs, even though the spleen contained substantial numbers of IgA ASCs. In contrast, IgM and IgG ASCs that localized in the lung were mainly from the spleen, even though relatively strong IgM and IgG responses were generated earlier in the MLN. Overall, these observations point towards fundamental differences between MLN and spleen in features of the B cell response to influenza infection.

Finally, for convenience, the modeling results are summarized and visualized in Fig. 4 for three types of ASCs considered in this study. The solid lines in Fig. 4 represent statistically significant parameter estimates, and the dashed lines are for negligible model terms.

In silico validation

A key question was whether limitations in the experimental data would significantly impact model predictions. In our analysis, the lymph node compartment was represented by ASC response data from the MLN, the major lymph node draining the lower respiratory tract. However, influenza X31 infection also elicits substantial ASC formation in lymph nodes draining the upper respiratory tract, predominantly in the group of cervical lymph nodes (CLN). The CLN are approximately 10-fold more cellular than the MLN throughout the response to X31 infection and, based on data from other studies, are likely to contribute up to 10-fold more virus-specific ASCs than does the MLN [4,32,33]. A limited analysis of virus-specific ASCs on days 5, 7, and 9 after influenza X31 infection demonstrated that the ratios of IgM, IgG, and IgA ASCs were similar in the CLN and MLN (Fig. S1 in Supporting Information). Another potential issue in our data was underestimation of the number of virus-specific ASCs that migrate to the lung. The results of other studies suggest that the use of an enzymatic digestion protocol might have increased our recovery of ASCs from lung tissue by up to 10-fold [1,3].

We therefore assessed the robustness of our best models (Table 2) to a combination of (i) a 10-fold increase in the number of ASCs generated in the lymph node compartment, and (ii) a 10-fold increase in the number of ASCs isolated from the lung. These increases were applied to the numbers of IgM, IgG, and IgA ASCs. The results of model fitting (Fig. S2 in Supporting Information) showed that all measures of ASC population dynamics shown in Table 3 were only marginally changed when calculated using the adjusted ASC counts. The plots shown in Fig. 3 also had the same patterns when the adjusted data set was used (Fig. S3 in Supporting Information). Recently, Anderson and colleagues [34] demonstrated that a high proportion of lymphocytes recovered from the perfused lung were located in the vasculature rather than in the lung tissue itself. Although a similar situation for ASCs has not been established, we also asked whether an overestimation of the number of ASCs that entered lung tissue would impact model predictions. We tested the robustness of our models using a 2-fold decrease in lung IgM, IgG, and IgA ASCs and a 10-fold increase in ASCs from the lymph node compartment. Model predictions in Fig. 3 were unchanged using the adjusted data sets. In summary, the in silico testing demonstrated that model predictions were unaffected by increased ASC numbers generated in the lymph node compartment in combination with an increase or decrease in lung ASC numbers.

We also conducted a sensitivity analysis by calculating the changes in model outputs (that is, the areas under the curves for B^N, B^S and B^L) corresponding to 1%, 5% or 10% changes in parameter values [35]. The results indicate that model outputs are not sensitive to perturbations in any parameter except for ρ^N (a 50% change in model outputs was observed for a 10% change in ρ^N). However, note that ρ^N primarily affects the magnitudes of ASC numbers in the lymph node and lung compartments and not ASC trafficking routes.

Discussion

Numerous studies have provided a general picture of the kinetics of virus-specific ASC formation and migration following primary influenza infection [1–5], but the quantitative dynamics of ASC populations have received little attention. For example, the relative population doubling times for IgM, IgG, and IgA ASCs have not been estimated, nor have their trafficking patterns during infection been studied in detail. In particular, the "burst size" or total number of virus-specific ASCs generated during the response in various lymphoid and non-lymphoid tissues has rarely been addressed. Part of the issue has been the difficulty in direct experimental measurement of population doubling times. We have addressed these issues by constructing a compartmental model that, for the first time, estimates ASC trafficking patterns, population doubling rates, and rates of disappearance from cell death, quiescence, or migration to other compartments.

Before discussing detailed model findings, it is important to recognize that estimates of population doubling times provide different and more informative information than estimates of activated ASC division times. There is much heterogeneity in B cell activation, differentiation and death times in immune responses. Thus, one population doubling time could model many different combinations of cells with different division times, without a way to discern the actual mixture experimentally. In order to estimate the total Ab secretion of ASCs contributing to influenza-specific serum Ab, one must have detailed information regarding the population heterogeneity and estimate several more parameters, integrating Ab secretion rates over the time of the immune response. Experimental validation of these additional parameters is quite difficult *in vivo*. In contrast, estimates of influenza-specific ASC population doubling time can be used directly to estimate changes in Ab concentration over time with a single parameter, and fewer identifiability issues. This actually leads to greater model precision, and is the primary reason we chose this parameterization of our model.

Our modeling estimates of population doubling times for IgM ASCs in MLN and spleen fit with the well-established concept of rapid IgM ASC formation preceding the IgG response. Interestingly, the population doubling time for IgA ASCs was comparable to that for IgM ASCs in the MLN but not in the spleen. This finding is consistent with previous studies that reported a rapid T cell-dependent IgA ASC response preceding IgG production in the MLN of influenza-infected mice [2,5]. Although both the IgA and IgG responses in this model of influenza infection are T cell-dependent, there are apparently key differences in the mechanisms of delivery of T cell help. In contrast to the situation for IgG production, T cell help for the early IgA response can be delivered in a non-antigen-specific manner to B cells deficient in major histocompatibility complex class II [2]. This may relate to the rapidity of the IgA response, but the mechanism is not understood. Early IgA ASCs in the MLN are almost exclusively specific for viral surface glycoproteins, with IgA ASCs specific for the internal nucleocapsid protein only appearing in the second week after infection [5]. Taken together, these observations have led to the proposal that the early IgA response is initiated when specific B

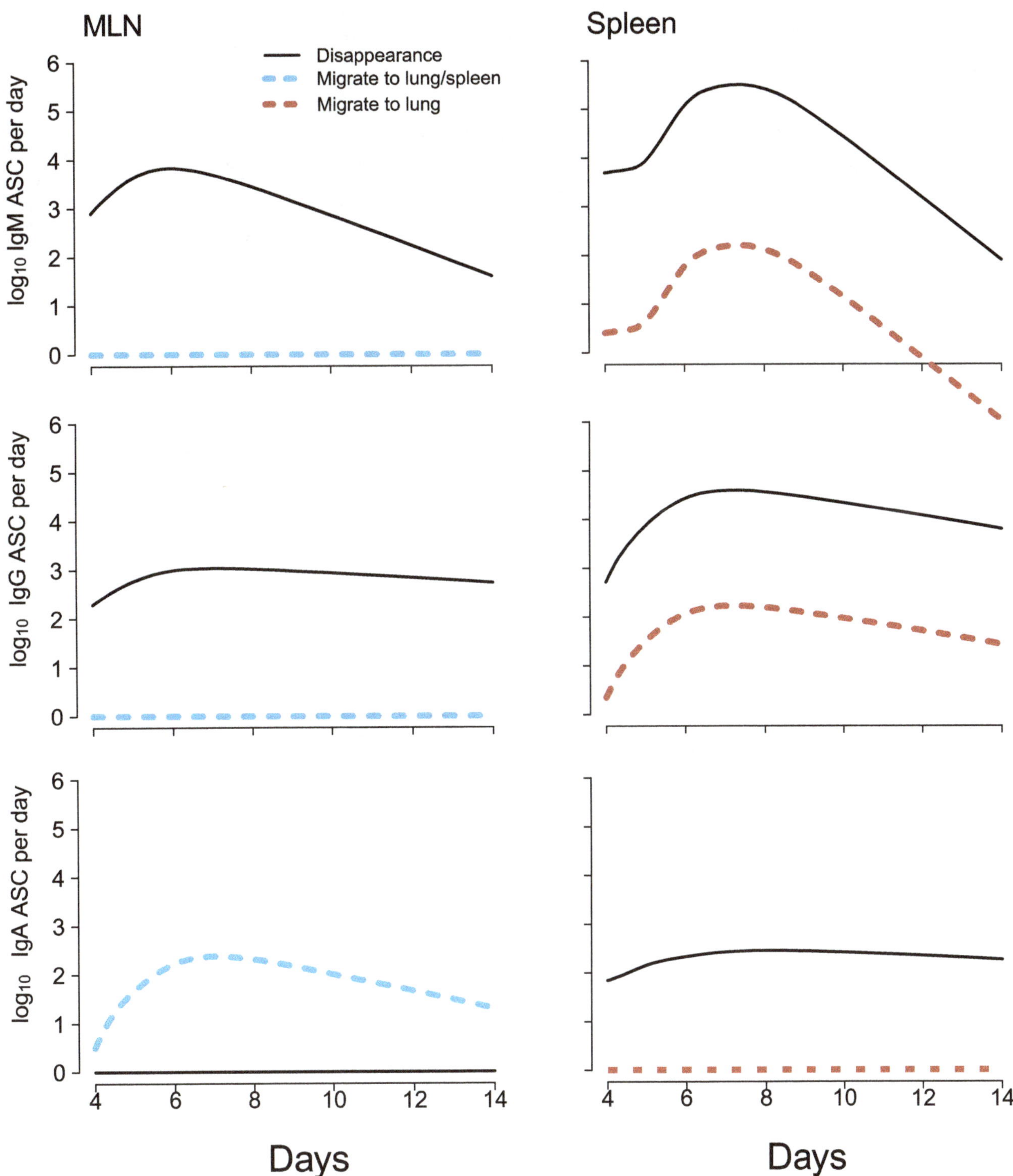

Figure 3. ASC disappearance compared with ASC migration from MLN and spleen. The term migration covers ASC trafficking from MLN to lung or spleen, or ASC trafficking from spleen to lung. Migration pathways reflect assumptions shown in Figure 1. The term disappearance covers ASC death or ASC migration to sites other than the lung or spleen.

cell clones recognize viral surface glycoproteins on infected DCs and is driven by soluble differentiation and class switching factors without the need for cognate T cell help [2,5].

One potential drawback to our model is our use of composite parameters for cell migration and disappearance. We use the term migration to include ASC trafficking from the MLN to spleen or lung, and from the spleen to lung; the term disappearance encompasses ASC loss from cell death, as well as migration to sites not sampled in our analysis. We used the composite parameter disappearance because both statistical and experimental methods

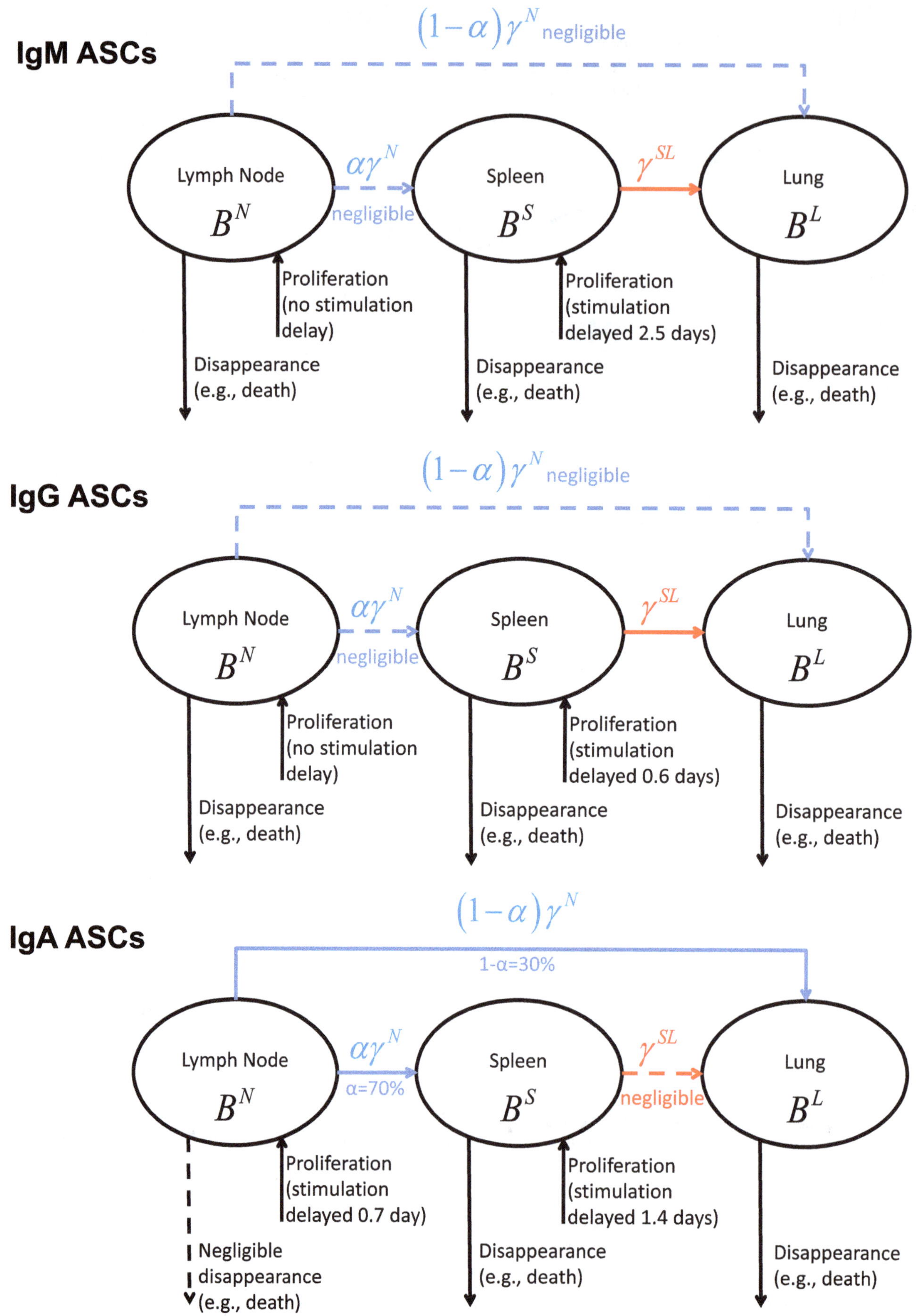

IgM ASCs
$(1-\alpha)\gamma^N$ negligible
Lymph Node
B^N
$\alpha\gamma^N$
negligible
Spleen
B^S
γ^{SL}
Lung
B^L
Proliferation (no stimulation delay)
Proliferation (stimulation delayed 2.5 days)
Disappearance (e.g., death)
Disappearance (e.g., death)
Disappearance (e.g., death)
IgG ASCs
$(1-\alpha)\gamma^N$ negligible
Lymph Node
B^N
$\alpha\gamma^N$
negligible
Spleen
B^S
γ^{SL}
Lung
B^L
Proliferation (no stimulation delay)
Proliferation (stimulation delayed 0.6 days)
Disappearance (e.g., death)
Disappearance (e.g., death)
Disappearance (e.g., death)
IgA ASCs
$(1-\alpha)\gamma^N$
1-α=30%
Lymph Node
B^N
$\alpha\gamma^N$
α=70%
Spleen
B^S
γ^{SL}
negligible
Lung
B^L
Proliferation (stimulation delayed 0.7 day)
Proliferation (stimulation delayed 1.4 days)
Negligible disappearance (e.g., death)
Disappearance (e.g., death)
Disappearance (e.g., death)

Figure 4. Visualization of the modeling results for the three types of ASCs, where the solid lines represent statistically significant parameter estimates and the dashed lines are for negligible parameter values.

were not able to separately estimate *in vivo* cell death and migration to other sites in multiple compartments. Accurately measuring *in vivo* cell death is difficult given the rapid clearance of apoptotic and necrotic cells [36]. Accounting for migration of ASCs to all unmeasured compartments is a difficult experimental challenge, requiring transgenic mouse systems and whole mouse imaging [37]. Definitive experiments would involve murine infection followed by simultaneous sampling of all lymph nodes within BcR transgenic mice to account for migration to non-draining lymph nodes, nasal mucosa and other mucosa-associated lymphoid tissues, as well as skin and liver. Novel radioactive labeling and imaging methods could be used as well. The numbers of mice and technical challenges for simultaneous daily collection of such data makes this a point of experimental investigation for future projects. However, the current manuscript demonstrates that the use of a composite parameter allows us to narrow down the mechanisms of cell disappearance while preserving model identifiability.

From about 7 days after influenza infection, virus-specific ASCs can be isolated from the tissues of the upper and lower respiratory tract. IgA ASCs predominate in the upper respiratory tract and are also numerous in the lung, together with IgG and (less consistently) IgM ASCs [3,4]. It is generally accepted that ASCs generated by influenza infection migrate to the respiratory tract from sites of formation in organized lymphoid tissues. Our modeling estimates extend this concept and indicate differences in ASC trafficking patterns that depend on site of formation and the expressed Ab class. For ASC populations in MLN and spleen, we estimated loss from migration or from disappearance. Notably, our modeling suggests that essentially all IgA ASC loss from the MLN results from migration to spleen or lung, with negligible IgA ASC migration from spleen to lung. This result points to a critical role for regional lymph nodes such as the MLN in the rapid generation of IgA ASCs that migrate to the respiratory tract in the course of influenza infection. These ASCs presumably take up residence in the lamina propria of the respiratory tract and secrete IgA that is transcytosed across epithelial cells and released at the mucosal surface. The kinetics of IgA ASC localization in the respiratory tract suggests that they contribute to the clearance of infectious virus. IgA with virus-neutralizing activity has been identified in nasal washings from mice on day 7 after influenza infection, a time when viral titers in the respiratory tract are declining [2,4].

In contrast to IgA ASCs, essentially all IgM and IgG ASC loss from the MLN occurred through disappearance and not from migration to spleen or lung. It seems unlikely that significant IgM and IgG ASC loss from the MLN during the period of our analysis resulted from migration to sites that were not sampled (encompassed by our use of the term disappearance). In addition to the respiratory tract, the major target site for ASC migration during the B cell response to influenza infection is the bone marrow. However, virus-specific ASCs are generally not detected in the bone marrow until 10 days or more after infection of the respiratory tract [4,14,38]. This points to cell death as the major reason for IgM and IgG ASC loss from the MLN. Presumably, these cells are products of the T cell-dependent extrafollicular pathway, which generates short-lived ASCs from activated B cells prior to the development of germinal centers. This is supported by evidence that virus-specific IgM, IgG, and IgA ASCs are present in the MLN before germinal center formation is first evident approximately 7–8 days after influenza infection [5,39,40]. Antiviral Abs produced via the extrafollicular pathway provide an early barrier to the spread of infection and also facilitate further virus-specific B cell activation [41].

Conventional dogma has cell death coinciding with contraction of the immune response. Our model suggests that ASC death begins early and continues throughout the B cell response. Our estimates indicate a more rapid death rate for IgM ASCs than for IgG ASCs, perhaps reflecting a large component of IgM ASC formation in the short-lived extrafollicular response or a survival advantage associated with IgG class switching signals. Apparently, the early IgA ASCs in the MLN are not susceptible to cell death like the IgM and IgG ASCs and, instead, leave the MLN and migrate to other sites. This fits with evidence discussed above that points to a mechanism of early IgA ASC generation that is distinct from the standard extrafollicular differentiation pathway [2,5]. Signals delivered to the developing IgA ASCs may promote survival and the expression of mucosal homing molecules [42].

Our modeling results suggest that the majority of IgM and IgG ASCs that migrate to the lung come from the spleen and not the MLN. This contrasts with the situation for IgA ASCs in the lung, most of which come from the MLN and not the spleen. An important factor may be the relative magnitude of the germinal center response in the spleen compared with the MLN. At the time of initial germinal center formation in the MLN and spleen on approximately day 8 after infection, the frequency of germinal center B cells (percentage of total cells) is similar in both locations. However, because of the cellularity of the spleen, this represents approximately 50-fold more germinal center B cells in the spleen [40]. It follows that the spleen is likely to generate substantial numbers of long-lived ASCs via the germinal center pathway at a stage of the response when the majority of IgM and IgG ASCs formed in the MLN are short-lived. ASCs generated in germinal centers typically express CXCR4 and traffic from sites of formation to the bone marrow where long-lasting populations are established. In addition, CXCR4-expressing ASCs may traffic to sites of inflammation, such as the influenza-infected lung, in response to local production of inflammatory chemokines. In particular, this may apply to a subset of IgM and IgG ASCs that express CXCR3, consistent with our modeling results [43,44]. The rates of ASC disappearance from the spleen measured in our analysis likely encompass not only cell death, as in the MLN, but also ASC movement into the circulation to seed the bone marrow. At times in our analysis, substantial numbers of IgA ASCs were present in the spleen, but our modeling indicated minimal migration of these cells from spleen to lung. The reason for this is unclear. Although some IgA ASCs in the spleen may have been generated by germinal center reactions, others with limited further migration potential may have trafficked to the spleen after formation in the MLN.

Our estimates of the half-life (more precisely the half-disappearance time) of ASC populations in the lung essentially only reflect cell death, since ASC migration from the lung is probably minimal. ASC migration to the lung in response to influenza infection establishes long-lasting populations [3,4,31]. It is therefore interesting that our half-disappearance time estimates for IgM, IgG, and IgA ASC populations in the lung were relatively short, indicating that these cells are not inherently long-lived. The longevity of ASCs in the lung, as in the bone marrow, may depend on a stable and supportive tissue environment that provides appropriate anchoring sites and survival factors [45]. Such an environment may not present in the lung during the periods of inflammation and tissue repair. Our modeling is consistent with a continuous influx of ASCs into the lung to maintain ASC population sizes, at least for a period of time after infection.

In summary, we have combined high frequency experimental data and mathematical modeling to provide estimates of ASC population dynamics that are difficult to measure experimentally. The results of our analysis of virus-specific ASC populations generated by primary influenza infection of the respiratory tract support existing concepts and, in addition, provide novel insights and identify directions for future experimentation. Most notably, our findings (i) emphasize the importance of the MLN in the early generation of IgA ASCs that migrate to the lung, (ii) point to key differences between mechanisms of IgA ASC formation and those of IgM and IgG ASC formation in the MLN that influence the longevity and migratory potential of early ASCs, and (iii) identify differences between MLN and spleen in their contribution to particular ASC populations in the lung. Further studies are required to provide a mechanistic understanding of the increasingly complex picture of ASC dynamics and trafficking that is emerging.

Supporting Information

Figure S1 Virus-specific ASC formation in the MLN and CLN following influenza infection. (A, B) Virus-specific ASC frequencies. (C, D) Proportions of virus-specific ASCs producing the IgM, IgG, and IgA Ab classes. B6 mice were infected intranasally with 10^5 EID_{50} of influenza X31. Virus-specific ASCs were enumerated by ELISpot assay at intervals after infection. The mean + SD is shown for 3–5 individual mice per group.

Figure S2 Fitted curves corresponding to a 10-fold increase in the ASC numbers in lymph node and lung.

Figure S3 ASC disappearance compared with ASC migration from MLN and spleen after a 10-fold increase in the ASC numbers in lymph node and lung.

Text S1 Derivation of the parametric form of a time-varying variable from data.

Text S2 Definition and use of a nonparametric time-varying parameter.

Author Contributions

Conceived and designed the experiments: MSZ MYS DT TRM AML. Performed the experiments: MYS DJT MSZ TRM AML SH. Analyzed the data: HM LZ JHW HW ASP. Contributed reagents/materials/analysis tools: MSZ MYS DJT. Wrote the paper: HM MYS SH JHW MSZ HW AML ASP DJT TRM.

References

1. Jones PD, Ada GL (1986) Influenza virus-specific antibody-secreting cells in the murine lung during primary influenza virus infection. J Virol 60: 614–619.
2. Sangster MY, Riberdy JM, Gonzalez M, Topham DJ, Baumgarth N, et al. (2003) An early CD4+ T cell-dependent immunoglobulin A response to influenza infection in the absence of key cognate T-B interactions. J Exp Med 198: 1011–1021.
3. Joo HM, He Y, Sangster MY (2008) Broad dispersion and lung localization of virus-specific memory B cells induced by influenza pneumonia. Proc Natl Acad Sci U S A 105: 3485–3490.
4. Liang B, Hyland L, Hou S (2001) Nasal-associated lymphoid tissue is a site of long-term virus-specific antibody production following respiratory virus infection of mice. J Virol 75: 5416–5420.
5. Sealy R, Surman S, Hurwitz JL, Coleclough C (2003) Antibody response to influenza infection of mice: different patterns for glycoprotein and nucleocapsid antigens. Immunology 108: 431–439.
6. Miao H, Hollenbaugh JA, Zand MS, Holden-Wiltse J, Mosmann TR, et al. (2010) Quantifying the early immune response and adaptive immune response kinetics in mice infected by influenza A virus Journal of Virology 84: 6687–6698.
7. Wolf AI, Mozdzanowska K, Quinn JW III, Metzgar M, Williams KL, et al. (2011) Protective antiviral antibody responses in a mouse model of influenza virus infection require TACI. The Journal of Clinical Investigation 121: 3954–3964.
8. Ho D, Neumann A, Perelson A, Chen W, Leonard J, et al. (1995) Rapid turnover of plasma virions and CD4 lymphocytes in HIV-1 infection. Nature 373: 123–126.
9. Kim H, Perelson AS (2006) Viral and latent reservoir persistence in HIV-1 infected patients on therapy. PLoS Comput Biol 2: e135.
10. Perelson AS, Essunger P, Cao Y, Vesanen M, Hurley A, et al. (1997) Decay characteristics of HIV-1-infected compartments during combination therapy. Nature 387: 188–191.
11. Perelson AS, Neumann AU, Markowitz M, Leonard JM, Ho DD (1996) HIV-1 dynamics in vivo: virion clearance rate, infected cell life-span, and viral generation time. Science 271: 1582–1586.
12. Smith AM, Adler FR, McAuley JL, Gutenkunst RN, Ribeiro RM, et al. (2011) Effect of 1918 PB1-F2 expression on influenza A virus infection kinetics. PLoS Comput Biol 7: e1001081.
13. Wu H, Kumar A, Miao H, Holden-Wiltse J, Mosmann TR, et al. (2011) Modeling of influenza-specific CD8+ T cells during the primary response indicates that the spleen is a major source of effectors. The Journal of Immunology 187: 4474–4482.
14. Sangster MY, Topham DJ, D'Costa S, Cardin RD, Marion TN, et al. (2000) Analysis of the virus-specific and nonspecific B cell response to a persistent B-lymphotropic gammaherpesvirus. J Immunol 164: 1820–1828.
15. Waffarn EE, Baumgarth N (2011) Protective B Cell Responses to Flu—No Fluke! The Journal of Immunology 186: 3823–3829.
16. Kallies A, Nutt SL (2010) Bach2: plasma-cell differentiation takes a break. The EMBO Journal 29: 3896–3897.
17. Belz GT, Smith CM, Kleinert L, Reading P, Brooks A, et al. (2004) Distinct migrating and nonmigrating dendritic cell populations are involved in MHC class I-restricted antigen presentation after lung infection with virus. Proceedings of the National Academy of Sciences of the USA 101: 8670–8675.
18. Belz GT, Wodarz D, Diaz G, Nowak MA, Doherty PC (2002) Compromised influenza virus-specific CD8(+)-T-cell memory in CD4(+)-T-cell-deficient mice. J Virol 76: 12388–12393.
19. Stock AT, Mueller SN, van Lint AL, Heath WR, Carbone FR (2004) Prolonged antigen presentation after herpes simplex virus-1 skin infection. The Journal of Immunology 173: 2241–2244.
20. Xia X, Moog CH (2003) Identifiability of nonlinear systems with application to HIV/AIDS models. Automatic Control, IEEE Transactions on 48: 330–336.
21. Miao H, Xia X, Perelson AS, Wu H (2011) On Identifiability of Nonlinear ODE Models and Applications in Viral Dynamics. SIAM Review 53: 3–39.
22. Walter E, Lecourtier Y (1981) Unidentifiable compartmental models: what to do? Mathematical Biosciences 56: 1–25.
23. Davies L, Gather U (1993) The identification of multiple outliers. Journal of the American Statistical Association 88: 782–792.
24. Motulsky H, Brown R (2006) Detecting outliers when fitting data with nonlinear regression - a new method based on robust nonlinear regression and the false discovery rate. BMC Bioinformatics 7: 123.
25. Moles CG, Banga JR, Keller K (2004) Solving nonconvex climate control problems: pitfalls and algorithm performances. Applied Soft Computing 5: 35–44.
26. Liang H, Miao H, Wu H (2010) Estimation of constant and time-varying dynamic parameters of HIV infection in a nonlinear differential equation model. Annals of Applied Statistics 4: 460–483.
27. Miao H, Jin X, Perelson A, Wu H (2012) Evaluation of Multitype Mathematical Models for CFSE-Labeling Experiment Data. Bulletin of Mathematical Biology 74: 300–326.
28. Efron B, Tibshirani RJ (1993) An introduction to the boostrap. Boca Raton, FL: Chapman & Hall/CRC.
29. Burnham KP, Anderson DR (2004) Multimodel inference: Understanding AIC and BIC in model selection. Sociological Methods Research 33: 261–304.
30. Smyth GK (2003) Pearson's Goodness of Fit Statistic as a Score Test Statistic. In: Goldstein DR, editor. Statistics and Science: A Festschrift for Terry Speed. Hayward, CA: Institute of Mathematical Statistics. pp. 115–126.
31. Jones PD, Ada GL (1987) Persistence of influenza virus-specific antibody-secreting cells and B-cell memory after primary murine influenza virus infection. Cell Immunol 109: 53–64.

32. Marshall D, Sealy R, Sangster M, Coleclough C (1999) TH cells primed during influenza virus infection provide help for qualitatively distinct antibody responses to subsequent immunization. J Immunol 163: 4673–4682.
33. Tamura S, Iwasaki T, Thompson AH, Asanuma H, Chen Z, et al. (1998) Antibody-forming cells in the nasal-associated lymphoid tissue during primary influenza virus infection. J Gen Virol 79 (Pt 2): 291–299.
34. Anderson KG, Sung H, Skon CN, Lefrancois L, Deisinger A, et al. (2012) Cutting Edge: Intravascular Staining Redefines Lung CD8 T Cell Responses. The Journal of Immunology 189: 2702–2706.
35. Saltelli A, Chan K, Scott EM (2000) Sensitivity analysis. New York: Wiley.
36. Elliott MR, Ravichandran KS (2010) Clearance of apoptotic cells: implications in health and disease. J Cell Biol 189: 1059–1070.
37. Reinhardt RL, Khoruts A, Merica R, Zell T, Jenkins MK (2001) Visualizing the generation of memory CD4 T cells in the whole body. Nature 410: 101–105.
38. Sangster M, Hyland L, Sealy R, Coleclough C (1995) Distinctive kinetics of the antibody-forming cell response to Sendai virus infection of mice in different anatomical compartments. Virology 207: 287–291.
39. Rothaeusler K, Baumgarth N (2010) B-cell fate decisions following influenza virus infection. Eur J Immunol 40: 366–377.
40. Boyden AW, Legge KL, Waldschmidt TJ (2012) Pulmonary infection with influenza A virus induces site-specific germinal center and T follicular helper cell responses. PLoS One 7: e40733.
41. Baumgarth N, Herman OC, Jager GC, Brown LE, Herzenberg LA, et al. (2000) B-1 and B-2 cell-derived immunoglobulin M antibodies are nonredundant components of the protective response to influenza virus infection. J Exp Med 192: 271–280.
42. McDermott MR, Bienenstock J (1979) Evidence for a common mucosal immunologic system. I. Migration of B immunoblasts into intestinal, respiratory, and genital tissues. J Immunol 122: 1892–1898.
43. Cyster JG (2003) Homing of antibody secreting cells. Immunol Rev 194: 48–60.
44. Kunkel EJ, Butcher EC (2003) Plasma-cell homing. Nat Rev Immunol 3: 822–829.
45. Chu VT, Berek C (2013) The establishment of the plasma cell survival niche in the bone marrow. Immunol Rev 251: 177–188.

12

The Effect of TIP on Pneumovirus-Induced Pulmonary Edema in Mice

Elske van den Berg[1]*, Reinout A. Bem[1], Albert P. Bos[1], Rene Lutter[2], Job B. M. van Woensel[1]

1 Pediatric Intensive Care Unit, Emma Children's Hospital, Academic Medical Center, Amsterdam, The Netherlands, **2** Department of Respiratory Medicine and Experimental Immunology, Academic Medical Center, Amsterdam, The Netherlands

Abstract

Background: Pulmonary edema plays a pivotal role in the pathophysiology of respiratory syncytial virus (RSV)-induced respiratory failure. In this study we determined whether treatment with TIP (AP301), a synthetic cyclic peptide that mimics the lectin-like domain of human TNF, decreases pulmonary edema in a mouse model of severe human RSV infection. TIP is currently undergoing clinical trials as a therapy for pulmonary permeability edema and has been shown to decrease pulmonary edema in different lung injury models.

Methods: C57BL/6 mice were infected with pneumonia virus of mice (PVM) and received TIP or saline (control group) by intratracheal instillation on day five (early administration) or day seven (late administration) after infection. In a separate set of experiments the effect of multiple dose administration of TIP versus saline was tested. Pulmonary edema was determined by the lung wet-to-dry (W/D) weight ratio and was assessed at different time-points after the administration of TIP. Secondary outcomes included clinical scores and lung cellular response.

Results: TIP did not have an effect on pulmonary edema in different dose regimens at different time points during PVM infection. In addition, TIP administration did not affect clinical severity scores or lung cellular response.

Conclusion: In this murine model of severe RSV infection TIP did not affect pulmonary edema nor course of disease.

Editor: Ian C. Davis, The Ohio State University, United States of America

Funding: The study was funded in part by APEPTICO GmbH, Vienna, Austria, which is the title holder of the TIP peptide AP301. Additional funding was received by the Janivo Foundation (reference 2011.063). The funders had no role in study design, data collection and analysis, decision to publish, or preparation of the manuscript.

Competing Interests: The study was funded in part by APEPTICO GmbH, Vienna, Austria, which is the titleholder of the TIP peptide AP301. APEPTICO had no role in study design, data collection and analysis, decision to publish, or preparation of the manuscript.

* Email: elske.vandenberg@amc.uva.nl

Background

Infection with the pneumovirus, respiratory syncytial virus (RSV) is an important cause of lower respiratory tract infection (LRTI) in young children [1]. The burden of RSV-induced LRTI is high and recently it was estimated that annually over 3.0 million young children with RSV-induced LRTI need to be admitted to the hospital worldwide. Despite years of research treatment for severe RSV-LRTI is limited to supportive care with oxygen and mechanical ventilation.

Histopathological studies of lungs of both animals and humans infected with respiratory syncytial virus show areas of pulmonary edema. Johnson *et al.* found mixtures of inflammatory cells, fibrin and edema in small airways of children with fatal RSV-LRTI [2]. In a study with baboons infected with human RSV massive pulmonary edema and vascular congestion was seen in lung tissue samples [3]. Several studies of mice infected with the pneumovirus pneumonia virus of mice (PVM), which is frequently used as a model for severe human RSV have shown that alveolar edema was present in lung tissue [4,5]. Based on these studies mechanical obstruction of the small airways and alveoli by edema appears to play a significant role in RSV-induced respiratory failure. Although clinical studies on the consequences of pulmonary edema in RSV disease are lacking pulmonary edema is associated with prolonged respiratory failure and a higher mortality in other pulmonary conditions such as acute respiratory distress syndrome (ARDS) [6–8].

The increased accumulation of alveolar fluid may inactivate surfactant, increase surface tension, promote inflammation, accelerate further flooding and thus may contribute to the characteristic oxygenation anomalies during severe RSV-LRTI [9]. The accumulation of fluid in the infected lung is caused, in part, by injury of the alveolar- and capillary barrier leading to increased permeability and, in addition, by compromised alveolar fluid clearance (AFC) [10]. AFC depends on vectorial transport of salt and water across the alveolar epithelium in part through apically located epithelial sodium channels (ENaC), followed by extrusion into the lung interstitium via a basolaterally located Na,K-ATPase [11]. In vivo and in vitro studies have shown that RSV directly affects alveolar fluid clearance by decreasing active epithelial Na+ transport in different lung epithelial cells such as tracheal epithelial cells and Clara cells [12–14].

Recently, the lectin-like domain of tumor necrosis factor alpha (TNF-alpha) [15], has been recognized as an important regulator of alveolar fluid balance. The synthetic peptide AP301 that mimics the lectin-like domain of TNF-alpha (designated TIP) has shown to be able to improve AFC *in situ* and *ex vivo* in a flooded rat lung injury model and *in vivo* when applied intratracheally [16,17] by both reducing vascular permeability and enhancing the absorption of excess alveolar fluid by up-regulating the sodium uptake. The same effect of TIP on AFC was found in an *in vivo* porcine broncho-alveolar lavage model of acute lung injury, in which nebulized TIP resulted in increased PaO_2/FiO_2 ratio and reduced extra vascular lung water index [18]. Vadász demonstrated that the effect of TIP was not limited to healthy lungs and found similar effects of TIP on alveolar liquid clearance in an *ex vivo* model of endo/exotoxin-induced lung injury [10]. Lucas *et al.* showed that in addition to its effect on pulmonary edema TIP also influenced inflammation by reducing neutrophil content and reactive oxygen species generation leading to improved lung function after lung transplantation in rats [19]. Together these studies suggest a promising role of TIP in treating pulmonary edema in several lung disease states and even the first safety studies in humans have been performed.

The aim of this study was to determine whether TIP reduces pulmonary edema in severe pneumovirus infection in mice. We used the pneumovirus PVM as a model of severe RSV infection in humans. PVM is capable of producing a form of respiratory disease in mice that is similar to severe RSV-LRTI in humans and has been shown to be a valuable alternative model of severe RSV infection to study the importance of virus-induced inflammatory responses in the development of severe respiratory virus disease [5,20].

Methods

Viral stock preparation

PVM strain J3666 originally was orignially obtained from Dr. A. J. Easton (University of Warwick, UK) and was kept virulent by continuous passage in mice [21]. Clarified lung supernatants containing PVM were prepared by pooling the lungs of eight BALB/c mice infected with PVM. The pooled lungs were homogenized in 8 mL Isove's modified Dulbecco's medium (IMDM, Life Technologies, Gaithersburg, MD) and spun at 13,000×g for 5 min at 4°C. The supernatant was stored in individual aliquots in liquid nitrogen. Titers of PVM virus stocks were determined by isolation of RNA directly from virions in suspension with the RNeasy Mini Kit (Qiagen, Venlo, The Netherlands) and reverse transcribed to cDNA (high-capacity cDNA kit; Applied Biosystems, Bleiswijk, The Netherland). Copies of the PVM *sh* gene (GenBank AY573815) were detected in qPCR reactions with specific primers and TAMRA probe and normalized for copies of the houskeeping gene GAPDH as described before [22]. The virus titer in the aliquots was 12×10^4 copies of PVM-*sh* per 10^9 copies of *gapdh*/µl. On the day of each experiment, one aliquot was thawed and diluted (1:1500) in RPMI medium (Invitrogen Ltd, Paisly, UK) for subsequent inoculation into the mice as described below.

AP301

The cyclic peptide AP301 was a kind gift of APEPTICO, Vienna, Austria. Details of the synthesis have been described previously [23].

Animal protocol

The animal protocols were approved by the Animal Care and Use Committee of the Academic Medical Center, University of Amsterdam, the Netherlands. Male C57BL/6J (C57) (Charles River laboratories, Someren, the Netherlands) aged 9- to 12-weeks-old received intratracheal instillations of 6×10^3 copies of PVM in a total volume of 80 µl. Briefly, the mice were anesthetized with inhaled isoflurane and intubated endotracheally with a 22-gauge Insyte angiocath (BD, Madrid, Spain). Placement of the catheter in the trachea was verified by visualizing the movement of a 100 µl bubble of water in an open syringe in response to respiratory efforts as described before [22]. Following the instillations of PVM the mice were returned to their cages with free access to water and food. For the administration of TIP the mice were intubated again under isoflurane anesthesia and received TIP intratracheally in different doses and instillation volumes depending on the experiment. At different time-intervals after the TIP instillation the mice were euthanized with intraperitoneal ketamin 252 mg/kg, dexdomitor 0.4 mg/kg and atropin 1 mg/kg and exsanguinated by carotid artery ligation. The left lung was removed and weighed (wet weight). Broncho-alveolar lavage (BAL) was performed of the right lung by instilling three separate aliquots of 0.4 ml 0.9% NaCl containing 0.6 mM EDTA. One aliquot of BAL fluid (BALF) was processed immediately for cell counts and differentials. After the BAL, the right lung was inflated and fixed with formalin and embedded in paraffin for subsequent histological studies.

Experimental design

The PVM-infected mice mice received TIP dissolved in normal saline intratracheally (dose, instillation volume and timing depending on the experiment as indicated) under isoflurane anesthesia. In all experiments control mice received saline without TIP in equal volumes.

Measurements

Clinical score. The mice were monitored daily for clinical distress using weight loss and a specific score system as previously described [4]: 1 = healthy, no signs of illness, 2 = subtle ruffled fur, 3 = evident ruffled fur with hunched posture, 4 = evident lethargy with abnormal breathing pattern, 5 = moribund, 6 = death [modified from Cook et al. [24]. The end point for sacrifice used in this study was a score of 4 and/or loss of >20% of starting body weight.

Lung cellular response. The total number of BALF leukocytes was counted in a Bürker Bright line counting chamber. Cytospin preparations (20,000 cells per slide) were stained with the Diff-quick method (Fisher Scientific Company L.L.C., Kalamazoo, MI), and differential cell counts were obtained by counting 200 leukocytes using a standard light microscope.

Lung permeability. BALF total protein was measured with the bicinchoninic acid method (BCA assay, Pierce, Rockford, IL). The high molecular weight protein IgM was measured in BALF by ELISA (Bethyl Laboratories, West Chester, PA).

Pulmonary edema. We assessed pulmonary edema formation using the lung wet-to-dry (W/D) weight ratio [25]. The left lung was removed, quickly blotted dry and weighed (wet weight) on an analytical balance. Subsequently the lung was dried in a 65°C stove for seven days and weighed again (dry weight). In addition, the location of pulmonary edema was determined on hematoxylin and eosin (H&E) stained lung tissue sections.

Statistical analysis

The data were analyzed using GraphPad Prism 4.0 software (GraphPad, San Diego, CA). Comparisons between multiple groups were performed using a two-way factorial analysis of variance (ANOVA), unless otherwise stated. Significance between groups was determined with the Bonferroni post hoc test. A p value of <0.05 was considered statistically significant. Data are reported as means ± standard error of the mean.

Results

Clinical response and pulmonary edema development during pneumovirus infection

The first clinical signs of PVM disease in C57 mice appeared on day 6 after PVM infection and consisted of mild weight loss. The condition of the mice rapidly deteriorated and by day 8 the mice reached a clinical score of more than 4 and lost more than 10% of their body weight (Fig. 1*A*). Pulmonary edema was first detected on day 6 after infection, by an increase in lung W/D weight ratio of infected mice as compared to baseline (Fig. 1*B*), which reached significance on day 8 after infection (6.85 ± 0.25 vs 4.27 ± 0.61, $p< 0.01$). The increase in pulmonary edema was paralleled by an increase in lung permeability as measured by an increase of the high molecular weight protein IgM in BALF of PVM-infected mice, which reached significance on day 7 and 8 after infection (day 0: 84.3 ± 6.2 vs day 7: 1092.0 ± 266.6, $p<0.01$ and vs day 8: 1248.0 ± 266.7, $p<0.001$) (Fig. 1*C*). Thus, intratracheal instillation of PVM in C57 mice led to measurable clinical disease that was paralleled by an increase in pulmonary edema and lung permeability. Based on disease severity and the level of pulmonary edema on day eight we chose day 7 for our first intervention experiment with TIP.

Intratracheal administration of TIP in different dose regimens did not affect pulmonary edema formation in PVM-infected mice

Based on previous studies using TIP in mice infected intranasally with influenza strain A/PR8/34 (H. Fischer et al., unpublished data), we first studied the effect of 20 µg TIP in 30 µl saline. No difference in lung W/D weight ratio was found between PVM-infected mice that were treated with TIP and control animals at any time-point (2, 4, and 6 hours after installation of TIP (Fig. 2*A*). To determine if the lack of an effect of 20 µg TIP was due to either a low dose of TIP or a small instillation volume, we repeated the experiments with a higher dose of TIP (80 µg) in an instillation volume of 60 µl of saline. Again, no significant difference in lung W/D weight ratio between TIP treated mice and controls was found at any time point (Fig. 2*B*).

Because TIP was given late during the course of disease the benefits of TIP might be limited due to overwhelming disease. Therefore we determined the effect of early administration of TIP on pulmonary edema formation during PVM infection. Mice received 80 µg TIP in 60 µl saline on day 5 after PVM infection (before the increase of the lung W/D weight ratio, see Fig 1*B*). No significant difference was found in lung W/D weight ratio 24, 48 or 72 hours after instillation between PVM-infected mice that received TIP as compared to control mice (Fig. 2*C*).

Finally, in order to test if a multiple-dose regimen of TIP would prevent or reduce pulmonary edema formation during PVM infection, mice received intratracheal instillation of 20 µg TIP in 30 µl of saline on day 0, 2, 4 and 6 after PVM infection. The mice were euthanized 24 hours after the last TIP instillation. No difference was found in the lung W/D ratio between the mice that received TIP and control mice (Fig. 2*D*).

Effects of instillation volume (up to 60 µl) and isoflurane anesthesia on pulmonary edema were ruled out in separate experiments (data not shown).

To determine if the lack of effect of TIP could be explained by the location of pulmonary edema, H&E stained lung tissue sections were examined. Similar to previous studies [4,5], we observed protein-rich edema fluid in the alveoli in H&E-stained lung sections of PVM-infected mice, the same area where TIP is thought to affect ENaC-mediated Na^+ transport. In line with our W/D ratio results we found no difference between TIP or saline treatment in these histological examinations (Fig. 3).

Thus, early or late intratracheal administration of 80 µg (single dose regimen) or 20 µg (single or multiple dose regimen) TIP in an instillation volume of 30–60 µl did not have an effect on pulmonary edema as measured by the lung W/D weight ratio of PVM-infected C57 mice.

Administration of TIP during PVM infection did not have an effect on clinical disease progression or pulmonary inflammation

In the first experiment the mice were analyzed 2, 4 and 6 hours after the instillation of TIP on day 7 after PVM infection. No change in weight loss or clinical score was observed, as expected during this short time frame. In the second experiment the mice received TIP on day 5 after infection and were analyzed on day 6, 7 and 8. No difference in weight loss or clinical score was seen between TIP treated animals and controls on day 6 and 7 (Fig. 4A and B). An unexpected significantly higher clinical score was seen in the TIP-treated mice compared to controls on day 8 after PVM infection. However this was not paralleled by an increase in weight loss. Weight loss and clinical score were not different between PVM-infected mice that received multiple doses of TIP as compared to controls (data not shown).

Because Lucas et al. found a decreased number of alveolar neutrophils in transplanted lungs that were pretreated with TIP [19], we also measured the number of neutrophils in the BALF, but no significant difference between the mice that were treated with TIP and control mice was found in any of the experiments (Fig. 4C).

Discussion

The aim of this study was to determine whether TIP reduces pulmonary edema in mice infected with PVM as a model for severe RSV infection in humans. We found that endotracheal administration of TIP in different dose regimens at different time points during the infection did not have an effect on pulmonary edema. In addition, TIP administration did not affect disease progression or lung cellular response.

Based on several histopathological studies [2–4,26] on lungs of human and animals infected with the pneumoviruses RSV or PVM pulmonary edema is present and appears to be important in the disease pathogenesis. Pulmonary edema formation depends on disruption of both the pulmonary capillary endothelium and the alveolar epithelial barrier in combination with insufficient alveolar fluid clearance mechanisms. RSV can have potentially deleterious effects at each step of this process. The endothelial junction protein vascular endothelial (VE) cadherin is critical for maintenance of endothelial barrier integrity in lung microvessels. Leukocyte signaling cytokines and chemokines like interleukin (IL)-6 and IL-8 and destabilizing agonists such as VEGF are found in elevated levels in the airways of RSV-infected patients and it has

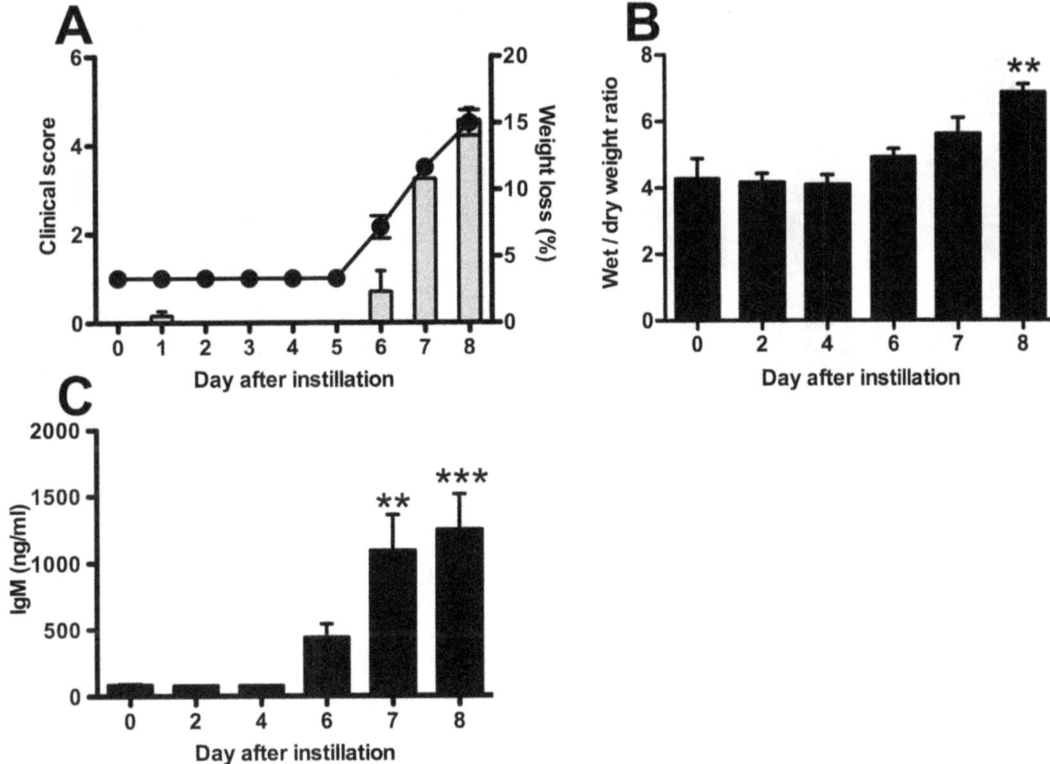

Figure 1. C57BL/6 mice intratracheally infected with 6×10^3 copies of PVM develop clinical signs, increased alveolar permeability and pulmonary edema. *A*: mean clinical scores (left y-axis, line) and weight loss (right y-axis, bar) during infection with PVM. *B*: lung wet-to-dry weight ratio of C57BL/6 mice during PVM infection. *C*: IgM concentration in bronchoalveolar lavage fluid (BALF) of PVM-infected C57BL/5 mice. The graphs represent the mean of 4 mice at each time-point (± SEM). **$p<0.01$, ***$p<0.001$, as compared to uninfected mice (t = 0).

been suggested that these mediators may contribute to edema formation by interrupting VE-cadherin bonds [27,28]. In vivo mice studies and in vitro studies with respiratory epithelium have demonstrated that replicating RSV virus directly affects fluid clearance in the lungs in experimental models by inhibiting ENaC via uridine triphosphate (UTP) release in the airspace lining fluid [12,13,29,30]. The mechanism behind the RSV induced UTP release is not known, but depends on active RSV replication. Various strategies to increase alveolar fluid clearance during RSV infection have been studied, but so far only treatment with leflunomide, an immunosuppressive agent that can decrease levels of UTP have shown promising effects in *in vivo* studies [13,31]. Aerolized or intravenous beta-adrenergic agonist, which have shown to stimulate lung edema clearance in hyperoxic injured rat lungs by upregulating apical Na^+ channels and basolateral N^+/K^+-ATPase treatment, failed to improve alveolar liquid clearance in RSV-infected mice [9]. In addition, in a trial in mechanically ventilated children with severe RSV infection investigating the effect of the immunomodulating drug dexamethasone, which besides anti-inflammatory effects also is known to increase α-ENaC mRNA expression *in vivo* and *vitro* [32,33], no beneficial clinical effect was seen [34,35].

This is the first *in vivo* study determining the effect of TIP on pulmonary edema in a viral infectious model. The lectin-like domain of TNF-α, mimicked by the 17 amino acid TIP peptide has been found to decrease hydrostatic pulmonary edema and endo/exotoxin-induced permeability edema in *in situ* and *ex vivo* animal studies [10,16,17]. TIP decreased vascular permeability and increased transepithelial Na^+ transport and thus alveolar fluid clearance by upregulating both amiloride-sensitive Na^+ channels and Na,K-ATPase in the epithelium in injured isolate rabbit lungs [10]. We hypothesized that TIP would decrease pulmonary edema in an *in vivo* murine model of pneumovirus induced lung injury. However, in contrast to the previous studies in other models and settings we did not find an effect of TIP in several regimens including various dosing and timing studies on pulmonary edema as measured by the lung W/D weight ratio or on clinical disease progression and lung cellular response in PVM-infected C57 mice.

There may be several explanations for the lack of an effect of TIP in our study. Firstly, the degree of endothelial and epithelial dysfunction differ between the PVM model and the experimental models in which TIP was studied before, eg hydrostatic and endo/exotoxin induced permeability edema. Studies using intra-alveolar and intravenous LPS demonstrated that endotoxin exposure increases lung vascular permeability, but does not affect the epithelial barrier or alveolar fluid transport [36,37]. In contrast the PVM model is characterized by increased alveolar epithelial barrier permeability and decreased fluid transport as shown by an increased lung permeability as measured by an increase of the high molecular weight protein IgM in BALF. This might be an important difference, as interstitial edema resulting from disruption of the endothelial barrier will not lead to alveolar flooding unless the lung epithelial barrier, which is normally much tighter than the endothelium, also is compromised. This might affect the efficacy of TIP in the PVM model, as alveolar flooding might overwhelm any transport capacity of the epithelium. Secondly, Chen *et al.* found that RSV directly inhibits alveolar fluid clearance in human and rodent tracheal epithelial and human Clara cells through the release of UTP levels inhibiting Na^+ transport [12]. The effect of RSV infection on AFC of the alveolar

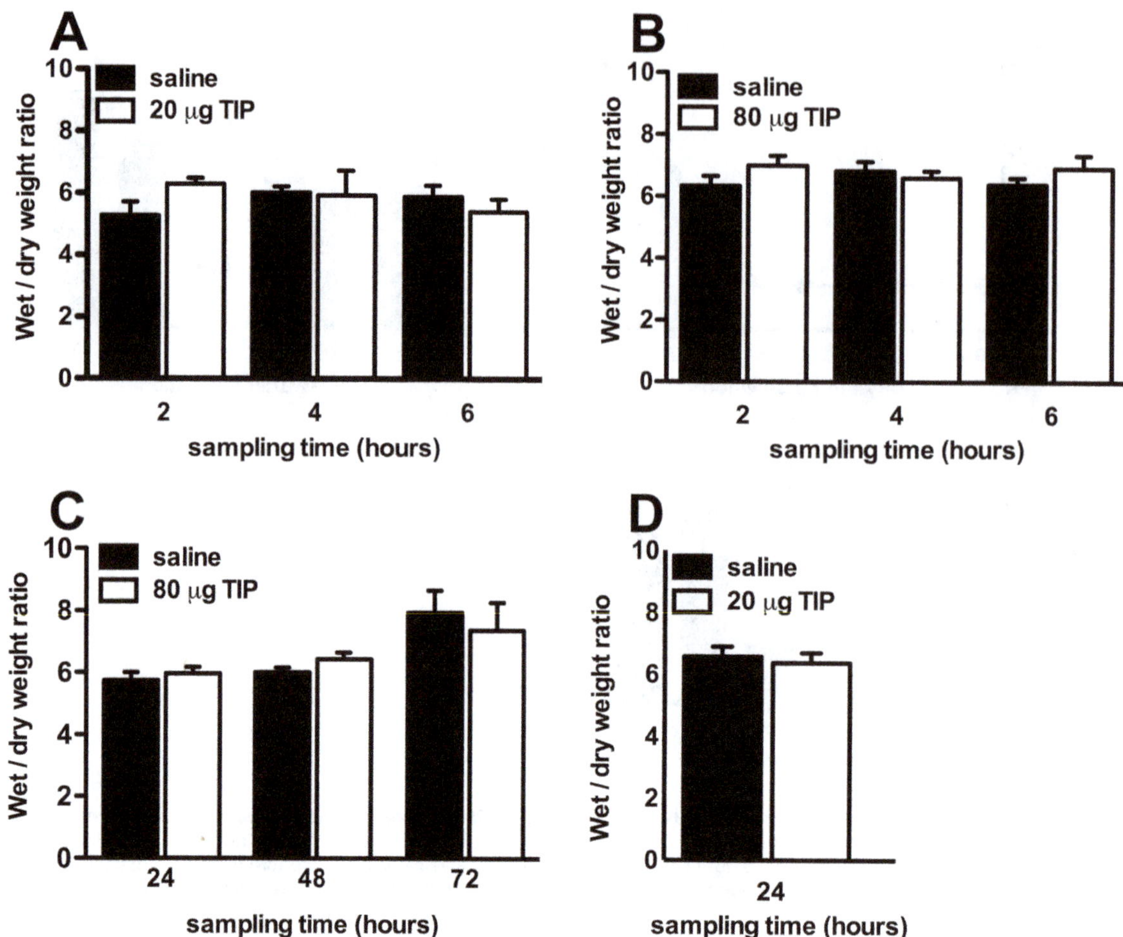

Figure 2. Intratracheal administration of TIP to PVM-infected C57BL/6 mice in different dose regimens and time schedules did not have an effect on pulmonary edema formation. *A*: Lung wet-to-dry weight ratio of the left lung of PVM-infected mice that received 20 μg of TIP in 30 μl saline or 30 μl saline on day seven after infection and were studied two, four or six hours later. *B*: Lung wet-to-dry weight ratio of the left lung of PVM-infected mice that received 80 μg of TIP in 60 μl saline or 60 μl saline (control) on day seven after infection and were studied two, four or six hours later. *C*: Lung wet-to-dry weight ratio of the left lung of PVM-infected mice that received 80 μg of TIP in 60 μl saline or 60 μl saline (control) on day 5 after infection and were studied 24, 48 and 72 hours later. *D*: Lung wet-to-dry weight ratio of the left lung of PVM-infected mice that received 20 μg TIP in 30 μl of saline or 30 μl saline on day zero, two, four and six after infection and were studied on day seven after infection. The graphs represent the mean of 4–8 mice at each time-point (± SEM).

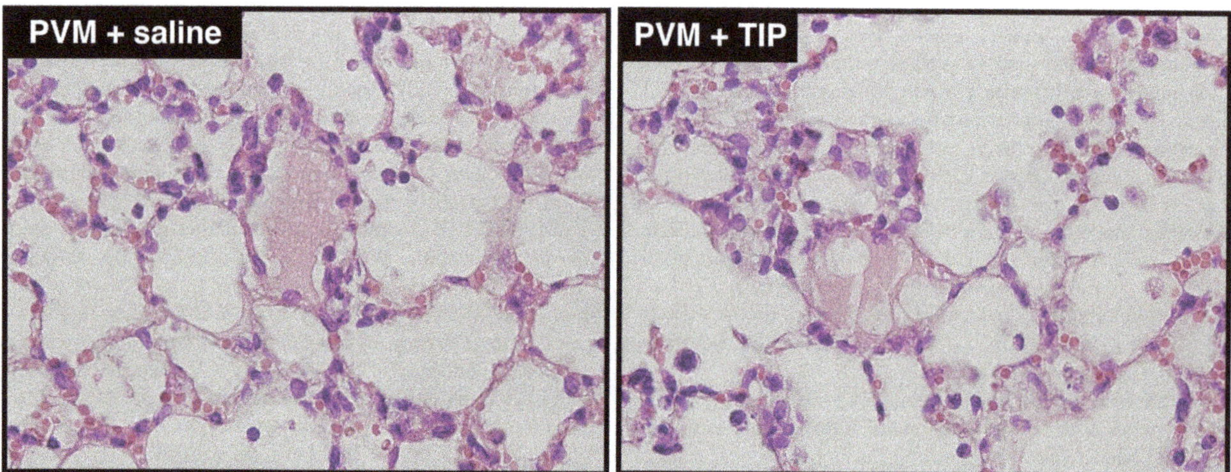

Figure 3. H&E staining of lung tissue from PVM-infected mice treated with TIP or saline. Representative H&E stained lung tissue sections from PVM-infected mice that were treated with 20 μg TIP in 30 μl saline (*right*) or 30 μl saline (*left*) on day seven after infection. The mice were studied two hours after the instillation of TIP or saline.

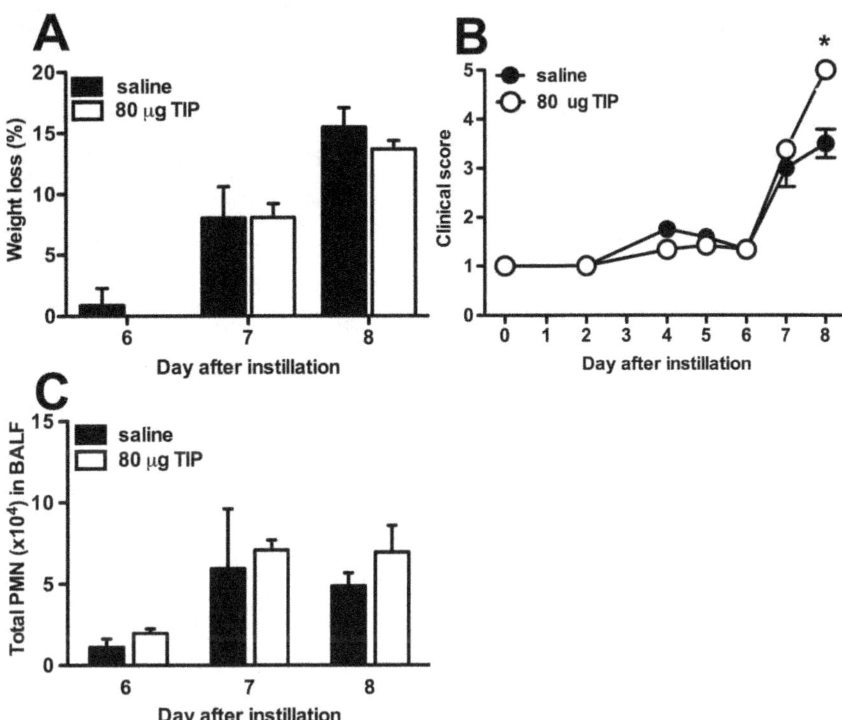

Figure 4. Single or multiple-dose regimen of TIP in PVM infection did not have an effect on weight loss, clinical score and lung cellular response. *A*: Change in body weight expressed as the percentage of the original weight of PVM-infected mice that received 80 μg of TIP in 60 μl saline (black bars) or saline (white bars) on day 5 after infection with PVM. *B*: Mean clinical score of PVM-infected mice that received 80 μg of TIP in 60 μl or saline on day 5 after infection with PVM, examined at daily intervals according to a standardized scoring system. *C*: Total polymorhonuclear neutrophils (PMN) measured in bronchoalveolar lavage fluid of PVM-infected mice that received 80 μg of TIP in 60 μl saline or saline on day 5 after infection with PVM. The graphs represent the mean of 4–6 mice at each time-point (± SEM). *p<0.05, **p<0.01, as compared to PVM-infected mice that received saline.

epithelial cells, the most important cell of oxygen transport in the lung, has to our best knowledge not been studied in detail. One could hypothesize that pneumovirus-induced UTP release is, among other mechanisms, also an important mechanism that influences AFC in alveolar epithelial cells and that as such up regulation of sodium uptake by TIP alone might not be sufficient to decrease pulmonary edema. Finally, ongoing viral replication and inflammation might have influenced the effectiveness of TIP in our model. Several studies investigating new treatment options in RSV disease have shown that dysregulated inflammation is an important process in the pathogenesis of pneumovirus disease [38]. Next studies should determine if TIP is more effective together with appropriate control of the ongoing inflammatory response or even with (new) antiviral agents.

The results of our study should be interpreted with caution. Pulmonary edema was assessed gravimetrically using the lung W/D weight ratio. Although, this method is common used method for pulmonary edema measurement it is sensitive for evaporative loss, regional heterogeneity or inclusion of blood in the wet lung weight [25,39]. However, the W/D weight measurements were consistent and repeatable and were confirmed by the evaluation of the clinical response that did not show a difference between TIP-treated mice and controls.

Conclusions

In conclusion we found no effect of TIP on pulmonary edema and clinical signs in a mouse model of severe RSV infection in humans. Further studies should focus on the effect of TIP on pulmonary edema in combination with anti-inflammatory agents and/or antiviral agents during pneumovirus disease.

Acknowledgments

We thank Dr. R. Lucas, Associate Professor Pharmacology and Toxicology of the Vascular Biology Center, Georgia Regents University, USA, for his careful reading of the manuscript and his detailed comments and suggestions for further improvement. In addition we thank Lydia Wolterman, Niels Kamp, Michael van der Sanden and Bert van Urk for expert technical assistance.

Author Contributions

Conceived and designed the experiments: EB RB AB RL JW. Performed the experiments: EB. Analyzed the data: EB. Contributed reagents/materials/analysis tools: RL JW. Wrote the paper: EB RB JW.

References

1. van Woensel JB, van Aalderen WM, Kimpen JL (2003) Viral lower respiratory tract infection in infants and young children. BMJ (Clinical Research ed.) 327: 36–40.
2. Johnson JE, Gonzales RA, Olson SJ, Wright PF, Graham BS (2007) The histopathology of fatal untreated human respiratory syncytial virus infection. Mod Pathol 20: 108–119.

3. Papin JF, Wolf RF, Kosanke SD, Jenkins JD, Moore SN, et al. (2013) Infant baboons infected with respiratory syncytial virus develop clinical and pathological changes that parallel those of human infants. Am J Physiol Lung Cell Mol Physiol 304: L530–539.
4. Bem RA, van den Berg E, Suidgeest E, van der Weerd L, van Woensel JB, et al. (2013) Cardiac dysfunction in pneumovirus-induced lung injury in mice. Pediatr Crit Care Med 14: e243–249.
5. Dyer KD, Garcia-Crespo KE, Glineur S, Domachowske JB, Rosenberg HF (2012) The Pneumonia Virus of Mice (PVM) model of acute respiratory infection. Viruses 4: 3494–3510.
6. Matthay MA, Robriquet L, Fang X (2005) Alveolar epithelium: role in lung fluid balance and acute lung injury. Proc Am Thorac Soc 2: 206–213.
7. Matthay MA, Wiener-Kronish JP (1990) Intact epithelial barrier function is critical for the resolution of alveolar edema in humans. Am Rev Respir Dis 142: 1250–1257.
8. Matthay MA, Zimmerman GA (2005) Acute lung injury and the acute respiratory distress syndrome: four decades of inquiry into pathogenesis and rational management. Am J Respir Cell Mol Biol 33: 319–327.
9. Nitta K, Kobayashi T (1994) Impairment of surfactant activity and ventilation by proteins in lung edema fluid. Respir Physiol 95: 43–51.
10. Vadasz I, Schermuly RT, Ghofrani HA, Rummel S, Wehner S, et al. (2008) The lectin-like domain of tumor necrosis factor-alpha improves alveolar fluid balance in injured isolated rabbit lungs. Crit Care Med 36: 1543–1550.
11. Mutlu GM, Sznajder JI (2005) Mechanisms of pulmonary edema clearance. Am J Physiol Lung Cell Mol Physiol 289: L685–695.
12. Chen L, Song W, Davis IC, Shrestha K, Schwiebert E, et al. (2009) Inhibition of Na+ transport in lung epithelial cells by respiratory syncytial virus infection. Am J Respir Cell Mol Biol 40: 588–600.
13. Davis IC, Lazarowski ER, Hickman-Davis JM, Fortenberry JA, Chen FP, et al. (2006) Leflunomide prevents alveolar fluid clearance inhibition by respiratory syncytial virus. Am J Respir Crit Care Med 173: 673–682.
14. Song W, Wei S, Matalon S (2010) Inhibition of epithelial sodium channels by respiratory syncytial virus in vitro and in vivo. Ann N Y Acad Sci 1203: 79–84.
15. Lucas R, Magez S, De Leys R, Fransen L, Scheerlinck JP, et al. (1994) Mapping the lectin-like activity of tumor necrosis factor. Science 263: 814–817.
16. Braun C, Hamacher J, Morel DR, Wendel A, Lucas R (2005) Dichotomal role of TNF in experimental pulmonary edema reabsorption. J Immunol 175: 3402–3408.
17. Elia N, Tapponnier M, Matthay MA, Hamacher J, Pache J-C, et al. (2003) Functional Identification of the Alveolar Edema Reabsorption Activity of Murine Tumor Necrosis Factor-alpha. Am J Respir Crit Care Med 168: 1043–1050.
18. Hartmann EK, Boehme S, Duenges B, Bentley A, Klein KU, et al. (2013) An inhaled tumor necrosis factor-alpha-derived TIP peptide improves the pulmonary function in experimental lung injury. Acta Anaesthesiol Scand 57: 334–341.
19. Hamacher J, Stammberger U, Roux J, Kumar S, Yang G, et al. (2010) The lectin-like domain of tumor necrosis factor improves lung function after rat lung transplantation–potential role for a reduction in reactive oxygen species generation. Crit Care Med 38: 871–878.
20. Bem RA, Domachowske JB, Rosenberg HF (2011) Animal models of human respiratory syncytial virus disease. Am J Physiol Lung Cell Mol Physiol 301: L148–156.
21. Domachowske JB, Bonville CA, Gao JL, Murphy PM, Easton AJ, et al. (2000) The chemokine macrophage-inflammatory protein-1 alpha and its receptor CCR1 control pulmonary inflammation and antiviral host defense in paramyxovirus infection. J Immunol 165: 2677–2682.
22. van den Berg E, van Woensel JB, Bos AP, Bem RA, Altemeier WA, et al. (2011) Role of the Fas/FasL system in a model of RSV infection in mechanically ventilated mice. Am J Physiol Lung Cell Mol Physiol 301: L451–460.
23. Hazemi P, Tzotzos SJ, Fischer B, Andavan GS, Fischer H, et al. (2010) Essential structural features of TNF-alpha lectin-like domain derived peptides for activation of amiloride-sensitive sodium current in A549 cells. J Med Chem 53: 8021–8029.
24. Cook PM, Eglin RP, Easton AJ (1998) Pathogenesis of pneumovirus infections in mice: detection of pneumonia virus of mice and human respiratory syncytial virus mRNA in lungs of infected mice by in situ hybridization. J Gen Virol 79 (Pt 10): 2411–2417.
25. Parker JC, Townsley MI (2004) Evaluation of lung injury in rats and mice. Am J Physiol Lung Cell Mol Physiol 286: L231–246.
26. Rosenberg HF, Domachowske JB (2008) Pneumonia virus of mice: severe respiratory infection in a natural host. Immunol Lett 118: 6–12.
27. Ali MH, Schlidt SA, Chandel NS, Hynes KL, Schumacker PT, et al. (1999) Endothelial permeability and IL-6 production during hypoxia: role of ROS in signal transduction. Am J Physiol 277: L1057–1065.
28. Lee CG, Yoon HJ, Zhu Z, Link H, Wang Z, et al. (2000) Respiratory syncytial virus stimulation of vascular endothelial cell growth Factor/Vascular permeability factor. Am J Respir Cell Mol Biol 23: 662–669.
29. Davis IC, Lazarowski ER, Chen FP, Hickman-Davis JM, Sullender WM, et al. (2007) Post-infection A77-1726 blocks pathophysiologic sequelae of respiratory syncytial virus infection. Am J Respir Cell Mol Biol 37: 379–386.
30. Davis IC, Sullender WM, Hickman-Davis JM, Lindsey JR, Matalon S (2004) Nucleotide-mediated inhibition of alveolar fluid clearance in BALB/c mice after respiratory syncytial virus infection. Am J Physiol Lung Cell Mol Physiol 286: L112–120.
31. Dunn MC, Knight DA, Waldman WJ (2011) Inhibition of respiratory syncytial virus in vitro and in vivo by the immunosuppressive agent leflunomide. Antivir Ther 16: 309–317.
32. Champigny G, Voilley N, Lingueglia E, Friend V, Barbry P, et al. (1994) Regulation of expression of the lung amiloride-sensitive Na+ channel by steroid hormones. EMBO J 13: 2177–2181.
33. Tchepichev S, Ueda J, Canessa C, Rossier BC, O'Brodovich H (1995) Lung epithelial Na channel subunits are differentially regulated during development and by steroids. Am J Physiol 269: C805–812.
34. van Woensel JB, van Aalderen WM, de Weerd W, Jansen NJ, van Gestel JP, et al. (2003) Dexamethasone for treatment of patients mechanically ventilated for lower respiratory tract infection caused by respiratory syncytial virus. Thorax 58: 383–387.
35. van Woensel JB, Vyas H (2011) Dexamethasone in children mechanically ventilated for lower respiratory tract infection caused by respiratory syncytial virus: a randomized controlled trial. Crit Care Med 39: 1779–1783.
36. Pittet JF, Wiener-Kronish JP, McElroy MC, Folkesson HG, Matthay MA (1994) Stimulation of lung epithelial liquid clearance by endogenous release of catecholamines in septic shock in anesthetized rats. J Clin Invest 94: 663–671.
37. Wiener-Kronish JP, Albertine KH, Matthay MA (1991) Differential responses of the endothelial and epithelial barriers of the lung in sheep to Escherichia coli endotoxin. J Clin Invest 88: 864–875.
38. Rosenberg HF, Domachowske JB (2012) Inflammatory responses to respiratory syncytial virus (RSV) infection and the development of immunomodulatory pharmacotherapeutics. Curr Med Chem 19: 1424–1431.
39. Matute-Bello G, Downey G, Moore BB, Groshong SD, Matthay MA, et al. (2011) An official American Thoracic Society workshop report: features and measurements of experimental acute lung injury in animals. Am J Respir Cell Mol Biol 44: 725–738.

13

Infection with Host-Range Mutant Adenovirus 5 Suppresses Innate Immunity and Induces Systemic CD4+ T Cell Activation in Rhesus Macaques

Huma Qureshi[1,2], Meritxell Genescà[1,2], Linda Fritts[1], Michael B. McChesney[1], Marjorie Robert-Guroff[3], Christopher J. Miller[1,2]*

1 Center for Comparative Medicine, University of California Davis, Davis, California, United States of America, **2** California National Primate Research Center, University of California Davis, Davis, California, United States of America, **3** Vaccine Branch, National Cancer Institute, National Institutes of Health, Bethesda, Maryland, United States of America

Abstract

Ad5 is a common cause of respiratory disease and an occasional cause of gastroenteritis and conjunctivitis, and seroconversion before adolescence is common in humans. To gain some insight into how Ad5 infection affects the immune system of rhesus macaques (RM) 18 RM were infected with a host-range mutant Ad5 (Ad5hr) by 3 mucosal inoculations. There was a delay of 2 to 6 weeks after the first inoculation before plasmacytoid dendritic cell (pDC) frequency and function increased in peripheral blood. Primary Ad5hr infection suppressed IFN-γ mRNA expression, but the second Ad5hr exposure induced a rapid increase in IFN-gamma mRNA in peripheral blood mononuclear cells (PBMC). Primary Ad5hr infection suppressed CCL20, TNF and IL-1 mRNA expression in PBMC, and subsequent virus exposures further dampened expression of these pro-inflammatory cytokines. Primary, but not secondary, Ad5hr inoculation increased the frequency of CXCR3+ CD4+ T cells in blood, while secondary, but not primary, Ad5hr infection transiently increased the frequencies of Ki67+, HLADR+ and CD95+/CCR5+ CD4+ T cells in blood. Ad5hr infection induced polyfunctional CD4 and CD8+ T cells specific for the Ad5 hexon protein in all of the animals. Thus, infection with Ad5hr induced a complex pattern of innate and adaptive immunity in RM that included transient systemic CD4+ T cell activation and suppressed innate immunity on re-exposure to the virus. The complex effects of adenovirus infection on the immune system may help to explain the unexpected results of testing Ad5 vector expressing HIV antigens in Ad5 seropositive people.

Editor: Jason D. Barbour, University of Hawaii Manoa, United States of America

Funding: P01 AI82278-01 from the National Institutes of Health, National Institute of Allergy and Infectious Disease to CJM. The funders had no role in study design, data collection and analysis, decision to publish, or preparation of the manuscript.

Competing Interests: The authors have declared that no competing interests exist.

* Email: cjmiller@ucdavis.edu

Introduction

Since the initial description in the 1950s, adenoviruses have been known as a cause of common childhood respiratory illnesses [1–4]. In immunocompetent patients, most of these infections are asymptomatic, mild, or self-limited. The prevalence of Ad5 in North American and other populations has been assessed serologically; almost all subjects tested have Ad5-specific binding antibodies, of which 30–60% also have neutralizing antibody responses [5–7]. Adenoviruses infect a broad range of animals in a relatively species-specific manner and adenoviruses can be persistently shed in respiratory secretions and stool [8–11]. Adenoviruses isolated from macaque monkey species (rhesus, cynomologus) are in a different phylogenetic group from the human adenoviruses and do not segregate with human Ad5 or other Group C adenoviruses [11].

The biology of wild type adenoviruses is considerably different from adenoviral vectors designed for gene therapy or as vaccine vectors. Adenoviral vectors carry gene deletions to create space for transgenes and/or to attenuate replication, and they are known to induce strong inflammatory responses following administration in humans and animal models [12,13]. In contrast, infection with wild type Ads suppress host inflammation [14–17], a property that may help the viruses establish persistent infection. Adenovirus infections and adenoviral vectors induce neutralizing antibodies and T cell immunity in nonhuman primates (NHP) and humans [10,18–25]. Pre-existing immunity to simian Ads does not affect Ad vector testing in NHP as the immune responses to simian Ads do not cross-reactive with Ad5 [10]. However, very little is known about modulation of innate immunity or immune activation following adenovirus infection in humans or NHP.

Understanding the immune effects of wild type adenovirus infection is of interest because of the prevalence of adenoviruses in humans and the continued development of adenoviruses as gene therapy and vaccine vectors for use in humans [26]. There have been several reports that the immunity to adenoviruses acquired through infection alters the immune response to vaccines in many people [27–30]. In the present study, we characterized innate and adaptive immune responses of RM after mucosal infection with a human host range Ad5 mutant (Ad5hr) adapted to replicate in nonhuman primates [31]. We found that Ad5hr infection, after repeated mucosal inoculation, had transient effects on blood plasmacytoid dendritic cell (pDC) frequency and function and altered the mRNA levels of antiviral and pro-inflammatory cytokines in PBMC. Further, Ad5hr infection affected the frequency of Ki67+CD4+, HLADR+ CD4+ and CCR5+ CD4+ T cells and putative CD4+ Treg cells in blood. Finally, Ad5hr infection induced Ad5 hexon-specific T cell responses in blood. Thus, Ad5hr infection of RM affects the host immune system in a dramatic manner that could affect the immune responses to subsequent vaccination with adenoviral vectors.

Results

Ad5hr shedding and neutralizing antibody responses in RM

As previously reported [32], 18 male RM were inoculated with Ad5hr orally and intranasally at week 0, then intratracheally at weeks 8 and 12. Ad5 DNA was shed in the nasal secretions of all animals for several days after the first inoculation, and in several animals after the 2nd and 3rd inoculations. By 18 weeks after the first Ad5 hr inoculation, Ad5 neutralizing antibody titers >200 had developed in all but 1 animal [32].

Delayed increase in number and function of pDC in blood after Ad5hr infection

To assess the effect of Ad5hr infection on pDC ($CD3^-$, $CD14^-$, $CD16^-$, $CD19^-$, $CD20^-$, $CD56^-$, HLA-DR^{++}, and $CD123^+$) frequency and function, the absolute number of pDC in blood and the ability of blood pDC to produce IFN-alpha in response to in-vitro stimulation with herpes simplex virus were determined [33,34]. There was a significant increase in the mean number of pDC in blood of the Ad5hr infected RM relative to pre-infection levels at 2 weeks ($p<0.01$, Fig 1A) and 18 weeks ($p<0.05$, Fig 1A) after the first Ad5hr inoculation. Relative to pre-infection levels, there was a significant increase in the mean number of IFN-alpha-producing pDCs in the blood of the Ad5hr infected RM 6 weeks ($p<0.05$, Fig 1B) and 18 weeks after the first Ad5hr inoculation ($p<0.01$, Fig 1B).

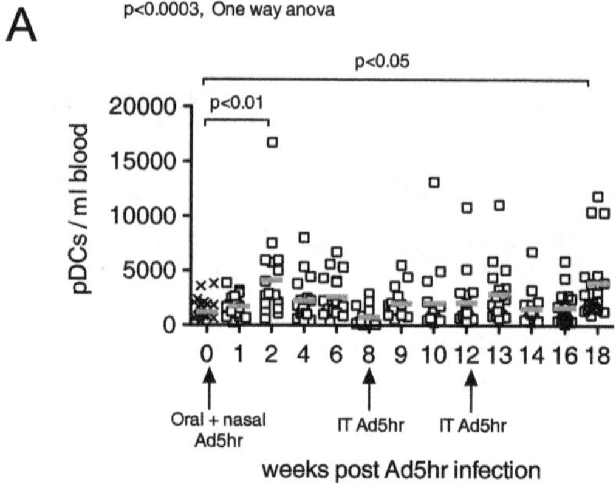

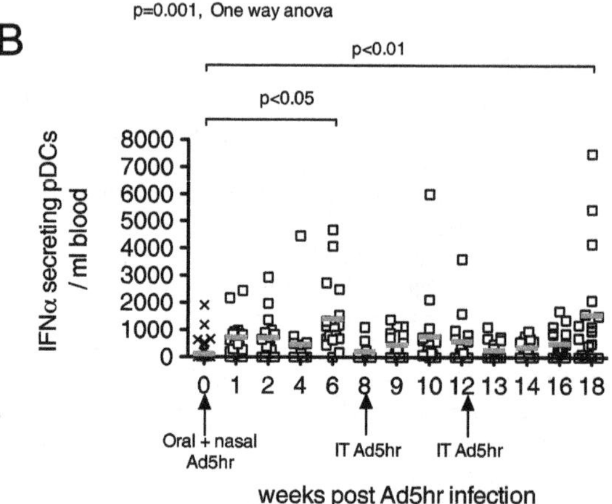

Figure 1. Effect of Ad5hr infection on the number and function of circulating pDC. A) number of pDC per ml of blood. B) number of IFN-α secreting pDCs per ml of blood. Arrows on the X axis indicate the time of Ad5hr inoculation. The mean values for all animals are indicated by blue bars. P values ≤0.05 from the ANOVA and Dunnetts's post-hoc tests are shown.

Increased frequencies of putative regulatory T cells (Tregs) in blood after Ad5hr infection

To assess the effect of Ad5hr infection on CD4+ regulatory T cells, we evaluated the frequency of CD4+ Treg (Foxp3+/CD25hi) and a CD4+ Treg subset expressing CTLA4 (Foxp3+/CTLA4+/CD25hi) that is thought to be particularly immunosuppressive, as CTLA4 is required for suppression by Tregs [35]. There was a significant increase in frequency of CD4+ Treg at 4, 12 and 18 weeks ($p<0.001$, Fig 2A) and CTLA4+/CD4+ Treg frequency at 1, 12 and 18 weeks ($p<0.05$, Fig 2B) after the first Ad5hr inoculation. After each increase, the frequency of both Treg subsets decreased to the pre-infection levels (Fig. 2).

Increased frequencies of CCR5+ CD4+ T cells, HLADR+ CD4+ T cells and Ki67+ CD4+T cells in blood after the second Ad5hr re-infection

The frequency of CCR5+ CD4+ T memory cells in blood increased at week 1 after primary Ad5hr infection ($p<0.01$, Fig 3A), then returned to pre-infection levels. However, after the second and third Ad5hr inoculations at weeks 8 and 12, the frequency of circulating CCR5+ CD4+ T cells at weeks 9, 10, 12 and 13 ($p<0.001$–0.05, Figure 3A) were elevated. After the second and third Ad5hr inoculations, there were also significant increases in the frequency of HLADR+CD4+ T cells at week 9 ($p<0.001$, Fig 3B) and week 16 ($p<0.05$, Fig 3B). We also found that the frequency of activated/proliferating Ki67+ CD4+ T cells was increased at week 9 ($p<0.001$, Fig 3C) and week 14 ($p<0.01$, Fig3C), after the second and third Ad5hr inoculations.

Reduced expression of proinflammatory cytokine and chemokine mRNAs in PBMC after Ad5hr infection

The mRNA levels of IFN-gamma, IFN-alpha, IL-1, CCL20 and TNF in PBMC were variably affected by the primary Ad5hr infection (Fig 4 A–E), but IL-1, CCL20 and TNF were significantly decreased after subsequent Ad5 exposures (Fig 4). In contrast, there were small but significant increases in IFN-gamma mRNA expression in PBMC ($p<0.05$, Fig 4 A) after the second Ad5hr exposure (weeks 9 & 12), which decreased following the 3rd exposure.

Ad5hr infection induced polyfunctional hexon-specific T cell responses in blood

We evaluated the T cell responses in PBMCs of the Ad5hr - inoculated RM to 3 pools of overlapping peptides representing the

A

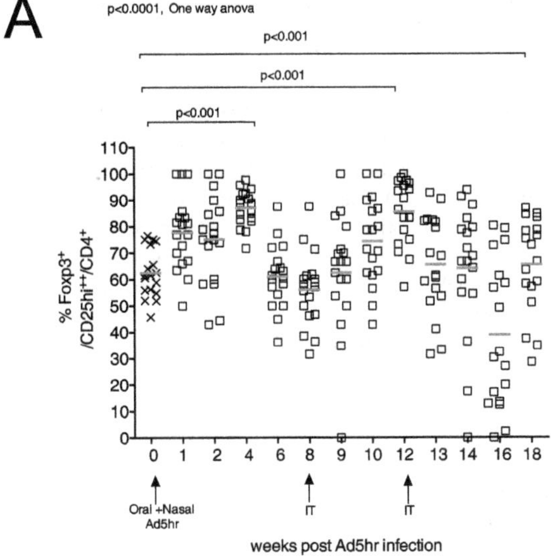

B

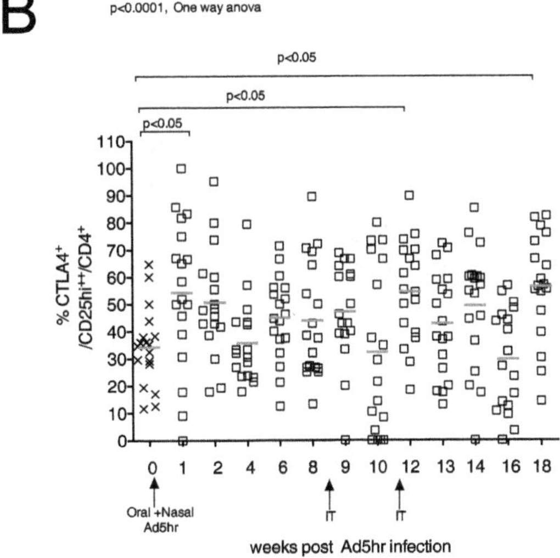

C

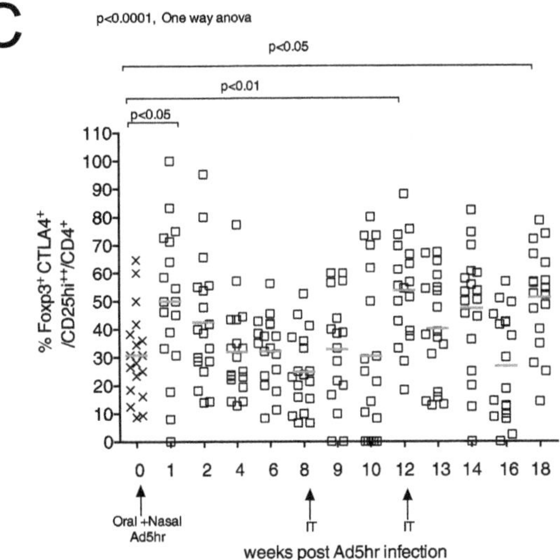

Figure 2. Effect of Ad5hr infection on CD4+ Treg frequency. A) The frequency of FOXP3$^+$/CD4$^+$ T cells that express a high level of CD25 in blood. B) The frequency of CTLA4$^+$/CD25^{hi}/ CD4$^+$ T cells in blood. C) The frequency of FOXP3$^+$/CTLA4+/CD25^{hi}/ CD4$^+$ T cells in blood. Arrows on the X axis indicate the time of Ad5hr inoculation. The mean values for all animals are indicated by blue bars. P values £ 0.05 from the ANOVA and Dunnetts's post-hoc tests are shown.

aa sequence of the Ad5 hexon protein. Moderate Ad5 hexon-specific CD8+ and CD4+ T cell responses (>2 fold increase vs pre-infection) were detected in about half of the RM at week 2 (Table 1). The hexon-specific T cells induced after primary Ad5hr infection produced 1–3 of the cytokines measured (Fig 5). Subsequent Ad5hr exposures (week 8 and 12) led to detectable hexon-specific CD4+ T cell responses in about 77% of RM (Table 1). By week 14, after 3 mucosal Ad5hr exposures, the hexon-specific CD4+ and CD8+T cell responses were more polyfunctional than the hexon-specific T cells detected at week 2 (Fig 5). Of note, the breadth of the hexon-specific T cell responses, as measured by the number of peptide pools eliciting positive responses, was maximum at week 10 after the second Ad5hr inoculation and most restricted at week 14 after 3 Ad5hr inoculations (Table 1).

Discussion

We previously showed that after RM are inoculated with Ad5hr, virus is consistently shed in feces and respiratory secretions after the first Ad5hr inoculation but shedding is intermittent after the second and third inoculations [32]. The pattern of virus shedding in Ad5hr-infected RM mirrors Ad5hr shedding in humans. Adenovirus shedding from the lower GI tract is common in children during symptomatic and asymptomatic infections and it also occurs in healthy adults [36–39]. A recent study found adenoviruses in 7.1% of approximately12,000 respiratory samples from pediatric populations with respiratory symptoms, and there was a high rate of adenovirus co-infection (21.7%) with multiple serotypes in many positive samples [40]. Although Ad5 infected RM and humans develop potent neutralizing antibody responses and Ad5-specific T cells responses [10,18–25,32], the pattern of virus shedding suggests that this immunity does not prevent re-infection. Further anti-Ad5 immunity is often incapable of completely clearing Ad5 infections as the virus can persist in mucosal surfaces of humans [8] and RM [9] for months.

The tropism of Ad5hr in RM and Ad5 in humans is similar and could explain how Ad5 infection affects innate immunity. The coxsakie virus adenovirus receptor (CAR) which binds to the knob domain of the fiber protein, is described as the primary receptor for human adenoviruses [41,42]. However, a number of cells that do not express CAR support adenovirus replication. In fact CAR has been shown to play a minor role in Ad5 infection of many cell types including epithelial cells. Further, human monocytes and dendritic cells (DCs) are susceptible to Ad5 infection despite their lack of CAR expression [43,44]. Although Langerhans cells and dermal DCs from skin express CAR, blocking CAR does not block Ad5 infection, indicating that other receptor pathways mediate viral entry into these cells [45]. Ad5hr in rhesus macaques and Ad5 in humans target lung and gut macrophages and dendritic cells [9]. Thus biology of Ad5hr infection of RM and Ad5 infection of humans are very similar. The affinity of Ad5 for long-lived antigen presenting cells, macrophages and DC in mucosal sites may partially explain the ability of these infections to suppress innate immunity and induce systemic CD4+ T cell activation.

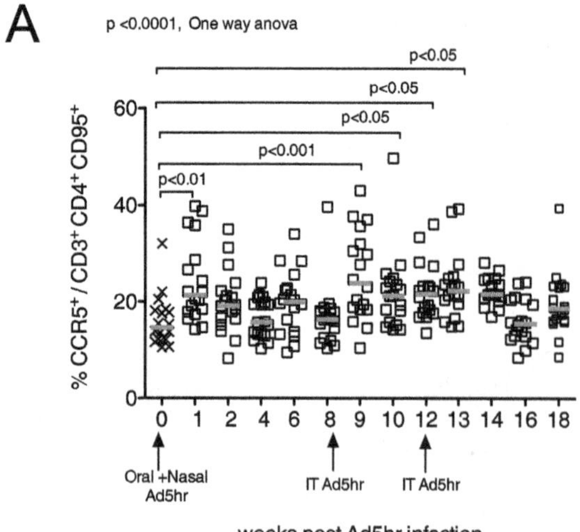

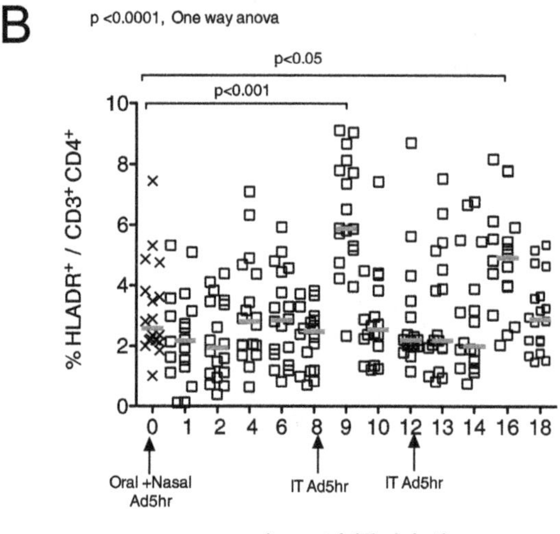

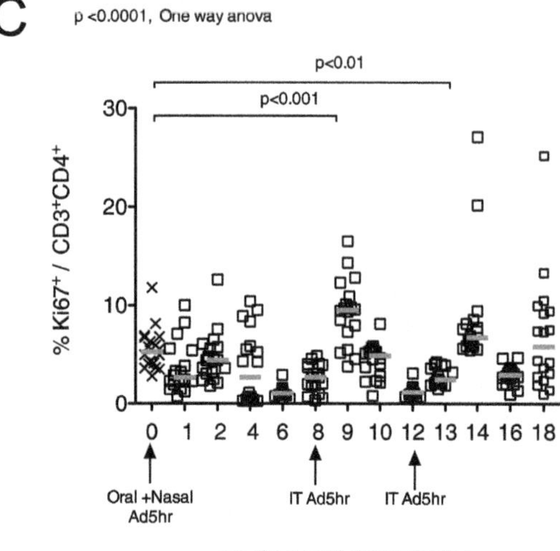

Figure 3. Effect of Ad5hr infection on the frequency of circulating CD4+T cells expressing activation markers. A) The percentage of CD95+/CD3+/CD4+ cells expressing CCR5. B) The percentage of CD3+/CD4+ cells expressing a high level of HLA-DR. C) The percentage of CD3+/CD4+ cells expressing Ki67. Arrows on the X axis indicate the time of Ad5hr inoculation. The mean values for all animals are indicated by blue bars. P values ≤0.05 from the ANOVA and Dunnetts's post-hoc tests are shown.

Here we find report that Ad5hr infection affects the RM immune system in a variety of ways, with repeated exposures having complex and additive effects. The host innate immune system was suppressed by Ad5hr infection as evidenced by changes in the number and function of pDC in blood and decreased expression of pro-inflammatory and immunoregulatory cytokines and chemokine mRNAs in PBMC. Ad5hr infection also altered the adaptive immune system of the host, transiently increasing the frequency of activated T cells and CD4+ T cells expressing Treg markers in blood.

There was a transient increase in pDC frequency and function 2 weeks after the initial Ad5hr exposure (Fig 1A& 1B); however, there was no change from pre-inoculation levels in the pDC frequency or function at week 1 after Ad5hr inoculation while viral replication was at its peak. Thus primary Ad5hr exposure did not appear to induce strong antiviral pDC immune responses in blood. To further understand the Ad5hr induced effects on the immune system, we characterized the antiviral/proinflammatory cytokine and chemokine mRNA expression levels in PBMCs of Ad5hr-infected RM. There was little change in cytokine or chemokine mRNA levels in PBMC at week 1 after the first Ad5hr exposure. Thus, at the gene expression level primary Ad5hr exposure did not induce, and may have suppressed, strong antiviral and pro-inflammatory immune responses in blood 7 days after oral inoculation. In contrast, 7- 14 days after subsequent Ad5hr exposures there was a very transient increase in IFN-gamma mRNA in PBMCs. Although IFN-gamma is a key molecule of antiviral defenses [46,47], it also increases the levels of immune activation and inflammation in response to infection [48,49]. Thus the expression of molecules associated with innate antiviral response was suppressed in PBMC by primary Ad5 infection and, with the exception of IFN-gamma, secondary Ad5 infections/ exposures reinforced and broadened this effect.

Human pDC infected *in vitro* with Ad5 or other Group C adenoviral strains do not produce inflammatory cytokines, in contrast to Group B and E strains [10], and in marked contrast to E1-deleted Ad5 vectors [50]. It seems likely that the inhibition of pDC responses and antiviral/proinflammatory cytokine and chemokine responses that we found in PBMCs of RM infected with Ad5hr is due to the expression of immunomodulatory viral gene products in the initial stages of infection when viral replication is unrestricted by host immunity. The viral proteins, E1 & E3, are the most likely mediators of this immunomodulation. These viral proteins suppress NFκB activation and the subsequent inflammatory response following Ad5 infection [14–16]. However, after the second and third Ad5hr inoculations, Ad5hr-specific immune responses may have blunted virus replication, with reduced expression of E1 & E3 and less suppression of interferon but not other innate immune responses.

After primary Ad5hr infection there was an increased frequency of activated CD4+ T cells in blood, although the levels of these cells quickly returned to baseline. However, subsequent Ad5hr exposures induced recurrent CD4+T cell activation, including expression of Ki67, a marker associated with T cell proliferation. Thus, as with IFN-gamma expression in PBMC, repeated Ad5hr exposure was necessary to induce systemic CD4+ T cell activation, which although not sustained, recurred upon re-exposure to Ad5. Similar transient CD4+ T cell activation was observed in RM after vaccination with an E1-deleted, replication defective Ad 5 vector [51]. As people are likely to be repeatedly exposed to Ad5,

A) IFN-gamma

p<0.0001, One way anova

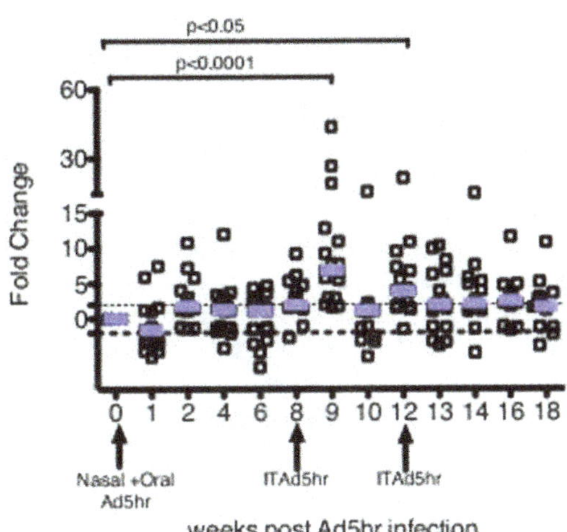

B) IFN-alpha

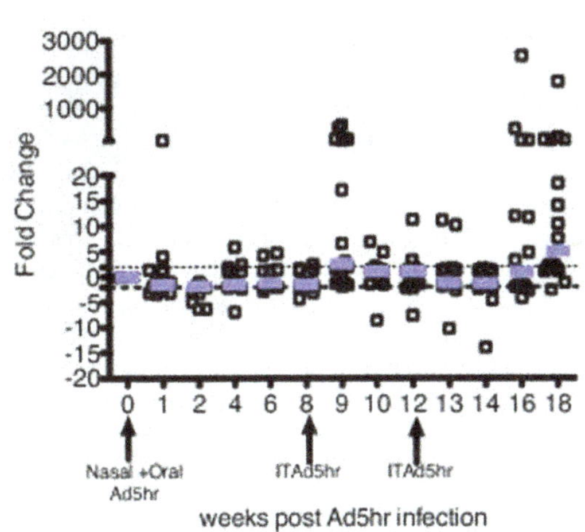

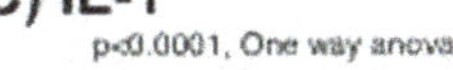

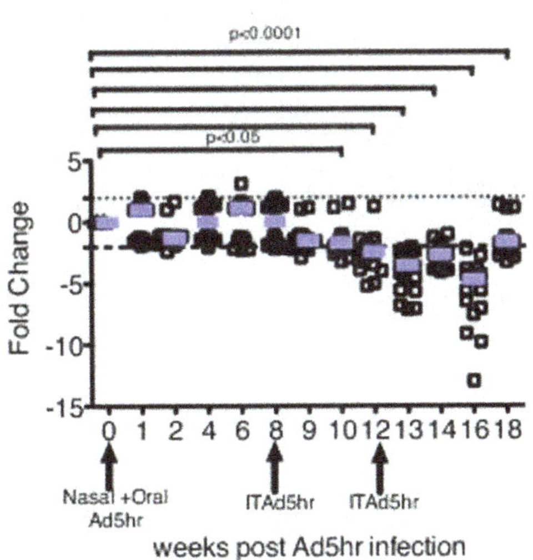

D) TNF

p<0.0001, One way anova

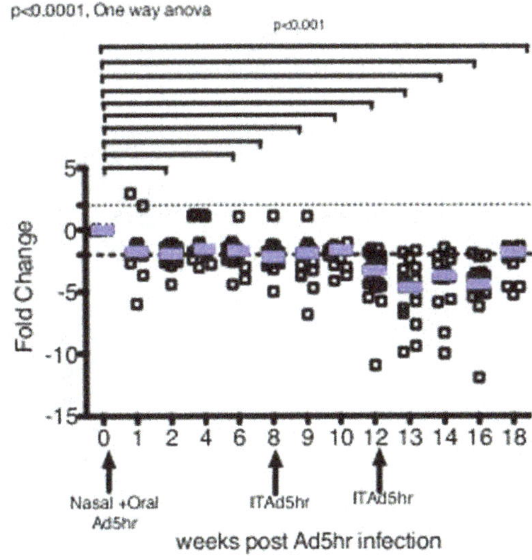

E) CCL20 (LARC)

p<0.0001, One way anova

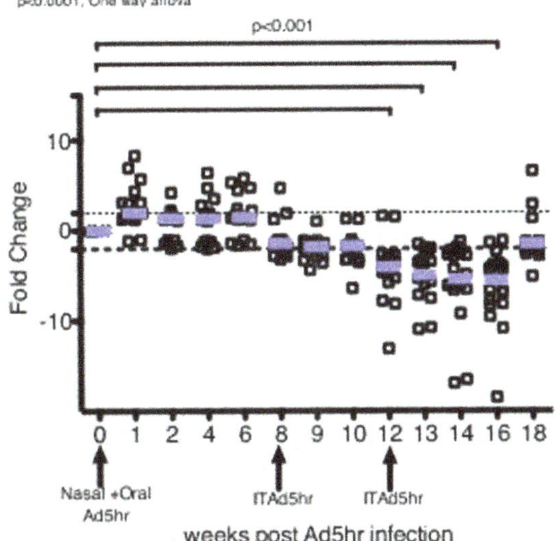

Figure 4. Effect of Ad5hr infection on proinflammatory cytokine and chemokine gene expression in PBMC. A) The fold-change of IFN-gammamRNA in PBMCs; B) IFN-α; C) IL-1; D) TNF and E) CCL20. The fold-change in target gene mRNA levels in study animals post-Ad5hr infection relative to the same target gene mRNA level before Ad5hr infection was calculated as described in Materials and Methods. Arrows on the X axis indicate the time of Ad5hr inoculation. The mean values for all animals are indicated by blue bars P values ≤0.05 from the ANOVA and Dunnetts's post-hoc tests are shown.

frequent periods of transient T cell activation probably occur with some frequency in Ad5 seropositive individuals.

A recent report showed that Ad5 immune complexes interact with Fc receptors on DC to enter the endosomal compartment where Ad5 genomic DNA interacts with TLR9 [52]. This TLR9 ligation activates DCs and results in production of proinflammatory cytokines. If this type of interaction occurs *in vivo*, it could activate Ad5-specifc and bystander T cells after secondary Ad5hr exposures. Because as we previously reported Ad5hr infection of RM induces Ad5-specific antibodies [32], this phenomenon could explain the enhanced virus transmission after Ad5 seropositive individuals were immunized with rAd5 Merck Step vaccine.

The frequency of Tregs in blood after the primary Ad5hr infection increased (Fig 2). This response to Ad5hr infection by RM is not unique, as upregulation of Tregs early after pathogen infection [53–55] with concomitant modulation of pathogen-specific immunity has been recently reported [54,56]. Furthermore, CTLA4 expression on Tregs is associated with Treg-mediated immune suppression 36 [57]. It has been shown that Tregs promote pathogen persistence in leishmania and TB infection [53,55].

After Ad5hr infection RM develop weak and variable hexon-specific CD4+ and CD8+ T cell responses in the blood. These hexon-specific T cells predominantly secreted 1–3 cytokines in various combinations (Table 1, Fig 5). Secondary Ad5hr exposures expanded hexon-specific CD4+ T cell responses (Table 1) with increases in polyfunctional T cells; especially IFN-gamma +/TNF+/IL-2+ CD4+ T cells (Fig 5). Similarly Ad5-specific CD4+ and CD8+ T cells are found in humans and CD4+ T cell responses are focused on the hexon protein [21,23].

Although, preexisting Ad5 specific immunity does not prevent infection, it does affect the immunogenicity of Ad5-based vaccines in RM and humans [27–30,32]. Adenovirus Immunity at the time of immunization with the Step vaccine modified T helper cell cytokine responses to the vaccine [28], reduces innate immune responses [30] and is associated with relatively poor HIV-specific T cell responses in both human and RM Step vaccine recipients [27,32]. Ad5-immunity present in the host prior to Ad5 vaccine immunization result in weaker HIV or SIV-specific T cell responses in that less vaccinees respond, and the magnitude, antigenic breadth and cytokine functions of the HIV/SIV-specific T cells were reduced compared to their Ad5 seronegative counterparts [27,32]. How the pre-existing Ad5 immunity affects the responses to vaccines has not been rigorously determined. The lower immune responses to HIV antigens in Ad5 seropositive people immunized with an Ad5 vector is assumed to be due to the killing of these APC as they express HIV and Ad5 antigens by pre-existing Ad5-specific memory cytotoxic T cells. In addition, preexisting Ad5-specific antibodies could form immune complexes with Ad5 vaccine virus that activate and expand Ad5-specific memory T cell responses. These Ad5-specific T cells, in turn, could limit HIV-specific immune responses to the vaccine by killing the DCs co-expressing Ad5 and HIV antigens [52].

The results reported here further demonstrate that Ad5hr infection alters the host immune system in complex ways that could affect the host response to subsequent vaccination, particularly if an immunization was given just before, or after, a secondary Ad5 infection/exposure. The Step Trial HIV vaccine resulted in enhanced infection in some Ad5-seropositive, uncircumcised vaccinees [58]. A vaccine study in macaques that modeled the Step Trial recapitulated the lack of protection and a greater risk of infection in immunized macaques with pre-existing Ad5 seropositivity [32]. In both the Step trial and the monkey study, enhanced susceptibility to infection was only seen in individuals with a prior or ongoing Ad5 infection. However, there is no evidence from these studies, or from HVTN 505 (the most recent efficacy trial of a HIV vaccine using a replication defective Ad5 vector in Ad5 seronegative men), that a replication defective Ad5 vector vaccine can enhance HIV transmission in individuals that are not, or have not been, infected with Ad5. Further, Ad5 infection alone is not associated with increased risk of HIV infection AIDS [59]. Thus the results reported here, taken together with the results of the clinical trials, raise the possibility that Ad5 infection alters the responses to immunizations in general. Additional experiments are needed to determine the relative contributions of the Ad5 vector and Ad5 infections to the

Table 1. Adenovirus hexon-specific T cell responses in PBMCs after Ad5hr infection.

	Week 2		Week 10		Week 14	
Peptides/T cell	# events*	% positive†	# events	% positive	# events	% positive
Pool 1/CD4	101±36	44	175±41‡	78	68±19	56
Pool 2/CD4	92±30	44	264±48‡	72	65±16	56
Pool 3/CD4	106±75‡	50	164±29‡	72	110±25‡	78
Pool 1/CD8	186±76‡	33	85±14	67	73±18	28
Pool 2/CD8	73±34	44	99±14	61	43±12	56
Pool 3/CD8	122±52‡	28	113±35‡	61	97±28‡	56

* Flow cytometric events (mean ±SE) normalized to 10^5 $CD3^+$ T cells.
† Percentage of responders /18 animals tested.
‡ Responses that were ≥ two-fold compared to pre-infection levels were considered strongly positive.

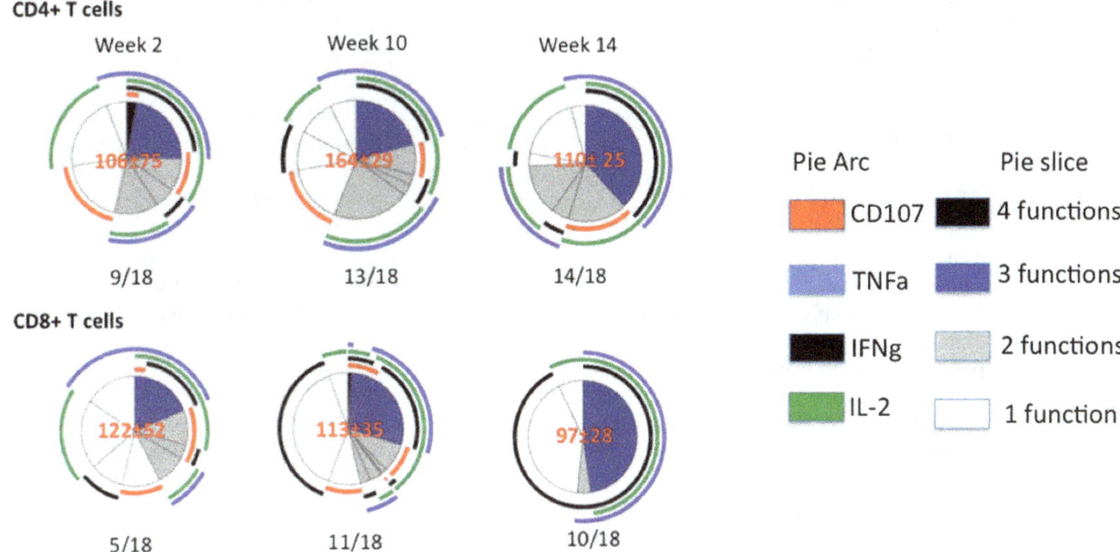

Figure 5. Ad5 hexon-specific T cell responses in PBMCs after Ad5hr infection as detected by multiparameter flow cytometry. Pie charts present the average CD4+ or CD8+T cell responses for all positive animals at weeks 2, 10 and 14 from the first Ad5hr inoculation, as described in Materials and Methods. Pie slice colors denote the number of positive functions (expression of IL-2, IFN-γ, TNF and CD107 degranulation). Pie arc colors denote the 4 functions separately. Red numbers in the center of pie charts are the mean ± standard deviation of hexon-specific T cells normalized to 10^5 CD3+ T cells. Fractional numbers below a pie chart refer to the number of animals in a group of 18 that responded.

unexpected outcomes of the Step trial and nonhuman primate studies.

Materials and Methods

Ethics Statement

As previously reported [32], the captive-bred 4–9 year old male rhesus macaques (Macaca mulatta) used in this study were from the California National Primate Research Center and they were housed in accordance with the recommendations of the Association for Assessment and Accreditation of Laboratory Animal Care International Standards and with the recommendations in the Guide for the Care and Use of Laboratory Animals of the National Institutes of Health. The Institutional Animal Use and Care Committee of the University of California, Davis, approved these experiments (Protocol # 15835). When immobilization was necessary, the animals were injected intramuscularly with 10 mg/kg of ketamine HCl (Parke-Davis, Morris Plains N.J.). All efforts were made to minimize suffering. Details of animal welfare and steps taken to ameliorate suffering were in accordance with the recommendations of the Weatherall report, "The use of non-human primates in research". Animals were housed in an air-conditioned facility with an ambient temperature of 21–25°C, a relative humidity of 40%–60% and a 12 h light/dark cycle. Animals were individually housed in suspended stainless steel wire-bottomed cages and provided with a commercial primate diet. Fresh fruit was provided once daily and water was freely available at all times. A variety of environmental enrichment strategies were employed including housing of animals in pairs, providing toys to manipulate and playing entertainment videos in the animal rooms. In addition, the animals were observed twice daily and any signs of disease or discomfort were reported to the veterinary staff for evaluation. For sample collection, animals were anesthetized with 10 mg/kg ketamine HCl (Park-Davis, Morris Plains, NJ, USA) or 0.7 mg/kg tiletamine HCl and zolazepan (Telazol, Fort Dodge Animal Health, Fort Dodge, IA) injected intramuscularly. The animals were sacrificed by intravenous administration of barbiturates prior to the onset of any clinical signs of disease.

Ad5hr infection

As previously reported [32], 18 RM were infected with 1.5×10^9 infectious particles/dose/route of Ad5hr [31], by nasal & oral routes at week 0 and by the intratracheal route at week 8 and 12.

Isolation of lymphocytes from blood

PBMCs were isolated from heparinized blood using Lymphocyte Separation Medium (ICN Biomedicals). PBMC samples were frozen in 10% dimethyl sulfoxide (DMSO; Sigma-Aldrich) and 90% fetal bovine serum (Gemini BioProducts), stored in liquid nitrogen until future use in immunological assays [32].

T cell phenotyping in blood

Blood samples were surface stained with 4 color panels of antibodies. Panel 1; anti-CD3 PerCP clone no. SP34, anti-CD4 APC clone no. M-T477, anti-CD95 FITC clone no. DX2 and anti-CCR5 PE clone no. 3A9. Panel 2; anti-CD3 PerCP clone no. SP34, anti-CD8 APC clone no. SK1, anti-CD38 PE clone OKT10, anti-HLADR FITC clone no G46-6. Surface stained samples were fixed with Q prep (Beckman Coulter). All antibodies were purchased from Pharmingen/Becton-Dickinson, San Diego, CA, unless specified. Data were acquired using a FACS Calibur cytometer (Becton Dickinson), and analyzed using FlowJo software (Treestar, Inc.) and a Macintosh G5 computer (Apple, Inc.). At least 100,000 small lymphocyte events were collected from each tube analyzed.

Intracellular staining for Ki-67 in blood

Blood samples were surfaced stained with the following antibodies; anti-CD3-Pacific Blue (Clone SP3F2), anti-CD4-

Amcyan (Clone L200), anti-CD8-Cy7APC (Clone SK1) and anti-CXCR3-PE (clone 1C -6). Thereafter, surface stained samples were washed and permeabilized with 0.5% saponin for intracellular staining, and then stained with Ki67-FITC (Clone B56) for 20 min. Ki67- stained samples were washed with the permeabilizing buffer and fixed with 1% paraformaldehyde.

Intracellular staining for cytokine and degranulation markers

As previously described in detail [32], for intracellular staining of PBMCs, cryopreserved samples were thawed and rested overnight at 37°C, in 5% CO2 atmosphere, in RPMI media (Gibco, Invitrogen Inc.) containing 10% fetal calf serum. To stimulate cells, 3 peptide pools spanning the hexon protein, 20mer peptides overlapping by 10 residues (Anaspec, Inc.), were prepared at 5 μg/ml/peptide in DMSO. The negative control contained co-stimulatory molecules and DMSO, and the positive control was staphylococcal enterotoxin B (0.2 μg/ml, Sigma-Aldrich). At least 100,000 events in the forward scatter/side scatter lymphocyte gate were acquired. Further, samples that had a large discrepancy between the number of events in the negative control and the peptide-stimulated tubes were eliminated. The background level of cytokine staining varied from sample to sample. Samples were considered positive in which, after subtracting the negative control, there were at least 5 positive events for a single functional marker, 3 positive events for two or more functional markers, and the sum of the different combinations of responses represented at least 10 events. In addition, a sample was not considered positive for a particular combination of functions if the frequency of T cells responding with that particular combination of functions was lower than 0.02%. The software program Simplified Presentation of Incredibly Complex Evaluations (SPICE; a gift from M. Roederer, Vaccine Research Center, NIAID/NIH) was used to create the pie charts that represent the average of all positive responses [60].

Relative quantification of cytokine/ chemokine mRNA expression levels in PBMC

The mRNA levels were determined by real-time PCR as described previously [61,62] for IL-1, IFN-alpha, IFN-gamma, TNF and CCL20. The comparative threshold cycle (Ct) method was used for quantification of mRNA levels (User Bulletin No. 2, ABI PRISM 7700 Sequence Detection System, Applied Biosystems). GAPDH was used as the reference gene and all samples were tested in duplicate. A ΔCt value was generated by subtracting the Ct value of GAPDH from the Ct value of the target mRNA. To compare the target gene mRNA levels pre- and post- Ad5hr infection, the mean ΔCt of a target gene at a pre-infection time point in an individual animal was used as a reference value to generate the ΔΔCt for the same target gene in the that particular animal at post-infection time points [63]. Thus, the ΔΔCt value of a target gene in study animals at post-infection time point is equal to difference between ΔCt value of the target gene in the study animal at a post-infection time point and the ΔCt value of the target gene in that animal at the pre-infection time point. The fold-change in target gene mRNA levels in study animals post-Ad5hr infection relative to target gene mRNA levels in the study animals pre-Ad5hr infection was calculated using one of 2 formulas based on the ΔΔCt:

1) Fold change of decreased mean mRNA level $= -1/2^{-\Delta\Delta Ct}$ (If the ΔΔCt was positive).
2) Fold change of increased mean mRNA level $= 2^{-\Delta\Delta Ct}$ (If the ΔΔCt was negative).

pDC enumeration and assessment of IFN-alpha production

Plasmacytoid DCs were phenotyped using a lineage marker Ab cocktail (CD3, CD14, CD16, CD19, CD20, CD56) and anti-CD123, as previously described [34].

Statistical analyses

Data are reported as the median and the standard error of the mean (SEM) for each animal group using Prism 5.0 software (GraphPad Software). Statistical analyses were performed by one-way ANOVA with Dunnetts's multiple comparison test if more than two groups were compared. The flow cytometric data analysis program, SPICE, was used to analyze T cell responses detected by polychromatic flow cytometry. A P value of <0.05 was considered significant.

Acknowledgments

We thank the Primate Services Unit at the CNPRC. Zhong-Min Ma, Jun Li and Tracy Rourke provided excellent technical assistance.

Author Contributions

Conceived and designed the experiments: CJM MRG. Performed the experiments: HQ MG LF CJM. Analyzed the data: HQ MG CJM MRG MBM. Contributed reagents/materials/analysis tools: MRG. Contributed to the writing of the manuscript: HQ MG CJM MRG MBM.

References

1. Chany C, Lepine P, Lelong M, Le TV, Satge P, et al. (1958) Severe and fatal pneumonia in infants and young children associated with adenovirus infections. Am J Hyg 67: 367–378.
2. Edwards KM, Thompson J, Paolini J, Wright PF (1985) Adenovirus infections in young children. Pediatrics 76: 420–424.
3. Evans AS (1958) Adenovirus infections in children and young adults; with comments on vaccination. N Engl J Med 259: 464–468.
4. Rowe WP, Huebner RJ, Gilmore LK, Parrott RH, Ward TG (1953) Isolation of a cytopathogenic agent from human adenoids undergoing spontaneous degeneration in tissue culture. Proc Soc Exp Biol Med 84: 570–573.
5. Barouch DH, Kik SV, Weverling GJ, Dilan R, King SL, et al. (2011) International seroepidemiology of adenovirus serotypes 5, 26, 35, and 48 in pediatric and adult populations. Vaccine 29: 5203–5209.
6. Nwanegbo E, Vardas E, Gao W, Whittle H, Sun H, et al. (2004) Prevalence of neutralizing antibodies to adenoviral serotypes 5 and 35 in the adult populations of The Gambia, South Africa, and the United States. Clin Diagn Lab Immunol 11: 351–357.
7. Thorner AR, Vogels R, Kaspers J, Weverling GJ, Holterman L, et al. (2006) Age dependence of adenovirus-specific neutralizing antibody titers in individuals from sub-Saharan Africa. J Clin Microbiol 44: 3781–3783.
8. Alkhalaf MA, Guiver M, Cooper RJ (2013) Prevalence and quantitation of adenovirus DNA from human tonsil and adenoid tissues. J Med Virol 85: 1947–1954.
9. Patterson LJ, Kuate S, Daltabuit-Test M, Li Q, Xiao P, et al. (2012) Replicating adenovirus-simian immunodeficiency virus (SIV) vectors efficiently prime SIV-specific systemic and mucosal immune responses by targeting myeloid dendritic cells and persisting in rectal macrophages, regardless of immunization route. Clin Vaccine Immunol 19: 629–637.
10. Calcedo R, Vandenberghe LH, Roy S, Somanathan S, Wang L, et al. (2009) Host immune responses to chronic adenovirus infections in human and nonhuman primates. J Virol 83: 2623–2631.
11. Roy S, Calcedo R, Medina-Jaszek A, Keough M, Peng H, et al. (2011) Adenoviruses in lymphocytes of the human gastro-intestinal tract. PLoS One 6: e24859.
12. Muruve DA (2004) The innate immune response to adenovirus vectors. Hum Gene Ther 15: 1157–1166.

13. Higginbotham JN, Seth P, Blaese RM, Ramsey WJ (2002) The release of inflammatory cytokines from human peripheral blood mononuclear cells in vitro following exposure to adenovirus variants and capsid. Hum Gene Ther 13: 129–141.
14. Friedman JM, Horwitz MS (2002) Inhibition of tumor necrosis factor alpha-induced NF-kappa B activation by the adenovirus E3-10.4/14.5K complex. J Virol 76: 5515–5521.
15. Jefferies WA, Burgert HG (1990) E3/19K from adenovirus 2 is an immunosubversive protein that binds to a structural motif regulating the intracellular transport of major histocompatibility complex class I proteins. J Exp Med 172: 1653–1664.
16. Lesokhin AM, Delgado-Lopez F, Horwitz MS (2002) Inhibition of chemokine expression by adenovirus early region three (E3) genes. J Virol 76: 8236–8243.
17. Schaack J, Bennett ML, Colbert JD, Torres AV, Clayton GH, et al. (2004) E1A and E1B proteins inhibit inflammation induced by adenovirus. Proc Natl Acad Sci U S A 101: 3124–3129.
18. Bradley RR, Lynch DM, Iampietro MJ, Borducchi EN, Barouch DH (2012) Adenovirus serotype 5 neutralizing antibodies target both hexon and fiber following vaccination and natural infection. J Virol 86: 625–629.
19. Bradley RR, Maxfield LF, Lynch DM, Iampietro MJ, Borducchi EN, et al. (2012) Adenovirus serotype 5-specific neutralizing antibodies target multiple hexon hypervariable regions. J Virol 86: 1267–1272.
20. Cheng C, Gall JG, Nason M, King CR, Koup RA, et al. (2010) Differential specificity and immunogenicity of adenovirus type 5 neutralizing antibodies elicited by natural infection or immunization. J Virol 84: 630–638.
21. Hutnick NA, Carnathan D, Demers K, Makedonas G, Ertl HC, et al. (2010) Adenovirus-specific human T cells are pervasive, polyfunctional, and cross-reactive. Vaccine 28: 1932–1941.
22. Kessler T, Hamprecht K, Feuchtinger T, Jahn G (2010) Dendritic cells are susceptible to infection with wild-type adenovirus, inducing a differentiation arrest in precursor cells and inducing a strong T-cell stimulation. J Gen Virol 91: 1150–1154.
23. Leen AM, Christin A, Khalil M, Weiss H, Gee AP, et al. (2008) Identification of hexon-specific CD4 and CD8 T-cell epitopes for vaccine and immunotherapy. J Virol 82: 546–554.
24. Onion D, Crompton LJ, Milligan DW, Moss PA, Lee SP, et al. (2007) The CD4+ T-cell response to adenovirus is focused against conserved residues within the hexon protein. J Gen Virol 88: 2417–2425.
25. Tang J, Olive M, Champagne K, Flomenberg N, Eisenlohr L, et al. (2004) Adenovirus hexon T-cell epitope is recognized by most adults and is restricted by HLA DP4, the most common class II allele. Gene Ther 11: 1408–1415.
26. Baden LR, Walsh SR, Seaman MS, Johnson JA, Tucker RP, et al. (2014) First-in-Human Evaluation of a Hexon Chimeric Adenovirus Vector Expressing HIV-1 Env (IPCAVD 002). J Infect Dis.
27. Frahm N, DeCamp AC, Friedrich DP, Carter DK, Defawe OD, et al. (2012) Human adenovirus-specific T cells modulate HIV-specific T cell responses to an Ad5-vectored HIV-1 vaccine. J Clin Invest 122: 359–367.
28. Pine SO, Kublin JG, Hammer SM, Borgerding J, Huang Y, et al. (2011) Pre-Existing Adenovirus Immunity Modifies a Complex Mixed Th1 and Th2 Cytokine Response to an Ad5/HIV-1 Vaccine Candidate in Humans. PLoS One 6: e18526.
29. Priddy FH, Brown D, Kublin J, Monahan K, Wright DP, et al. (2008) Safety and immunogenicity of a replication-incompetent adenovirus type 5 HIV-1 clade B gag/pol/nef vaccine in healthy adults. Clin Infect Dis 46: 1769–1781.
30. Zak DE, Andersen-Nissen E, Peterson ER, Sato A, Hamilton MK, et al. (2012) Merck Ad5/HIV induces broad innate immune activation that predicts CD8(+) T-cell responses but is attenuated by preexisting Ad5 immunity. Proc Natl Acad Sci U S A 109: E3503–3512.
31. Klessig DF, Grodzicker T (1979) Mutations that allow human Ad2 and Ad5 to express late genes in monkey cells map in the viral gene encoding the 72K DNA binding protein. Cell 17: 957–966.
32. Qureshi H, Ma ZM, Huang Y, Hodge G, Thomas MA, et al. (2012) Low-dose penile SIVmac251 exposure of rhesus macaques infected with adenovirus type 5 (Ad5) and then immunized with a replication-defective Ad5-based SIV gag/pol/nef vaccine recapitulates the results of the phase IIb step trial of a similar HIV-1 vaccine. J Virol 86: 2239–2250.
33. Chung E, Amrute SB, Abel K, Gupta G, Wang Y, et al. (2005) Characterization of virus-responsive plasmacytoid dendritic cells in the rhesus macaque. Clin Diagn Lab Immunol 12: 426–435.
34. Abel K, Wang Y, Fritts L, Sanchez E, Chung E, et al. (2005) Deoxycytidyl-Deoxyguanosine Oligonucleotide Classes A, B, and C Induce Distinct Cytokine Gene Expression Patterns in Rhesus Monkey Peripheral Blood Mononuclear Cells and Distinct Alpha Interferon Responses in TLR9-Expressing Rhesus Monkey Plasmacytoid Dendritic Cells. Clin Diagn Lab Immunol 12: 606–621.
35. Wing K, Onishi Y, Prieto-Martin P, Yamaguchi T, Miyara M, et al. (2008) CTLA-4 control over Foxp3+ regulatory T cell function. Science 322: 271–275.
36. Buimovici-Klein E, Lange M, Ong KR, Grieco MH, Cooper LZ (1988) Virus isolation and immune studies in a cohort of homosexual men. J Med Virol 25: 371–385.
37. Cinek O, Witso E, Jeansson S, Rasmussen T, Drevinek P, et al. (2006) Longitudinal observation of enterovirus and adenovirus in stool samples from Norwegian infants with the highest genetic risk of type 1 diabetes. J Clin Virol 35: 33–340.
38. Hillis WD, Cooper MR, Bang FB (1973) Adenovirus infections in West Bengal. I. Persistence of viruses in infants and young children. Indian J Med Res 61: 980–988.
39. Lew JF, Moe CL, Monroe SS, Allen JR, Harrison BM, et al. (1991) Astrovirus and adenovirus associated with diarrhea in children in day care settings. J Infect Dis 164: 673–678.
40. Wong S, Pabbaraju K, Pang XL, Lee BE, Fox JD (2008) Detection of a broad range of human adenoviruses in respiratory tract samples using a sensitive multiplex real-time PCR assay. J Med Virol 80: 856–865.
41. Bergelson JM, Cunningham JA, Droguett G, Kurt-Jones EA, Krithivas A, et al. (1997) Isolation of a common receptor for Coxsackie B viruses and adenoviruses 2 and 5. Science 275: 1320–1323.
42. Tomko RP, Xu R, Philipson L (1997) HCAR and MCAR: the human and mouse cellular receptors for subgroup C adenoviruses and group B coxsackieviruses. Proc Natl Acad Sci U S A 94: 3352–3356.
43. Cheng C, Gall JG, Kong WP, Sheets RL, Gomez PL, et al. (2007) Mechanism of ad5 vaccine immunity and toxicity: fiber shaft targeting of dendritic cells. PLoS Pathog 3: e25.
44. Lore K, Adams WC, Havenga MJ, Precopio ML, Holterman L, et al. (2007) Myeloid and plasmacytoid dendritic cells are susceptible to recombinant adenovirus vectors and stimulate polyfunctional memory T cell responses. J Immunol 179: 1721–1729.
45. Rozis G, de Silva S, Benlahrech A, Papagatsias T, Harris J, et al. (2005) Langerhans cells are more efficiently transduced than dermal dendritic cells by adenovirus vectors expressing either group C or group B fibre protein: implications for mucosal vaccines. Eur J Immunol 35: 2617–2626.
46. Maraskovsky E, Chen WF, Shortman K (1989) IL-2 and IFN-gamma are two necessary lymphokines in the development of cytolytic T cells. J Immunol 143: 1210–1214.
47. Giovarelli M, Santoni A, Jemma C, Musso T, Giuffrida AM, et al. (1988) Obligatory role of IFN-gamma in induction of lymphokine-activated and T lymphocyte killer activity, but not in boosting of natural cytotoxicity. J Immunol 141: 2831–2836.
48. Abel K, La Franco-Scheuch L, Rourke T, Ma ZM, De Silva V, et al. (2004) Gamma Interferon-Mediated Inflammation Is Associated with Lack of Protection from Intravaginal Simian Immunodeficiency Virus SIVmac239 Challenge in Simian-Human Immunodeficiency Virus 89.6-Immunized Rhesus Macaques. J Virol 78: 841–854.
49. Reinhart TA, Fallert BA, Pfeifer ME, Sanghavi S, Capuano S, 3rd, et al. (2002) Increased expression of the inflammatory chemokine CXC chemokine ligand 9/monokine induced by interferon-gamma in lymphoid tissues of rhesus macaques during simian immunodeficiency virus infection and acquired immunodeficiency syndrome. Blood 99: 3119–3128.
50. Varnavski AN, Zhang Y, Schnell M, Tazelaar J, Louboutin JP, et al. (2002) Preexisting immunity to adenovirus in rhesus monkeys fails to prevent vector-induced toxicity. J Virol 76: 5711–5719.
51. Sun Y, Bailer RT, Rao SS, Mascola JR, Nabel GJ, et al. (2009) Systemic and mucosal T-lymphocyte activation induced by recombinant adenovirus vaccines in rhesus monkeys. J Virol 83: 10596–10604.
52. Perreau M, Pantaleo G, Kremer EJ (2008) Activation of a dendritic cell-T cell axis by Ad5 immune complexes creates an improved environment for replication of HIV in T cells. J Exp Med 205: 2717–2725.
53. Belkaid Y, Piccirillo CA, Mendez S, Shevach EM, Sacks DL (2002) CD4+ CD25+ regulatory T cells control Leishmania major persistence and immunity. Nature 420: 502–507.
54. Fulton RB, Meyerholz DK, Varga SM (2010) Foxp3+ CD4 regulatory T cells limit pulmonary immunopathology by modulating the CD8 T cell response during respiratory syncytial virus infection. J Immunol 185: 2382–2392.
55. Scott-Browne JP, Shafiani S, Tucker-Heard G, Ishida-Tsubota K, Fontenot JD, et al. (2007) Expansion and function of Foxp3-expressing T regulatory cells during tuberculosis. J Exp Med 204: 2159–2169.
56. Shafiani S, Tucker-Heard G, Kariyone A, Takatsu K, Urdahl KB (2010) Pathogen-specific regulatory T cells delay the arrival of effector T cells in the lung during early tuberculosis. J Exp Med 207: 1409–1420.
57. Tai X, Van Laethem F, Pobezinsky L, Guinter T, Sharrow SO, et al. (2012) Basis of CTLA-4 function in regulatory and conventional CD4(+) T cells. Blood 119: 5155–5163.
58. Buchbinder SP, Mehrotra DV, Duerr A, Fitzgerald DW, Mogg R, et al. (2008) Efficacy assessment of a cell-mediated immunity HIV-1 vaccine (the Step Study): a double-blind, randomised, placebo-controlled, test-of-concept trial. Lancet 372: 1881–1893.
59. Curlin ME, Cassis-Ghavami F, Magaret AS, Spies GA, Duerr A, et al. (2011) Serological immunity to adenovirus serotype 5 is not associated with risk of HIV infection: a case-control study. AIDS 25: 153–158.
60. Genesca M, Skinner PJ, Hong JJ, Li J, Lu D, et al. (2008) With minimal systemic T-cell expansion, CD8+ T Cells mediate protection of rhesus macaques immunized with attenuated simian-human immunodeficiency virus SHIV89.6 from vaginal challenge with simian immunodeficiency virus. J Virol 82: 11181–11196.
61. Wang Y, Abel K, Lantz K, Krieg AM, McChesney MB, et al. (2005) The Toll-like receptor 7 (TLR7) agonist, imiquimod, and the TLR9 agonist, CpG ODN, induce antiviral cytokines and chemokines but do not prevent vaginal transmission of simian immunodeficiency virus when applied intravaginally to rhesus macaques. J Virol 79: 14355–14370.

14

Increased Risk of Dementia in Patients Exposed to Nitrogen Dioxide and Carbon Monoxide: A Population-Based Retrospective Cohort Study

Kuang-Hsi Chang[1,2], Mei-Yin Chang[3], Chih-Hsin Muo[4], Trong-Neng Wu[1], Chiu-Ying Chen[1], Chia-Hung Kao[5,6]*

1 Department of Public Health, China Medical University, Taichung, Taiwan, **2** Department of Medical Research, Taichung Veterans General Hospital, Taichung, Taiwan, **3** Department of Medical Laboratory Science and Biotechnology, School of Medical and Health Sciences, Fooyin University, Kaohsiung, Taiwan, **4** Management Office for Health Data, China Medical University Hospital, Taichung, Taiwan, **5** Graduate Institute of Clinical Medical Science, College of Medicine, China Medical University, Taiwan, **6** Department of Nuclear Medicine and PET Center, China Medical University Hospital, Taichung, Taiwan

Abstract

Background: The air pollution caused by vehicular emissions is associated with cognitive decline. However, the associations between the levels of nitrogen dioxide (NO_2) and carbon monoxide (CO) exposure and dementia remain poorly defined and have been addressed in only a few previous studies.

Materials and Methods: In this study, we obtained data on 29547 people from the National Health Insurance Research Database (NHIRD) of Taiwan, including data on 1720 patients diagnosed with dementia between 2000 and 2010, and we evaluated the risk of dementia among four levels of air pollutant. Detailed data on daily air pollution were available from January 1, 1998 to December 31, 2010. Yearly average concentrations of pollutants were calculated from the baseline to the date of dementia occurrence, withdrawal of patients, or the end of the study, and these data were categorized into quartiles, with Q1 being the lowest level and Q4 being the highest.

Results: In the case of NO_2, the adjusted hazard ratios (HRs) of dementia for all participants in Q2, Q3, and Q4 compared to Q1 were 1.10 (95% confidence interval (CI), 0.96–1.26), 1.01 (95% CI, 0.87–1.17), and 1.54 (95% CI, 1.34–1.77), and in the case of CO, the adjusted HRs were 1.07 (95% CI, 0.92–1.25), 1.37 (95% CI, 1.19–1.58), and 1.61 (95% CI, 1.39–1.85).

Conclusion: The results of this large retrospective, population-based study indicate that exposure to NO_2 and CO is associated with an increased risk of dementia in the Taiwanese population.

Editor: Gianluigi Forloni, "Mario Negri" Institute for Pharmacological Research, Italy

Funding: The study was supported in part by China Medical University (CMU102-BC-2), Taiwan Ministry of Health and Welfare Clinical Trial and Research Center of Excellence (MOHW103-TDU-B-212-113002), Taiwan Ministry of Health and Welfare Cancer Research Center for Excellence (MOHW103-TD-B-111-03), and International Research-Intensive Centers of Excellence in Taiwan (I-RiCE) (NSC101-2911-I-002-303). The funders had no role in study design, data collection and analysis, decision to publish, or preparation of the manuscript.

Competing Interests: The authors have declared that no competing interests exist.

* Email: d10040@mail.cmuh.org.tw

Introduction

Ambient air pollution includes solid and gaseous pollutants [1,2]. Most of the studies that have investigated the effects of pollutants on cognitive functions have examined the influence of solid pollutants [3–8]. However, exposure to ambient gaseous pollutants such as nitrogen dioxide (NO_2) is known to increase the risk of cerebrovascular and neurodegenerative diseases and ischemic stroke [9–12]. Cerebrovascular disease is the principal contributor to dementia [13,14], and Alzheimer's disease (AD) is the most common neurodegenerative disease. Moreover, a population-base study reported that dementia often developed after the occurrence of an ischemic stroke [15]. Several previous studies have suggested negative associations between NO_2 exposure and cognitive development in children, including preschool children [16–18], and animal studies have indicated that NO_2 exposure inhibits the recovery of nerve function after a stroke [19,20]. In addition, one animal study reported that nitration can induce beta-amyloid aggregation and plaque formation [21]; beta-amyloid aggregation is a pathologic hallmark of AD. However, a literature search indicated that only a few studies have been conducted to address the link between NO_2 exposure and cognitive function in adults. In a recent study conducted on 1496 middle-aged people living in Los Angeles, no statistically significant correlation was detected between the level of NO_2 exposure and cognitive functions [22]. Therefore, we conducted a retrospective cohort study to determine the association between NO_2 and dementia risk. Furthermore, in this study, we evaluated the influence of carbon monoxide (CO), because acute CO poisoning may cause headache, nausea, malaise, and fatigue [23], and chronic CO exposure has been linked to depression, confusion, memory loss, and cognitive decline [24,25]. Comparison between this study with other environmental study of Taiwan NHRID, the main difference is the residential area definition. In previous studies, the residential area is as the insurance area [26]. In present study, we defined the residential areas as the location of clinics which subjects sought treatment for acute upper respiratory infections.

Materials and Methods

Data sources and study population

In March 1995, the Taiwan National Health Insurance (NHI) program, which is a single-payer, compulsory social insurance system that has provided insurance coverage to almost every citizen in Taiwan, was established. The NHI covered approximately 99% of the 22.96 million citizens in Taiwan at the end of 2007 [27]. To protect patient privacy, the data on patient identities are encrypted in the National Health Insurance Research Database (NHIRD), and the database is accessible to researchers and the public in Taiwan. In this study, we used a subset of the NHIRD data containing comprehensive health-care data, including files on ambulatory care claims, inpatient claims, and prescriptions received by 1000000 people who were randomly selected from all insured beneficiaries. These data files can be linked through an encrypted but unique personal identification number and, thus, provide a longitudinal medical history of each patient. The health status of each person was identified according to the International Classification of Disease, Ninth Revision, Clinical Modification (ICD-9-CM).

Exposure assessment

Across Taiwan, 74 ambient air quality monitoring stations are located based on population density. Air quality data are maintained by Taiwan Environmental Protection Administration. [28]. A database containing daily NO_2 and CO concentrations measured at the monitoring stations was available for the period from January 1, 1998 to December 31, 2010. The people included in this study were assigned pollutant-exposure values based on the data obtained from the monitoring station present in the residential district in which the clinic where the people most frequently sought treatment for acute upper respiratory infection was located (ICD-9-CM Code 460). Yearly average concentrations of pollutants were calculated from the baseline to the date of dementia occurrence, the withdrawal of patients, or the end of the study period, and the data were categorized into quartiles.

Study patients

We identified 29547 people who were aged 50 years or older and for whom estimable air pollution data were available, but who did not present a history of head injury (ICD-9-CM Codes 800.804, 850.854.1, 310.2, and 959.01), stroke (ICD-9-CM Codes 430–438), or dementia (ICD-9-CM Codes 290.0–290.4, 294.1, and 331.0) before 2000.

Data Availability Statement

All data and related metadata are deposited in an appropriate public repository: The study population's data were from Taiwan NHIRD (http://w3.nhri.org.tw/nhird//date_01.html) are maintained by Taiwan National Health Research Institutes (http://nhird.nhri.org.tw/) [27]. The National Health Research Institutes (NHRI) is a non-profit foundation established by the government. Air quality data were from Taiwan Air Quality Monitoring Network (http://taqm.epa.gov.tw/taqm/en/PsiMap.aspx) in Taiwan Environmental Protection Administration (http://www.epa.gov.tw/) [28].

Ethics statement

Because identification numbers of patients had been encrypted, patient consent was not required for this study. This study was approved by the Research Ethic Committee at China Medical University (CMU-REC-101-012). The committee waived the requirement for consent.

Statistical analysis

We used x^2 tests to examine the distributions of sex, monthly income (New Taiwan Dollar<14 400, 14 400–18 300, 18 301–21 000, and >21 000), diabetes (DM, ICD-9-CM Code 250), ischemic heart disease (IHD, ICD-9-CM Codes 410–414), hypertension (HT, ICD-9-CM Codes 401–405),chronic obstructive pulmonary disease(COPD, ICD-9-CM Codes 490–496), alcoholism (ICD-9-CM Codes 303.305.0andV113),and the quartiles of NO_2 concentration (ppb; <6652.3, 6652.3–8349.0, 8349.1–9825.5,>9825.5) and CO concentration (ppm; <196.2, 196.2–241.6, 241.7–296.9, >296.9). A one-way analysis of variance (ANOVA) was performed to compare the age among the quartiles of NO_2 and CO concentrations. We calculated the incidence density rates of dementia in person-years in each quarter stratified according to sex. The incidence rate ratio (IRR) was estimated using a Poisson regression. Univariate and multivariate Cox proportional hazard regression analyses were performed to calculate the hazard ratios (HRs) and 95% confidence intervals (CIs) of the risk of dementia in association with pollutant levels. Multiple models were tested by controlling for age, sex, monthly income, DM, HT, IHD, COPD, alcoholism, and urbanization. Plots of the Kaplan-Meier analysis were used to determine the probability of people remaining without dementia, and the log-rank test was used to evaluate the differences among quartiles of pollutant concentrations. All analyses were performed using SAS 9.2 software (SAS Institute Inc., Cary, NC, USA), and the Kaplan-Meier survival curve was plotted using the Statistical Package for the Social Sciences (Version 15.1; SPSS Inc, Chicago, IL, USA). All tests were considered statistically significant when two-tailed P values were <.05.

Results

We obtained a total of 29547 and 29537 data on daily NO_2 and CO exposure, respectively. Dementia was not present at the baseline (2000), and 1720 people developed dementia after follow-up (yearly CO data were available for 1718 people). We categorized the NO_2 and CO levels into quartiles, with Q1 being the lowest level and Q4 being the highest. The people included in this study had a mean age of 61.4 years (SD 8.5 y). In both the NO_2 and CO groups, the highest level of the quartiles was associated with the people being slightly younger, more frequently earning a high monthly income, and living in a highly urbanized residential area, but less frequently exhibiting IHD and COPD compared with other quartiles (Tables 1 and 2). Table 3 shows the associations between the gaseous pollutant levels and the risk of dementia. Among the quartiles Q1, Q2, Q3, and Q4 of NO_2 in all patients, the IRRs in Q2, Q3, and Q4 compared with that in Q1 were 1.05, 0.90, and 1.35, and the adjusted HRs of dementia were 1.10 (95% CI, 0.96–1.26), 1.01 (95% CI, 0.87–1.17), and 1.54 (95% CI, 1.34–1.77), respectively. Among men, we determined that the IRRs in Q2, Q3, and Q4 compared with that in Q1 were 1.08, 0.79, and 1.28, and the adjusted HRs were 1.16 (95% CI, 0.95–1.43), 0.89 (95% CI, 0.71–1.11), and 1.52 (95% CI, 1.23–1.88), respectively. Among women, the IRRs in Q2, Q3, and Q4 compared with that in Q1 were 1.05, 1.11, and 1.56, and the adjusted HRs were 1.05 (95% CI, 0.87–1.27), 1.11 (95% CI, 0.92–1.35), and 1.56 (95% CI, 1.29–1.87), respectively. When the data on sex were stratified or merged for analysis, statistically significant correlations of IRRs and adjusted HRs were measured in Q4 compared with those in Q1.

Among the quartiles of CO concentration, the IRRs in Q2, Q3, and Q4 compared with that in Q1 were 0.96, 1.23, and 1.36, and the adjusted HRs were 1.07 (95% CI, 0.92–1.25), 1.37 (95% CI,1.19–1.58),and 1.61 (95% CI, 1.39–1.85), respectively, in all people included in the study. Among men, the IRRs in Q2, Q3, and Q4 compared with that in Q1 were 0.97, 1.18, and 1.28, and the adjusted HRs were 1.16 (95% CI, 0.93–1.45), 1.28 (95% CI, 1.04–1.58), and 1.57 (95% CI, 1.26–1.94), respectively. Among women, the IRRs in Q2, Q3, and Q4 compared with that in Q1 were 0.95, 1.28, and 1.43, and the adjusted HRs were 1.01 (95% CI, 0.82–1.24), 1.46 (95% CI, 1.21–1.77), and 1.64 (95% CI, 1.36–1.98), respectively. A clear trend that was detected was an increase in the risk of dementia as CO exposure increased. Figures 1 and 2 show the Kaplan-Meier curves of freedom that were calculated for dementia and are separated according to pollutant level. Statistically significant differences in the occurrence of dementia were observed among the quartiles of NO_2 and CO concentrations (log-rank test, $P<.001$).

Discussion

The major finding of previous animal study was that nitration was highly correlated with beta-amyloid aggregation and plaque formation, and beta-amyloid aggregation is a pathologic hallmark of AD [21]. Another animal study indicated that NO_2 expose can exacerbate the ultra structural impairment of synapses in stroke rats, and induce neuronal damage in healthy rats [29]. The apolipoprotein E (APOE) e4 allele was a well know genetic risk factor or AD, and a randomized clinical trial has found CO poisoning can induce APOE e4 carriers suffer greater morbidity [30].

The major finding of our study was that increased exposure to NO_2 (Q4) is associated with an enhanced risk of dementia in men and women. The probability of dementia occurrence was increased by 52%–56% in Q4 compared with Q1. A similar trend was observed in the CO group, and the results collectively showed that increasing levels of the 2 pollutants increased the risk of dementia in a dose-dependent manner.

This study was a national population-based investigation on ambient air pollution and dementia. Therefore, collecting individual exposure data was not feasible. To obtain exposure data associated with study patients, previous studies have identified the residential areas of patients by employing a GIS-based system. To protect the privacy of patients, the NHIRD does not provide patients' addresses. Therefore, we identified the residential areas of the patients based on the location of the clinic at which the patients most frequently sought treatment for acute upper respiratory tract infection. In the United States, upper respiratory tract infections are the most common type of infectious disease, and each adult experiences approximately 3 respiratory infections annually [31]. Identifying residential areas in the accessible medical resources, as we did in this study, is more accurate than listing patients according to insurance area [32,33].

Previous studies have suggested that smoking and drinking alcohol are highly correlated with the risk of AD [34–40]. Because of the limitations of the NHIRD, we could not obtain data on the smoking or drinking status of the patients. Therefore, we performed multivariate analysis with COPD and alcoholism adjusted in accordance with previous studies that indicated that smoking is a major causative factor in the development of COPD, and in which alcoholism was diagnosed based on drinking patterns and the attitudes of patients [41–43]. In Taiwan, women are not encouraged to smoke or drink alcohol, as reflected in the low prevalence of these behaviors among women (3% and 1%, respectively) [44,45]. We were able to overcome this limitation by stratifying and adjusting the data according to sex [46].

We adjusted for urbanization in the multivariate analysis. The level of urbanization was determined according to population density (number of people/km^2), the population ratio of people with a college-level education or higher, the population ratio of people aged over 65 years, the population ratio of agricultural workers, and the number of physicians per 100000 people [47]. The 359 communities in Taiwan were classified into 7groups: highly urbanized area, moderately urbanized area, boomtown, general town, aging town, agricultural town, and remote town. This classification method has been used in several studies [48–50].

In addition, we obtained results contrasting those related to dementia, as shown in Tables 1 and 2: the frequency of IHD and COPD were low at the highest level of the pollutants. These results agree with the explanation provided by previous studies suggesting that patients who are highly educated and earn a high monthly income live in areas where the level of air pollutants is high [6,22].

The strengths of this study are the following. First, this study was based on a long follow-up period, which allowed the possible occurrence of dementia to be assessed. Second, Taiwan launched a national health insurance (NHI) in 1995, operated by a single-buyer, the government. All insurance claims should be scrutinized by medical reimbursement specialists and peer review. The diagnoses of dementia were based on the ICD-9 code determined by qualified clinical neurology physicians under strict audit in the reimbursement process. Therefore the diagnoses and codes for dementia should be accurate and reliable. Third, this study was conducted using a large population derived from the NHIRD. In Taiwan, the government is the only compulsory social insurance provider; approximately 99% of the 23.74 million citizens of Taiwan are enrolled in the NHI program. Because this was a nationwide study, we considered urbanized towns throughout Taiwan. Lastly, in this study, cerebrovascular and cardiovascular diseases were considered and the association between pollutants and dementia was evaluated. We excluded subjects with cardiovascular before the index date in this study because cardiovascular was a widely known predictor for dementia. IHD increased 27% risk for dementia in both model 1 and model 2. (Table S1).

Certain limitations of this study should be considered. First, the evidence derived from a retrospective cohort study is generally lower in statistical quality than that obtained from randomized trials because, in such retrospective studies, potential biases exist that are related to the adjustment of confounding variables. Despite our meticulous study design and the measures adopted to control for confounding factors, bias resulting from unknown confounders may have affected our results. Second, all data in the

Table 1. Comparison of Baseline Characteristics among quartiles of NO_2 yearly average.

	Quartiles of NO_2 yearly average								p	Total (n = 29547)	
	Q1 (n = 7349)		Q2 (n = 7425)		Q3 (n = 7572)		Q4 (n = 7201)				
Dementia	406	5.5	425	5.7	374	4.9	515	7.2	<0.001	1720	5.8
Age (mean, SD)	61.8	8.4	61.4	8.5	61.0	8.4	61.4	8.8	<0.001†	61.4	8.5
Male	3365	45.8	3469	46.7	3474	45.9	3298	45.8	0.611	13606	46.0
Monthly income											
<14400	1481	20.2	1814	24.4	2004	26.5	1991	27.7	<0.001	7290	24.7
14400–18300	1054	14.3	1324	17.8	1511	20.0	1480	20.6		5369	18.2
18301–21000	3255	44.3	2399	32.3	1992	26.3	1785	24.8		9431	31.9
>21000	1559	21.2	1887	25.4	2062	27.2	1944	27.0		7452	25.2
DM	845	11.5	837	11.3	916	12.1	850	11.8	0.421	3448	11.7
IHD	1347	18.3	1354	18.2	1295	17.1	1222	17.0	0.047	5218	17.7
HT	2899	39.4	2906	39.1	2889	38.2	2785	38.7	0.391	11479	38.8
COPD	2612	35.5	2608	35.1	2579	34.1	2376	33.0	0.005	10175	34.4
Alcoholism	19	0.3	19	0.3	22	0.3	10	0.1	0.250	70	0.2
Urbanization											
Highly urbanization	1330	18.1	1668	22.5	2503	33.1	3720	51.7	<0.001	9221	31.2
Moderate urbanization	2157	29.4	2782	37.5	2908	38.4	1828	25.4		9675	32.7
Boomtown	907	12.3	986	13.3	1485	19.6	1126	15.6		4504	15.2
General town	1692	23.0	1160	15.6	412	5.4	298	4.1		3562	12.1
Aging town	304	4.1	56	0.8	68	0.9	72	1.0		500	1.7
Agricultural town	658	9.0	321	4.3	111	1.5	88	1.2		1178	4.0
Remote town	301	4.1	452	6.1	85	1.1	69	1.0		907	3.1

Chi-square test;
†T-test;

Table 2. Comparison of Baseline Characteristics among quartiles of CO yearly average.

	Quartiles of CO yearly average								p	Total (n = 29537)	
	Q1 (n = 7565)		Q2 (n = 6428)		Q3 (n = 7681)		Q4 (n = 7863)				
Dementia	391	5.2	321	5.0	476	6.2	530	6.7	<0.001	1718	5.8
Age (mean, SD)	61.8	8.3	61.1	8.3	61.4	8.6	61.3	8.8	<0.001†	61.4	8.5
Male	3532	46.7	2882	44.8	3587	46.7	3597	45.7	0.084	13598	46.0
Monthly income											
<14400	1477	19.5	1477	23.0	2190	28.5	2144	27.3	<0.001	7288	24.7
14400–18300	1074	14.2	1189	18.5	1513	19.7	1591	20.2		5367	18.2
18301–21000	3401	45.0	2095	32.6	1887	24.6	2046	26.0		9429	31.9
>21000	1613	21.3	1667	25.9	2088	27.2	2080	26.5		7448	25.2
DM	862	11.4	712	11.1	918	12.0	954	12.1	0.173	3446	11.7
IHD	1430	18.9	1054	16.4	1394	18.1	1339	17.0	<0.001	5217	17.7
HT	2980	39.4	2455	38.2	3021	39.3	3017	38.4	0.306	11473	38.8
COPD	2785	36.8	2189	34.1	2607	33.9	2587	32.9	<0.001	10168	34.4
Alcoholism	19	0.3	15	0.2	24	0.3	12	0.2	0.232	70	0.2
Urbanization											
Highly urbanization	912	12.1	1697	26.4	2694	35.1	3918	49.8	<0.001	9221	31.2
Moderate urbanization	2388	31.6	2615	40.7	2323	30.2	2346	29.8		9672	32.7
Boomtown	1084	14.3	819	12.7	1576	20.5	1024	13.0		4503	15.2
General town	1684	22.3	772	12.0	781	10.2	322	4.1		3559	12.0
Aging town	336	4.4	22	0.3	65	0.8	74	0.9		497	1.7
Agricultural town	699	9.2	253	3.9	120	1.6	106	1.3		1178	4.0
Remote town	462	6.1	250	3.9	122	1.6	73	0.9		907	3.1

Chi-square test;
†T-test;

Table 3. Comparisons of difference dementia incidences and associated hazard ratios among four levels of air pollutants by gender stratification.

			Dementia	PY	Incidence rate#	IRR*	95%CI	aHR†	95%CI
NO_2	Total	Q1	406	75461.4	5.38	1.00		1.00	
		Q2	425	75246.1	5.65	1.05	0.92, 1.20	1.10	0.96, 1.26
		Q3	374	77576.5	4.82	0.90	0.78, 1.03	1.01	0.87, 1.17
		Q4	515	71461.0	7.21	1.35	1.18, 1.54	1.54	1.34, 1.77
	Male	Q1	186	33853.8	5.49	1.00		1.00	
		Q2	206	34587.2	5.96	1.08	0.89, 1.32	1.16	0.95, 1.43
		Q3	152	34973.3	4.35	0.79	0.64, 0.98	0.89	0.71, 1.11
		Q4	224	31976.0	7.01	1.28	1.05, 1.56	1.52	1.23, 1.88
	Female	Q1	220	41607.6	5.29	1.00		1.00	
		Q2	219	40658.9	5.39	1.02	0.85, 1.23	1.05	0.87, 1.27
		Q3	222	42603.2	5.21	0.99	0.82, 1.19	1.11	0.92, 1.35
		Q4	291	39485.0	7.37	1.41	1.18, 1.67	1.56	1.29, 1.87
CO	Total	Q1	391	77816.4	5.02	1.00		1.00	
		Q2	321	66509.7	4.83	0.96	0.83, 1.11	1.07	0.92, 1.25
		Q3	476	77215.4	6.16	1.23	1.08, 1.41	1.37	1.19, 1.58
		Q4	530	78172.7	6.78	1.36	1.19, 1.55	1.61	1.39, 1.85
	Male	Q1	182	35681.8	5.10	1.00		1.00	
		Q2	145	29334.5	4.94	0.97	0.78, 1.20	1.16	0.93, 1.45
		Q3	212	35371.7	5.99	1.18	0.97, 1.44	1.28	1.04, 1.58
		Q4	227	34977.3	6.49	1.28	1.05, 1.55	1.57	1.26, 1.94
	Female	Q1	209	42134.6	4.96	1.00		1.00	
		Q2	176	37175.2	4.73	0.95	0.78, 1.16	1.01	0.82, 1.24
		Q3	264	41843.8	6.31	1.28	1.07, 1.54	1.46	1.21, 1.77
		Q4	303	43195.4	7.01	1.43	1.20, 1.70	1.64	1.36, 1.98

Incidence rate#, per 1,000 person-years;
IRR*, incidence rate ratio;
Adjusted HR† : multiple analysis including age, sex, monthly income, DM, IHD, HT, COPD, alcoholism and urbanization.

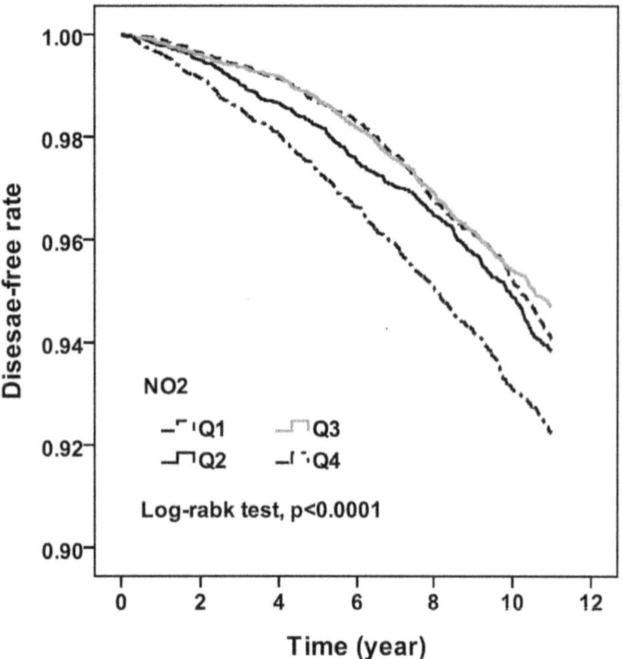

Figure 1. Probability free of dementia among quartiles of yearly average concentration in NO_2.

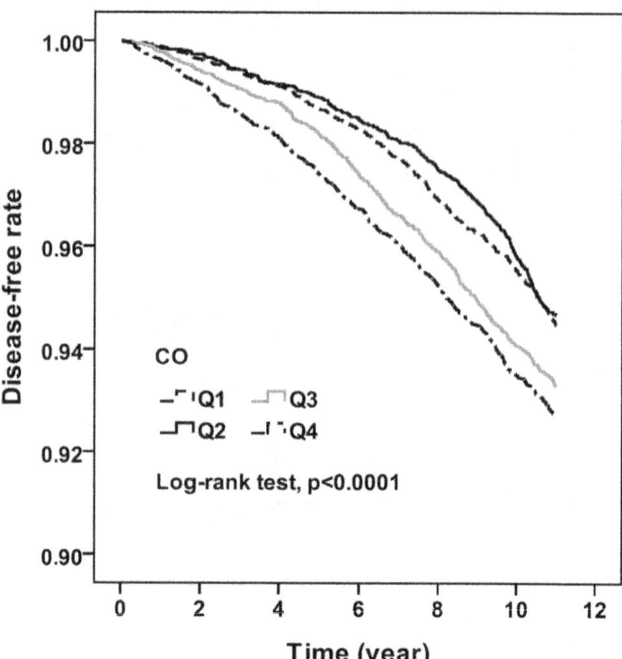

Figure 2. Probability free of dementia among quartiles of yearly average concentration in CO.

NHIRD are anonymous. Thus, relevant clinical variables, such as imaging results and pathology findings, were unavailable for the patient cases included in this study. Third, the participants were assigned to residential districts based on the clinic where they most frequently sought treatment for acute upper respiratory infection. Therefore, the resident who has no acute upper respiratory infection during study period had being excluded in this study. In our opinion, the resident without respiratory infection related medical record exposed to low level air pollutants. It might under the estimated risk of dementia. Nevertheless, the data on air pollutants and dementia diagnoses were reliable.

Conclusions

Understanding the regional distribution of human health statuses can facilitate the investigation of the spread of diseases and the related risk factors as well as the assessment of medical resources and the planning of the use of these resources. In future research, animal studies can be conducted to further examine the association between air pollutants and neurological disorders.

Author Contributions

Study concept and design: KHC CHK. Acquisition of data: KHC MYC CHM TNW CYC CHK. Analysis and interpretation of data: KHC CHM CHK. Drafting of the manuscript: KHC MYC CHM TNW CYC CHK. Critical revision of the manuscript for important intellectual content: KHC CHM CHK. Statistical analysis: CHM. Obtained funding: CHK. Administrative, technical, or material support: KHC MYC CHM TNW CYC CHK. Study supervision: CHK.

References

1. Dickey JH, Part VII (2000) Air pollution: overview of sources and health effects. Dis Mon 46:566–89.
2. Lewtas J (2007) Air pollution combustion emissions: characterization of causative agents and mechanisms associated with cancer, reproductive, and cardiovascular effects. Mutat Res 636:95–133.
3. Weuve J, Puett RC, Schwartz J, Yanosky JD, Laden F, et al. (2012) Exposure to particulate air pollution and cognitive decline in older women. Arch Intern Med 172:219–27.
4. Srám RJ, Benes I, Binková B, Dejmek J, Horstman D, et al. (1996) Teplice program–the impact of air pollution on human health. Environ Health Perspect 104 Suppl 4:699–714.
5. Suglia SF, Gryparis A, Wright RO, Schwartz J, Wright RJ (2008) Association of black carbon with cognition among children in a prospective birth cohort study. Am J Epidemiol 167:280–6.
6. Chen JC, Schwartz J (2009) Neurobehavioral effects of ambient air pollution on cognitive performance in US adults. Neurotoxicology 30:231–9.
7. Ranft U, Schikowski T, Sugiri D, Krutmann J, Krämer U (2009) Long-term exposure to traffic-related particulate matter impairs cognitive function in the elderly. Environ Res 109:1004–11.
8. Power MC, Weisskopf MG, Alexeeff SE, Coull BA, Spiro A 3rd, et al. (2011) Traffic-related air pollution and cognitive function in a cohort of older men. Environ Health Perspect 119:682–7.
9. Lisabeth LD, Escobar JD, Dvonch JT, Sánchez BN, Majersik JJ, et al. (2008) Ambient air pollution and risk for ischemic stroke and transient ischemic attack. Ann Neurol 2008;64:53–9.
10. Migliore L, Coppedè F (2009) Environmental-induced oxidative stress in neurodegenerative disorders and aging. Mutat Res 674:73–84.
11. Turin TC, Kita Y, Rumana N, Nakamura Y, Ueda K, et al (2012) Ambient air pollutants and acute case-fatality of cerebro-cardiovascular events: Takashima Stroke and AMI Registry, Japan (1988–2004). Cerebrovasc Dis 34(2):130–9.
12. Andersen ZJ, Kristiansen LC, Andersen KK, Olsen TS, Hvidberg M, et al. (2012) Stroke and long-term exposure to outdoor air pollution from nitrogen dioxide: a cohort study. Stroke 43:320–5.
13. Knopman DS (2007) Cerebrovascular disease and dementia. Br J Radiol 80 :S121–7.
14. O'Brien JT (2006) Vascular cognitive impairment. Am J Geriatr Psychiatry 14:724–33.

15. Kokmen E, Whisnant JP, O'Fallon WM, Chu CP, Beard CM (1996) Dementia after ischemic stroke: a population-based study in Rochester, Minnesota (1960–1984). Neurology 46:154–9.
16. Morales E, Julvez J, Torrent M, de Cid R, Guxens M, et al. (2009) Association of early-life exposure to household gas appliances and indoor nitrogen dioxide with cognition and attention behavior in preschoolers. Am J Epidemiol 169:1327–36.
17. Freire C, Ramos R, Puertas R, Lopez-Espinosa MJ, Julvez J, et al. (2010) Association of traffic-related air pollution with cognitive development in children. J Epidemiol Community Health 64:223–8.
18. Clark C, Crombie R, Head J, van Kamp I, van Kempen E, et al. (2012) Does traffic-related air pollution explain associations of aircraft and road traffic noise exposure on children's health and cognition? A secondary analysis of the United Kingdom sample from the RANCH project. Am J Epidemiol 176:327–37.
19. Zhu N, Li H, Han M, Guo L, Chen L, et al. (2012) Environmental nitrogen dioxide (NO2) exposure influences development and progression of ischemic stroke. Toxicol Lett 214:120–30.
20. Li H, Xin X (2013) Nitrogen dioxide (NO(2)) pollution as a potential risk factor for developing vascular dementia and its synaptic mechanisms. Chemosphere 92:52–8.
21. Kummer MP, Hermes M, Delekarte A, Hammerschmidt T, Kumar S, et al. (2011) Nitration of tyrosine 10 critically enhances amyloid β aggregation and plaque formation. Neuron 71:833–44.
22. Gatto NM, Henderson VW, Hodis HN, St John JA, Lurmann F, et al. (2013) Components of air pollution and cognitive function in middle-aged and older adults in Los Angeles. Neurotoxicology 40C:1–7.
23. Blanco F, Alkorta I, Solimannejad M, Elguero J (2009) Theoretical study of the 1:1 complexes between carbon monoxide and hypohalous acids. J Phys Chem A 113:3237–44.
24. Roberts GP, Youn H, Kerby RL (2004) CO-sensing mechanisms. Microbiol Mol Biol Rev 68:453–73, table of contents.
25. Chen HL, Chen PC, Lu CH, Hsu NW, Chou KH, et al. (2013) Structural and cognitive deficits in chronic carbon monoxide intoxication: a voxel-based morphometry study. BMC Neurol 13:129.
26. Jung CR, Lin YT, Hwang BF (2013) Air pollution and newly diagnostic autism spectrum disorders: a population-based cohort study in Taiwan. PLoS One 8:e75510.
27. National Health Insurance Research Database (NHIRD): Introduction to the National Health Insurance Research Database (NHIRD), Taiwan (2010) Available: http://w3.nhri.org.tw/nhird//date_01.html
28. Taiwan Air Quality Monitoring Network in Taiwan Environmental Protection Administration. Available: http://taqm.epa.gov.tw/taqm/en/PsiMap.aspx
29. Li H, Xin X (2013) Nitrogen dioxide (NO (2)) pollution as a potential risk factor for developing vascular dementia and its synaptic mechanisms. Chemosphere 92:52–8
30. Hopkins RO, Weaver LK, Valentine KJ, Mower C, Churchill S, et al. (2007) Apolipoprotein E genotype and response of carbon monoxide poisoning to hyperbaric oxygen treatment. Am J Respir Crit Care Med 176: 1001–6.
31. Garibaldi RA (1985) Epidemiology of community-acquired respiratory tract infections in adults. Incidence, etiology, and impact. Am J Med 78:32–7.
32. Kuo SS, Chang RE (2010) Geographical analysis of ESRD incidence and environment [Dissertation]. Taipei: Graduate Institute of Health Care Organization Administration, National Taiwan University. [In Chinese: English abstract]
33. Ministry of the Interior, R.O.C. (Taiwan). Monthly bulletin of interior statistics. Available at: http://sowf.moi.gov.tw/stat/month/list.htm. Accessed 2011 March 3. [In Chinese: English abstract]
34. Cataldo JK, Prochaska JJ, Glantz SA (2010) Cigarette smoking is a risk factor for Alzheimer's Disease: an analysis controlling for tobacco industry affiliation. J Alzheimers Dis 19:465–80.
35. Deng J, Shen C, Wang YJ, Zhang M, Li J, et al. (2010) Nicotine exacerbates tau phosphorylation and cognitive impairment induced by amyloid-beta 25–35 in rats. Eur J Pharmacol 637:83–8.
36. Oddo S, Caccamo A, Green KN, Liang K, Tran L, et al. (2005) Chronic nicotine administration exacerbates tau pathology in a transgenic model of Alzheimer's disease. Proc Natl Acad Sci U S A 102:3046–51.
37. Juan D, Zhou DH, Li J, Wang JY, Gao C, et al. (2004) A 2-year follow-up study of cigarette smoking and risk of dementia. Eur J Neurol 11:277–82.
38. Peters R, Peters J, Warner J, Beckett N, Bulpitt C (2008) Alcohol, dementia and cognitive decline in the elderly: a systematic review. Age Ageing 37:505–12.
39. Deng J, Zhou DH, Li J, Wang YJ, Gao C, et al. (2006) A 2-year follow-up study of alcohol consumption and risk of dementia. Clin Neurol Neurosurg 108:378–83.
40. Anstey KJ, Mack HA, Cherbuin N (2009) Alcohol consumption as a risk factor for dementia and cognitive decline: meta-analysis of prospective studies. Am J Geriatr Psychiatry 17:542–55.
41. Pauwels RA, Rabe KF (2004) Burden and clinical features of chronic obstructive pulmonary disease (COPD). Lancet 364:613–20.
42. Patel BD, Loo WJ, Tasker AD, Screaton NJ, Burrows NP, et al. (2006) Smoking related COPD and facial wrinkling: is there a common susceptibility? Thorax 61:568–571.
43. Enoch MA, Goldman D (2002) Problem drinking and alcoholism: diagnosis and treatment. Am Fam Physician 65:441–8.
44. Liang CY, Chou TM, Ho PS, Shieh TY, Yang YH (2004) Prevalence Rates of Alcohol Drinking in Taiwan. Taiwan Journal of Oral Medicine & Health Sciences 20:91–104
45. Chuang YC, Chuang KY (2008) Gender differences in relationships between social capital and individual smoking and drinking behavior in Taiwan. Soc Sci Med 67:1321–30.
46. Chang KH, Chung CJ, Lin CL, Sung FC, Wu TN, et al. (2014) Increased risk of dementia in patients with osteoporosis: a population-based retrospective cohort analysis. Age (Dordr) 36:967–75.
47. Liu C, Hung Y, Chuang Y, Chen Y, Weng W, et al. (2006) Incorporating development stratification of Taiwan townships into sampling design of large scale health interview survey. Journal of Health Management 4:1–22 [in Chinese].
48. Chiang PH, Chang YC, Lin JD, Tung HJ, Lin LP, et al. (2013) Healthcare utilization and expenditure analysis between individuals with intellectual disabilities and the general population in Taiwan: a population-based nationwide child and adolescent study. Res Dev Disabil 34:2485–92.
49. Lin YJ, Tian WH, Chen CC (2011) Urbanization and the utilization of outpatient services under National Health Insurance in Taiwan. Health Policy 103:236–43.
50. Lin HC, Lin YJ, Liu TC, Chen CS, Lin CC (2007) Urbanization and place of death for the elderly: a 10-year population-based study. Palliat Med 21:705–11.

Avian Influenza A H7N9 Virus Induces Severe Pneumonia in Mice without Prior Adaptation and Responds to a Combination of Zanamivir and COX-2 Inhibitor

Can Li[1]ⓢ, Chuangen Li[1]ⓢ, Anna J. X. Zhang[1,2,3]*, Kelvin K. W. To[1,2,3], Andrew C. Y. Lee[1], Houshun Zhu[4], Hazel W. L. Wu[1,2], Jasper F. W. Chan[1,2,3], Honglin Chen[1,2,3,6,7], Ivan F. N. Hung[3,4], Lanjuan Li[5,6,7], Kwok-Yung Yuen[1,2,3,6,7]*

1 Department of Microbiology, The University of Hong Kong, Hong Kong, China, **2** State Key Laboratory of Emerging Infectious Diseases, The University of Hong Kong, Hong Kong, China, **3** Research Centre of Infection and Immunology, The University of Hong Kong, Hong Kong, China, **4** Department of Medicine, The University of Hong Kong, Hong Kong, China, **5** State Key Laboratory for Diagnosis and Treatment of Infectious Diseases, the First Affiliated Hospital, College of Medicine, Zhejiang University, Hangzhou, China, **6** Collaborative Innovation Center for Diagnosis and Treatment of Infectious Diseases, Hangzhou, China, **7** Zhejiang University, Hangzhou, China

Abstract

Background: Human infection caused by the avian influenza A H7N9 virus has a case-fatality rate of over 30%. Systematic study of the pathogenesis of avian H7N9 isolate and effective therapeutic strategies are needed.

Methods: BALB/c mice were inoculated intranasally with an H7N9 virus isolated from a chicken in a wet market epidemiologically linked to a fatal human case, (A/chicken/Zhejiang/DTID-ZJU01/2013 [CK1]), and with an H7N9 virus isolated from a human (A/Anhui/01/2013 [AH1]). The pulmonary viral loads, cytokine/chemokine profiles and histopathological changes of the infected mice were compared. The therapeutic efficacy of a non-steroidal anti-inflammatory drug (NSAID), celecoxib, was assessed.

Results: Without prior adaptation, intranasal inoculation of 10^6 plaque forming units (PFUs) of CK1 caused a mortality rate of 82% (14/17) in mice. Viral nucleoprotein and RNA expression were limited to the respiratory system and no viral RNA could be detected from brain, liver and kidney tissues. CK1 caused heavy alveolar inflammatory exudation and pulmonary hemorrhage, associated with high pulmonary levels of proinflammatory cytokines. In the mouse lung cell line LA-4, CK1 also induced high levels of interleukin-6 (IL-6) and cyclooxygenase-2 (COX-2) mRNA. Administration of the antiviral zanamivir did not significantly improve survival in mice infected with CK1, but co-administration of the non-steroidal anti-inflammatory drug (NSAID) celecoxib in combination with zanamivir improved survival and lung pathology.

Conclusions: Our findings suggested that H7N9 viruses isolated from chicken without preceding trans-species adaptation can cause lethal mammalian pulmonary infection. The severe proinflammatory responses might be a factor contributing to the mortality. Treatment with combination of antiviral and NSAID could ameliorate pulmonary inflammation and may improve survival.

Editor: Kevan L. Hartshorn, Boston University School of Medicine, United States of America

Funding: This work was supported by the Providence Foundation Ltd, in memory of the late Lui Hac Minh, and a donation from Larry Chi-Kin Yung. The funders had no role in study design, data collection and analysis, decision to publish, or preparation of the manuscript.

Competing Interests: The authors have declared that no competing interests exist.

* Email: kyyuen@hkucc.hku.hk (K-YY); zhangajx@hku.hk (AJXZ)

ⓢ These authors contributed equally to this work.

Background

Avian influenza A H7N9 virus infecting human first emerged in China in February 2013 [1–3]. It is associated with a crude case-fatality rate of over 30% in humans despite of oseltamivir treatment [4]. Severe human infections were characterized by rapidly progressive acute community-acquired pneumonia, multi-organ dysfunction and cytokine dysregulation, which did not respond to treatment with antibiotics against typical and atypical pneumonic pathogens [5]. Similar to the influenza A H5N1 and other avian influenza viruses, most patients with H7N9 infection had a history of direct or occupational contact with poultry or visits to wet market [1,6–8]. Phylogenetic analysis showed that this H7N9 virus is a novel triple reassortant virus comprising of hemagglutinin (HA) gene from H7N3, neuraminidase (NA) gene from H7N9 and internal genes from H9N2 [9,10]. Some of the human isolates already harboured genetic mutations of the polymerase PB2 gene which favour mammalian adaptation, and mutations of the hemagglutinin (HA) gene which increase its binding affinity for human type α-2,6 sialic acid linked receptors [3]. Novel reassortants have emerged in Southern China, which contained additional potential virulence markers [11].

Since most patients had poultry contact and the internal gene segments are closely related to H9N2 isolated from domestic poultries, it has been postulated that H7N9 virus from wild birds first entered the domestic poultry population, reassorted with other avian influenza viruses, acquired the characteristics for adaptation to humans and finally infected humans [3,12,13]. One major question is whether H7N9 virus isolated from poultry can directly infect humans. Mice and ferrets have been used as surrogates to study the pathogenicity of the 2013 H7N9 viruses in mammals. Several studies have shown that the human H7N9 virus A/Anhui/1/2013 (AH1), which was isolated from a fatal human case [2], could cause death in mice without prior adaptation [14–18], while another human H7N9 virus A/Shanghai/2/2013 did not lead to death in mice [19]. On the other hand, H7N9 viruses isolated from poultries or wild birds appeared to be less virulent in mouse models. H7N9 viruses isolated from one chicken and two pigeons of China in 2013 did not cause any signs of disease [18]. H7N9 viruses isolated from a duck of Japan in 2011 and from a shoveler of Egypt in 2007 caused fatal disease in mice, but the 50% mouse lethal doses (MLD_{50}) were much higher than that of the human H7N9 isolates [14,17].

In our previous study, we have isolated an H7N9 virus from a chicken (A/chicken/Zhejiang/DTID-ZJU01/2013 [CK1]) in a wet market epidemiologically linked to a patient with fatal H7N9 infection [1]. Since the patient likely acquired the H7N9 virus from the market, we postulate that CK1 may cause severe disease in mammals without further adaptation. In this study, we assessed the viral tropism and replication, histopathological changes and the host cytokine/chemokine response in CK1-infected mice. The human virus AH1 was used for comparison. Furthermore, we studied the treatment effect of a combination of neuraminidase inhibitor zanamivir and non-steroidal anti-inflammatory drug (NSAID) celecoxib in a BALB/c mouse model because combination treatment of zanamivir and celecoxib improved the survival of mice infected with H5N1 virus whereas zanamivir alone was significantly less effective [20].

Results

Chicken H7N9 virus CK1 caused severe lung inflammation and fatal outcome in mice without prior adaptation

CK1 and AH1 were propagated in chicken embryos, and the viral titres in the allantoic fluid were determined in Madin Darby canine kidney (MDCK) cells. The viral titres were $10^{8.2}$ tissue culture infective doses ($TCID_{50}$) per ml and $10^{7.66}$ plaque forming units (PFU) per ml for CK1, and $10^{8.8}$ $TCID_{50}$ per ml and $10^{8.4}$ PFU per ml for AH1. Next, we determined the MLD_{50} of CK1 in BALB/c mice, and compared to that of AH1. CK1 caused lethal infection with a mortality rate of 83% (5/6) at inoculation dose of 10^6 PFU which was the highest dose that could be tested in this study, but no mice died when infected with 10^5, 10^4 or 10^3 PFU. The MLD_{50} dose of CK1 could only be assumed to be between 10^5-10^6 PFU, while the MLD_{50} dose for AH1 was determined to be $10^{4.8}$ PFU. This indicated that CK1 is less virulent in mice than AH1. Since 10^6 PFU of CK1 and 10^5 PFU of human AH1 caused similar rate of mortality in mice, we used these doses in the subsequent experiments for the study of pathogenesis.

As shown in Fig. 1, significant morbidity and mortality were observed in CK1-infected mice during the 14-day study period. Two to three days after infection, the mice started to show disease symptoms of ruffled fur before developing laboured breathing and loss of body weight (Fig. 1a). The mortality rates were 82% (14/17) for CK1 and 90% (18/20) for AH1 (Fig. 1b).

Histopathological findings of lung tissues from infected mice were examined, scored, and compared with those of non-infected mice (Fig. 2). At day 2 post-infection (p.i.), CK1-infected mouse lungs showed a typical and severe viral pneumonia with focal perivascular and peribronchiolar interstitial lymphocytes, monocyte/macrophages infiltration and vascular congestion. One notable feature was the widely distributed bronchial and bronchiolar epithelial cells necrosis (Fig. 2c and 2d). At day 4 p.i., the inflammatory and necrotic changes affected larger areas of the lung including walls of alveoli (Fig. 2e and 2f). These changes became more severe at day 6 p.i., and were accompanied by alveolar hemorrhage (Fig. 2g and 2h). Pulmonary vascular endothelial damage, vascular thrombosis and perivascular edema could be seen in some of the infected lungs (data not shown). The type of pulmonary pathological changes in CK1 was similar to AH1-infected mouse lungs. There was no significant difference in the semi-quantitative histological scores between CK1 and AH1 infection (Table 1).

CK1 infected multiple cell types in the mouse respiratory tract

To determine the tissue tropism of CK1, immunostaining was performed using antibody targeting the influenza nucleoprotein (NP). AH1-infected mice were used as the control. Immunostaining of lung tissues from uninfected mice with mouse anti-NP antibody showed that there was no non-specific staining (Fig. 3A, a and b). CK1 and AH1 infected various cell types in the mouse respiratory tract from trachea to the alveoli (Fig. 3A, c to h). NP-positive stainings were seen in the epithelial cells of the trachea (Fig. 3A, e and f), bronchioles and alveolar pneumocytes (Fig. 3A, g and h). Morphologically, NP-positive cells in alveoli were mainly type II pneumocytes. No differences in the distribution and cell types of NP-positive cells were observed between CK1- and AH1-infected lungs. However, even at 10-times higher inoculation dose, CK1-infected mice had a persistently lower pulmonary viral load from day 2 p.i. to day 6 p.i when compared to those infected by AH1 using both quantitative reverse transcriptase-polymerase chain reaction (RT-PCR) and $TCID_{50}$ assay ($P<0.01$ or <0.05, Fig. 3B). This may suggest that CK1 did not replicate as efficiently as AH1 in mouse lungs.

To determine whether chicken H7N9 virus could disseminate outside the respiratory system, viral RNA detection was performed by quantitative RT-PCR in brain, liver and kidney tissues. No viral genome RNA was detectable in these tissues, suggesting the absence of extrapulmonary viral replication. But on day 6 p.i., degenerative changes in liver, heart and kidney including hepatocytes degeneration and focal cells necrosis (Fig. 4b and 4c), kidney tubular epithelial cells degeneration and peri-tubular vessels congestion (Fig. 4e and 4f), and myocardial cell swelling with red blood cells infiltrating between myocardial fibers, were observed (Fig. 4h and 4i).

CK1 induced high level of pulmonary proinflammatory cytokines and chemokines

To study the cytokine/chemokine response after CK1 infection, the pulmonary protein levels of proinflammatory cytokine interleukin-1β (IL-1β) and IL-6, anti-inflammatory cytokine interleukin-10 (IL-10), and the chemokine "regulated on activation normal T cell expressed and presumably secreted" (RANTES)

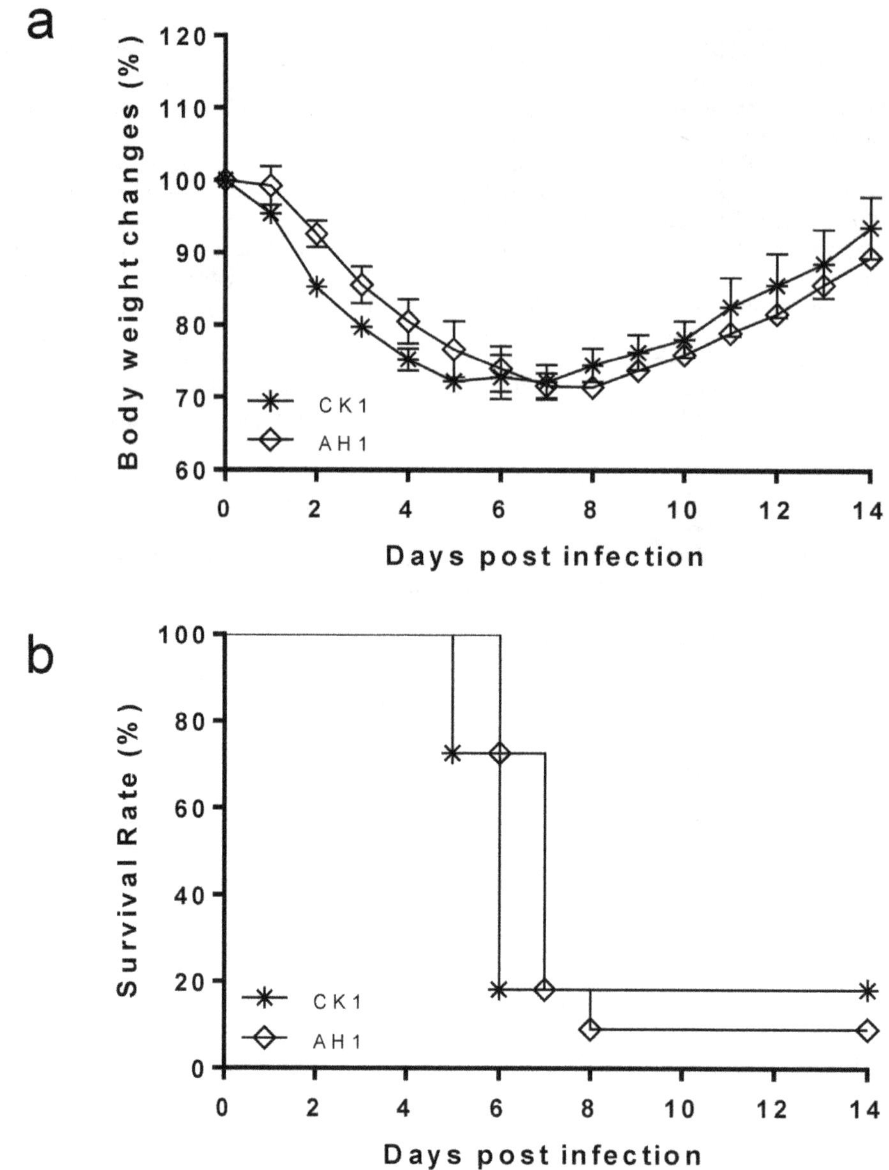

Figure 1. Body weight changes (a) and survival rate (b) of the BALB/c mice infected with 10^6 PFU of A/chicken/Zhejiang/DTID-ZJU01/2013(H7N9) (CK1, ✳) or 10^5 PFU of A/Anhui/1/2013(H7N9) (AH1, ◇) via intranasal route. Body weight and survival were monitored for 14 days after virus infection. Data shown are the average of three experiments (n = 17 for CK1 and n = 20 for AH1 group).

Table 1. Average histological score of CK1- and AH1-infected mouse lung tissues*.

Histological changes	CK1			AH1		
	Day 2 p.i. (n = 3)	Day 4 p.i. (n = 3)	Day 6 p.i. (n = 3)	Day 2 p.i. (n = 3)	Day 4 p.i. (n = 3)	Day 6 p.i. (n = 3)
Necrosis	2.6	3.3	2.6	2.3	3.3	3.6
Infiltration	2.6	3.8	4.0	3.0	3.1	4.0
Hemorrhage	1.0	2.3	2.6	1.0	1.6	2.0

p.i.: post-infection.
*Details of the histological scores are presented in Table 2.

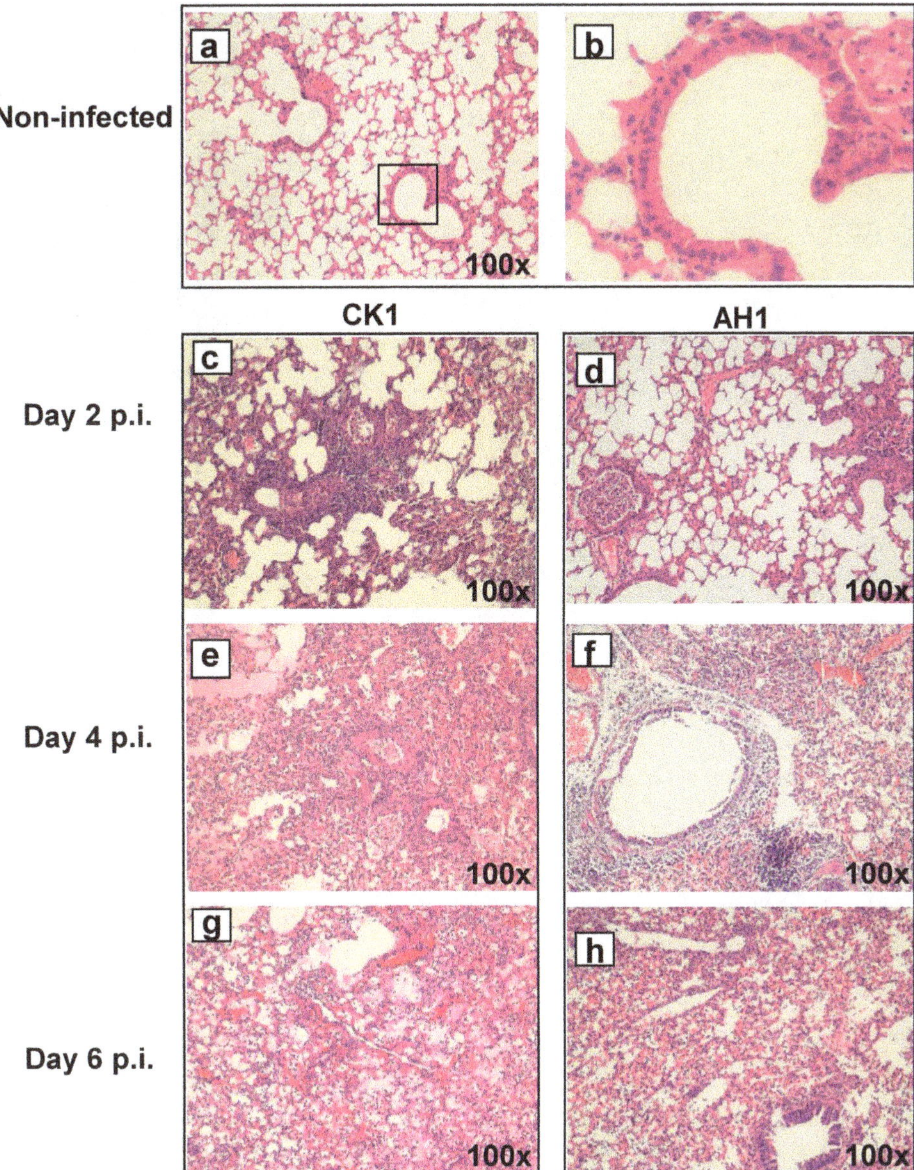

Figure 2. Histopathological changes in the lung tissue infected with CK1 or AH1. Representative histological images of haematoxylin and eosin (H&E) stained lung tissue sections of normal mouse lung (a, and amplified image b) and infected mouse lung at various time points post infection (c-h). Mouse lung at day 2 p.i. showed peribronchiolar interstitial infiltration, bronchiole epithelial cell necrosis and necrotic cell debris within alveolar lumens (c, CK1 infection; d, AH1 infection). At day 4 p.i, mouse lung showed alveolar space exudation, bronchiole epithelial cell necrosis, alveolar cell necrosis and destruction of alveolar wall (e and f). At day 6 p.i., alveolar exudation, infiltration, hyaline membrane formation and alveolar hemorrhage with red blood cells within the alveolar space (*g* and *h*). Original magnification ×100.

were determined by enzyme immunoassay. CK1 induced high pulmonary levels of proinflammatory cytokine IL-1β, IL-6 and chemokine RANTES at all studied time points after infection (Fig. 5A). Compared to AH1, CK1 induced significantly higher IL-1β and IL-6 on day 4 p.i ($P<0.05$). The anti-inflammatory cytokine IL-10 only increased on day 6 p.i in both AH1 and CK1 infection, but at a significantly lower level in CK1-infected mice ($P<0.05$).

Since the detection of interferon production is not sensitive enough by enzyme immunoassay, we determined the mRNA levels of interferon-α (IFN-α), interferon-β (IFN-β) and interferon-γ (IFN-γ) in mouse lung homogenates using quantitative RT-PCR [21]. On day 2 p.i, more than 50-fold increase of IFN-β mRNA levels were observed in CK1-infected mice, which was significantly higher than that of AH1-infected mice ($p<0.05$). There was no significant difference in the IFN-α and IFN-γ mRNA levels between CK1 and AH1 (Fig. 5B).

We have previously reported that upregulation of cyclooxygenase 2 (COX-2) gene played an important role in the pathogenesis of avian H5N1 virus infection [20]. Therefore, we tested the COX-2 gene expression in mouse lungs after H7N9 infection. There was a surge of the level of COX-2 mRNA on day 1 p.i. with about 20-fold increase in CK1-infected lung tissues (Fig. 5B). However, the difference in COX-2 mRNA levels between CK1 and AH1-infected samples did not reach statistical significance.

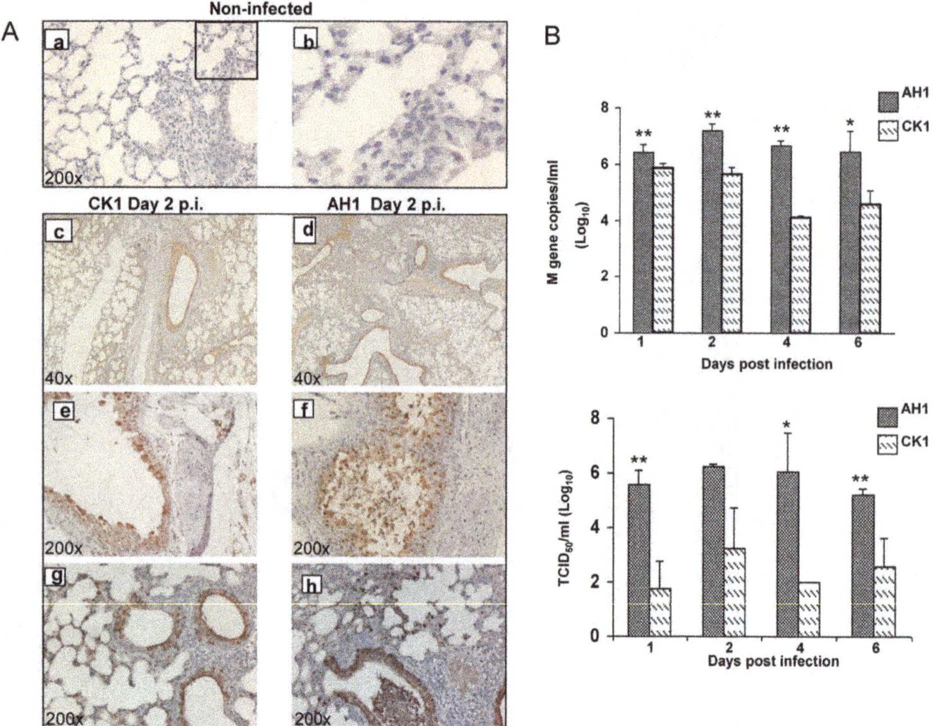

Figure 3. CK1 and AH1 replication profile in mouse lung. A. Representative images of immunohistochemically stained influenza nucleoprotein (NP) in formalin fixed mouse lung tissue infected with CK1 or AH1 at day 2 p.i. Viral NP protein was labeled brown by 3,3′-diaminobenzidine (DAB). Uninfected mouse lung as negative control *(a)*, amplified image (b); Representative images of CK1(c) and AH1 (d) infected mouse lung stained NP positive at 40x magnification. Trachea epithelial cells (e and f), bronchiole epithelial and alveolar epithelial cells (g and h) were stained positive for viral NP protein. (Original magnification ×200). B. Viral load in infected mouse lung homogenates. Mice were infected with 10^5 of AH1 or 10^6 PFU of CK1, at day 1, 2, 4 and 6 p.i., 3–5 mice from each group were sacrificed. The left side of the lung was homogenized in 1 ml of MEM culture medium. Viral loads were determined by amplification of viral M gene copy numbers by real time RT-PCR (top panel), and infectious viral titre were determined by $TCID_{50}$ assay on MDCK cells (bottom panel). $^{**}P<0.01$; $^{*}P<0.05$.

The above findings suggest that although CK1 did not replicate as efficiently as AH1 in mouse lung, CK1 induced higher levels of proinflammatory response in infected mice than that of AH1. To test this finding, we performed an *in vitro* study using mouse lung epithelial cell line LA-4. After virus inoculation, CK1 and AH1 replicated to a comparable level in LA-4 cells (Fig. 5C, top panel), but CK1 induced significantly higher expression mRNA levels of IL-6 and COX-2 at 6 and 9 hours p.i. than AH1 ($P<0.05$).

Combination of celecoxib and zanamivir could ameliorate lung inflammation and improve survival

Most H7N9 isolates are susceptible to neuraminidase inhibitors in enzymatic assay [14,15], but the efficacy is poor in patients with delayed treatment. Mouse experiments demonstrated that neuraminidase inhibitor was only effective when administered within 24 hours after virus infection [14,15]. We investigated whether COX-2 inhibitor celecoxib with or without neuraminidase inhibitor, zanamivir, could lower the overwhelming inflammatory responses and improve survival in mice infected with CK1 as in the case of H5N1 infection. When administered at 48 hours p.i., treatment with celecoxib-zanamivir combination had the highest survival rate, with 70% (7/10) survival and a mean survival time (MST) of 12.6 days, while the untreated control mice only had 18% (3/17) survival ($p = 0.0059$) (Fig. 6a). The survival rate of the celecoxib-zanamivir combination group was significantly higher than that of zanamivir alone ($p = 0.0013$) or celecoxib alone ($p = 0.0037$). All the mice in the zanamivir alone group and celecoxib alone group succumbed to the infection. At day 4 p.i., all three treatment groups (zanamivir and celecoxib combination, zanamivir alone or celecoxib alone group) showed a trend of reduction in the pulmonary levels of proinflammatory cytokine IL-6, IL-1β and RANTES although this reduction was not statistically significant (Fig. 7a). There was no difference in the pulmonary viral load among all groups at day 4 p.i. (Fig. 7b). Compared with the diffuse alveolar infiltration and exudation in untreated mice (Fig. 7c), mice in the celecoxib-zanamivir combination group showed mainly mild bronchiolitis with peribronchiolar lymphocytic infiltration, adjacent mild alveolitis and vascular congestion. Pathological changes were also ameliorated with zanamivir and/or celecoxib treatment (Fig. 7d).

Discussion

The 2013 H7N9 viruses isolated from poultry and human in China are closely related phylogenetically [1,22], but H7N9 virus isolated from poultries often lacks important genetic signature for mammalian adaptation. For example, CK1 did not possess either the PB2 627K or 701N mutation, which is found in most H7N9 isolates from human [1,3]. In this study, we assessed the virulence of CK1 using a well-established influenza mouse model [20,23–25]. We have shown that CK1 could cause lethal infection in mice, and the MLD_{50} was <2 log higher than that of the human H7N9 virus AH1. Mice infected with 10^6 PFU of CK1 exhibited similar mortality rate, body weight loss, and pulmonary damage as those infected with 10^5 PFU of AH1. Our data suggests that CK1 may

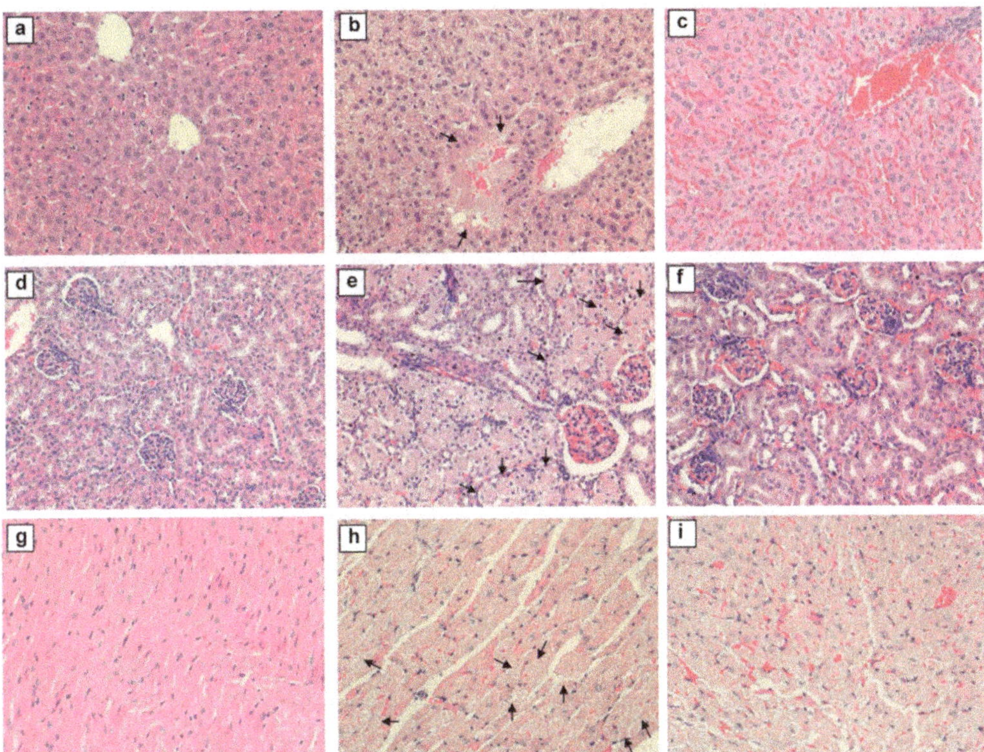

Figure 4. Liver, kidney and heart tissue degenerative changes in CK1-infected mice at day 6 post infection. Representative images of haematoxylin and eosin (H&E) stained tissue sections are presented. The liver (a), kidney (d), heart (g) of uninfected mice were shown for comparison. CK1-infected mice at day 6 p.i. showed liver hepatocytes degeneration, focal cells necrosis (arrows, b) and hemorrhagic changes (c); kidney tubular epithelial cells degenerative changes (arrows, e) and peritubular vessels congestion (f). Mild myocardial cell swelling (arrows, h) and red blood cells infiltrating between degenerative myocardial fibers (i) were seen in the heart. Original magnification ×200.

also be virulent in humans without further adaptations. CK1 may be more virulent in mice than other poultry H7N9 virus isolates tested in other studies. Zhang *et al* compared the virulence of three poultry isolates of 2013 H7N9 virus (A/chicken/Shanghai/S1053/2013, A/pigeon/Shanghai/S1069/2013 and A/pigeon/Shanghai/S1421/2013) with AH1 [18]. Mice inoculated with ≥ 10^4 50% egg infectious dose of AH1 had significant weight loss; while mice inoculated with the chicken or pigeon H7N9 isolates did not have any weight loss. Similarly, Belser *et al* inoculated mice with A/shoveler/Egypt/00215-NAMRU3/07 at a dose >100 times higher than the MLD_{50} for AH1, but no mice died [17]. Watanabe *et al* found that the MLD_{50} was about 3 logs higher for A/duck/Gunma/466/2011 (H7N9) than that of AH1 [14]. When compared to three poultry isolates with low virulence in mice, there are several unique substitutions found in CK1 in the haemagglutinin, neuraminidase and NS1 protein (table S1). For instance, CK1 HA gene contains avian type 217Q (226 in H3 numbering) rather than the 217L that is found among the majority of H7N9 human and avian isolates. This may favour the infection in mouse respiratory tract which predominantly expresses α-2,3 linked sialic acids receptors. Future studies comparing CK1 with the other poultry H7N9 viruses with low virulence in mice may help us to understand specific mutations that contribute to high virulence in mammals.

Immunohistochemical staining with anti-NP antibody showed that, similar to AH1, CK1 infected the middle and lower respiratory tract. A similar phenomenon was seen in H5N1 viruses originating from Hong Kong, in which both avian and human viruses led to similar extent of infection in the respiratory tract of mice [26]. On the other hand, the pulmonary viral loads were higher in the AH1 group than the CK1 group even inoculation dose of CK1 was 10-time higher than AH1, suggesting that AH1 replicates better in the mammalian respiratory tract than CK1. One possibility is that CK1 can induce a higher level of IFN-β than AH1, which may suppress the viral replication better. Another possibility is that CK1 lacks the PB2 E627K substitution which is associated with more efficient replication at a lower body temperature, a characteristic of mammalian adaptation when compared with the situation in avian species [1,27,28]. This finding is also similar to that of H5N1 virus, in which strains with PB2 627K can replicate to a higher titre in mice lungs than strains with PB2 627E [29,30].

Cytokine dysregulation is a feature of severe influenza in humans and animal models. Patients with severe H5N1 and 2009 pandemic H1N1 had very high levels of IL-6 [31,32]. Our previous study comparing the wild type 2009 pandemic H1N1 and its more virulent mutant with D225G substitution in the haemagglutinin showed that the levels of IL-6 and IL-1β were higher in mice infected with mutant virus than those with wild type virus [24]. CK1 had a significantly lower level of pulmonary viral load when compared to AH1-infected mice, but CK1 induced a more pronounced proinflammatory cytokine/chemokine response. One exception is that CK1 had a lower IL-10 level than that of AH1 on day 6 p.i. In another study comparing different 2009 pandemic H1N1 isolates in mice, more virulent viral isolates induced higher levels of IL-6, but lower levels of IL-10 [33]. As the viral load was lower in the CK1 group, the difference in cytokine/chemokine cannot be explained by the difference in the initial viral

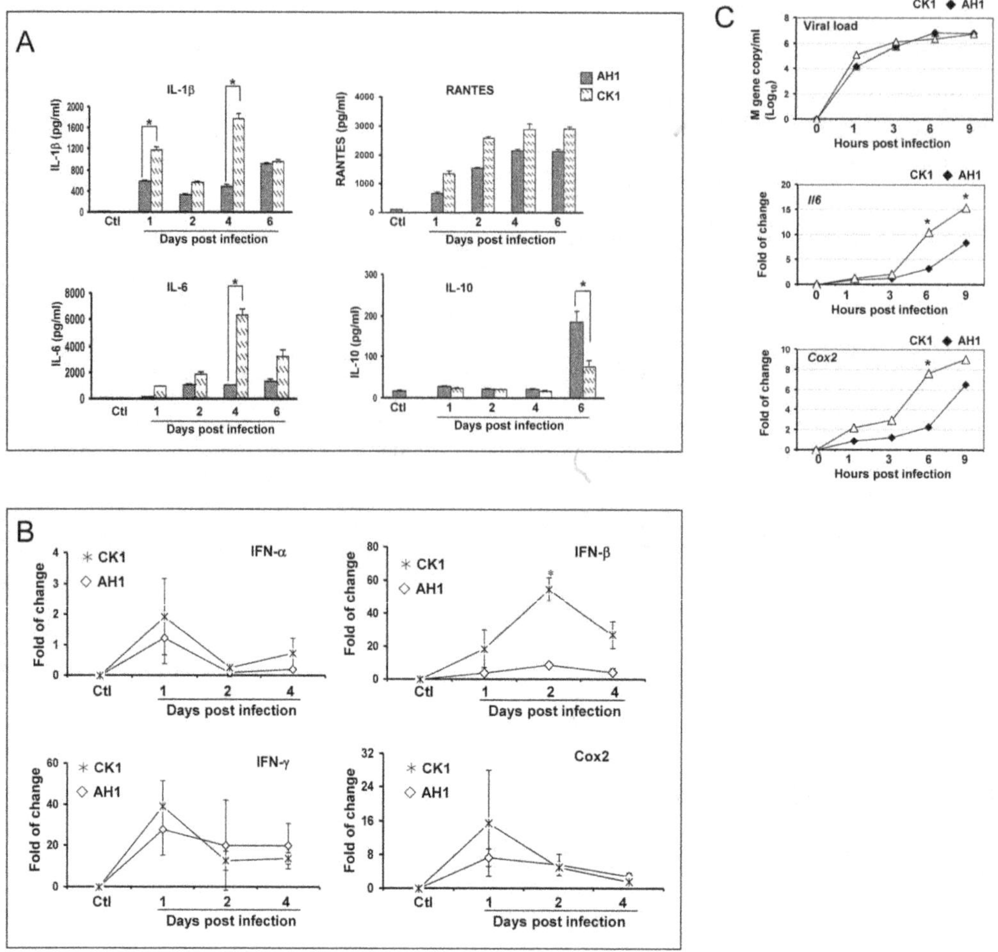

Figure 5. Cytokines and COX-2 expression in infected mice lung and mouse lung epithelial cell line LA-4. (A) The protein levels of cytokines IL-1β, IL-6, RANTES and IL-10 presented in mouse lung homogenates were determined by ELISA. On day 1, 2, 4 and 6 p.i., the left lungs from infected mice (3–5 mice from each group) were homogenized in 1 ml of MEM medium. Clarified homogenates were used for cytokine detection. Non-infected mouse lung specimens were used as baseline controls. (B) mRNA level of IFN-α, IFN-β, IFN-γ and COX-2 genes in mouse lung were determined by real time RT-PCR. Mouse β-actin mRNA was used for RNA concentration normalization. Error bar indicates ±SD. * $P<0.05$. C. viral load, IL-6 and COX-2 mRNA levels in CK1- and AH1-infected mouse lung epithelial cell line LA-4 determined by real time RT-PCR. 2×10^5 cells/per well in 12-well plate were infected with AH1 or CK1 at M.O.I of 2. At indicated times post virus infection, the cells were harvested for RNA extraction and real time RT-PCR detection of viral M gene (top panel) and IL-6 (middle panel) and COX-2 (bottom panel) mRNA. β-actin was used as RNA concentration normalization, and the data presented are the average of two experiments. * $P<0.05$.

inoculation dose. In human, more severe cytokine dysregulation has been demonstrated in fatal than non-fatal cases of influenza virus infection [1,31]. NS1 has been shown to be important in the induction of host inflammatory response [34]. NS1 may affect the innate immune response through the interaction between RIG-I [35] and host proteins containing the PDZ domain [36]. There is one amino acid difference in the NS1 proteins of AH1 and CK1 at amino acid position 3 (serine in AH1 and phenylalanine in CK1), but the significance of this difference remains to be determined.

The type of histopathological changes induced by CK1 was similar to that of AH1. Extrapulmonary involvement in infected mice was limited to histopathological changes without virological evidence of direct infection which is consistent with AH1 infection in ferrets [37]. The degenerative changes in the heart, liver and kidney during the later stage of infection may be related to the hypoxic and immune-related damage triggered by the cytokine dysregulation as seen in severe influenza [1,24,31,32]. In ferrets, AH1 could cause hepatic lipidosis [37]. The lack of extrapulmonary viral dissemination is compatible with our recent clinical study showing lack of viremia and absence of viruses in tissues from patients [5]. This is in contrast to H5N1 infection, in which extrapulmonary spread is commonly seen in mouse models [38]. One major characteristic of H5N1 virus is the presence of multibasic amino acid at the cleavage site of HA, which renders it susceptible to cleavage by a wide range of tissue proteases [7], whereas H7N9 virus with only one arginine at this cleavage site may have limited its tropism to the respiratory tissues [1,2]. The lack of extrapulmonary spread in our mouse model is similar to another mouse model using SH2 [19], but different from the ferret model, in which SH2 was detected outside the respiratory tract, including the central nervous system[39]. However, the difference in virus strain and animal host makes a direct comparison difficult. In another study, AH1 caused disseminated infection in mouse, but the infectious dose ($10^{6\text{-}8}$ $TCID_{50}$) was higher than that in our study [16].

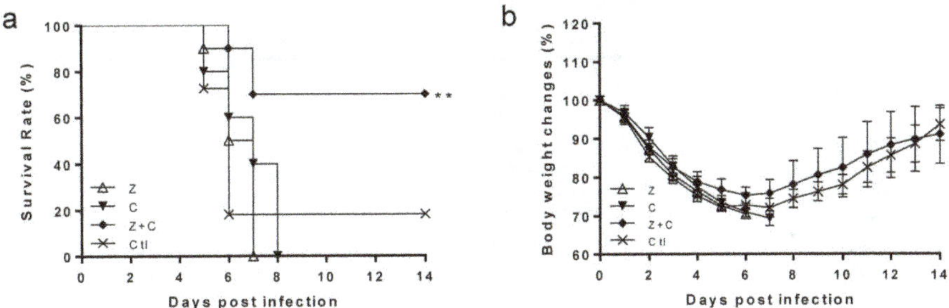

Figure 6. Survivals and body weight changes of mice treated with combination of zanamivir and celecoxib, zanamivir or celecoxib alone by intraperitoneal injection. The mice were infected with 10^6 PFU of CK1 and treated with (1) combination treatment (♦): celecoxib 2 mg daily from day 2 to day 4 p.i., and zanamivir 2mg twice daily from day 2 to day 8 p.i; (2) zanamivir alone (Δ): zanamivir 2mg twice daily from day 2 to day 8 p.i; (3) celecoxib alone (▼): celecoxib 2 mg daily from day 2 to day 4 p.i., (4) control group (×): Celecoxib solven (1% DMSO/PBS) 200ul from day 2 to day 4 p.i. The survival (a) and body weight change (b) were observed for 14 days after infection. Data shown are the average of two experiments (in total, n = 10 for each treatment group, n = 17 for control group). *$P<0.05$ as compared to untreated control group.

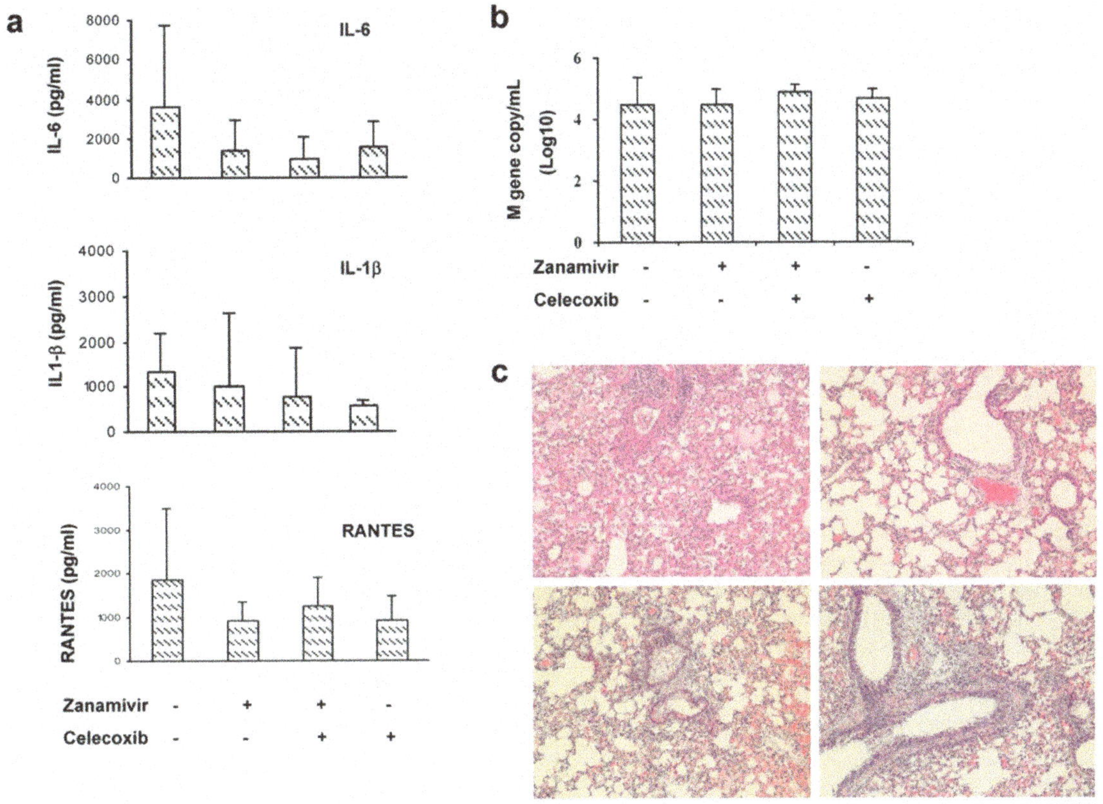

d

Lung histology score				
	untreated (n=3)	zanamivir (n=5)	celecoxib (n=5)	combination (n=5)
necrosis	3.3	1.7 *	1.7 *	1.2 *
infiltration	3.8	2.9 *	1.7 *	2 *
haemorrhage	2.3	1.9	1.9	0.7 *

* *P* value <0.05 when compared to untreated controls

Figure 7. Changes of cytokines and viral loads in the lungs of CK1-infected mice after treatments. At day 4 p.i., mice from different treatment groups were sacrificed. Left-side lungs were homogenized and the clarified homogenate were used for IL-6, IL-1β and RANTES determination by EIA (a) and the viral loads were determined by real time quantitative RT-PCR (b). n = 5 for each group. Error bar indicates ±SD. (c) Representative histological images of H&E stained lung tissues of untreated mice (top left panel), treated with celecoxib-zanamivir combination (top right panel), zanamivir alone (bottom left panel), and celecoxib alone (bottom right panel). Original magnification ×100. (d) Average histology score of mouse lung tissues with different treatment.

Table 2. Mouse lung tissue histological score.

Histological changes	Airway and alveolar cells necrosis (necrosis)	Cell infiltration and alveolar hyaline membrane formation (infiltration)	Alveolar hemorrhage (hemorrhage)
Score 0	Normal lung	Normal lung	Normal lung
Score 1	Airway epithelial cell necrosis limited in one lung lobe	Infiltration cells only on vessel wall or peribronchiolar in one lobe	Hemorrhage restricted in one small area (one 20x field)
Score 2	Airway epithelial cell necrosis in more than one lung lobes, with cell debris congested in airway lumens	Few cells (1–5 cells) in air space but in focal area of one lobe	Hemorrhage in one larger area (more than one 20x field) in one lobe
Score 3	Airway epithelial cell necrosis in more than one lung lobes; small area of alveolar wall collapse	More cells in air space in more than one lobe; and alveolar space hyaline membrane formation in focal area	Hemorrhage in more than one lung lobes, with focal area of alveolar space congested with RBC
Score 4	Airway epithelial cell necrosis in more than one lung lobes alveolar wall collapse in more than one lobes	Severe infiltration with air space congested; large area of hyaline formation in more that one lobes	All 4 lobes showed focal or diffuse hemorrhage

Celecoxib, a COX-2 inhibitor, reduced pulmonary inflammation and improved survival in this study when combined with zanamivir despite their delayed administration at 48 hr p.i. which is similar to a previous study of H5N1 infection [20]. The beneficial effect of the addition of celecoxib may also be related to the suppression of viral replication [40]. However, the cytokine/chemokine profile and viral loads were similar to zanamivir alone, celecoxib alone, or even the untreated control group at day 4 p.i. Our results are similar to that of another study using oseltamivir in the treatment of H7N9 infection in mice [15]. The lack of reduction in the pulmonary viral loads suggests that our treatment regimens had little antiviral effect in the lungs during the early period of infection. This indicated other mechanisms may be involved in the improvement of the survival of CK1-infected mice. Currently, there are no human studies on the use of celecoxib despite its frequent clinical use for many years as an anti-inflammatory medication. As the mortality remains high despite the use of neuraminidase inhibitor in H7N9 infections and that some strains of H7N9 viruses are resistant to neuraminidase inhibitors [1,2,14], celecoxib-zanamivir combination should be further investigated in randomized clinical trials for treating severe influenza.

In this study, we have used zanamivir instead of oseltamivir in the treatment experiments for several reasons. Firstly, zanamivir has low IC_{50} against H7N9 virus, even for those with R294K mutations which confer resistance to oseltamivir [9,14]. Secondly zanamivir can be given intravenously in humans, while oseltamivir can only be given via the oral route or through nasogastric tubes which may not be feasible in some patients with severe H7N9 infection. Furthermore, intravenous route is not affected by absorption in the gastrointestinal tract. Intravenous zanamivir also results in a very high systemic drug concentration. After one single dose of 600 mg intravenous zanamivir, the C_{max} is above 30 μg/ml, which is much higher than the IC_{50} of H7N9 virus, even for strains with R294K mutations [41]. Intravenous zanamivir has been used in H7N9 patients with favourable outcome [11]. We used the intraperitioneal route in mice to mimic the intravenous route in humans.

There are several limitations to our study. Firstly only one chicken isolate of H7N9 was studied. Further studies should be performed for more poultry viral isolates with and without epidemiological link to human cases. Secondly, although the mouse model is a well-established mammalian model for influenza, important differences exist between mice and humans which may affect clinical relevance.

Conclusion

We have demonstrated that chicken H7N9 virus can cause lethal disease in mice, which was associated with severe pulmonary and extrapulmonary pathologies, and cytokine dysregulation. Although the chicken H7N9 isolate had a lower viral replication in the lung, it has triggered a more intense proinflammatory cytokine/chemokine response. Celecoxib and zanamivir appear to ameliorate pulmonary inflammation and improve survival.

Materials and Methods

Viral isolates and animals

The H7N9 virus CK1, isolated from a chicken, and AH1, isolated from a fatal human case, were used in this study [1,2]. The viruses were propagated in 10-day-old specific-pathogen-free (SPF) chicken embryos at 37°C for 48 hours as described previously without serial passage. Allantoic fluid was titrated in MDCK cells for the determination of $TCID_{50}$ and PFU as described previously [42]. Aliquots of virus stock were stored at −80°C until use. HA, NA, PB2 and NS genes of the CK1 stock were sequenced and found no additional mutations other than the sequence data deposited in the GeneBank. Female BALB/c mice at 6–8 weeks old were obtained from the Laboratory Animal Unit, the University of Hong Kong. The animals were housed in SPF-free facilities with 12-hour light-dark cycles and standard pellet feed and water *ad libitum*. Virus challenge experiments were carried out in biosafety level 3 animal facilities. All animal-related experiments were performed according to the standard operating procedures as previously described [20] and were approved by the University of Hong Kong committee on the use of live Animals in teaching and research.

Virus inoculation and drug treatment

For the determination of MLD_{50}, groups of six BALB/c mice were inoculated with 50 µL 10-fold dilutions of CK1 or AH1 via intranasal route under ketamine (100 mg/kg given intraperitoneally) and xylazine (10 mg/kg given intraperitoneally) anaesthesia. Mortality was observed for 14 days. MLD_{50} titres were calculated by the method of Reed and Muench. For pathogenesis study, groups of BALB/c mice were inoculated via intranasal route with 10^6 PFU of CK1 or 10^5 PFU of AH1 under ketamine (100 mg/kg) and xylazine (10 mg/kg) anaesthesia. The body weights, symptoms, and survivals of the mice were monitored daily for 14 days after virus inoculation. Disease severity was scored (Table S2). As a humane endpoint, the animals were euthanized by intraperitoneal injection of pentobarbital sodium (100mg/kg) when the disease score was 4, or when the disease score was 3 with a weight loss exceeding 30%. For sample collection on 1, 2, 4 and 6 days p.i., three to five mice from each group were sacrificed to collect their blood, brain, heart, liver, kidneys and lungs. The collected organs were separated into two sets, one set being frozen at −80°C for RNA and protein extraction, and the other set being fixed in 10% neutral formalin for histopathological study. Drug treatment was modified from our previous study for H5N1 [20]. Celecoxib (Sigma-Aldrich, St. Louis, MO, USA) was dissolved in 10% dimethyl sulfoxide at 100 mg/ml; and zanamivir (GlaxoSmithKline Australia Pty LTD, Boronia, Australia) was dissolved in phosphate buffered saline (PBS) at 10 mg/ml. Mice were inoculated with 10^6 PFU of CK1. Ten mice in each treatment group and 17 in control group were observed for 14 days to monitor survival. An additional five mice in each treatment group and 3 mice in control group were sacrificed on day 4 p.i. for pathological study. The celecoxib-zanamivir combination group was treated with intraperitoneal injection of celecoxib at 2 mg/day from day 2 to day 4 p.i. and intraperitoneal injection of zanamivir 2 mg twice daily from day 2 to day 8 p.i. The zanamivir alone group was treated with zanamivir twice daily from day 2 to day 8 p.i. Celecoxib alone group was treated with celecoxib at 2 mg/day from day 2 to day 4 p.i. Untreated control group received same volume of solvents for celecoxib.

Determination of viral load in homogenized specimens

The left lungs, left hemispheres of the brain, left kidneys, and 0.2 g of liver were homogenized separately in 1 ml of cold minimum essential medium (MEM) supplemented with 1% penicillin and streptomycin. Clarified samples of homogenate supernatant were stored in aliquots at −80°C until use. For quantitative real-time RT-PCR detection of viral gene expression, total RNA were extracted from 350 µl of clarified tissue homogenates using Qiagen RNeasy Mini kit (Qiagen, Germantown, MD, USA) as we described previously [20,23]. Reverse transcription was performed using Superscript RT II enzyme (Life Technology, CA, USA) using influenza specific UNI12 primer (5′-AGCAAAAGCAGG-3′). The cDNA was amplified by real-time PCR performed on LightCycler 480 system (Roche Applied Sciences) using SYBR Green I Master (Roche). Influenza A M gene was used as the target gene with forward primer 5′-CTTCTAACCGAGGTCGAAACG-3′ and reverse primer 5′-GGCATTTTGGACAAAKCGTCTA-3′. The pcDNA3.1 plasmid containing the cloned M gene fragment was applied as standard. The detection limit of this assay was 100 copies of the viral M gene per ml of tissue homogenates. Viral titres were also determined by $TCID_{50}$ assay as we described previously [42].

Determination of interferons and cytokines in homogenized lung specimens

The pulmonary expression levels of IFN-α, IFN-β, IFN-γ, and COX-2 mRNA were determined by real-time RT-PCR using oligodT transcribed-cDNA from lung tissue homogenates. The expression of β-actin was quantified by real-time RT-PCR and used for RNA normalization, and a ΔΔCt method was used to estimate the differential gene expression between samples. Primers for real-time PCR: IFN-α forward primer: 5′-ARSYTGTSTGATGCARCAGGT-3′, IFN-α reverse primer: 5′-GGWACACAGTGATCCTGTGG; IFN-β-forward primer: 5′-AGCTCCAAGAAAGGACGAACAT-3′, IFN-β-reverse primer, 5′-GCCCTGTAGGTGAGGTTGATCT-3′; IFN-γ-forward primer: 5′-ARSYTGTSTGATGCARCAGGT-3′, IFN-γ-reverse primer: 5′-GGWACACAGTGATCCTGTGG-3′; Mouse β-actin-forward primer: 5′-TCACCCACACTGTGCCCATCTACGA-3′, Mouse β-actin-reverse primer: 5′-GGATGCCACAGGATTCCATACCCA-3′; COX-2 forward primer: 5′-TCTGGAACATTGTGAACAACATC-3′, reverse primer: 5′-AAGCTCCTTATTTCCCTTCACAC-3′.

Protein levels of IL-1β, IL-6, IL-10, and RANTES in clarified lung homogenates were determined by enzyme immunoassay (R&D system, Inc., Minneapolis, MN, USA) as described previously [23]. The detection limits of these assays were 7.8 pg/ml for IL-1β, IL-6 and RANTES, and 16 pg/ml for IL-10.

Histopathological and immunohistochemical staining of influenza nucleoprotein in lung tissue

To examine pathological changes of infected mouse lung at different time after infection, right side of the lung were fixed in 10% formalin. All 4 lung lobes were embedded in paraffin and sectioned at 5µm for haematoxylin and eosin (H&E) staining. All lung fields of the 4 lobes were examined at 20x magnification for each sample. The severity of histological changes was graded according to a semiquantitative scoring system (Table 2) [17,43,44].

For influenza NP staining, de-paraffinized and rehydrated tissue sections were treated with Antigen Unmasking Solution according the manufacturer's instructions (Vector Laboratories Inc. Burlingame, CA, USA) to unmask the antigens. After blocking with 1% bovine serum albumin, the sections were incubated with mouse anti-influenza NP-antibody (HB65, ATCC) at 4°C overnight, followed by biotin-conjugated goat anti-mouse IgG (Calbiochem, Darmstadt, Germany) for 30 min at room temperature. Streptavidin/peroxidase complex reagent (Vector Laboratories, Burlingame, CA) was then added and incubated at room temperature for 30 min. Colour development was performed with 3, 3′-diaminobenzidine (DAB, Vector Laboratories, Burlingame, CA, USA) and images were captured with Nikon80i imaging system with the help of Spot-advance computer software.

In vitro infection of mouse lung epithelial cells and detection of viral load, IL-6 and COX-2 mRNA level by quantitative real time RT-PCR

Mouse lung epithelial cell line LA-4 (ATCC # CCL-196) was seeded in 12-well plates at 2×10^5 cells per well and incubated overnight at 37°C with 5% CO_2. The cells were incubated with CK1 or AH1 at a multiplicity of infection of 2 for 1 h at 37°C. The cells were washed twice with PBS after removing the virus,and further incubated for 1, 3, 6, and 9 hours. At each time point after infection, the cells were harvested. Total RNA extraction, cDNA transcription and real-time RT-PCR determination of viral M gene copies, IL-6 and COX-2 mRNA level were performed as described above.

Statistical analysis

Mouse survival rates were analyzed by the Kaplan-Meier method and Log-rank test using SPSS 17.0 for Windows (SPSS Inc., Chicago, IL). Pulmonary viral loads, cytokine, chemokine profiles, and histology scores were analyzed by Student's t-test. A P value of <0.05 was considered statistically significant.

Supporting Information

Table S1 Unique substitutions in sequence of CK1 virus when compared to other H7N9 poultry isolates with low pathogenicity in mice.

Table S2 H7N9 infected mouse disease severity scoring system.

Author Contributions

Conceived and designed the experiments: AJXZ KKWT HC IFNH LL KYY. Performed the experiments: Can Li Chuangen Li ACYL HZ HW. Analyzed the data: AJXZ KKWT JFWC HC IFNH LL KYY. Contributed reagents/materials/analysis tools: LL. Contributed to the writing of the manuscript: Can Li Chuangen Li AJXZ KKWT ACYL HZ HW JFWC HC IFNH LL KYY.

References

1. Chen Y, Liang W, Yang S, Wu N, Gao H, et al. (2013) Human infections with the emerging avian influenza A H7N9 virus from wet market poultry: clinical analysis and characterisation of viral genome. Lancet 381: 1916–1925.
2. Gao R, Cao B, Hu Y, Feng Z, Wang D, et al. (2013) Human infection with a novel avian-origin influenza A (H7N9) virus. N Engl J Med 368: 1888–1897.
3. To KK, Chan JF, Chen H, Li L, Yuen KY (2013) The emergence of influenza A H7N9 in human beings 16 years after influenza A H5N1: a tale of two cities. Lancet Infect Dis 13: 809–821.
4. European Centre for Disease Prevention and Control Rapid risk assessment. Human infection with avian influenza A viruses, China. 24 February 2014. Stockholm: ECDC; 2014.
5. Yu L, Wang Z, Chen Y, Ding W, Jia H, et al. (2013) Clinical, virological, and histopathological manifestations of fatal human infections by avian influenza A(H7N9) virus. Clin Infect Dis 57: 1449–1457.
6. Yuen KY, Chan PK, Peiris M, Tsang DN, Que TL, et al. (1998) Clinical features and rapid viral diagnosis of human disease associated with avian influenza A H5N1 virus. Lancet 351: 467–471.
7. To KK, Ng KH, Que TL, Chan JM, Tsang KY, et al. (2012) Avian influenza A H5N1 virus: a continuous threat to humans. Emerg Microbes Infect 1: e25.
8. Gao HN, Lu HZ, Cao B, Du B, Shang H, et al. (2013) Clinical findings in 111 cases of influenza A (H7N9) virus infection. N Engl J Med 368: 2277–2285.
9. To KK, Chan JF, Yuen KY (2014) Viral lung infections: epidemiology, virology, clinical features, and management of avian influenza A(H7N9). Curr Opin Pulm Med 20: 225–232.
10. Lam TT, Wang J, Shen Y, Zhou B, Duan L, et al. (2013) The genesis and source of the H7N9 influenza viruses causing human infections in China. Nature 502: 241–244.
11. To KK, Song W, Lau SY, Que TL, Lung DC, et al. (2014) Unique reassortant of influenza A(H7N9) virus associated with severe disease emerging in Hong Kong. J Infect 69: 60–68.
12. Liu D, Shi W, Gao GF (2014) Poultry carrying H9N2 act as incubators for novel human avian influenza viruses. Lancet.
13. Yu X, Jin T, Cui Y, Pu X, Li J, et al. (2014) Influenza H7N9 and H9N2 viruses: coexistence in poultry linked to human H7N9 infection and genome characteristics. J Virol 88: 3423–3431.
14. Watanabe T, Kiso M, Fukuyama S, Nakajima N, Imai M, et al. (2013) Characterization of H7N9 influenza A viruses isolated from humans. Nature 501: 551–555.
15. Baranovich T, Burnham AJ, Marathe BM, Armstrong J, Guan Y, et al. (2013) The Neuraminidase Inhibitor Oseltamivir Is Effective Against A/Anhui/1/2013 (H7N9) Influenza Virus in a Mouse Model of Acute Respiratory Distress Syndrome. J Infect Dis.
16. Xu L, Bao L, Deng W, Zhu H, Chen T, et al. (2013) The mouse and ferret models for studying the novel avian-origin human influenza A (H7N9) virus. Virol J 10: 253.
17. Belser JA, Gustin KM, Pearce MB, Maines TR, Zeng H, et al. (2013) Pathogenesis and transmission of avian influenza A (H7N9) virus in ferrets and mice. Nature 501: 556–559.
18. Zhang Q, Shi J, Deng G, Guo J, Zeng X, et al. (2013) H7N9 influenza viruses are transmissible in ferrets by respiratory droplet. Science 341: 410–414.
19. Mok CK, Lee HH, Chan MC, Sia SF, Lestra M, et al. (2013) Pathogenicity of the novel A/H7N9 influenza virus in mice. MBio 4: pii: e00362–00313.
20. Zheng BJ, Chan KW, Lin YP, Zhao GY, Chan C, et al. (2008) Delayed antiviral plus immunomodulator treatment still reduces mortality in mice infected by high inoculum of influenza A/H5N1 virus. Proc Natl Acad Sci U S A 105: 8091–8096.
21. Zhang AJ, Li C, To KK, Zhu HS, Lee AC, et al. (2014) Toll-like receptor 7 agonist imiquimod in combination with influenza vaccine expedites and augments humoral immune responses against influenza A(H1N1)pdm09 virus infection in BALB/c mice. Clin Vaccine Immunol 21: 570–579.
22. Kageyama T, Fujisaki S, Takashita E, Xu H, Yamada S, et al. (2013) Genetic analysis of novel avian A(H7N9) influenza viruses isolated from patients in China, February to April 2013. Euro Surveill 18: 20453.
23. Zhang AJ, To KK, Li C, Lau CC, Poon VK, et al. (2013) Leptin mediates the pathogenesis of severe 2009 pandemic influenza A(H1N1) infection associated with cytokine dysregulation in mice with diet-induced obesity. J Infect Dis 207: 1270–1280.
24. Zheng B, Chan KH, Zhang AJ, Zhou J, Chan CC, et al. (2010) D225G mutation in hemagglutinin of pandemic influenza H1N1 (2009) virus enhances virulence in mice. Exp Biol Med (Maywood) 235: 981–988.
25. Chan KH, Zhang AJ, To KK, Chan CC, Poon VK, et al. (2010) Wild type and mutant 2009 pandemic influenza A (H1N1) viruses cause more severe disease and higher mortality in pregnant BALB/c mice. PLoS One 5: e13757.
26. Dybing JK, Schultz-Cherry S, Swayne DE, Suarez DL, Perdue ML (2000) Distinct pathogenesis of hong kong-origin H5N1 viruses in mice compared to that of other highly pathogenic H5 avian influenza viruses. J Virol 74: 1443–1450.
27. Steel J, Lowen AC, Mubareka S, Palese P (2009) Transmission of influenza virus in a mammalian host is increased by PB2 amino acids 627K or 627E/701N. PLoS Pathog 5: e1000252.
28. Gao Y, Zhang Y, Shinya K, Deng G, Jiang Y, et al. (2009) Identification of amino acids in HA and PB2 critical for the transmission of H5N1 avian influenza viruses in a mammalian host. PLoS Pathog 5: e1000709.
29. Morita M, Kuba K, Ichikawa A, Nakayama M, Katahira J, et al. (2013) The lipid mediator protectin D1 inhibits influenza virus replication and improves severe influenza. Cell 153: 112–125.
30. Shinya K, Hamm S, Hatta M, Ito H, Ito T, et al. (2004) PB2 amino acid at position 627 affects replicative efficiency, but not cell tropism, of Hong Kong H5N1 influenza A viruses in mice. Virology 320: 258–266.
31. To KK, Hung IF, Li IW, Lee KL, Koo CK, et al. (2010) Delayed clearance of viral load and marked cytokine activation in severe cases of pandemic H1N1 2009 influenza virus infection. Clin Infect Dis 50: 850–859.
32. de Jong MD, Simmons CP, Thanh TT, Hien VM, Smith GJ, et al. (2006) Fatal outcome of human influenza A (H5N1) is associated with high viral load and hypercytokinemia. Nat Med 12: 1203–1207.
33. Camp JV, Chu YK, Chung DH, McAllister RC, Adcock RS, et al. (2013) Phenotypic differences in virulence and immune response in closely related clinical isolates of influenza A 2009 H1N1 pandemic viruses in mice. PLoS One 8: e56602.
34. Moltedo B, Lopez CB, Pazos M, Becker MI, Hermesh T, et al. (2009) Cutting edge: stealth influenza virus replication precedes the initiation of adaptive immunity. J Immunol 183: 3569–3573.
35. Ruckle A, Haasbach E, Julkunen I, Planz O, Ehrhardt C, et al. (2012) The NS1 protein of influenza A virus blocks RIG-I-mediated activation of the noncanonical NF-kappaB pathway and p52/RelB-dependent gene expression in lung epithelial cells. J Virol 86: 10211–10217.
36. Zielecki F, Semmler I, Kalthoff D, Voss D, Mauel S, et al. (2010) Virulence determinants of avian H5N1 influenza A virus in mammalian and avian hosts: role of the C-terminal ESEV motif in the viral NS1 protein. J Virol 84: 10708–10718.
37. Kreijtz JH, Kroeze EJ, Stittelaar KJ, de Waal L, van Amerongen G, et al. (2013) Low pathogenic avian influenza A(H7N9) virus causes high mortality in ferrets upon intratracheal challenge: a model to study intervention strategies. Vaccine 31: 4995–4999.
38. Suguitan AL Jr., Matsuoka Y, Lau YF, Santos CP, Vogel L, et al. (2012) The multibasic cleavage site of the hemagglutinin of highly pathogenic A/Vietnam/1203/2004 (H5N1) avian influenza virus acts as a virulence factor in a host-specific manner in mammals. J Virol 86: 2706–2714.
39. Zhu H, Wang D, Kelvin DJ, Li L, Zheng Z, et al. (2013) Infectivity, transmission, and pathology of human-isolated H7N9 influenza virus in ferrets and pigs. Science 341: 183–186.
40. Lee SM, Gai WW, Cheung TK, Peiris JS (2011) Antiviral effect of a selective COX-2 inhibitor on H5N1 infection in vitro. Antiviral Res 91: 330–334.
41. Marty FM, Man CY, van der Horst C, Francois B, Garot D, et al. (2014) Safety and pharmacokinetics of intravenous zanamivir treatment in hospitalized adults

with influenza: an open-label, multicenter, single-arm, phase II study. J Infect Dis 209: 542–550.
42. Li IW, Chan KH, To KW, Wong SS, Ho PL, et al. (2009) Differential susceptibility of different cell lines to swine-origin influenza A H1N1, seasonal human influenza A H1N1, and avian influenza A H5N1 viruses. J Clin Virol 46: 325–330.
43. Xu T, Qiao J, Zhao L, He G, Li K, et al. (2009) Effect of dexamethasone on acute respiratory distress syndrome induced by the H5N1 virus in mice. Eur Respir J 33: 852–860.
44. Ehrentraut H, Clambey ET, McNamee EN, Brodsky KS, Ehrentraut SF, et al. (2013) CD73+ regulatory T cells contribute to adenosine-mediated resolution of acute lung injury. FASEB J 27: 2207–2219.

Spatial Analysis on Hepatitis C Virus Infection in Mainland China: From 2005 to 2011

Lu Wang[1], Jiannan Xing[1,2], Fangfang Chen[1], Ruixue Yan[1], Lin Ge[1], Qianqian Qin[1], Liyan Wang[1], Zhengwei Ding[1], Wei Guo[1], Ning Wang[1]*

1 National Center for AIDS/STD Control and Prevention, Chinese Center for Disease Control and Prevention, Beijing, China, 2 Beijing Human Resources and Social Security Bureau, Beijing, China

Abstract

Background: The burden of Hepatitis C virus (HCV) has become more and more considerable in China. A macroscopic spatial analysis of HCV infection that can provide scientific information for further intervention and disease control is lacking.

Methods: All geo-referenced HCV cases that had been recorded by the China Information System for Disease Control and Prevention (CISDCP) during 2005–2011 were included in the study. In order to learn about the changes of demographic characteristics and geographic distribution, trend test and spatial analysis were conducted to reflect the changing pattern of HCV infection.

Results: Over 770,000 identified HCV infection cases had specific geographic information during the study period (2005–2011). Ratios of gender (Male/Female, Z-value = −18.53, P<0.001), age group (≤30 years old/≥31 years old, Z-value = −51.03, P<0.001) and diagnosis type (Clinical diagnosis/Laboratory diagnosis, Z-value = −130.47, P<0.001) declined. HCV infection was not distributed randomly. Provinces Henan, Guangdong, Guangxi, Xinjiang, and Jilin reported more than 40,000 HCV infections during 2005 to 2011, accounting for 43.91% of all cases. The strength of cluster of disease was increasing in China during the study period. Overall, 11 provinces had once been detected as hotspots during 7 years, most of which were located in the central or border parts of China. Tibet, Qinghai, Jiangxi were the regions that had coldspots.

Conclusions: The number of clustering of HCV infection among older adults increased in recent years. Specific interventions and prevention programs targeting at main HCV epidemic areas are urgently in need in mainland China.

Editor: Wenzhe Ho, Temple University School of Medicine, United States of America

Funding: This study was supported by the mega-projects of national scientific research under the 12th Five-Year Plan of China (2012ZX10001001). The funders had no role in study design, data collection and analysis, decision to publish, or preparation of the manuscript.

Competing Interests: The authors have declared that no competing interests exist.

* Email: wangnbj@163.com

These authors contributed equally to this work.

Introduction

Hepatitis C virus (HCV) is known as the major cause of chronic liver disease, human hepatic cirrhosis, and even hepatocellular carcinoma [1]. The fact that more and more HCV infections or patients who living with HCV has become a severe public health problem [2]. WHO has estimated that there are more than 150 million people with chronic liver disease which were caused by HCV infection in 2012, and over 350,000 people has been dead from HCV-related diseases worldwide each year [3]. Due to lack of vaccine and unavailability of effective therapy, the prevention of HCV infection has been a great challenge, especially in China, which is the largest developing country and owns one-fifths of the world's population. The population of China had approached 1.35 billion at the end of 2011 [4]. Although the prevalence of HCV infection had been lower in China after mid-1990s and the overall prevalence of anti-HCV was less than 1% in recent years [5,6], the huge size of China population makes the absolute number of people infected with HCV enormous.

HCV infection is a public issue, which has an association with the interrelated social, geographic, historical and economic elements, just like other infectious diseases. Although various studies have already shown the prevalence of HCV infection varies with the different geographic positions in China [1,4,7], most of existing studies mainly focused on the spatial distribution of HCV genotypes and limited researches on the spatial distribution of HCV infection itself [8–10]. Shunquan Wu et al used spatial technique to work on the prevalence of HCV infection in Fujian province, and found that the HCV infection did have a relationship with spatial factors and the cluster of disease [11]. Apart from this study, the HCV infections in some provinces were more serious than other surrounding provinces, which might attribute to poor economy, inadequate primary health infrastructure, or inappropriate treatments [1]. In addition, HCV infection shares the same transmission routes with HIV infection, which had been already observed cluster of disease in studies [12,13]. Especially for the intravenous drug users (IDUs), the prevalence of co-infection of HIV and HCV are high [14], and the HIV epidemics have association with geographic factors [15].

Since there is a geographic indicator related to the HIV infection, a macroscopic spatial analysis of HCV infection in this country is needed to probe whether the distribution of HCV infection was randomly distributed or not, which might facilitate prevention and control for HCV epidemic. In this study, we utilize the data of HCV reported cases in mainland of China from the year of 2005 to 2011 to explore the potential relationship between HCV infection and geographic distribution by using geographical information systems (GIS) and spatial statistics, which including general spatial autocorrelation (a tool was used to measure and analyze the degree of dependency among observations in a geographic space) and local spatial autocorrelation (a tool was used to detect cluster of high-value or low-value of observations).

Methods

Data collection and management

In 2004, after the Severe Acute Respiratory Syndrome (SARS) outbreak, China has established a world's largest web-based disease reporting system, called China Information System for Disease Control and Prevention (CISDCP). Since then, all medical institutions should report diagnosed HCV infection cases to

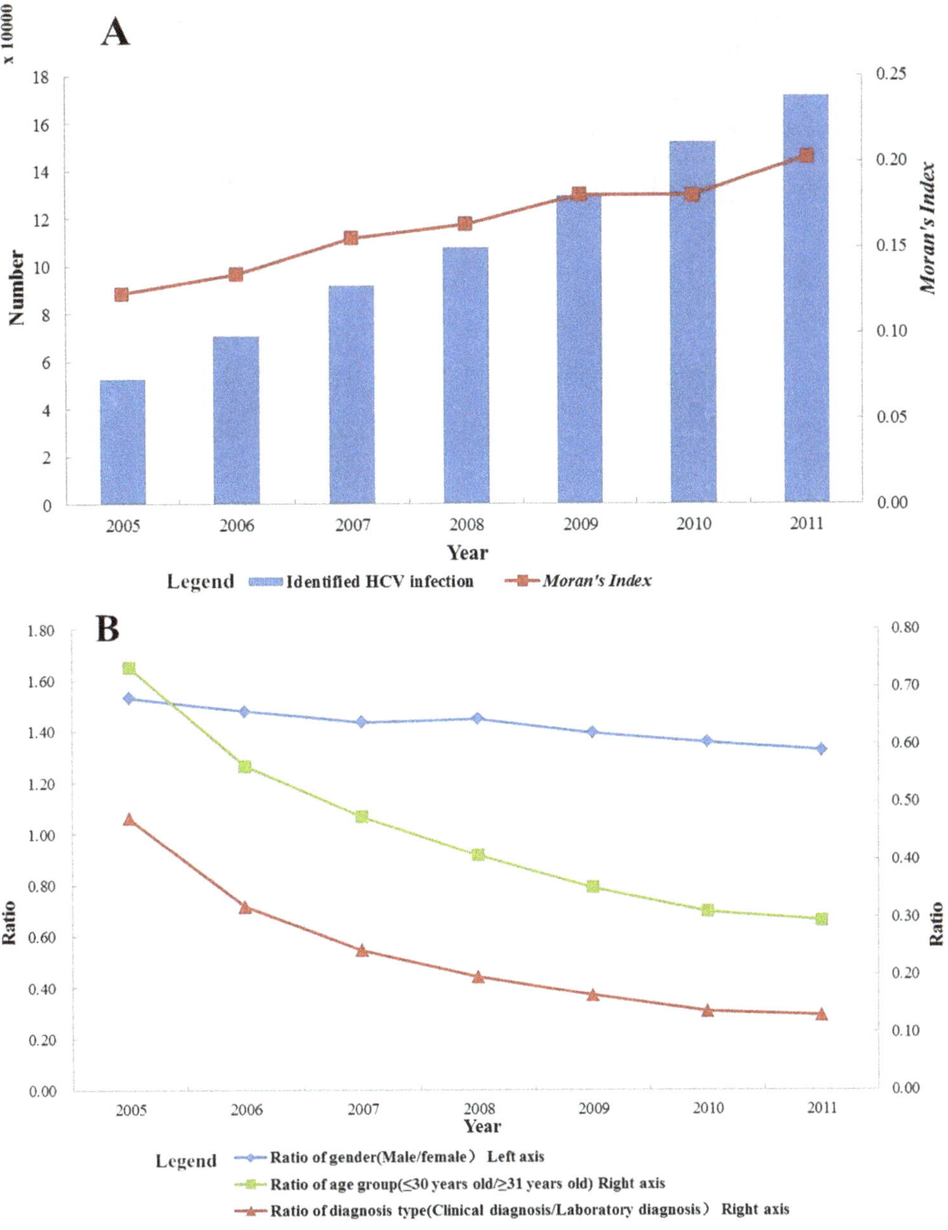

Figure 1. (A) Number and *Moran's Index* of identified HCV infection cases by year. (B) Ratio of gender, age group and diagnosis type of identified HCV infection cases by year.

specific local Center for Disease Control and Prevention (CDC) through CISDCP. Demographic information (age, gender, address, registered residency places, time of onset of the disease etc.) were collected using standardized case report forms (CRFs) by conducting private interviews. After being checked, confirmed case reports were saved in the web-based system. The procedure of reporting HCV case through CISDCP is consistent around the whole country. This comprehensive and well-organized system, CISDCP, can provide both the number of HCV infection cases and the spatial distribution information of these cases across the country.

All HCV infection cases, identified during 2005 to 2011 in CISDCP, were included. In order to identify the residential locations of the reported HCV infection cases, the corresponding national standard geocodes at city level were included in the analysis. Any personal identifiers which might reveal the privacy of the participants were removed before data analysis in this study. Electronic maps were obtained from China CDC (CCDC). ArcGIS 10.1 software (ESRI Inc., Redlands, CA, USA) was used to create electronic maps and SPSS18.0 software (IBM Inc., Armonk, NY, USA) was used to process and analyze the data.

The data in this study was based on HCV regular monitoring system in China, and related ethics committee and Chinese government have approved for the system to collect patient data. Since this study focused on population-level analyses only and did not access any individually identifiable patient data, ethics committee approval was not particularly required in this study.

Anyone can apply for using the data in ***The data-center of China public health science*** (http://www.phsciencedata.cn/Share/en/data.jsp?id=9906073c-200a-4b44-8ffe-0867bfa42557) or email to data@chinacic.cn.

Trend analysis

We used Cochran-Armitage trend test to analyze the changing patterns of demographic and other characteristics, by ratios of gender (male/female), age group (≤30 years old/≥31 years old) and diagnosis type (clinical diagnosis/laboratory diagnosis) of the identified HCV infection cases from 2005 to 2011. In the present study, $\alpha = 0.05$ has been selected as the level of significance for the test.

General spatial autocorrelation

General spatial autocorrelation test statistic is a technique which is able to measure and analyze the spatial clusters in the data, and calculate the degree of dependency among observations in the whole geographic space [16]. In our study, general Moran's Index was used to discover and measure the HCV infection clusters in

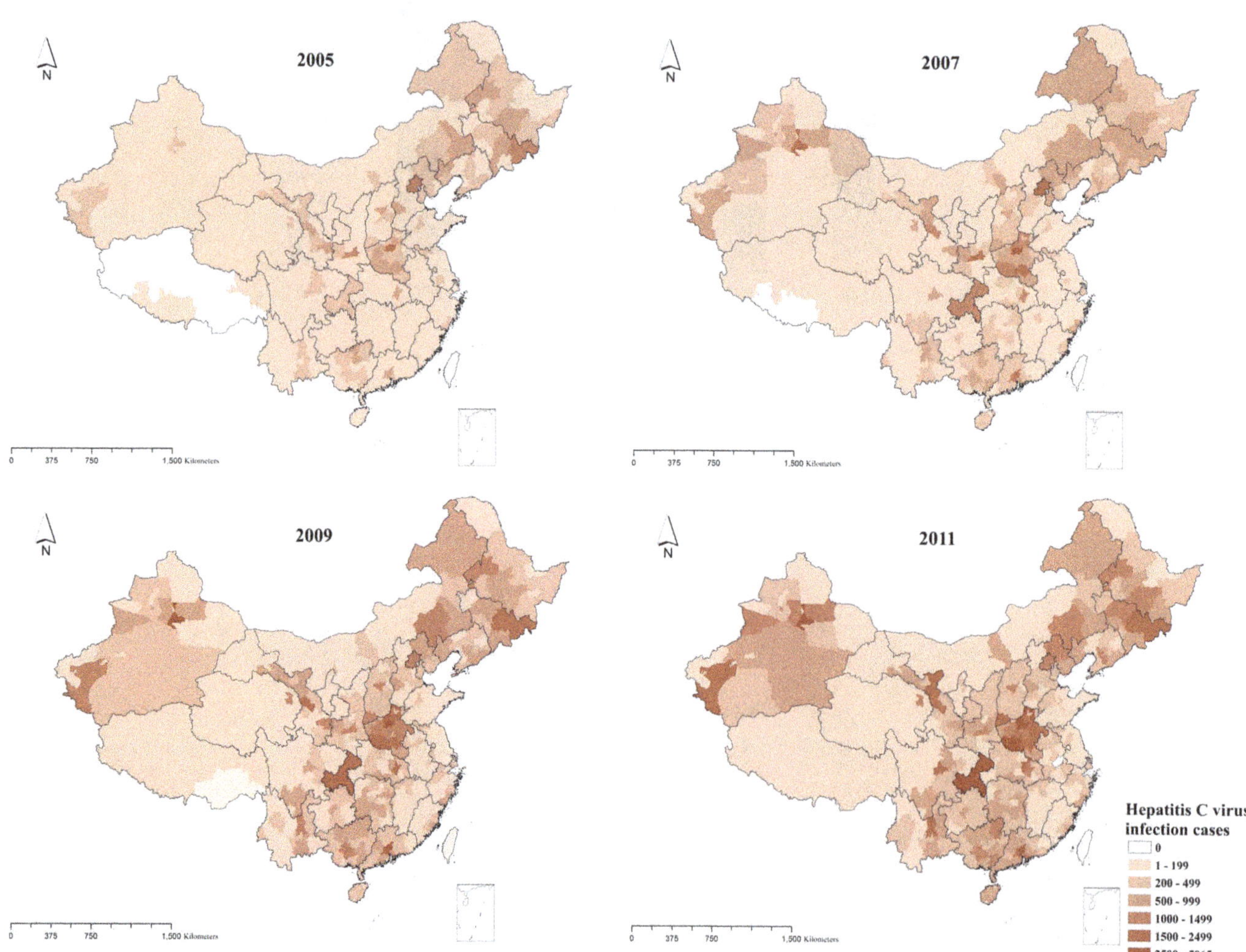

Figure 2. Geographical distribution of the number of identified HCV infection cases reported at city level in the years 2005, 2007, 2009 and 2011 in China.

Table 1. Results of general spatial autocorrelation of from 2005 to 2011.

Year	*Moran's Index*	*Z*-value	*P*-value
2005	0.123	9.497	<0.01
2006	0.134	10.458	<0.01
2007	0.155	11.983	<0.01
2008	0.163	12.528	<0.01
2009	0.180	13.771	<0.01
2010	0.180	13.789	<0.01
2011	0.203	15.460	<0.01
Total(2005–2011)	0.178	13.655	<0.01

mainland China. The value of Moran's Index was set between [−1, 1]. When the value of general Moran's Index was >0 and Z-value >1.96, or the general Moran's Index was <0 and Z-value <−1.96, it indicated that the distribution of identified HCV infection cases clustered in the whole area; otherwise, the distribution of the infection cases was random. The specific formula of general Moran's Index was calculated as: [12]:

$$I=\frac{n\sum_i\sum_j w_{ij}(x_i-\overline{x})(x_j-\overline{x})}{(\sum_i\sum_j w_{ij})\sum_i(x_i-\overline{x})^2}$$

Where n is the number of spatial units (cities), x_i and x_j were the observations from unit i to unit j about the phenomenon X; w_{ij} represents the adjacent weight matrix. If the unit i was adjacent to the unit j, then w_{ij} would be 1; otherwise, it would be 0. In order to avoid the human influence of distance band of matrix, the threshold distance between cities was used in this study.

Local spatial autocorrelation

This method, also name local indicator of spatial association (LISA), was initially created to detect the clustering of cases of rare diseases [17]. The method focused on detecting specific local clusters of cases without any preconception about their locations. In other words, the aim of local spatial autocorrelation is to recognize clusters which may not be identifiable by general spatial autocorrelation. The Getis statistics was chosen as the parameter to identify the local clusters in the present study, and the formula of it was showed as below [12]:

$$G_i(d)=\frac{\sum\limits_{i=1}^{n}\sum\limits_{j=1,j\neq i}^{n} w_{ij}(d)x_j}{\sum\limits_{i=1}^{n}\sum\limits_{j=1,j\neq i}^{n} x_i}(i\neq j)$$

The meaning of parameters are similar as general Moran's Index formula, Z-test was conducted for the Gi parameter. If Z-value was>1. 96, the local clusters were identified as high-value correlations (statistically significant hotspot, meaning the city had a high number of cases and was surrounded by other cities with high number of cases as well); and if Z-value was <−1.96, the local clusters can be identified as low-value correlation (statistically significant coldspot, meaning the city had a low number of cases).

We conducted local spatial autocorrelation at city level to detect the hotspots and coldspots of HCV infection in mainland China.

Results

Basic information

There were774,787 identified HCV infection cases that had accurate geographic information during the study period (2005–2011).7,568 cases(accounting for 0.98% of all identified) were excluded from the present study, due to lack of spatial information. Increased trend of number of identified HCV infection cases with years was observed (Figure 1A). During 2005–2011, the overall gender ratio (male/female) was 1.39; the mean age of all cases was 47.31 years (95%CI: 47.27 to 47.35) and, 16.51% of cases were ≤ 30 years. Almost 83.8%of HCV infection cases were identified by laboratory diagnosis and the rest were identified by clinical diagnosis.

Trend analysis

The ratio of gender (Male/Female) was generally decreasing, 1.53, 1.47, 1.43, 1.44, 1.39 and 1.35 from 2005 to 2011 respectively, Z-value =−18.53 (P<0.001). The ratio of age groups of cases (≤30 years old/≥31 years old) was 0.26 in 2005, while 0.16 in 2011. This trend also has statistical significance (Z-value =−51.03, P<0.001).

Clinically diagnosis case is defined as a patient was detected by clinically agencies when he/she seek for treatment, while laboratory diagnosis case was simply detected by laboratory. The ratio of diagnosis type (Clinical diagnosis/Laboratory diagnosis) was also presented decreasing trend during study period, from 0.47 in 2005 to 0.12 in 2011 (Z-value =−130.47, P<0.001). The trend analyses were described in Figure 1B.

Spatial analysis

The geographical distribution of identified HCV infection cases was found to be unbalanced in the mainland of China. As figure 2 presented, most cities have reported HCV infection cases during the study period, and the number of cities which have reported HCV infection cases were 339,341,341,342 in the year of 2005, 2007, 2009 and 2011, respectively. Henan province, Guangdong province, Guangxi Zhuang Autonomous Region, Xinjiang Uygur Autonomous Region and Jilin province have respectively reported more than 40,000 HCV infection cases during the period of 2005 to 2011. The total number of HCV identified cases in these five regions is 340,209, which accounted for 43.91% of all cases.

Firstly, general spatial autocorrelation was conducted for the cumulative number of HCV infection diagnosed between 2005

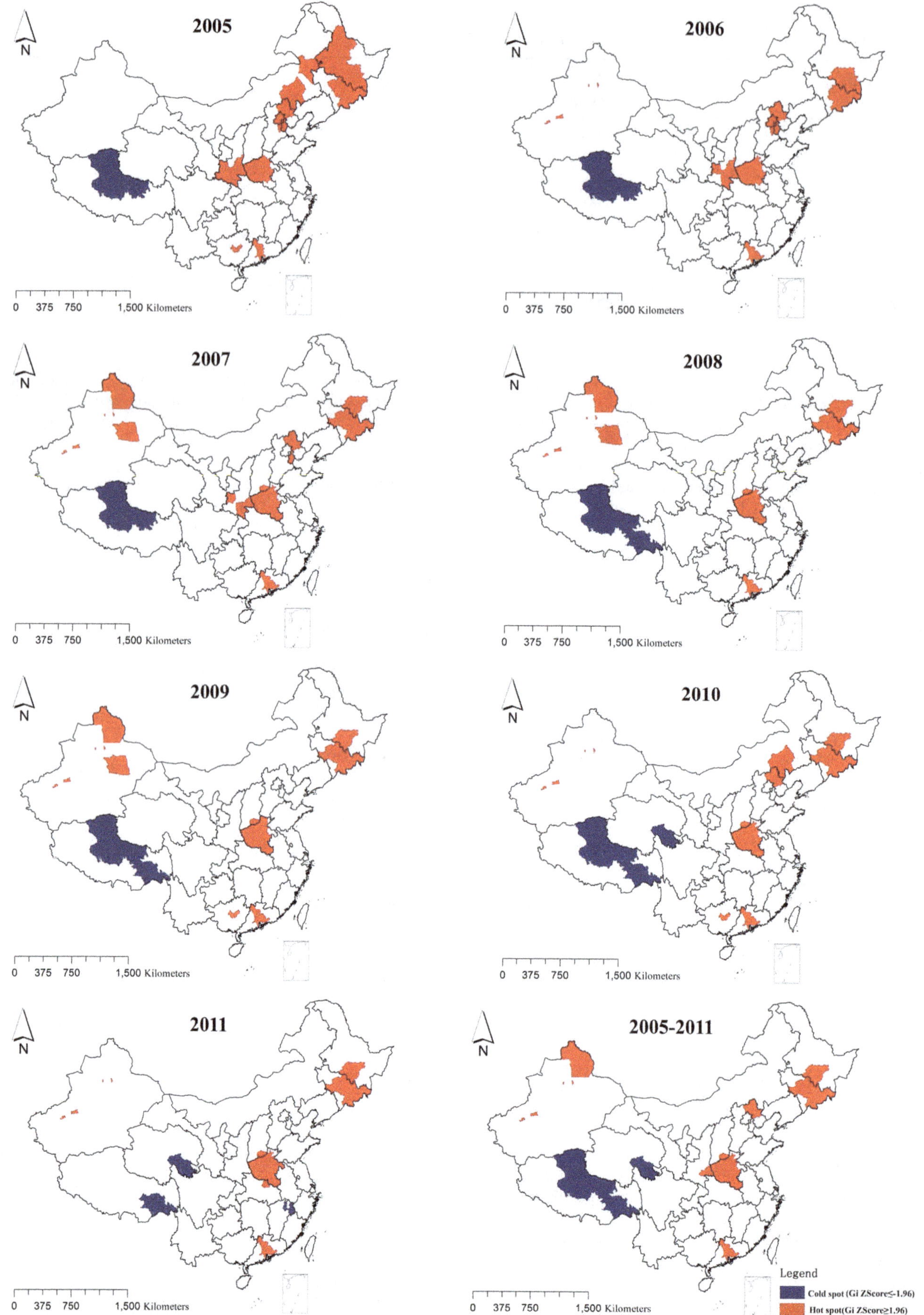

Figure 3. Hotspots and Coldspots of identified HCV infection cases at city level by year in China, 2005–2012.

and 2011 by using distance matrix, and the value of *Moran's Index* was 0.178 and $P<0.01$. Then we conducted general spatial autocorrelation for the number of identified HCV infection cases of each year from 2005 to 2011(Table 1). The results indicated that HCV epidemic clustered in the mainland of China for total year and by each year, and the value of *Moran's Index* was increasing from 2005 to 2011 in general, meaning the strength of clustering of HCV cases got severer year by year (Figure 1A).

In order to figure out whether the stronger clusters resulted from the possible hotspots or coldspots and then to find them in specific area, local spatial autocorrelation was conducted by using the same matrix as general spatial autocorrelation.

As figure 3 showed, in general, hotspots concentrated in the areas where there was huge number of HCV infection cases, for example, Henan province and Jilin province etc. However, new hotspots were also observed in Hebei, Beijing, Tianjin and other provinces in recent years.

The coldspots were mainly limited to three areas: Tibet, Qinghai and Jiangxi. Tibet was always one of the coldspots in each year from the 2005 to 2011. During this period, the number of hot spots at city level decreased from 42 in 2005 to 31 in 2011, however, the number of coldspots increased slightly at the same period. The result of local spatial autocorrelation for the cumulative number of HCV infection cases reported between 2005 and 2011 was little different from the results of each year during this period. The details of hotpots and coldspots were listed in Table 2, and the reason for listing hotspots in provincial level is we mainly discussed cluster in this level.

Discussion

Our study showed that not only the identified number of HCV cases in mainland China increased, but also the cases tended to more clustering, which means targeted interventions may be very helpful in China. After the implementation of the blood donation law (1998), and the law requiring mandatory screening for anti-HCV before blood donation (1993) [1,4] in China, HCV infected patients might have more opportunities to get tested, which could possibly lead to the increased number of detection of HCV infection cases.

According to the previous study [18], the reported incidence of HCV infection in China was gradually increased during 1997 to 2011, especially since CISDCP was established in 2004. The upsurge was observed in both the prevalent number of HCV infection and its incidence indicating the emerging HCV infection epidemic in China.

Due to risky behaviors male conduct, for example, intravenous drug use and paid-blood/plasma donation, males are prone to get infected by HCV compared with female. However, the gender ratio (male/female) of HCV cases was decreasing in the present study, which was consistent with other studies [11,19]. The equality of women's status, for example, more chances to involve into social connections and continuous improvement of mobility might be the reason. The ratio of age groups (≤30 years old/≥31 years old) and diagnosis types (Clinical diagnosis/Laboratory diagnosis) both showed a decreasing trend.

In the present study, the proportion of people aged more than 30 years old was increasing by year, so older people became more likely to get infected by HCV. Persistent HCV infection risk factors caused by the cumulative effect (the number and degrees of risk factors growing with the HCV-infected patient getting older) and more opportunities to assess to the clinical invasive treatment might explain this phenomenon.

Much more infection cases were diagnosed by laboratory, indicating that large-scaled improvement of laboratory testing capabilities has promoted early detection to explore more cases than ever, which also contributed to the growing number of identified number of HCV cases. Instead, some hospitals might not have adequate capabilities to detect infection.

The number of cities which reported HCV infection cases remained stable by year, with the number of infection cases increasing in the same period. However, spatial analysis indicated that the hotspots and coldspots existed, which indicated the HCV infection and epidemic was not randomly distributed.

Henan province, Guangdong province, Guangxi Zhuang Autonomous Region, Xinjiang Uygur Autonomous Region and Jilin province accounted for more than 40 percent of identified HCV infection cases in China during the study period. The illegal blood/plasma donation, intravenous drug use and poorer economy status etc. might be attributed to HCV infection

Table 2. Distribution of Hotspots and Coldspots of HCV infection in China from 2005 to 2011.

	Hotspots		Coldspots	
Year	Number (city level)	Province, Municipality or Autonomous region where the hotspots located	Number (city level)	Province, Municipality or Autonomous region where the coldspots located
2005	42	Henan, Jilin, Guangdong, Shaanxi, Inner Mongolia, Hebei, Tianjin, Beijing, Heilongjiang	1	Tibet
2006	36	Henan, Jilin, Xinjiang, Guangdong, Shaanxi, Hebei, Tianjin, Beijing, Heilongjiang	1	Tibet
2007	37	Henan, Jilin, Xinjiang, Guangdong, Shaanxi, Shanxi, Hebei, Tianjin, Heilongjiang	1	Tibet
2008	31	Henan, Jilin, Xinjiang, Guangdong, Shanxi, Heilongjiang	2	Tibet
2009	33	Henan, Jilin, Xinjiang, Guangdong, Guangxi, Shanxi, Heilongjiang	2	Tibet
2010	32	Henan, Jilin, Xinjiang, Guangdong, Guangxi, Inner Mongolia, Shanxi, Heilongjiang, Hebei	3	Tibet, Qinghai
2011	31	Henan, Jilin, Xinjiang, Guangdong, Hubei, Shanxi, Heilongjiang	3	Tibet, Qinghai, Jiangxi
2005–2011	32	Henan, Jilin, Xinjiang, Guangdong, Shaanxi, Shanxi, Hebei, Heilongjiang	3	Tibet, Qinghai

epidemic in these provinces. The northern and central areas reported more infection cases than the rest of regions in China during the study period. There are 11 provinces, municipalities or autonomous regions once had the hotspots located from 2005 to 2011, and the number of hotspots is decreasing by year. The central and border areas were the regions where the hotspots frequently located.

Owing to the poorer economy status, Henan province suffered from paid-blood/plasma donation since 1990s [20]. Although various interventions (voluntary donation, etc.) and blood donation law had been conducted for many years, the huge gap between demand and supplement motivates the blood mostly through employer-organized blood collection. However, the donors may not have been true volunteers, as they may be forced by the employer in some degrees [1]. In addition, the poor economy and low level of health status facilitated HCV infection in this area during the period (2005–2011).

Hotspots were observed in Guangdong province, Guangxi Zhuang Autonomous Region, and Xinjiang Uygur Region in most of 7 years. These provinces located in the heroin trafficking route, which begin from "Golden Triangle" and then go to the southwestern or west provinces in China [15]. The circulation of drug logically brings out some risky behaviors of HCV infection [21], for example, the needles or cottons sharing, which were also the major reasons for HIV infection [22]. The northern hotspots frequently located in Changchun (Jilin province), Harbin (Heilongjiang province), both of two cities are the provincial capitals, which bring together many of medical resources and there were more likely to have clinical infection than other areas. In addition, Yanbian Korean Autonomous prefecture (Jilin province) was another location that a lot of case clustered, nationality and sharing a household with someone who had hepatitis C are contributed to the infection, according to a case-control study [23]. The other cities which did not show hotspots might result from many reasons, for example, the report numbers of these cities were lower and distributed randomly. However, this part of work will be taken in the further researches to understand.

Comparing with the changing status of hotspots, the coldspots were confined to three provinces in this study, Tibet, Qinghai, and Jiangxi. Tibet owned coldspots during 2005 and 2011, and this phenomenon might due to life style and religion of Tibet. Expect for these factors, the poor health system to have enough capacity to detect HCV cases might also be a reason for that.

The large sample size and the use of GIS system for analyzing the geological distribution, hotspots and coldspots of the epidemic, might be considered as the important strengths of this study, however, our study has some limitations like other case-record based studies,

Firstly, our data relied on CISDCP and it has possibility that some provinces may underreport the numbers of infection cases. For example, some cases may have not been identified yet. However, with the rapid development of CISDCP and surveillance system, the influence of this bias in our study is weakened. Second, the number of identified HCV infection cases might be influenced by the intensity of anti-HCV test.

Even with the limitations, this study still demonstrated that there was an upsurge of HCV epidemic in China, and the randomly spatial distribution has not been reported in recent years. Given the rising number of HCV infection case identified, the decreasing number of cities of hotspots and the increasing number of cities of coldspots indicated the specialized intervention strategies and prevention programs which targeting highly epidemic areas seemed to be urgently required in China. Studies exploring the reason of cluster and the correlation between increasing number of cases and cluster might be a good research area for further studies.

Acknowledgments

The authors thank all staff members responsible for HCV case reporting in medical institutes in mainland China, and all participants involving in this project for their efforts.

Author Contributions

Conceived and designed the experiments: Lu Wang JX. Performed the experiments: Lu Wang JX. Analyzed the data: Lu Wang JX. Contributed reagents/materials/analysis tools: Lu Wang JX RY LG QQ Liyan Wang ZD WG NW. Wrote the paper: Lu Wang JX FC.

References

1. Gao XF, Cui Q, Shi X, Su J, Peng ZH, et al. (2011) Prevalence and trend of hepatitis C virus infection among blood donors in Chinese mainland: a systematic review and meta-analysis. BMC Infect Dis 11: 88.
2. Shepard CW, Finelli L, Alter MJ (2005) Global epidemiology of hepatitis C virus infection. Lancet Infect Dis 5: 558–567.
3. World Health Organization (July 2013) Hepatitis C fact sheet. Available: http://www.who.int/mediacentre/factsheets/fs164/en. Accessed 26 March 2014.
4. National Bureau of Statistics of China (2011). China statistical yearbook 2011. Beijing: Statistics Press.
5. Cui Y, Jia JD (2013) Update on epidemiology of hepatitis B and C in China. J Gastroenterol Hepatol 28 Suppl 1: 7–10.
6. Kuang YQ, Yan J, Li Y, Huang X, Wang Y, et al. (2013) Molecular epidemiologic characterization of a clustering HCV infection caused by inappropriate medical care in Heyuan city of Guangdong, China. PLoS One 8: e82304.
7. Li D, Long Y, Wang T, Xiao D, Zhang J, et al. (2013) Epidemiology of hepatitis C virus infection in highly endemic HBV areas in China. PLoS One 8: e54815.
8. Zeng G, Wang Z, Wen S, Jiang J, Wang L, et al. (2005) Geographic distribution, virologic and clinical characteristics of hepatitis B virus genotypes in China. J Viral Hepat 12: 609–617.
9. Lu L, Nakano T, He Y, Fu Y, Hagedorn CH, et al. (2005) Hepatitis C virus genotype distribution in China: predominance of closely related subtype 1b isolates and existence of new genotype 6 variants. J Med Virol 75: 538–549.
10. Xia XS, Lu L, Tee KK, Zhao WH, Wu JG, et al. (2008) The unique HCV genotype distribution and the discovery of a novel subtype 6u among IDUs co-infected with HIV-1 in Yunnan, China. J Med Virol 80: 1142–1152.
11. Wu SQ, Wu FQ, Hong RT, He J (2012) Incidence analyses and space-time cluster detection of hepatitis C in Fujian province of China from 2006 to 2010. PLoS One 7: e40872.
12. Peng ZH, Cheng YJ, Reilly KH, Wang L, Qin QQ, et al. (2011) Spatial distribution of HIV/AIDS in Yunnan province, People's Republic of China. Geospat Health 5: 177–182.
13. Jia ZW, Wang L, Chen RY, Li D, Wang L, et al. (2011) Tracking the evolution of HIV/AIDS in China from 1989–2009 to inform future prevention and control efforts. PLoS One 6: e25671.
14. Chen X, He JM, Ding LS, Zhang GQ, Zou XB, et al. (2013) Prevalence of hepatitis B virus and hepatitis C virus in patients with human immunodeficiency virus infection in Central China. Arch Virol 158: 1889–1894.
15. Beyrer C, Razak MH, Lisam K, Chen J, Lui W, et al. (2000) Overland heroin trafficking routes and HIV-1 spread in south and south-east Asia. AIDS 14: 75–83.
16. Tobler WR (1970) A computer movie simulating urban growth in the Detroit region. Economic geography 46: 234–240.
17. Ord JK, Getis A (1995) Local spatial autocorrelation statistics: distributional issues and an application. Geographical analysis 27: 286–306.
18. Hajarizadeh B, Grebely J, Dore GJ (2013) Epidemiology and natural history of HCV infection. Nat Rev Gastroenterol Hepatol 10: 553–562.
19. Qin QQ, Guo W, Wang LY, Yan RX, Ge L, et al. (2013) Epidemiological characteristics of hepatitis C in China, 1997–2011. Chinese J Epidemiol 34: 548–551, [In Chinese].
20. Tian D, Li L, Liu Y, Li H, Xu X, et al. (2012) Different HCV genotype distributions of HIV-infected individuals in Henan and Guangxi, China. PLoS One 7: e50343.
21. Williams CT, Liu W, Levy JA (2011) Crossing Over: Drug Network Characteristics and injection risk along the China-Myanmar border. AIDS Behav 15: 1011–1016.

17

Modes of Transmission of Influenza B Virus in Households

Benjamin J. Cowling[1]*, Dennis K. M. Ip[1], Vicky J. Fang[1], Piyarat Suntarattiwong[2], Sonja J. Olsen[3,4], Jens Levy[3], Timothy M. Uyeki[4], Gabriel M. Leung[1], J. S. Malik Peiris[1,5], Tawee Chotpitayasunondh[2], Hiroshi Nishiura[6¶], J. Mark Simmerman[7¶]

1 School of Public Health, Li Ka Shing Faculty of Medicine, The University of Hong Kong, Hong Kong Special Administrative Region, China, **2** Queen Sirikit National Institute of Child Health, Bangkok, Thailand, **3** Influenza Program, Thailand MOPH-US CDC Collaboration, Nonthaburi, Thailand, **4** Influenza Division, US Centers for Disease Control and Prevention, Atlanta, Georgia, United States of America, **5** Centre for Influenza Research, Li Ka Shing Faculty of Medicine, The University of Hong Kong, Hong Kong Special Administrative Region, China, **6** Graduate School of Medicine, The University of Tokyo, Bunkyo-ku, Tokyo, Japan, **7** Epidemiology and Medical Affairs, Sanofi Pasteur, Bangkok, Thailand

Abstract

Introduction: While influenza A and B viruses can be transmitted via respiratory droplets, the importance of small droplet nuclei "aerosols" in transmission is controversial.

Methods and Findings: In Hong Kong and Bangkok, in 2008–11, subjects were recruited from outpatient clinics if they had recent onset of acute respiratory illness and none of their household contacts were ill. Following a positive rapid influenza diagnostic test result, subjects were randomly allocated to one of three household-based interventions: hand hygiene, hand hygiene plus face masks, and a control group. Index cases plus their household contacts were followed for 7–10 days to identify secondary infections by reverse transcription polymerase chain reaction (RT-PCR) testing of respiratory specimens. Index cases with RT-PCR-confirmed influenza B were included in the present analyses. We used a mathematical model to make inferences on the modes of transmission, facilitated by apparent differences in clinical presentation of secondary infections resulting from aerosol transmission. We estimated that approximately 37% and 26% of influenza B virus transmission was via the aerosol mode in households in Hong Kong and Bangkok, respectively. In the fitted model, influenza B virus infections were associated with a 56%–72% risk of fever plus cough if infected via aerosol route, and a 23%–31% risk of fever plus cough if infected via the other two modes of transmission.

Conclusions: Aerosol transmission may be an important mode of spread of influenza B virus. The point estimates of aerosol transmission were slightly lower for influenza B virus compared to previously published estimates for influenza A virus in both Hong Kong and Bangkok. Caution should be taken in interpreting these findings because of the multiple assumptions inherent in the model, including that there is limited biological evidence to date supporting a difference in the clinical features of influenza B virus infection by different modes.

Editor: Gerardo Chowell, Arizona State University, United States of America

Funding: This project was supported by the National Institute of Allergy and Infectious Diseases under contract no. HHSN266200700005C, ADB No. N01-AI-70005 (NIAID Centers for Excellence in Influenza Research and Surveillance), the Harvard Center for Communicable Disease Dynamics from the National Institute of General Medical Sciences (grant no. U54 GM088558), and the Area of Excellence Scheme of the Hong Kong University Grants Committee (grant no. AoE/M-12/06). The household trials in Hong Kong and Bangkok were supported by the United States Centers for Disease Control and Prevention (cooperative nos. 1 U01 CI000439 and 5 U51 IP000345). HN received funding support from JST PRESTO. The funding bodies had no role in study design and analysis or the decision to publish, but the CDC was involved in the design of the original studies and the preparation of this manuscript. This work represents the views of the authors and does not reflect the official policy of their institutions, including the Centers for Disease Control and Prevention. The findings and conclusions in this report are those of the authors and do not necessarily represent the official position of the Centers for Disease Control and Prevention.

Competing Interests: BJC has received research funding from MedImmune Inc. and Sanofi Pasteur, and consults for Crucell NV. DKMI has received research funding from F. Hoffmann-La Roche Ltd. JSMP receives research funding from Crucell NV and serves as an ad hoc consultant for GlaxoSmithKline and Sanofi Pasteur. JMS has retired from the US CDC and now works with Sanofi Pasteur.

* Email: bcowling@hku.hk

¶ These authors are joint senior authors on this work.

Introduction

Influenza viruses are believed to be spread between humans through a number of modes of transmission, including primarily through inhalation of respiratory droplets containing infectious virus, and possible contact of respiratory secretions containing infectious virus with mucous membranes. A distinction is sometimes drawn between larger versus smaller respiratory droplets, as large droplets quickly fall to the ground [1,2], while droplet nuclei can remain suspended in the air for prolonged periods because of their low settling velocity [3]. However, aerosols are easily removed from the environment through ventilation, and infectious virus suspended in aerosols could be fragile and easily lose infectivity. The threshold for small particles is typically drawn in the range 5 μm to 20 μm [3–5]. Only a small number of pathogens are thought to transmit via aerosols, including varicella virus, *M. tuberculosis* and rubeola virus (measles) [6]. The potential for influenza virus to spread by aerosols remains controversial [3–5,7,8]. There is growing evidence that influenza A virus can spread by aerosols [3–5,8–10], but less discussion over the potential role of aerosols in influenza B virus transmission with limited published literature. Infectious influenza B virus can be detected in the aerosol fraction (particles <5 μm) of exhaled breath of subjects with influenza B virus infection [11].

Influenza B viruses can infect all age groups. Compared to influenza A viruses, infections with influenza B virus are more commonly identified in children compared to adults [12], perhaps because of slower evolutionary rates [13] leading to greater herd immunity among adults. Influenza B virus infections can cause severe illness in all ages [14], and the mortality impact of influenza B epidemics in populations is generally estimated to be comparable to the impact of influenza A(H1N1) epidemics but somewhat less than influenza A(H3N2) epidemics, with the majority of excess deaths occurring in the very young and very old [15–18].

Historical volunteer challenge studies reported a difference in clinical presentation of influenza A virus infections depending on the mode of infection [9]. In one classic study, 23 people were experimentally inoculated with aerosols, 7 subsequently had serologic evidence of infection and virus was recovered from one additional volunteer without serologic evidence of infection, and 4 of those 8 had typical ILI with fever [19].

In another study, 24 people were inoculated intranasally and had milder illness than people with naturally-acquired illness [20]. In some infectious diseases (e.g. smallpox, plague), the clinical severity is known to depend on the mode of acquisition, and this property has recently been termed 'anisotropic' infection [21]. We previously assumed that influenza A virus also has the anisotropic property, and based on that property, further assuming that hand hygiene and face masks act primarily against contact and large droplet transmission respectively, we estimated that up to 50% of influenza A virus transmission within households in Hong Kong and Bangkok occur via the aerosol route [9]. Here, we propose that the same anisotropic nature may hold for influenza B virus infections, specifically that the mode of exposure leading to an infection may affect the pattern in subsequent signs and symptoms [21], and we use the same modeling framework to infer the proportion of household transmission of influenza B virus that occurs via the aerosol route.

Methods

Sources of Data

During 2008–2011, large randomized controlled trials were conducted in Hong Kong and Bangkok to study the efficacy of hand hygiene and surgical face masks in reducing influenza virus transmission in households [22,23]. In each study, local residents who had acute respiratory illness and living in a household with at least 2 other people of whom none had reported acute respiratory illness in the preceding 14 days were enrolled. Pooled nasal and throat swab (NTS) specimens were collected from each participant for testing with the QuickVue Influenza A+B rapid diagnostic test (Quidel, San Diego, California). Participants with a positive rapid influenza test result were further followed up along with their household contacts. Households were randomly allocated in equal proportions into one of three intervention groups: (1) a control intervention, (2) control plus hand hygiene intervention, and (3)

Table 1. Minor differences between the study designs in Hong Kong and Bangkok.

Study component	Hong Kong	Bangkok
Recruitment locations	45 public and private outpatient clinics across Hong Kong (population 7 million).	Outpatient department of a large pediatric public hospital in Bangkok (population 8 million).
Study period	January 2008–June 2009	April 2008–February 2011
Age of index cases	Any age	Children 1 m to 15 y of age
Eligibility of index case (symptoms)	Presenting with at least two of: fever ≥37.8°C, cough, sore throat, headache, runny nose, phlegm, and myalgia; living with at least two other people.	For <2 years: fever >38°C *and* one or more of the following symptoms; nasal congestion, cough, conjunctivitis, respiratory distress, sore throat, new seizure. For >2 years: Presenting with influenza-like illness (fever plus cough or sore throat); living with at least two other people.
Exclusion criteria	Recent (within 14 d) acute respiratory illness in any household member	Recent (within 7 d) influenza-like illness in any household member; recent (within 12 m) influenza vaccination in any household member.
Hand hygiene intervention	Distribution of alcohol hand rub to each household member in addition to liquid hand soap to the household	Distribution of liquid hand soap to the household
Measurement of body temperature	All households were provided and instructed in the use of a free tympanic thermometer and asked to record their body temperature daily.	Thermometers were not provided to households, and participants recorded either measured body temperature or 'feverishness'.

Table 2. Characteristics of index cases with confirmed influenza B virus infection and their household contacts in Hong Kong, by intervention group.

	Control		Hand hygiene		Face mask+hand hygiene	
Characteristics	**n**	**(%)**	**n**	**(%)**	**n**	**(%)**
Index cases	*35*		*36*		*33*	
Age group						
≤5 y	5	(14%)	3	(8%)	4	(12%)
6–15 y	25	(71%)	21	(58%)	21	(64%)
>16 y	5	(14%)	12	(33%)	8	(24%)
Male	16	(46%)	19	(53%)	10	(30%)
Median household size (IQR)	4	(3, 5)	4	(3, 4)	4	(3, 5)
Household contacts	*112*		*101*		*106*	
Age group						
≤5 y	6	(5%)	1	(1%)	5	(5%)
6–15 y	13	(12%)	12	(12%)	12	(11%)
16–30 y	21	(19%)	17	(17%)	17	(16%)
31–50 y	58	(52%)	48	(48%)	51	(48%)
>50 y	14	(12%)	23	(23%)	21	(20%)
Male	39	(35%)	40	(40%)	46	(43%)
Received seasonal influenza vaccination in the previous 12 m	15	(13%)	12	(12%)	14	(13%)

control plus facemasks and hand hygiene interventions. A home visit was scheduled as soon as possible after randomization to implement the intervention, collect baseline demographic data and NTS specimens from all household contacts aged ≥2 years, and to describe the information to be recorded in daily symptom diaries. Further home visits were scheduled at 3 and 6 days after the first home visit to monitor adherence to intervention and to collect further NTS specimens from all household contacts regardless of illness. The two study protocols were very similar, and notable differences are summarized in Table 1.

All NTS specimens were tested by reverse-transcription polymerase chain reaction (RT-PCR) for influenza A and B

Table 3. Characteristics of index cases with confirmed influenza B virus infection and their household contacts in Bangkok, by intervention group.

	Control		Hand hygiene		Face mask+hand hygiene	
Characteristics	**n**	**(%)**	**n**	**(%)**	**n**	**(%)**
Index cases	*37*		*38*		*38*	
Age group						
≤5 y	12	(32%)	14	(37%)	10	(26%)
6–15 y	25	(68%)	24	(63%)	28	(74%)
>16 y	0	(0%)	0	(0%)	0	(0%)
Male	24	(65%)	23	(61%)	23	(61%)
Median household size (IQR)	2	(2, 3)	3	(2, 3)	3	(2, 5)
Household contacts	*84*		*91*		*89*	
Age group						
≤5 y	1	(1%)	5	(5%)	4	(4%)
6–15 y	10	(12%)	14	(15%)	10	(11%)
16–30 y	13	(15%)	18	(20%)	15	(17%)
31–50 y	49	(58%)	41	(45%)	37	(42%)
>50 y	11	(13%)	13	(14%)	23	(26%)
Male	35	(42%)	39	(43%)	33	(37%)
Received seasonal influenza vaccination in the previous 12 m	0	(0%)	0	(0%)	0	(0%)

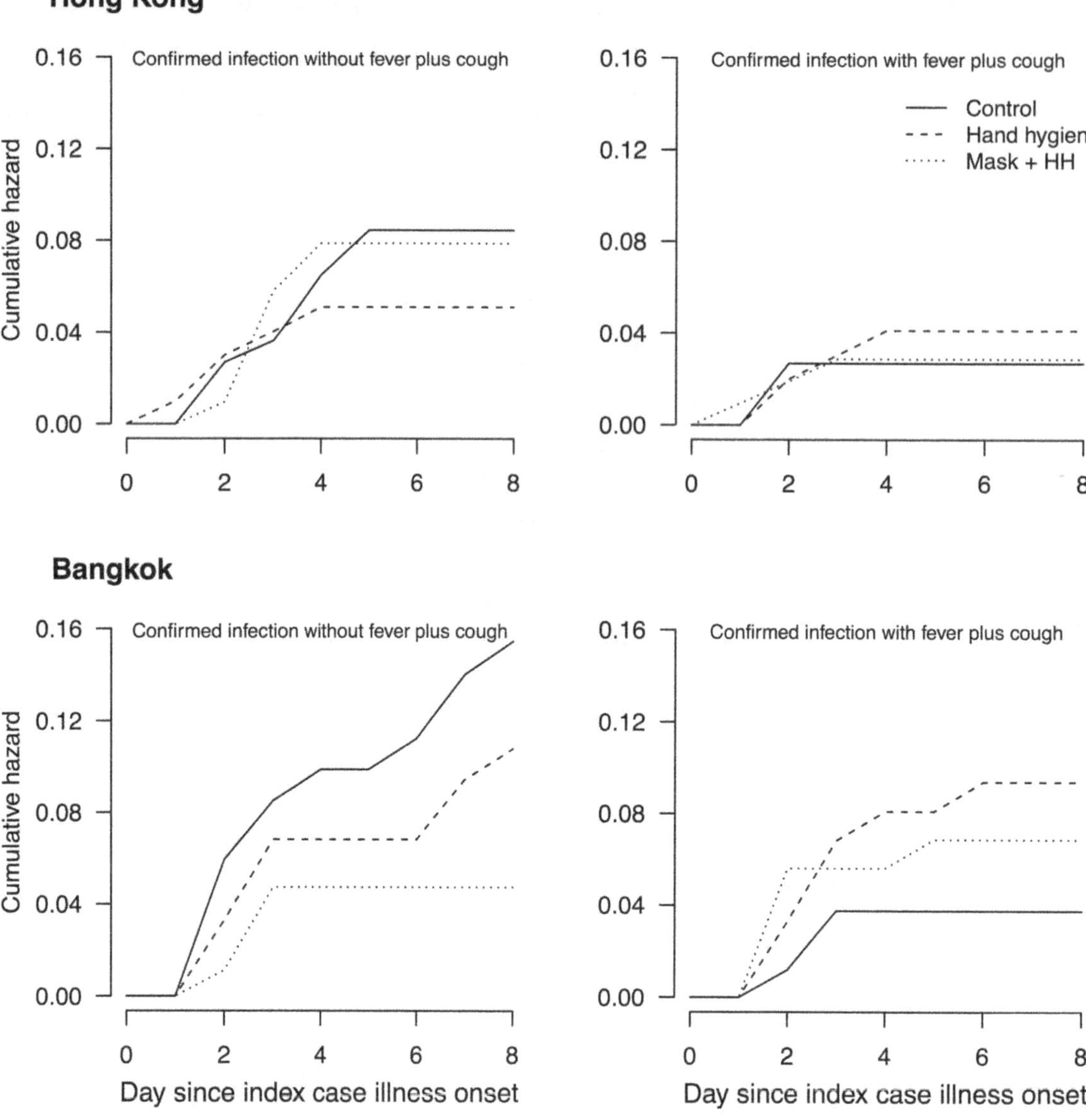

Figure 1. Cumulative hazards of RT-PCR-confirmed influenza B virus infections presenting with fever plus cough or not presenting with fever plus cough, among the household contacts in 104 and 113 households of index cases with RT-PCR-confirmed influenza B virus infection in Hong Kong and Bangkok, respectively.

viruses using standard methods as described elsewhere [22,23]. In the present analyses only the households of index cases with RT-PCR-confirmed influenza B virus infection are included; results for index cases with influenza A were reported elsewhere [9].

In the present analyses, we used data on influenza B virus transmission in families from the studies in Hong Kong and Bangkok. Specifically, we identified all index cases with confirmed influenza B virus infection, and their household contacts. We then determined which household contacts had RT-PCR confirmed infection, the corresponding times of illness onset, and whether fever and cough were reported. In the analyses we also used the allocated intervention group for each household, and the age of each household contact.

Ethics Statement

All subjects 18 years of age and older gave written informed consent, and proxy written consent was obtained from parents or legal guardians for children aged 17 years old or younger. The protocols for the studies in Hong Kong and in Bangkok were approved by Institutional Review Board of the University of Hong Kong, and the Institutional Review Board of Queen Sirikit Hospital Bangkok, respectively [22,23].

Statistical Analysis

We used the Nelson-Aalen non-parametric estimator of the cumulative hazards of infection with or without febrile disease plus cough in each intervention group [24]. We constructed a competing risks survival analysis model that accounted for the alternative modes of transmission and used it to infer the relative importance of alternative modes of transmission assuming that the risk of fever plus cough higher in aerosol transmission, compared with the other two modes. We assumed independent hazards over time of influenza transmission in households with one or more secondary cases. The cause-specific probability of aerosol trans-

Table 4. Point estimates and 95% credible intervals of model parameters under an exemplar plausible scenario that hand hygiene and surgical face masks reduced contact and droplet transmission respectively by 50% from the time of application of those interventions.

	Hong Kong (104 households with 319 contacts)		Bangkok (113 households with 264 contacts)	
Parameters	**Estimate**	**(95% CI)**	**Estimate**	**(95% CI)**
ϑ Shape of the Weibull distribution	2.16	(1.30, 3.12)	0.77	(0.39, 1.28)
λ_1 Force of contact transmission*	0.18	(0.01, 0.40)	0.16	(0.01, 0.48)
λ_2 Force of droplet transmission*	0.20	(0.01, 0.40)	0.07	(0.00, 0.24)
λ_3 Force of aerosol transmission*	0.22	(0.02, 0.38)	0.08	(0.00, 0.25)
π_1 Risk of fever plus cough for infections by contact route	23%	(1%, 66%)	25%	(1%, 63%)
π_2 Risk of fever plus cough for infections by droplet route	24%	(1%, 60%)	31%	(2%, 75%)
π_3 Risk of fever plus cough for infections by aerosol route	56%	(26%, 97%)	72%	(41%, 99%)
θ_1 Proportion of household adults immune or not exposed	90%	(85%, 94%)	65%	(45%, 79%)
θ_2 Proportion of household children immune or not exposed	69%	(54%, 82%)	61%	(34%, 82%)

*The forces of infection in combination with a shared shape parameter determine the hazard associated with each competing mode of transmission. The relative contribution of each mode *j* is calculated as the cause-specific probabilities $\lambda_j^{\phi}/\left(\lambda_1^{\phi}+\lambda_2^{\phi}+\lambda_3^{\phi}\right)$.

mission was estimated to measure the relative contribution of aerosol transmission among all three modes.

A mixture model was used to allow for a certain proportion (θ) of subjects to be immune or not exposed, with the density of infection described as $f(t)=(1-\theta)f_u(t)$, where $f_u(t)$ is the probability density function for the exposed and susceptible group. The time to infection (T) for each of three modes of transmission was assumed to follow a Weibull distribution with an identical shared shape parameter (ϕ) and mode-specific scale parameters (λ_j). The sub-hazards for modes of transmission, $j=1$, 2 and 3 representing contact, large droplets and aerosols respectively were written as follows:

$$h_{u1}(T_i,X_{hi},X_{mi})=\phi\lambda_1^{\phi}T_i^{\phi-1}\exp(\beta_1X_{hi}),\qquad where\ \beta_1=\log(1-r_1);$$
$$h_{u2}(T_i,X_{hi},X_{mi})=\phi\lambda_2^{\phi}T_i^{\phi-1}\exp(\beta_2X_{mi}),\qquad where\ \beta_2=\log(1-r_2);$$
$$h_{u3}(T_i,X_{hi},X_{mi})=\phi\lambda_3^{\phi}T_i^{\phi-1},$$

where X_{hi}/X_{mi} are the dichotomous indicator variables representing the allocation of hand hygiene/surgical mask interventions respectively to individual i, and r_1/r_2 represent the relative risk reductions in contact/large droplet transmission by hand hygiene/surgical masks respectively. We assumed that the risk of fever plus cough caused by infections follows a Bernoulli distribution with mean parameter π_j, $j=1$, 2, 3 for three arms, respectively. We estimated $\phi,\lambda_1,\lambda_2,\lambda_3,\pi_1,\pi_2,\pi_3,\theta_1,\theta_2$. We were unable to estimate r_1 and r_2 so we examined the estimates of the other parameters for a range of values of r_1 and r_2. Further technical details of the model are provided in an earlier publication [9].

We performed statistical inference under a Bayesian framework, using Markov chain Monte Carlo (MCMC) to obtain parameter estimates from the posterior distributions [25]. We specified flat priors for each parameter. For each MCMC chain we ran 120,000 iterations, discarding the first 20,000 iterations as burn-in, and drawing every tenth subsequent value to compose the posterior distribution. All the statistical analyses were conducted in R version 2.15.1 (R Foundation for Statistical Computing, Vienna, Austria).

Results

In Hong Kong and Bangkok there were 104 and 113 households, respectively, with an index case with RT-PCR-confirmed influenza B virus infection. The characteristics of index cases and their household contacts are shown in Tables 2 and 3 for Hong Kong and Bangkok respectively. We examined the cumulative hazard of RT-PCR-confirmed influenza B virus infections for household contacts, and found increases in the risk of infection with fever plus cough, and decreases in the risk of infection without fever plus cough, in the intervention arms compared to the control arm. The change was particularly apparent in the households in Bangkok (Figure 1). To be more specific, we found a statistically significant decrease in the risk of infection without fever plus cough, in the hand hygiene plus face masks arm compared to the control arm in the households in Bangkok.

Under the scenario where randomization to the hand hygiene intervention reduced contact transmission by 50% while randomization to face mask and hand hygiene interventions reduced both contact and droplet transmission by 50%, we fitted the transmission model to the Hong Kong and Bangkok data. We estimated that in the absence of interventions, aerosol transmission was responsible for 37% and 26% of secondary infections in Hong Kong and Bangkok, respectively (Table 4). We also varied the assumed efficacy of hand hygiene and face masks from 0% to 100% and estimated the relative importance of aerosol transmission in the absence of interventions, which ranged from approximately 20% to 80% in Hong Kong and 20% to 32% in Bangkok (Figure 2).

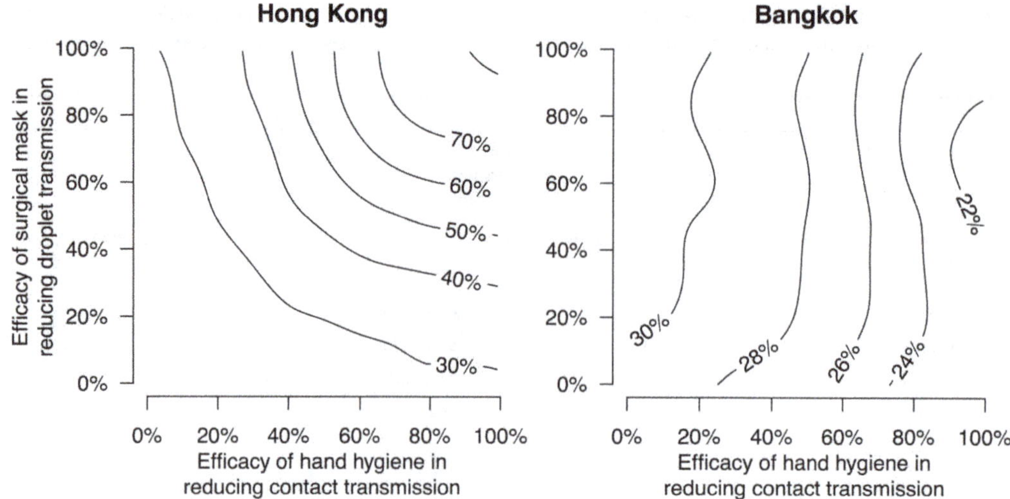

Figure 2. The relative importance (cause-specific probability) of aerosol transmission in households in Hong Kong and Bangkok. The contour lines show the proportion of secondary influenza B virus infections attributed to aerosol transmission in the control arm of each study, under varying assumptions about the efficacy of randomization to the hand hygiene and surgical mask interventions in reducing contact (x-axis) and droplet (y-axis) transmission respectively.

We compared the cause-specific probabilities of each mode of transmission as well as the associated illnesses in the control arm for influenza A and B virus infections, in Hong Kong and Bangkok respectively (Figure 3). Data for influenza A were extracted from a previous report [9]. Both influenza A and B virus infections attributed to aerosol transmission were associated with a higher risk of fever plus cough, compared with the other two modes of transmission. The point estimates of aerosol transmission were lower for influenza B compared to influenza A in both Hong Kong and Bangkok.

Discussion

We propose that the mode of spread associated with an influenza B virus infection affects the probability of experiencing fever plus cough for that infection. Based on that hypothesis, we estimated that approximately 37% and 26% of transmission was via the aerosol mode in households in Hong Kong and Bangkok, respectively. However, we should exercise caution in interpreting these findings because we have not been able to find literature supporting the anisotropic nature of influenza B virus infection, whereas we previously described literature supporting this

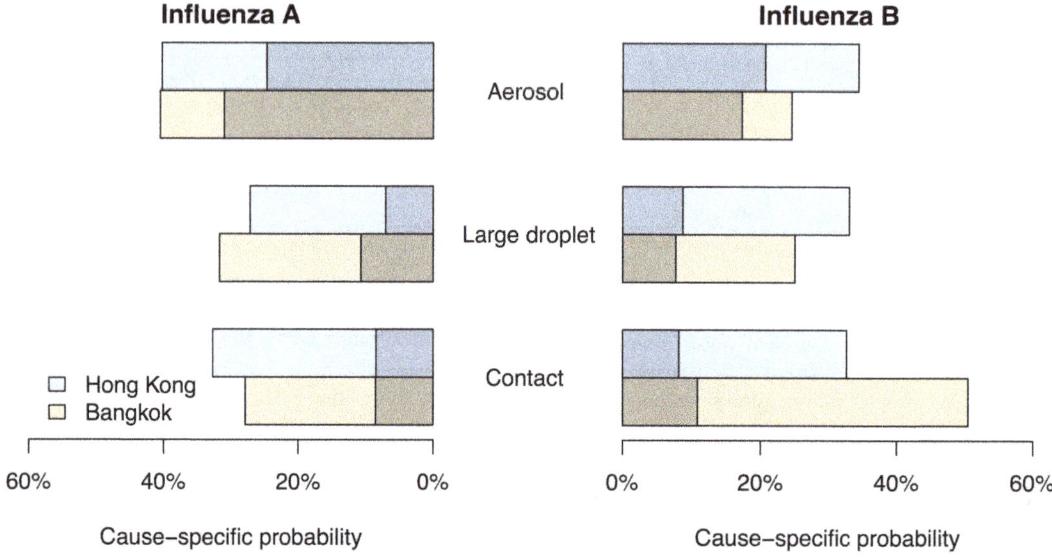

Figure 3. The proportion of all influenza A and B virus infections attributed to each mode in the control arms of the studies in Hong Kong (blue) and Bangkok (brown), and the infections associated with fever plus cough (darker shade) or not associated with fever plus cough (lighter shade). Data shown on influenza A were extracted from a previous study [9]. The contributions of the three modes sum to 100% within each geographic location and influenza type.

property for influenza A virus infections [9]. Nevertheless, patterns in secondary infections and disease in the controlled trials in Hong Kong and Bangkok were consistent with this hypothesis (Figure 1). This also implicitly suggested that though hand hygiene and face masks could reduce the risk of transmission through contact or large droplets, but meanwhile increase the risk of aerosol transmission, which was associated with a greater risk of illness with fever plus cough.

Whereas we previously estimated that approximately half of within-household transmission of influenza A virus could be associated with aerosols [9], here we estimated a slightly reduced importance of aerosols for influenza B virus (Figure 3). One explanation for such a difference could be the age mix of cases of influenza A versus B, if aerosol transmission were more important among adults than children. We did not have sufficient sample size in the present study to examine whether modes of transmission might vary by age, but this would be an interesting area for further exploration.

If aerosol transmission is indeed an important mode of spread of influenza B virus, this may have important implications for control efforts. In particular measures targeting contact transmission, such as hand hygiene, and measures targeting large respiratory droplet transmission, such as surgical face masks, may not be sufficient to substantially reduce the risk of transmission. Control measures that might reduce aerosol transmission indoors include improvement in ventilation [26], modification of humidity [27], or the use of personal protective equipment that is more effective against aerosols than surgical masks. While the use of N95 respirators may not be practical in community settings and fit-testing is unlikely although required for optimal performance, other types of face masks with improved filtration compared to standard surgical masks or procedure masks may be available in the future.

There are a number of limitations to our analysis. First, our model did not include the possibility of variability in infectiousness between index cases, variability in immunity to different modes of transmission, or variability in within-household transmissibility associated with physical dimensions of the home, ventilation rates etc, and inclusion of these or other factors potentially affecting transmission dynamics could be natural extensions to our model. Because interventions were allocated randomly among households, the possibility of confounding should be minimized. Second, our model implicitly assumes that only the first infectious exposure is relevant to susceptible contacts, and once infected by that first exposure, further exposures are unimportant. Our model could be modified to allow for multiple simultaneous exposures by one or more modes, if it were understood how this might affect the course of disease. Third, while we assumed that all infections of household contacts during the 7-day follow-up were acquired within the household, it is possible that some infections were acquired outside. However in a separate study with a similar design in Hong Kong we used molecular epidemiology analyses of virus sequence data to demonstrate that most secondary influenza cases acquired infection from within the household [28], and a similar observation was reported in a household transmission study in Canada [29]. Fourth, it is possible that some secondary influenza virus infections were not confirmed due to poor quality specimens collected during home visits, or if peak influenza B viral shedding in the respiratory tract occurred between home visits at 3-day intervals. We did include serological data although this could have provided additional information on infections among household contacts. Fifth, by recruiting in outpatient clinics and using a rapid test to screen index cases, we may have introduced selection bias towards index cases with more serious illness or higher levels of virus shedding, affecting the relative importance of different modes of transmission. Finally, we did not explicitly account for imperfect adherence to the interventions, although the parameters in our model account for moderate efficacy of interventions against specific modes of transmission. Further improvements in the model might be obtained by incorporating limited data on adherence that was mainly self-reported by participants.

In conclusion, we propose that the aerosol route may be an important mode of transmission of influenza B virus in households. Further studies of non-pharmaceutical interventions in households would be improved by more careful monitoring of viral contamination on surfaces [30,31] and in the air, and inclusion of this information in transmission models.

Acknowledgments

We thank Mark Dworkin, Heath Kelly, Yuguo Li, Marc Lipsitch, Don Milton, Jeffrey Shaman, Joe Wu, Peng Wu and Hui-Ling Yen for helpful discussions. We thank Lincoln Lau and Nancy Leung for technical assistance. We thank Rita Fung, Hau Chi So, Calvin Cheng, Winnie Wai, Joey Sin, Wing Hong Seto, Raymond Yung, Daniel Chu, Billy Chiu, Paco Lee, Ming Chi Chiu, Hoi Che Lee and Peter Houck for assistance with the Hong Kong trial and Suchada Kaewchana, Robert Gibbons, Richard Jarman, Wiwan Sanasuttipun, Susan Maloney, and Laurie Kamimoto for assistance with the Bangkok trial.

Author Contributions

Conceived and designed the experiments: BJC DKMI VJF HN. Analyzed the data: BJC VJF HN. Contributed to the writing of the manuscript: BJC DKMI VJF PS SJO JL TMU GML JSMP TC HN JMS. Interpreted data: PS SJO JL TMU GML JSMP TC JMS.

References

1. Gralton J, Tovey E, McLaws ML, Rawlinson WD (2011) The role of particle size in aerosolised pathogen transmission: a review. J Infect 62: 1–13.
2. Xie X, Li Y, Chwang AT, Ho PL, Seto WH (2007) How far droplets can move in indoor environments–revisiting the Wells evaporation-falling curve. Indoor Air 17: 211–225.
3. Tellier R (2006) Review of aerosol transmission of influenza A virus. Emerg Infect Dis 12: 1657–1662.
4. Weber TP, Stilianakis NI (2008) Inactivation of influenza A viruses in the environment and modes of transmission: a critical review. J Infect 57: 361–373.
5. Tellier R (2009) Aerosol transmission of influenza A virus: a review of new studies. J R Soc Interface 6 Suppl 6: S783–790.
6. Tang JW, Li Y, Eames I, Chan PK, Ridgway GL (2006) Factors involved in the aerosol transmission of infection and control of ventilation in healthcare premises. J Hosp Infect 64: 100–114.
7. Brankston G, Gitterman L, Hirji Z, Lemieux C, Gardam M (2007) Transmission of influenza A in human beings. Lancet Infect Dis 7: 257–265.
8. Cowling BJ (2012) Airborne transmission of influenza: implications for control in healthcare and community settings. Clinical infectious diseases 54: 1578–1580.
9. Cowling BJ, Ip DK, Fang VJ, Suntarattiwong P, Olsen SJ, et al. (2013) Aerosol transmission is an important mode of influenza A virus spread. Nat Commun 4: 1935.
10. Noti JD, Lindsley WG, Blachere FM, Cao G, Kashon ML, et al. (2012) Detection of infectious influenza virus in cough aerosols generated in a simulated patient examination room. Clin Infect Dis 54: 1569–1577.
11. Milton DK, Fabian MP, Cowling BJ, Grantham ML, McDevitt JJ (2013) Influenza virus aerosols in human exhaled breath: particle size, culturability, and effect of surgical masks. PLoS Pathog 9: e1003205.
12. Monto AS, Sullivan KM (1993) Acute respiratory illness in the community. Frequency of illness and the agents involved. Epidemiol Infect 110: 145–160.
13. Air GM, Gibbs AJ, Laver WG, Webster RG (1990) Evolutionary changes in influenza B are not primarily governed by antibody selection. Proc Natl Acad Sci U S A 87: 3884–3888.
14. Chan PK, Chan MC, Cheung JL, Lee N, Leung TF, et al. (2013) Influenza B lineage circulation and hospitalization rates in a subtropical city, Hong Kong, 2000–2010. Clin Infect Dis 56: 677–684.

15. Thompson WW, Shay DK, Weintraub E, Brammer L, Cox N, et al. (2003) Mortality associated with influenza and respiratory syncytial virus in the United States. JAMA 289: 179–186.
16. Goldstein E, Viboud C, Charu V, Lipsitch M (2012) Improving the estimation of influenza-related mortality over a seasonal baseline. Epidemiology 23: 829–838.
17. Wu P, Goldstein E, Ho LM, Yang L, Nishiura H, et al. (2012) Excess mortality associated with influenza A and B virus in Hong Kong, 1998–2009. Journal of Infectious Diseases 206: 1862–1871.
18. Simmerman JM, Chittaganpitch M, Levy J, Chantra S, Maloney S, et al. (2009) Incidence, seasonality and mortality associated with influenza pneumonia in Thailand: 2005–2008. PLoS One 4: e7776.
19. Alford RH, Kasel JA, Gerone PJ, Knight V (1966) Human influenza resulting from aerosol inhalation. Proc Soc Exp Biol Med 122: 800–804.
20. Little JW, Douglas RG, Jr., Hall WJ, Roth FK (1979) Attenuated influenza produced by experimental intranasal inoculation. J Med Virol 3: 177–188.
21. Milton DK (2012) What was the primary mode of smallpox transmission? Implications for biodefense. Front Cell Infect Microbiol 2: 150.
22. Cowling BJ, Chan KH, Fang VJ, Cheng CK, Fung RO, et al. (2009) Facemasks and hand hygiene to prevent influenza transmission in households: a randomized trial. Annals of Internal Medicine 151: 437–446.
23. Simmerman JM, Suntarattiwong P, Levy J, Jarman RG, Kaewchana S, et al. (2011) Findings from a household randomized controlled trial of hand washing and face masks to reduce influenza transmission in Bangkok, Thailand. Influenza and Other Respiratory Viruses 5: 256–267.
24. Aalen OO (1978) Nonparametric inference for a family of counting processes. Annals of Statistics 6: 701–726.
25. Gilks WR, Richardson S, Spiegelhalter DJ (1996) Markov Chain Monte Carlo in Practice. Boca Raton: Chapman & Hall/CRC.
26. Hobday RA, Dancer SJ (2013) Roles of sunlight and natural ventilation for controlling infection: historical and current perspectives. J Hosp Infect 84: 271–282.
27. Tamerius JD, Shaman J, Alonso WJ, Bloom-Feshbach K, Uejio CK, et al. (2013) Environmental predictors of seasonal influenza epidemics across temperate and tropical climates. PLoS Pathog 9: e1003194.
28. Poon LL, Chan KH, Chu DK, Fung CC, Cheng CK, et al. (2011) Viral genetic sequence variations in pandemic H1N1/2009 and seasonal H3N2 influenza viruses within an individual, a household and a community. J Clin Virol 52: 146–150.
29. Papenburg J, Baz M, Hamelin ME, Rheaume C, Carbonneau J, et al. (2010) Household transmission of the 2009 pandemic A/H1N1 influenza virus: elevated laboratory-confirmed secondary attack rates and evidence of asymptomatic infections. Clin Infect Dis 51: 1033–1041.
30. Simmerman JM, Suntarattiwong P, Levy J, Gibbons RV, Cruz C, et al. (2010) Influenza virus contamination of common household surfaces during the 2009 influenza A (H1N1) pandemic in Bangkok, Thailand: implications for contact transmission. Clin Infect Dis 51: 1053–1061.
31. Levy JW, Suntarattiwong P, Simmerman JM, Jarman RG, Johnson K, et al. (2014) Increased hand washing reduces influenza virus surface contamination in Bangkok households, 2009–2010. Influenza Other Respir Viruses 8: 13–16.

18

Comorbidities and Disease Severity as Risk Factors for Carbapenem-Resistant *Klebsiella pneumoniae* Colonization: Report of an Experience in an Internal Medicine Unit

Antonio Nouvenne[1,2]*, Andrea Ticinesi[1,2], Fulvio Lauretani[3], Marcello Maggio[2], Giuseppe Lippi[4], Loredana Guida[1], Ilaria Morelli[1], Erminia Ridolo[1,2], Loris Borghi[1,2], Tiziana Meschi[1,2]

1 Internal Medicine and Critical Subacute Care Unit, Parma University Hospital, Parma, Italy, **2** Department of Clinical and Experimental Medicine, University of Parma, Parma, Italy, **3** Geriatrics Unit, Parma University Hospital, Parma, Italy, **4** Laboratory of Clinical Chemistry and Hematology, Parma University Hospital, Parma, Italy

Abstract

Background: Carbapenem-resistant *Klebsiella pneumoniae* (CRKP) is an emerging multidrug-resistant nosocomial pathogen, spreading to hospitalized elderly patients. Risk factors in this setting are unclear. Our aims were to explore the contribution of multi-morbidity and disease severity in the onset of CRKP colonization/infection, and to describe changes in epidemiology after the institution of quarantine-ward managed by staff-cohorting.

Methods and Findings: With a case-control design, we evaluated 133 CRKP-positive patients (75 M, 58 F; mean age 79±10 years) and a control group of 400 CRKP-negative subjects (179 M, 221 F; mean age 79±12 years) admitted to Internal Medicine and Critical Subacute Care Unit of Parma University Hospital, Italy, during a 10-month period. Information about comorbidity type and severity, expressed through Cumulative Illness Rating Scale-CIRS, was collected in each patient. During an overall 5-month period, CRKP-positive patients were managed in an isolation ward with staff cohorting. A contact-bed isolation approach was established in the other 5 months. The effects of these strategies were evaluated with a cross-sectional study design. CRKP-positive subjects had higher CIRS comorbidity index (12.0±3.6 vs 9.1±3.5, $p<0.0001$) and CIRS severity index (3.2±0.4 vs 2.9±0.5, $p<0.0001$), along with higher cardiovascular, respiratory, renal and neurological disease burden than control group. CIRS severity index was associated with a higher risk for CRKP-colonization (OR 13.3, 95%CI6.88–25.93), independent of comorbidities. Isolation ward activation was associated with decreased monthly incidence of CRKP-positivity (from 16.9% to 1.2% of all admissions) and infection (from 36.6% to 22.5% of all positive cases; $p=0.04$ derived by Wilcoxon signed-rank test). Mortality rate did not differ between cases and controls (21.8% vs 15.2%, $p=0.08$). The main limitations of this study are observational design and lack of data about prior antibiotic exposure.

Conclusions: Comorbidities and disease severity are relevant risk factors for CRKP-colonization/infection in elderly frail patients. Sanitary measures may have contributed to limit epidemic spread and rate of infection also in internal medicine setting.

Editor: Hiroshi Nishiura, The University of Tokyo, Japan

Funding: The authors have no support or funding to report.

Competing Interests: The authors have declared that no competing interests exist.

* Email: antonio.nouvenne@alice.it

Introduction

In the era of antibiotic resistance and multi-drug resistant bacteria, the emergence and spread of carbapenem-resistant *Klebsiella pneumoniae* (CRKP), also known as carbapenemase-producing *Klebsiella pneumoniae*, has rapidly become a major health concern for hospitalized patients in industrialized countries [1]. Carbapenemases are β-lactamases that can hydrolyze carbapenems. Their outbreak in clinical isolates of Gram negative bacteria has been appreciated since the late 1990 s, with an increasing number of carbapenem-affine types identified ever since [2–3]. *Klebsiella pneumoniae* is the most frequent bacterial species associated with production of high-affinity carbapenemases. Their genes typically reside on transferable plasmids and are conventionally known as KPC. The first in vivo isolation of a CRKP strain dates back to 2000 in an intensive care unit of North Carolina [4]. During the following years, CRKP has been responsible of a large number of nosocomial outbreaks in many hospitals of Northeastern United States, causing a large number of deaths due to septic shock [5]. CRKP had reached all developed countries worldwide by the end of the 2000 s. In Europe, CRKP has an heterogeneous distribution, with some countries such as Poland and Greece, where CRKP infection is currently considered as endemic, and others such as Sweden and Portugal, where only few sporadic cases have been identified [6]. The first Italian CRKP isolation was recorded in Florence in 2009 in a patient with complicated intra-abdominal infection [7]. Since then, CRKP has rapidly spread throughout the country. This explains why Italy, that was classified only a few years ago as a nation with sporadic isolations, has been recently upgraded to an endemic country [6,8]. Moreover, recent national data showed that CRKP is more frequently isolated from patients outside intensive care units (ICU), often admitted to geriatric or internal medicine wards [9–11].

CRKP is generally transmitted by contact and primarily colonizes lower intestinal tract and inguinal or perineal skin, so that active microbiological screening is regarded as an effective measure to prevent the onset of infection [12]. The main risk factors for colonization or infection identified in literature are critical illness and chronic diseases such as respiratory failure, prior antibiotic therapy and prior hospitalization [13–15]. When the infection occurs, it is generally associated with a bloodstream bacteremia followed by quick development of septic shock. Blood culture isolation of CRKP is an independent predictor of death, and the overall mortality ranges from 41% to 80% despite the establishment of appropriate antibiotic therapy [16–18]. Therapeutic options are indeed very limited, and include aminoglycosides, tigecycline, colistin, fosfomycin or even carbapenems themselves, when the minimal inhibitory concentrations (MICs) are ≤4 mg/L [19–21].

Few studies have investigated the characteristics of CRKP outbreaks in populations of elderly frail hospitalized patients with multi-morbidity. However, the quick spread of this pathogen in general internal medicine and geriatric wards around the globe may suggest that chronic diseases could play a major role as risk factors.

Aims

We carried out a case-control study to explore the contribution of multi-morbidity and disease severity, measured through literature-validated indexes, in the onset of CRKP colonization/infection in a population of hospitalized, elderly and frail patients. With a cross-sectional study design, we have then described the changes in CRKP epidemic trend and rate of infection occurred after the institution of special sanitary measures, namely quarantine ward with staff cohorting management.

Setting and Methods

The University Hospital of Parma, Italy, is a 1218-bed tertiary referral facility with approximately 51300 admissions per year. From August 2011 to May 2012, it has been the scenario of a pandemic outbreak of CRKP colonization and infection. This phenomenon especially involved older patients admitted to general internal medicine units. In order to limit the diffusion of CRKP, Healthcare Hospital Direction arranged an immediate transfer of all patients with a CRKP positivity to Internal Medicine and Critical Subacute Care Unit. This unit, a 94-bed large internal medicine area, split in smaller wards and organized by intensity of care, is mainly dedicated to the care of elderly frail patients.

All CRKP-positive patients were managed by contact isolation precautions. They received antibiotic therapy only in the presence of clinical or laboratory signs of infection. Colonized patients with no signs of infection were not treated.

Following the recommendations issued by Italian Health Ministry and Emilia-Romagna Region Health Authority [22], all high-risk patients admitted to our unit and all patients with clinical signs of infection underwent an active microbiological surveillance program consisting of a weekly rectal swab for CRKP detection. A patient was considered at high risk of CRKP infection if he/she had been transferred from another hospital or from a community nursing home, hospitalized in the previous 60 days, transferred from an intensive care unit, in contact (i.e., in the same room) with a CRKP-positive patient or completely bedridden for at least 3 days. In case of clinical signs of infection, other microbiological tests, such as blood or urine culture, were prescribed whenever appropriate and according to the clinical characteristics of each patient. Surveillance was continued until the patient was discharged or had 3 consecutive rectal swabs negative for CRKP detection.

Moreover, given the high number of CRKP-positive patients, from October 2011 (two months after the beginning of the outbreak) to February 2012, under the indication of Healthcare Hospital Direction, a 14-bed isolation ward with a staff-cohorting management was activated. This ward was reserved only to CRKP-positive patients with dedicated health care professionals that could not come to contact with other CRKP-negative patients. A simple model validated in the literature and already used to control multi-drug resistant infection outbreaks was used [23–24]. This 14-bed isolation ward was closed at the end of February 2012, since its maintenance was considered no longer cost-effective by Healthcare Hospital Direction, due to the rapid and consistent decrease of new cases of CRKP positivity. Colonized or infected patients admitted thereafter were only managed by contact isolation precautions until the end of the observation period. Active microbiological surveillance was continued throughout the study period, regardless of the management by staff cohorting or contact isolation.

To assess whether comorbidity number and severity is a risk factor for CRKP colonization/infection, we carried out a case-control study (Figure 1). We reviewed all clinical records of patients admitted to our unit from August 2011 to May 2012 (1897 subjects) to check CRKP status. CRKP positivity was defined as the presence of at least one biological sample positive for CRKP. All patients admitted to our unit who failed to meet the requirements for epidemiological surveillance program or who had microbiological analysis (i.e., all rectal swabs) negative for CRKP were considered as CRKP-negative. For the study purposes, all consecutive CRKP-positive patients (133 subjects) who were identified during the study period were considered as cases. We also randomly selected 400 clinical records of CRKP-negative patients and considered them as controls.

Moreover, subjects in whom CRKP was isolated only in rectal swabs performed for epidemiological surveillance reasons and with other biological samples resulted negative for CRKP, were considered as CRKP-colonized. Subjects who had clinical signs of infection and at least one biological sample, other than rectal swab, positive for CRKP were considered as CRKP-infected, irrespective of their rectal swab status.

In both cases and controls, a well-trained physician recorded age, primary diagnosis, type and severity of comorbidities according to the Cumulative Illness Rating Scale (CIRS) score [25], overall hospital length of stay, biological sample of CRKP isolation and genotypic characteristics when available, possible clinical signs of CRKP infection and final outcome (discharge or death).

To describe changes in epidemiologic trend after the institution of the staff cohorting quarantine ward, we also carried out a cross-sectional study (Figure 1). We considered only CRKP-positive patients, classified as colonized or infected according to the above criteria. Incidence of CRKP-positivity was calculated as the number of newly diagnosed cases per month related to the overall number of admissions in the same month. Outbreak control was defined as a persistent decline or stability in the trend of monthly

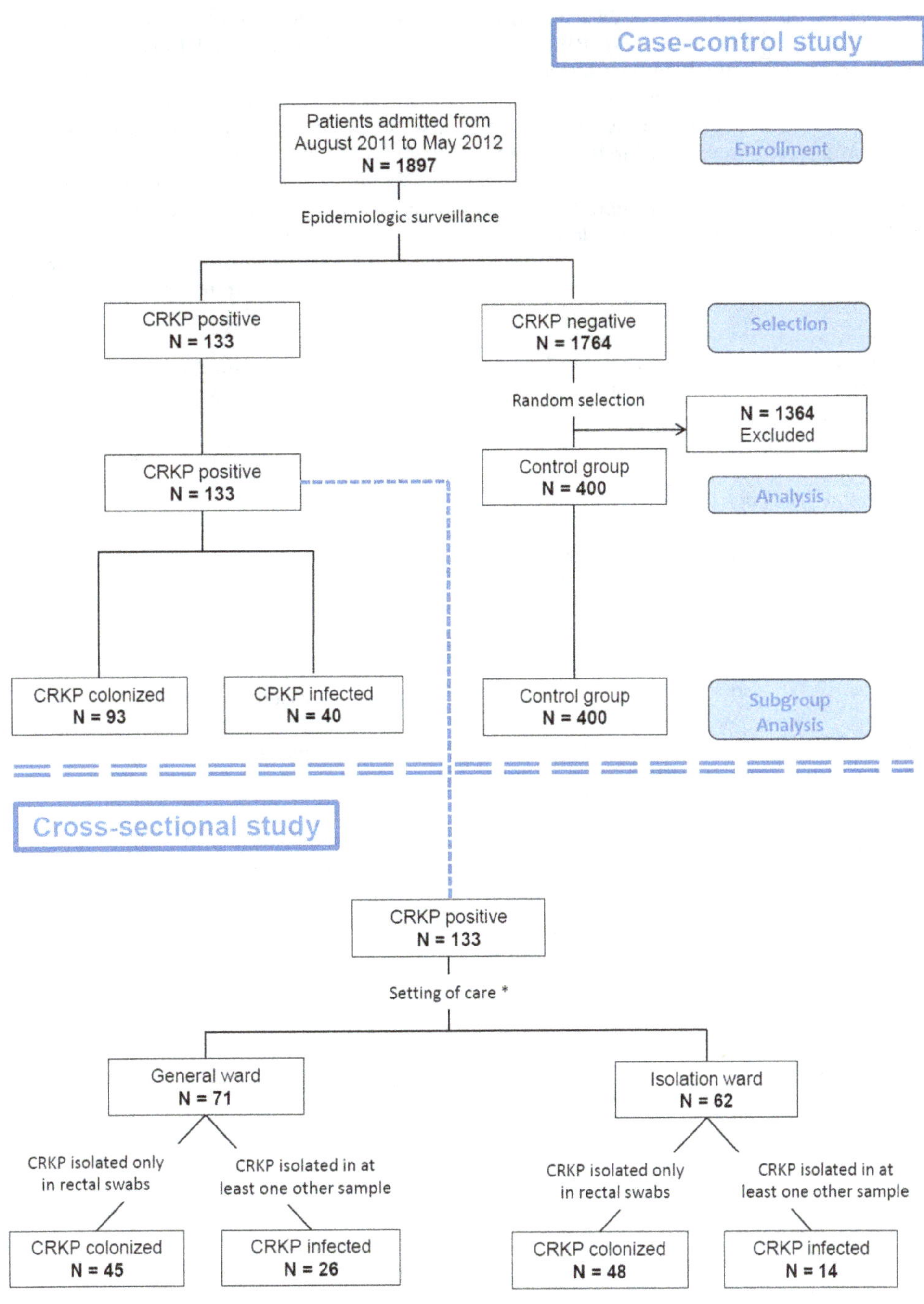

Figure 1. Summary of the study design.

incidence. The rate of infection was calculated as the percentage of CRKP-infected patients related to the overall number of CRKP-positive patients. Data about CRKP genotype was also recorded for each patient whenever available.

The protocol was authorized by the Ethics Committee of Healthcare Hospital Direction of Parma University Hospital, that is also supported by a Scientific Research Board and a specific Research Plan approved by Geriatric-Rehabilitation Department. All patients signed a specific informed consent form at time of admission, stating that the patient authorizes personal and clinical data treatment and analysis in aggregate way for scientific-statistic research purposes according to Italian legislation. All the clinical investigations were performed according to the principles expressed in the Declaration of Helsinki.

For descriptive purposes, baseline characteristics of cases and controls were compared using a χ^2 test (Mantel-Haenszel method) and ANOVA model for categorical and continuous variables, respectively.

Bivariate tests were used: χ^2 for dichotomic variables was used to test the significance of categorical covariates. Parametric (ANOVA) and non-parametric test, the Wilcoxon signed-rank test, were used to assess the significance of continuous covariates. Logistic regression analysis was used to examine the relationship between CIRS category in the case group compared to control group.

All analyses were performed using SAS (version 8.2, SAS Institute, Inc., Cary, NC) with a statistical significance level set at $p<0.05$.

Results

The total number of CRKP-positive patients observed from August 2011 to May 2012 (42 weeks) was 133 (75 M, 58 F; mean age 79±12 years). The control group (400 patients) included 179 males and 221 females, with a mean age of 79±10 years. In the same period, the overall number of patients admitted to our unit was 1897, so that the overall incidence of CRKP positivity was 7%.

As also shown in Figure 1, 93 patients out of 133 cases (70%), were classified as simply CRKP-colonized, while 40 patients (30%) were CRKP-infected. The biological samples, other than rectal swabs, in which CRKP was first isolated in infected subjects were blood or vascular catheters in 21 cases (52.5%), urine in 13 cases (32.5%), phlegm in 3 cases (7.5%) and surgical wound swabs in other 3 cases (7.5%).

CRKP-positive patients had a large number of comorbidities with a high degree of clinical complexity, as attested by high values of CIRS comorbidity and CIRS severity indexes (Table 1). Both indexes were significantly higher in CRKP-positive patients than in controls (comorbidity index 12.0±3.6 vs 9.1±3.5; $p<0.0001$; severity index 3.2±0.4 vs 2.9±0.5; $p<0.0001$) (Table 1). The comparison of the mean values of each CIRS score item between cases and controls is shown in Table 2. CRKP-positive patients had a significantly higher burden of cardiovascular, respiratory, renal, neurological and musculoskeletal disorders than CRKP-negative patients. Cardiovascular and respiratory diseases were indeed the most frequent among the case group, with a prevalence of 64% and 54%, respectively. The role of cardiovascular, respiratory, neurological and renal diseases as risk factors for CRKP colonization was confirmed by logistic regression analysis, and appeared to be independent of age, sex, head and neck, upper and lower gastrointestinal, hepatic, urological, endocrine and psycho-behavioral diseases (Table 3). Moreover, a high CIRS severity index was found to be the leading risk factor for CRKP positivity (odds ratio 13.3; 95% CI 6.88–25.93; $p<0.0001$).

A subgroup analysis performed on infected vs colonized patients showed that neither the CIRS comorbidity score (11.5±3.1 vs 12.2±3.8, $p=0.36$), nor the CIRS severity index (3.1±0.3 vs 3.2±0.4, $p=0.55$) were statistically different between these two groups.

Mean hospital length of stay was significantly longer in CRKP-positive patients than in the control group (35±24 vs 18±12 days, $p<0.001$), as also shown in Table 1.

Twenty-nine CRKP-positive patients out of 133 died during hospitalization (21.8%). However, the mortality rate was not significantly different compared to that observed in the control group (61/400 subjects, 15%; $p=0.08$). When only CRKP-infected patients were considered, the hospital mortality rate was 47.5%, while it was much lower in CRKP-colonized patients (10 patients out of 93; 10.7%).

A total number of 71 CRKP-positive patients was managed in the general medical ward with simple contact bed isolation precautions (from August to September 2011 and from March to May 2012). Sixty-two CRKP-positive patients were managed with staff cohorting approach in the isolation ward (from October 2011 to February 2012), as shown in Figure 1. The highest monthly incidence was observed in the first two months of the epidemic outbreak (23 and 18 new cases per month, with a 16.9% and a 13.2% monthly incidence, respectively). After the activation of the staff cohorting isolation ward, a net decrease in incidence of new cases was observed, with an average of 8 cases per month (range 3–13). A statistical analysis performed with Wilcoxon signed-rank test demonstrated that the decrease between the first (August-September 2011) and the second period (October 2011–February 2012) was statistically significant ($p=0.04$). After closure of the quarantine ward at the end of February 2012, an increased incidence of new CRKP cases was recorded, although not statistically significant (second period October 2011–February 2012 vs third period March–May 2012, $p=0.08$). The overall monthly incidence trend is shown in Figure 2. The mean monthly incidence during the period of quarantine ward management was 4.0%, whereas it was 10.3% in the period of general ward management. This difference was statistically significant ($p=0.03$), as also shown in Figure 3.

The rate of CRKP-infected patients was similar in the subgroup managed by contact isolation approach in general ward (26 subjects out of 71, 36.6%) and in the subgroup managed by staff cohorting approach in isolation ward (14 subjects out of 62, 22.5%, $p=0.07$ with Mantel-Haenszel chi-square). Mortality was also not statistically different in the two groups (16.1% in quarantine ward vs 26.7% in general ward, $p=0.14$ with Mantel-Haenszel chi-square).

Information about the CRKP genotype was available in 102 out of 133 patients. In 76 patients (74%) the strain was positive for blaKPC or other type A carbapenemases, in 12 patients (12%) the strain was positive for type B carbapenemases, namely New Delhi metallo-beta-lactamase (NDM-1), whereas in the remaining 14 patients (14%) the isolated CRKP strain was genotypically classified as not carbapenemase producer. The infection and mortality rates were higher in patients positive for NDM-1-producing strains (50% and 42%, respectively) than in patients positive for type A carbapenemase-producing strains (25% and 17%, respectively) and in patients positive for non-carbapenemase-producing strains (29% and 7%, respectively). The groups exhibited also similar CIRS comorbidity score and severity index.

Discussion

CRKP has rapidly emerged as a notable cause of nosocomial infections in Italy, with a high potential for developing large pandemic outbreaks [9,11,18,26–28]. In this study, we have demonstrated that chronic comorbidities, namely cardiovascular, respiratory, renal and neurological impairments, along with disease severity, play a relevant role as risk factors for CRKP colonization/infection in elderly hospitalized subjects. To our knowledge, this is the first study in a population of frail elderly with a large number of comorbidities admitted to an internal medicine setting. The present investigation is also one of the few that considered this health issue from a genuine clinical perspective, more focused on disease-related risk factors for CRKP colonization/infection rather than on microbiological or molecular issues. The main limitations are the retrospective design, the lack of data about prior antibiotic exposure and functional status of patients before admission. Moreover, comorbidities were assessed through CIRS, which is not completely objective even when performed by a trained physician, although well-validated in medical literature.

Table 1. Characteristics of the study population.

	CASES n = 133	CONTROLS n = 400	p*
Age (years) (mean ± SD)	79±12	79±10	0.50
Men (n, %)	75 (56.4)	221 (55.3)	0.94
CIRS comorbidity Score**	**12.0±3.6**	**9.1±3.5**	**<0.0001**
CIRS severity Index***	**3.2±0.4**	**2.9±0.5**	**<0.0001**
Number of comorbidities****	**3.8±1.2**	**3.3±1.5**	**<0.0001**
Hospital length of stay (days)	**35±24**	**18±12**	**<0.0001**

* Age- and sex-adjusted (where possible).
** CIRS comorbidity Score was calculated as the sum of each of the first 13 items of organ or system disease, excluding only psycho-behavioral disease item. For each item, a score ranging from 0 to 4 can be given. 0 means absence of disease, while 4 means a potential life-threatening disease.
*** CIRS severity Index represents the number of times that a patient ranks 3 or 4 points in each of the 14 items of CIRS (psycho-behavioral disease included).
**** Number of comorbidities was calculated as the number of acute or chronic illnesses that were recorded during the hospital stay for each patient.
CIRS = Cumulative Index Rating Scale.

Some risk factors for CRKP colonization and infection have already been investigated in the literature. For example, the importance of prior antibiotic exposure, especially to carbapenems, has been earlier emphasized [13–15].

Few studies have assessed the role of specific comorbidities as risk factors for developing a CRKP colonization or infection. There is actually only one study, performed in an ICU setting, that has associated a specific chronic disease, namely chronic obstructive pulmonary disease (COPD), with the risk of CRKP positivity [14]. Our data seem to confirm this finding, since CRKP-positive patients do have a higher degree of respiratory impairment than control subjects, although we also showed that cardiovascular, neurological and kidney disease may represent other substantial risk factors. Therefore, in our experience, a high number of comorbidities is an outstanding element influencing the risk of becoming CRKP-positive (Tables 2–3).

As also shown in an ICU context [13–16], disease severity is another relevant risk factor, irrespective of the number of comorbidities. According to our data, patients with a high CIRS severity index actually have an impressive 13-fold risk of becoming CRKP-positive, regardless of single organs or systems involved in disease. Thus, we can argue that CRKP, both in ICUs and in internal medicine wards, mainly affects frail complex patients with severe prognosis. In this subset of patients, in whom the clinical course is often difficult to manage, CRKP provides a new, sometimes fatal, element of clinical complexity. However, it is also noteworthy that a higher risk for infection is a finding common to resistant organisms in these patients. CRKP has actually epidemiologic features similar to the ones of other emerging nosocomial pathogens.

Therefore, it should be no longer only considered a typical ICU concern, but also a pathogen that internal medicine health care professionals and physicians need to deal with.

Table 2. Differences between singular CIRS categories in the cases compared to controls.

CIRS CATEGORY*	CASES n = 133	CONTROLS n = 400	p**
Heart disease	**2.12±1.52**	**1.13±1.42**	**<0.0001**
Hypertension	**1.34±1.12**	**0.73±0.91**	**<0.0001**
Vascular, hematological disease	0.84±1.55	0.67±1.31	0.20
Respiratory disease	**1.97±1.78**	**1.05±1.54**	**<0.0001**
Eye, ear, nose, and throat disease	0.12±0.68	0.10±0.43	0.73
Upper gastrointestinal disease	0.30±1.02	0.37±0.99	0.53
Lower gastrointestinal disease	0.47±1.23	0.50±1.22	0.76
Liver disease	0.12±0.67	0.15±0.62	0.62
Kidney disease	**1.03±1.55**	**0.61±1.23**	**0.001**
Other genitourinary disease	0.14±0.71	0.21±0.74	0.28
Musculoskeletal, skin disease	**0.27±1.00**	**0.58±1.23**	**0.009**
Neurological disease	**1.30±1.72**	**0.96±1.51**	**0.03**
Endocrine, metabolic disease	0.72±1.20	0.77±1.44	0.70
Psychiatric or cognitive disease	1.30±1.81	1.29±1.53	0.73

* All the single CIRS items are listed in this Table. For each item, a score ranging from 0 to 4 can be given. 0 means absence of disease, while 4 means a potential life-threatening disease.
** Age- and sex-adjusted.
CIRS = Cumulative Index Rating Scale.

Table 3. Odds of association between CIRS category in the case group (n = 133) compared to control group (n = 400).

	ODDS RATIO	95% CI	p*
CIRS severity Index	**13.3**	**6.88–25.93**	**<0.0001**
Hypertension	1.96	1.43–2.70	<0.0001
Heart disease	1.68	1.36–2.09	<0.0001
Respiratory disease	1.46	1.25–1.70	<0.0001
Vascular, hematological disease	1.39	1.16–1.66	0.0004
Kidney disease	1.37	1.14–1.64	<0.0001
Neurological disease	1.33	1.12–1.57	0.001

* Also adjusted for age; sex; eye, ear, nose and throat disease; upper and lower gastrointestinal disease; liver disease; other genitourinary diseases; endocrine and metabolic disease; psychiatric and cognitive diseases.
CIRS = Cumulative Index Rating Scale.

However, despite the high comorbidity burden of our patients, the recorded mortality rate was surprisingly not as high as that reported in literature [16–18]. As a matter of fact, the number of deaths was not significantly different in all CRKP-positive patients than those recorded in the control group of CRKP-free patients. However, when the CRKP infection occurs, the mortality rises due to the high risk of fatal septic shock. The mortality rate that we have recorded in CRKP-infected subjects is actually very similar to that previously reported in our country by Tumbarello and colleagues in a multicenter study [18]. We can hypothesize that simple rectal colonization by CRKP does not significantly modify the clinical course of frail elderly patients with multiple comorbidities. However, when the infection occurs, it significantly threatens survival of these patients, similarly to what has been shown in ICU patients. Further research is needed to better understand factors that induce the transformation of colonization into infection, both in intensive care and internal or geriatric medicine settings.

In our experience, we have also observed the effects of an isolation ward activation with a staff cohorting management, as an attempt to limit the contacts of CRKP-negative patients with colonized or infected patients. However, the cross-sectional design of the study does not allow to establish whether or not the variations in incidence of CRKP positivity are causally related to different management strategies. Moreover, patients were managed by staff cohorting or by contact bed precautions on a temporal basis and not on a random assignment. However, the remarkable decrease of monthly incidence observed after the institution of these measures, combined with the new increase detected after the isolation ward was closed (Figure 2), indirectly suggests that this approach may be related to a decrease in the incidence of new cases. Our data also indicate that this strategy may help reducing the rate of CRKP-positive patients that develop a clinical infection by CRKP. Further research is needed to confirm these hypotheses. Staff cohorting management is a simple sanitary measure, which was proven effective in other nosocomial pandemics [24–25]. Some recent studies in Greece demonstrated that the implementation of basic hand hygiene and contact precautions by health care professionals, isolation of CRKP-positive patients in dedicated rooms and staff cohorting are effective, either alone or in combination, to limit the spread of CRKP, although in surgical and intensive care settings [29–30]. There are also reports in which even more strict hygienic measures have been applied, such as daily chlorhexidine baths for positive patients, environmental surveillance for CRKP detection on surfaces at high risk for contamination and meticulous daily environmental cleaning [31–32]. These measures are obviously

CONTACT BED ISOLATION | 14-BED WARD ACTIVATION WITH STAFF COHORTING | CONTACT BED ISOLATION

MONTHLY INCIDENCE

18% 15% 12% 9% 6% 3% 0%

16,9% 13,2% 6,2% 5,6% 2,6% 1,2% 4,3% 4,5% 8,8% 8,2%

AUGUST '11 SEPTEMBER '11 OCTOBER '11 NOVEMBER '11 DECEMBER '11 JANUARY '12 FEBRUARY '12 MARCH '12 APRIL '12 MAY '12

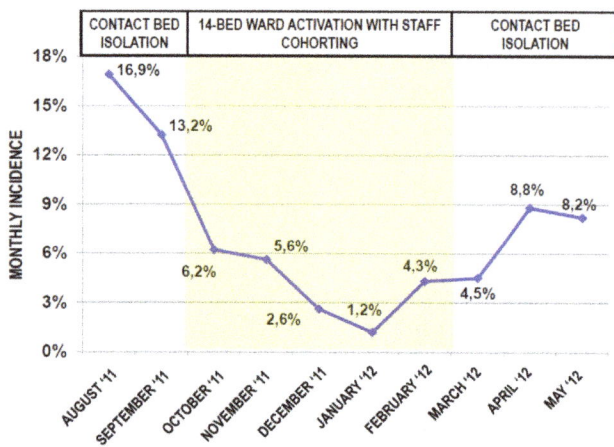

Figure 2. Trend in monthly incidence of CRKP positive cases in the period studied. (CRKP = Carbapenemase-resistant *Klebsiella pneumoniae*).

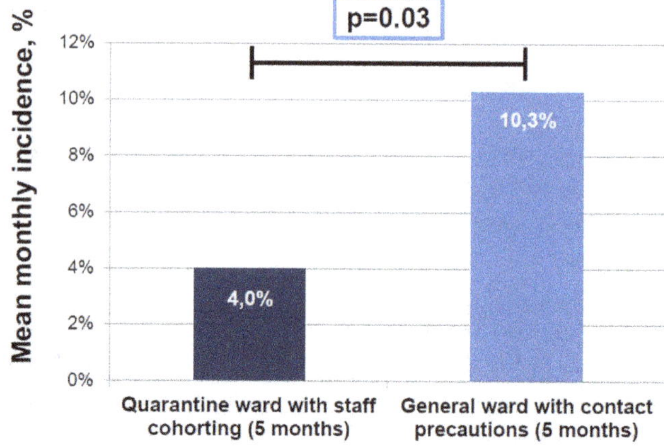

Figure 3. Comparison of mean monthly incidence of new cases of CRKP positivity between quarantine ward management period and general ward management period. Statistical analysis performed with analysis of variance. (CRKP = Carbapenemase-resistant *Klebsiella pneumoniae*).

more difficult to be established in a non-ICU setting. Nevertheless, it is plausible that the higher number of hygienical precautions are established, the more effective is the prevention protocol for limiting multi-drug resistant outbreaks, even in geriatric frail patients.

However, possible biases should also be taken into account for the interpretation of our results. For example, considering that the lowest incidence in our experience was reported during winter months, we cannot exclude that CRKP colonization/infection outbreaks exhibit a seasonal periodicity. Our data are in agreement with those from a large multicenter epidemiologic study that some years ago evaluated non-multidrug-resistant *Klebsiella pneumoniae* strains [33]. Interestingly, opposite data emerged from a subsequent study conducted in a temperate climate area of the United States [34].

Conclusions

CRKP outbreaks are becoming a relevant health issue, not only in an intensive care setting, but also in internal medicine and geriatric wards. Special sanitary measures, such as epidemiologic surveillance with weekly rectal swabs, bed isolation and quarantine ward activation with staff cohorting management may play a role in controlling the epidemic spread.

Our experience clearly suggests that a high number of comorbidities, and particularly cardiovascular, respiratory, renal and neurological disease, and high disease severity represent relevant risk factors for colonization and infection in elderly frail patients. Therefore these data open new scenarios for the most suitable strategies for issuing effective preventive measures in those patients at higher risk, not only admitted in ICU setting but also in general internal medicine wards. The clinicians' awareness and knowledge of this problem will therefore be crucial in the future for management of these severe hospital pandemics. Future research is needed to assess the relationships between the domains of frailty and chronic illness and the risk for CRKP colonization or infection.

Acknowledgments

We are grateful to Prof. Matteo Goldoni for his smart advice in the phase of manuscript preparation and revision.

Author Contributions

Conceived and designed the experiments: AN AT LB TM. Performed the experiments: LG IM ER. Analyzed the data: AN AT FL MM. Wrote the paper: AN AT GL TM.

References

1. Chen LF, Anderson DJ, Paterson DL (2012) Overview of the epidemiology and the threat of *Klebsiella pneumoniae* carbapenemases (KPC) resistance. Infect Drug Resist 5: 133–141.
2. Nordmann P, Poirel L (2002) Emerging carbapenemases in Gram-negative aerobes. Clin Microbiol Infect 8: 321–331.
3. Cornaglia G, Giamarellou H, Rossolini GM (2011) Metallo-β-lactamases: a last frontier for β-lactams? Lancet Infect Dis 11: 381–393.
4. Yigit H, Queenan AM, Anderson GJ, Domenech-Sanchez A, Biddle JW, et al. (2001) Novel carbapenem-hydrolyzing β-lactamase, KPC-1, from a carbapenem-resistant strain of *Klebsiella pneumoniae*. Antimicrob Agents Chemother 45: 1151–1161.
5. Lomaestro BM, Tobin EH, Shang W, Gootz T (2006) The spread of *Klebsiella pneumoniae* carbapenemase-producing *K. pneumoniae* to upstate New York. Clin Infect Dis 43: e26–e28.
6. Munoz-Price LS, Poirel L, Bonomo RA, Schwaber MJ, Daikos GL, et al. (2013) Clinical epidemiology of the global expansion of *Klebsiella pneumoniae* carbapenemases. Lancet Infect Dis 13: 785–796.
7. Giani T, D'Andrea MM, Pecile P, Borgianni L, Nicoletti P, et al. (2009) Emergence in Italy of *Klebsiella pneumoniae* sequence type 258 producing KPC-3 carbapenemase. J Clin Microbiol 47: 3793–3794.
8. Nordmann P, Cuzon G, Naas T (2009) The real threat of *Klebsiella pneumoniae* carbapenemase-producing bacteria. Lancet Infect Dis 9: 228–236.
9. Gaibani P, Ambretti S, Berlingeri A, Gelsomino F, Bielli A, et al. (2011) Rapid increase of carbapenemase-producing Klebsiella pneumoniae strains in a large Italian hospital: surveillance period 1 March-30 September 2010. Euro Surveill 12: pii 19800.
10. Giani T, Pini B, Arena F, Conte V, Bracco S, et al. (2013) Epidemic diffusion of KPC carbapenemase-producing *Klebsiella pneumoniae* in Italy: results of the first countrywide survey, 15 May to 30 June 2011. Euro Surveill 18: pii 20489.
11. Gagliotti C, Ciccarese V, Sarti M, Giordani S, Barozzi A, et al. (2013) Active surveillance for asymptomatic carriers of carbapenemase-producing *Klebsiella pneumoniae* in a hospital setting. J Hosp Infect 83: 330–332.
12. Nordmann P, Gniadkowski M, Giske CG, Poirel L, Woodford N, et al. (2012) Identification and screening of carbapenemase-producing *Enterobacteriaceae*. Clin Microbiol Infect 18: 432–438.
13. Gasink LB, Edelstein PH, Lautenbach E, Synnestevedt M, Fishman NO (2009) Risk factors and clinical impact of *Klebsiella pneumoniae* carbapenemase-producing *K. pneumoniae*. Infect Control Hosp Epidemiol 30: 1180–1185.
14. Papadimitriou-Olivgeris M, Marangos M, Fligou F, Christofidou M, Bartzavali C, et al. (2012) Risk factors for KPC-producing *Klebsiella pneumoniae* enteric colonization upon ICU admission. J Antimicrob Chemother 67: 2976–2981.
15. Armand-Lefèvre L, Angebault C, Barbier F, Hamelet E, Defrance G, et al. (2013) Emergence of imipenem-resistant Gram-negative bacilli in intestinal flora of intensive care patients. Antimicrob Agents Chemother 57: 1488–1495.
16. Mouloudi E, Protonotariou E, Zagorianou A, Iosifidis E, Karapanagiotou A, et al. (2010) Bloodstream infections caused by metallo-β-lactamase/*Klebsiella pneumoniae* carbapenemase-producing *K. pneumoniae* among intensive care unit patients in Greece: risk factors for infection and impact of type of resistance on outcomes. Infect Control Hosp Epidemiol 31: 1250–1256.
17. Zarkotou O, Pournaras S, Tselioti P, Dragoumanos V, Pitiriga V, et al. (2011) Predictors of mortality in patients with bloodstream infections caused by KPC-producing *Klebsiella pneumoniae* and impact of appropriate antimicrobial treatment. Clin Microbiol Infect 17: 1798–1803.
18. Tumbarello M, Viale P, Viscoli C, Trecarichi EM, Tumietto F, et al. (2012) Predictors of mortality in bloodstream infections caused by *Klebsiella pneumoniae* carbapenemase-producing *K. pneumoniae*: importance of combination therapy. Clin Infect Dis 55: 943–950.
19. Livermore DM, Warner M, Mushtaq S, Doumith M, Zhang J, et al. (2011) What remains against carbapenem-resistant Enterobacteriaceae? Evaluation of chloramphenicol, ciprofloxacin, colistin, fosfomycin, minocycline, nitrofurantoin, temocillin and tigecycline. Int J Antimicrob Agents 37: 415–419.
20. Hirsch EB, Guo B, Chang KT, Cao H, Ledesma KR, et al. (2013) Assessment of antimicrobial combinations for *Klebsiella pneumoniae* carbapenemase-producing *K. pneumoniae*. J Infect Dis 207: 786–793.
21. Daikos GL, Markogiannakis A (2011) Carbapenemase-producing *Klebsiella pneumoniae*: (when) might we still consider treating with carbapenems? Clin Microbiol Infect 17: 1135–1141.
22. Gagliotti C, Cappelli V, Carretto E, Pan A, Sarti M, et al. Indicazioni pratiche e protocolli operativi per la diagnosi, la sorveglianza e il controllo degli enterobatteri produttori di carbapenemasi nelle strutture sanitarie e socio-sanitarie. Regione Emilia-Romagna, Agenzia Sanitaria e Sociale Regionale. Bologna, January 2013. http://assr.regione.emilia-romagna.it/it/servizi/pubblicazioni/rapporti-documenti. Accessed on December 2nd, 2013. Italian language.
23. Jochimsen EM, Fish L, Manning K, Young S, Singer DA, et al. (1999) Control of vancomycin-resistant enterococci at a community hospital: efficacy of patient and staff cohorting. Infect Control Hosp Epidemiol 20: 106–109.
24. Chitnis AS, Caruthers PS, Rao AK, Lamb J, Lurvey R, et al. (2012) Outbreak of carbapenem-resistant Enterobacteriaceae at a long-term acute care hospital: sustained reductions in transmission through active surveillance and targeted interventions. Infect Control Hosp Epidemiol 33: 984–992.
25. Miller MD, Paradis CF, Houck PR, Mazumdar S, Stack JA, et al. (1992) Rating chronic medical illness burden in geropsychiatric practice and research: application of the Cumulative Illness Rating Scale. Psychiatry Res 41: 237–248.
26. Agodi A, Voulgari E, Barchitta M, Politi L, Koumaki V, et al. (2011) Containment of an outbreak of KPC-3-producing *Klebsiella pneumoniae* in Italy. J Clin Microbiol 49: 3986–3989.
27. Giuffrè M, Bonura C, Geraci DM, Saporito L, Catalano R, et al. (2013) Successful control of an outbreak of colonization by *Klebsiella pneumoniae* carbapenemase-producing *K. pneumoniae* sequence type 258 in a neonatal intensive care unit, Italy. J Hosp Infect 85: 233–236.
28. Aschbacher R, Giani T, Corda D, Conte V, Arena F, et al. (2013) Carbapenemase-producing Enterobacteriaceae during 2011-12 in the Bolzano area (Northern Italy): incresing diversity in a low-endemicity setting. Diagn Microbiol Infect Dis 77: 354–356.
29. Spysa V, Psichogiou M, Bouzala GA, Hadjihannas L, Hatzakis A, et al. (2012) Transmission dynamics of carbapenemase-producing Klebsiella pneumoniae

and anticipated impact of infection control strategies in a surgical unit. PLoS One 7: e41068.

30. Poulou A, Voulgari E, Vrioni G, Xidopoulos G, Pliagkos A, et al. (2012) Imported *Klebsiella pneumoniae* carbapenemase-producing *K. Pneumoniae* clones in a Greek hospital: impact of infection control measures for restraining their dissemination. J Clin Microbiol 50: 2618–2623.
31. Munoz-Price LS, Hayden MK, Lolans K, Won S, Calvert K, et al. (2010) Successful control of an outbreak of *Klebsiella pneumoniae* carbapenemase-producing *K. pneumoniae* at a long-term acute care hospital. Infect Control Hosp Epidemiol 31: 341–347.
32. Munoz-Price LS, De La Cuesta C, Adams S, Wyckoff M, Cleary T, et al. (2010) Successful eradication of a monoclonal strain of *Klebsiella pneumoniae* carbapenemase-producing *K. pneumoniae* outbreak in a surgical intensive care unit in Miami, Florida. Infect Control Hosp Epidemiol 31: 1074–1077.
33. Anderson DJ, Richet H, Chen LF, Spelman DW, Hung YJ, et al. (2008) Seasonal variation in *Klebsiella pneumoniae* bloodstream infection on 4 continents. J Infect Dis 197: 752–756.
34. Al-Hasan MN, Lahr BD, Eckel-Passow JE, Baddour LM (2010) Epidemiology and outcome of *Klebsiella* species bloodstream infection: a population-based study. Mayo Clin Proc 85: 139–144.

Immune Biomarkers Predictive of Respiratory Viral Infection in Elderly Nursing Home Residents

Jennie Johnstone[1]*, Robin Parsons[2], Fernando Botelho[2], Jamie Millar[2], Shelly McNeil[3], Tamas Fulop[4], Janet McElhaney[5], Melissa K. Andrew[6], Stephen D. Walter[1], P. J. Devereaux[1,7], Mehrnoush Malekesmaeili[8], Ryan R. Brinkman[8,9], James Mahony[10,11], Jonathan Bramson[2,10,11]¶, Mark Loeb[1,7,10,11]*¶

1 Department of Clinical Epidemiology and Biostatistics, McMaster University, Hamilton, Ontario, Canada, **2** McMaster Immunology Research Centre, McMaster University, Hamilton, Ontario, Canada, **3** Canadian Center for Vaccinology, IWK Health Centre and Capital Health, Dalhousie University, Halifax, Nova Scotia, Canada, **4** Department of Medicine, Geriatrics Division, Research Center on Aging, University of Sherbrooke, Sherbrooke, Quebec, Canada, **5** Department of Medicine, Northern Ontario School of Medicine, Sudbury, Ontario, Canada, **6** Department of Medicine, Dalhousie University, Halifax, Nova Scotia, Canada, **7** Department of Medicine, McMaster University, Hamilton, Ontario, Canada, **8** Terry Fox Laboratory, British Columbia Cancer Agency, Vancouver, British Columbia, Canada, **9** Department of Medical Genetics, University of British Columbia, Vancouver, British Columbia, Canada, **10** Department of Pathology and Molecular Medicine, McMaster University, Hamilton, Ontario, Canada, **11** Institute for Infectious Disease Research, McMaster University, Hamilton, Ontario, Canada

Abstract

Objective: To determine if immune phenotypes associated with immunosenescence predict risk of respiratory viral infection in elderly nursing home residents.

Methods: Residents ≥65 years from 32 nursing homes in 4 Canadian cities were enrolled in Fall 2009, 2010 and 2011, and followed for one influenza season. Following influenza vaccination, peripheral blood mononuclear cells (PBMCs) were obtained and analysed by flow cytometry for T-regs, CD4+ and CD8+ T-cell subsets (CCR7+CD45RA+, CCR7-CD45RA+ and CD28-CD57+) and CMV-reactive CD4+ and CD8+ T-cells. Nasopharyngeal swabs were obtained and tested for viruses in symptomatic residents. A Cox proportional hazards model adjusted for age, sex and frailty, determined the relationship between immune phenotypes and time to viral infection.

Results: 1072 residents were enrolled; median age 86 years and 72% female. 269 swabs were obtained, 87 were positive for virus: influenza (24%), RSV (14%), coronavirus (32%), rhinovirus (17%), human metapneumovirus (9%) and parainfluenza (5%). In multivariable analysis, high T-reg% (HR 0.41, 95% CI 0.20–0.81) and high CMV-reactive CD4+ T-cell% (HR 1.69, 95% CI 1.03–2.78) were predictive of respiratory viral infection.

Conclusions: In elderly nursing home residents, high CMV-reactive CD4+ T-cells were associated with an increased risk and high T-regs were associated with a reduced risk of respiratory viral infection.

Editor: Christine Bourgeois, INSERM, France

Funding: This work was supported by Canadian Institutes of Health Research (CIHR), Public Health Agency of Canada (PHAC)/CIHR Influenza Research Network (PCIRN), National Institues of Health (R01 EB008400/EB/NIBIB), Natural Sciences and Engineering Research Council of Canada. The funders had no role in study design, data collection and analysis, decision to publish, or preparation of the manuscript.

Competing Interests: The authors have declared that no competing interests exist.

* Email: johnsj48@mcmaster.ca (JJ); loebm@mcmaster.ca (ML)

¶ JB and ML are co-senior authors on this work.

Introduction

The burden of respiratory viral infection in elderly nursing home residents is high [1]. With active surveillance the incidence of respiratory viral infection is estimated to range from 1.4–2.8 per 1000 resident days [2]. Influenza and respiratory syncytial virus (RSV) are the viruses commonly responsible for morbidity and mortality associated with infection, but other respiratory viruses including parainfluenza, human metapneumovirus, coronavirus and rhinovirus can also cause severe disease in this population [1,3–7]. It is a widely held belief that immunosenescence, the waning of immune function associated with old age, is responsible for this increased risk and severity of infection [8]; however, only sparse data exist to substantiate this position [9].

As a first step towards the identification of immune biomarkers predictive of respiratory viral infection in elderly nursing home residents, we characterized immune phenotypes in elderly nursing home residents [10]. Whole blood analysis of circulating CD4+ and CD8+ T-cell subsets was performed in a cross-sectional study involving 262 nursing home elderly participants and immune phenotypes were compared to immune phenotypes from healthy adults. In addition, we explored how individual immune phenotypes were influenced by age, sex, frailty and nutritional status in the nursing home elderly [10]. We observed lower naïve CD8+ T-cells (CD8+CD45RA+CCR7+) and higher terminally differentiated memory T-cells (CD8+CD45RA+CCR7-) and senescent T-cells (CD8+CD28−) when compared to healthy adults [10], consistent with prior findings in elderly people [11–14]. It is hypothesized that the reduced numbers of naïve CD8+ T-cells observed in the elderly due to thymic involution, coupled with an accumulation of poorly functioning terminally differentiated memory T-cells and senescent cells possibly arising from chronic antigenic stimulation by cytomegalovirus (CMV) [15,16], predisposes elderly people to infection [17].

Supporting this hypothesis, senescent CD8+ T-cells and high titres of CMV antibody have been found to be associated with influenza vaccine failure in older people [18–20]. Whether these same CD4+ T-cell subsets are associated with infection is less clear. The accumulation of a separate class of T-cell, the regulatory CD4+ T-cell (T-regs) in elderly people has also been observed in elderly nursing home residents [10] and community dwelling elderly people [21]. While T-regs are known to be responsible for controlling the magnitude of CD4+ and CD8+ T-cell responses to viral infections [22], whether the accumulated T-regs in the elderly lead to impairment of host control of infection is not known.

To our knowledge, the relationship between immune phenotypes associated with immunosenescence and risk of respiratory viral infection has not been studied. If a relationship is established, this could help identify elderly nursing home residents at highest risk of become ill and could provide more focused care through targeted prevention. To this end, we sought to identify immune biomarkers predictive of respiratory viral infection during the ensuing respiratory viral season, in an elderly nursing home cohort.

Methods

Subjects and Setting

In this prospective cohort study, elderly participants were recruited from 32 nursing homes in 4 Canadian cities (Halifax, Nova Scotia, Sherbrooke, Quebec, Hamilton, Ontario and Vancouver, British Columbia) in September and October 2009, 2010 and 2011. Residents recruited for a separate study [10] were also eligible for inclusion in this study. Residents ≥65 years of age were eligible for the study. Exclusion criteria included individuals: not planning to be vaccinated against influenza, receiving immunosuppressive medications (including cancer chemotherapy, oral corticosteroid use >21 days, methotrexate, post-transplant medications and/or anti-cytokine or B-lymphocyte depletion therapies), or expected to die within 30 days, as determined by the supervising physician. Written informed consent was obtained from all participants or their legally appointed guardian in the event they were not competent to provide consent themselves. The study protocol was approved by the Research Ethics Board at each participating institution and nursing home.

Trained research personnel abstracted baseline demographics from the participants based on an interview, examination and chart review. Frailty was rated according to the Clinical Frailty Scale, an 8-point scale ranging from 1–8 as follows: (1) very fit, (2) well, (3) well with treated comorbid illness, (4) apparently vulnerable, (5) mildly frail defined as dependence in instrumental activities of daily living (ADL), (6) moderately frail defined as required assistance with basic ADL, (7) severely frail defined as completely dependent on others for ADL and (8) very severely frail [23]. The Clinical Frailty Scale has been validated in the nursing home population [23]. Participants received the seasonal influenza vaccine, typically in October or November, by public health nurses in accordance with guideline recommendations for the given year [24–26]. Peripheral blood mononuclear cells (PBMCs) were drawn from participants 21 days post vaccination.

Residents were actively followed by research staff for the influenza season immediately following the PBMC draw. The influenza season was defined as spanning from the first week ≥5% of specimens submitted to the local public health laboratory for viral testing were positive for influenza and ending when <5% were positive for influenza for 2 consecutive weeks. The influenza season was chosen as the period of follow-up as the rate of respiratory viral infection is highest during the winter months [2]. Trained research personnel reviewed each participant for the presence of symptoms or signs of respiratory illness twice weekly or more often if notified of symptoms by nursing home staff. Nasopharyngeal swabs (Copan ESwab, Copan Diagnostics Inc., Murrieta, California) were obtained by the research staff when a resident had one or more of the following new symptoms or signs: fever (≥38°Celsius), worsening cough, nasal congestion, sore throat, headache, sinus problems, muscle aches, fatigue, ear ache or infection, chills, not otherwise explained by an alternative diagnosis.

Peripheral Blood Mononuclear Cell Analysis and Flow Cytometry

Blood was obtained from participants between 0700 and 1000 hours and hand delivered to the research laboratory for immediate processing. PBMCs were isolated and frozen using a validated common standard operating procedure [27].

T-cell immune phenotypes were determined by thawing patient PBMCs as previously described [28]. Viability of the PBMCs was found to range between 87% and 98% and the average viability was 94.6%. An aliquot ($0.5–16\times10^6$ cells/stain) was placed in round-bottom 96-well plates with anti-CD3-Qdot605, anti-CD8-Alexa Flour 700, anti-CD4-Pacific Blue, anti-CD45RA-PE Texas Red, anti-CD28-PE, anti-CD57-FITC, anti-CCR7-PE Cy7. T-regs were identified using anti-CD3-FITC, anti-CD4-Pacific Blue, anti-CD127-PerCP-Cy5.5, anti-CD25-PE, and anti-FoxP3-Alexa-Fluor700. The following antibodies were purchased from BD Bioscience: anti-CD4-Pacific Blue, anti-CD28-PE, anti-CCR7-PE-Cy7 and anti-CD25-PE. The following antibodies were purchased from eBioscience: anti-CD3-FITC, anti-CD127-PerCP-Cy5.5, anti-FoxP3-AlexaFluor700. The anti-CD3-Qdot605 was purchased from Invitrogen. The anti-CD57-FITC and anti-CD45RA-PE-TexasRed antibodies were purchased from Beckman Coulter. We defined the T-cell subsets as follows: naïve (CD45RA+CCR7+), terminally differentiated (CD45RA+CCR7-) and senescent (CD28-CD57+). T-regs were defined as CD4+CD25^{hi}CD127^{lo}Foxp3+. CD4+ and CD8+ immune phenotypes and T-regs were expressed as a percentage of CD3+. Antibody staining was performed using a Beckman Coulter Biomek NX^{P} Laboratory Automation Workstation (Beckman Coulter, Ontario) as previously described [29], followed by analysis using an LSR II flow cytometer with a high-throughput sampler (BD Biosciences, NJ, USA). T-regs were analyzed using FlowJo 9.6 (Treestar Inc, Ashland, OR). T-cell subset analysis employed an automated gating pipeline using the flowDensity algorithm [30]. This approach uses customized threshold calculations for the different cell subsets to mimic a manual gating scheme based on expert knowledge of hierarchical gating order and 1D density information. Population identification is individually tuned to each cell population in a data driven manner. T-cell subpopulations were identified using characteristics of their density distribution such as the number of peaks, height and width of each peak, change of the slope in the distribution curve, standard deviation, and median density (Figure S1). CD45RA thresholds were estimated based on control samples, which where then applied automatically to stimulated samples. CCR7 thresholds were estimated based on CD57+ populations given the explicit instruction that CD57+ cells are CCR7- (Figure S1). A total of 17 populations identified by this approach using high performance computing resources at the Michael Smith Genome Sciences Centre in order to reduce computational time.

CMV-reactive T-cells were identified by stimulating PBMCs with a pool of overlapping peptides spanning the immunodominant pp65 protein of CMV (PepTivator pp65, Miltenyi Biotec) according to our published protocols [28]. Briefly, thawed PBMCs were cultured overnight at 37°C and stimulated with CMV peptides (2 ug/ml) for 1 hr at 37°C. A matched set of PBMCs were stimulated with DMSO as a negative control. Brefeldin A (BD Biosciences) was then added according to the manufacturer's instructions and the cells were incubated for an additional 4 hours. The cells were stained with anti-CD4-PacificBlue and anti-CD8-AlexaFluor700, permeabilized and finally stained with anti-IFN-γ-APC, anti-TNF-α-FITC and anti-CD3-QDot605. CMV-reactive T-cells were identified as CD3+ (CD4+ or CD8+) IFN-γ+ TNF-α+.

Respiratory Virus Detection

Using 200 ul of nasopharyngeal swab material, nucleic acid was extracted by the bioMerieux easyMAG automated extractor. Specimens were tested using the xTAG Respiratory Virus Panel (RVP) assay for influenza A (subtype H1 and H3), influenza B, RSV (subtype A and B), parainfluenza (1–4), coronavirus (NL63, OC43, HKU1 and 229E), human metapneumovirus, entero-rhinovirus, and adenovirus as per the manufacturer's protocol (Luminex Molecular Diagnostics, Inc., Toronto, Ontario).

Statistical analysis

The immune phenotype distributions as well as the age distribution were skewed, and so the distributions of these continuous variables were summarized as medians and inter-quartile ranges (IQR). The age and sex for those who had PBMCs obtained and those who did not were compared using Mann-Whitney U and chi-square test as appropriate. Complete case analysis of immune phenotypes was planned if there was <10% missing data for each parameter [31].

Unadjusted hazard ratios (HR) and 95% confidence intervals (CIs) using Cox proportional hazards model were first constructed to explore the relationship between immune phenotypes and time to symptomatic respiratory viral infection. In the event a resident had multiple respiratory viral infections, only the first infection was included as an outcome. If a participant died prior to a respiratory viral infection, their time was censored on the date of death. We hypothesized that the following immune phenotypes associated with immunosenescence would be associated with increased risk of infection [12–17,21]: low CD4+ and CD8+ naïve T-cells and high CD4+ and CD8+ terminally differentiated and senescent T-cells as well as high CMV-reactive CD4+ and CD8+ T-cells and high T-regs. Low was defined as immune phenotypes in the first quartile of the distribution and high was defined as immune phenotypes in the fourth quartile of the distribution. *A priori*, it was decided that age, sex and frailty would be included in the final model, given their potential for confounding with the effects of primary interest in this population [32]. Immune phenotypes with a p-value <0.20 in univariable analysis were included in the final multivariable model. The final model was determined using backwards elimination. A sandwich variance estimator was used to account for the clustering effect at the level of the nursing homes [33]. The proportional hazards assumption for continuous variables was explored graphically by plotting partial residuals against time to event and tested by regressing the partial residuals against time. The proportional hazards assumption for categorical variables was examined by a log-minus-log graph to ensure the plotted lines remained parallel. The presence of multicollinearity was examined using the variance inflation factor (VIF); presence of multicollinearity was defined as VIF >5.

P-values and 95% CIs were constructed using 2-tailed tests. P-values <0.05 were considered statistically significant. Statistical analyses were performed using R, version 3.0.2 [34].

Results

Nursing Home Cohort

In total, 1165 residents were enrolled in the study and of these, and PBMC were obtained from 1087 (93%). Reasons for not obtaining PBMCs were either refusal of influenza vaccine or refusal of blood draw. There was no statistically significant difference in age (median, 86 (IQR 80–90) versus 85 (IQR 79–89) without PBMCs, p = 0.42) or sex (%female, 72% versus 64% without PBMCs, p = 0.12) between those that did and did not have PBMCs obtained. Fifteen participants (1%) withdrew before the end of the study, leaving 1072 as our final sample size. Seventy-three participants died before a respiratory viral infection could be identified.

Baseline Characteristics

Baseline characteristics of the final cohort are summarized in Table 1. The median age was 86 years (IQR 80–90 years) and the ages ranged from 65–102 years. Eight persons were ≥100 years. Most (93%) had at least one co-morbidity, and almost half (44%) scored either 7 or 8 on the Clinical Frailty Scale, which is defined as severely and very severely frail respectively. Figures 1, 2 and 3 describe the gating strategies used to define the immune phenotypes. The medians and corresponding IQRs for each immune cell type tested in this study can be found in Table 1.

Respiratory Virus Infection

In total, 269 swabs were obtained from 233 symptomatic people. Nasopharyngeal swabs were positive for viruses in 87 symptomatic residents (Table 2). Coronavirus (32%), influenza (24%), rhinovirus (17%) and RSV (14%) were the most common viruses found. One nasopharyngeal swab positive for influenza A also had rhinovirus present.

Predictors of Respiratory Virus Infection

We subsequently investigated whether a relationship existed between specific immune cell populations and respiratory virus infection. The proportional hazards assumption was satisfied for all covariates included in the model and there was no concerning evidence of multicollinearity (all VIFs were <3). In univariable analyses, low naïve CD8+ T-cell% (HR 0.69, 95% CI 0.51–0.95) and high T-reg% (HR 0.47, 95% CI 0.26–0.85) were associated with a reduced risk of respiratory viral infection and high terminally differentiated CD8+ T-cell% (HR 1.57, 95% CI 1.10–2.24), high senescent CD8+ T-cell% (HR 1.55, 95% CI 1.11–2.17) and high CMV-reactive CD4+ T-cell% (HR 1.82, 95% CI 1.13–2.94), were associated with an increased risk of respiratory viral infection (Table 3). In multivariable analysis adjusted for age, sex and frailty, only high T-reg% (HR 0.41, 95% CI 0.20–0.81) and high CMV-reactive CD4+ T-cell% (HR 1.69, 95% CI 1.03–

Table 1. Baseline characteristics of the nursing home elderly.

	Total n = 1072
Demographics [n(%)]	
Age (years)	
65–74	131 (12)
75–84	337 (31)
85–94	508 (47)
≥95	96 (9)
Sex (F)	776 (72)
Prior co-morbidity	
COPD	186 (17)
Coronary artery disease	346 (32)
Diabetes	290 (27)
Heart failure	148 (14)
Stroke	273 (25)
Dementia	511 (48)
≥5 medications	966 (90)
Frailty	
4	76 (7)
5	174 (16)
6	354 (33)
7	460 (43)
8	8 (1)
Immune Phenotypes [median (IQR)]	
CD8+ T-cell	
Naïve CD8+ T-cell%	1.10 (0.60–1.82)
Terminally differentiated CD8+ T-cell%	8.95 (4.72–14.80)
Senescent CD8+ T-cell%	5.87 (2.40–11.58)
CD8+ CMV T-cell%	0.32 (.03–1.53)
CD4+ T-cell	
Naïve CD4+ T-cell%	13.2 (6.90–22.85)
Terminally differentiated CD4+ T-cell%	8.46 (4.93–14.04)
Senescent CD4+ T-cell%	1.66 (0.28–4.54)
CD4+ CMV T-cell%	0.06 (0.006–0.40)
T-reg	
T-reg%	2.73 (2.12–3.45)

2.78) remained predictive of respiratory viral infection in the final model (Table 3 and Figure 4).

Discussion

In this prospective cohort study of elderly nursing home residents, CD4+ T cells, in particular T-regs and CMV-reactive CD4+ T-cells were predictive of respiratory viral infection during the ensuing respiratory viral season in multivariable analysis. In contrast, CD8+ T-cells were not found to be predictive in multivariable analysis. To our knowledge, this is the first study to identify immune biomarkers predictive of respiratory viral infection in elderly people.

T-regs are responsible for creating the balance between the immune response to pathogens and the harmful sequelae of inflammation that arises with this response [35]. High T-regs have been consistently observed in elderly people when compared to healthy adults [10,21], and it has been hypothesized that this shift may be associated with increased risk of infection seen in the elderly [21,36]. It is intriguing that in our study higher levels of circulating T-regs were associated with reduced risk of symptomatic respiratory virus infection. We did not systematically test all residents in our study for respiratory virus throughout the study, so we cannot determine whether the association between high T-regs and reduced risk of infection was due to absence of infection or whether there was a higher incidence of asymptomatic infections in the high T-reg group. Little is known about the role of T-regs in preventing acute respiratory viral infection in humans [35]. In mice, a robust T-reg response has been observed during influenza [37] and RSV infection [38] and depletion of T-regs delays RSV viral clearance from lungs [38] suggesting that T-regs play an important role in controlling the immune response to respiratory

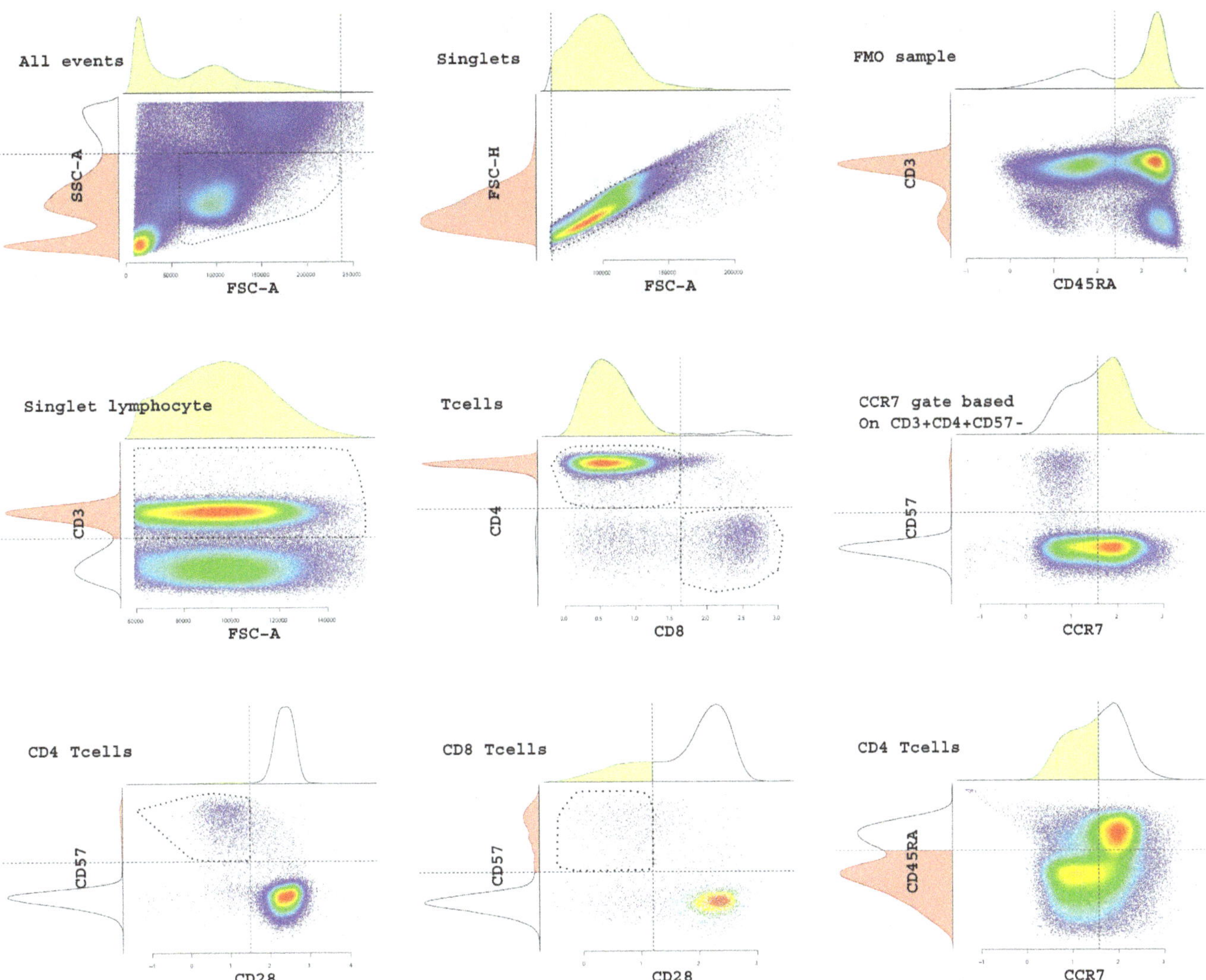

Figure 1. Gating strategy for T-cell phenotypes. T cell phenotypes were defined using the flowDensity software package. Lymphocytes were first gated from non-margin events, and then singlets were gated. CD45RA thresholds were calculated based on singlet lymphocytes FMO. CD3+ cells were gated and then separated into CD4+CD8- and CD4-CD8+. Expression of CD57, CD28, CD45RA and CCR7 was analyzed on either CD4+CD8- or CD8-CD4+.

viral infection. In aged mice, higher percentages of T-regs are observed at baseline and during acute influenza infection when compared to younger mice, and their presence is thought to contribute to a decrease and delay of CD8+ T-cell response during acute influenza infection [39]. In consideration of the murine data, we speculate that elevated levels of T-regs may suppress immune pathology associated with anti-viral immunity.

CMV has been proposed as the chronic antigenic stimulus responsible for accelerated immunosenescence, including the accumulation of senescent CD8+ T-cells [40,41]. There have been at least three studies looking at the association between CMV infection and influenza vaccine response in the elderly [20,42,43]. In one, CMV was associated with influenza vaccine non-response [20], however two other studies found no association [42,43]. In contrast to the reports on seropositivity, we focused on the T-cell response to CMV and observed that elevated frequencies of CMV-reactive CD4+ T-cells, but not CMV-reactive CD8+ T-cells, were associated with an increased risk of respiratory viral infection. We are unaware of any other study linking CMV-reactive CD4+ T-cells to increased risk of respiratory viral infection. It is difficult to speculate on the possible biological relationship between the CMV-reactive CD4+ T cells and susceptibility to infection. Given the observation that CD4+ T-regs also correlate with susceptibility, we interpret these collective data as an indication that the distribution of functional cells (i.e. effector, suppressor, Th1, Th2, etc...) within the CD4+ T cell compartment has a strong influence on host resistance in the elderly. Most research to date has focused on CD8+ T-cells in the elderly and these observation strongly support a new line of research in the elderly to understand how and why skewing of the CD4+ T-cell compartment contributes significantly to the outcome of respiratory infection.

Low naïve CD8+ T-cells, high terminally differentiated CD8+ T-cells and senescent CD8+ T-cells have been described in elderly populations [10–14] and have been hypothesized to predict risk of infection [9,17]. Although there were associations between these immune phenotypes and risk of respiratory viral infection in univariable analyses, after adjustment for known confounders such

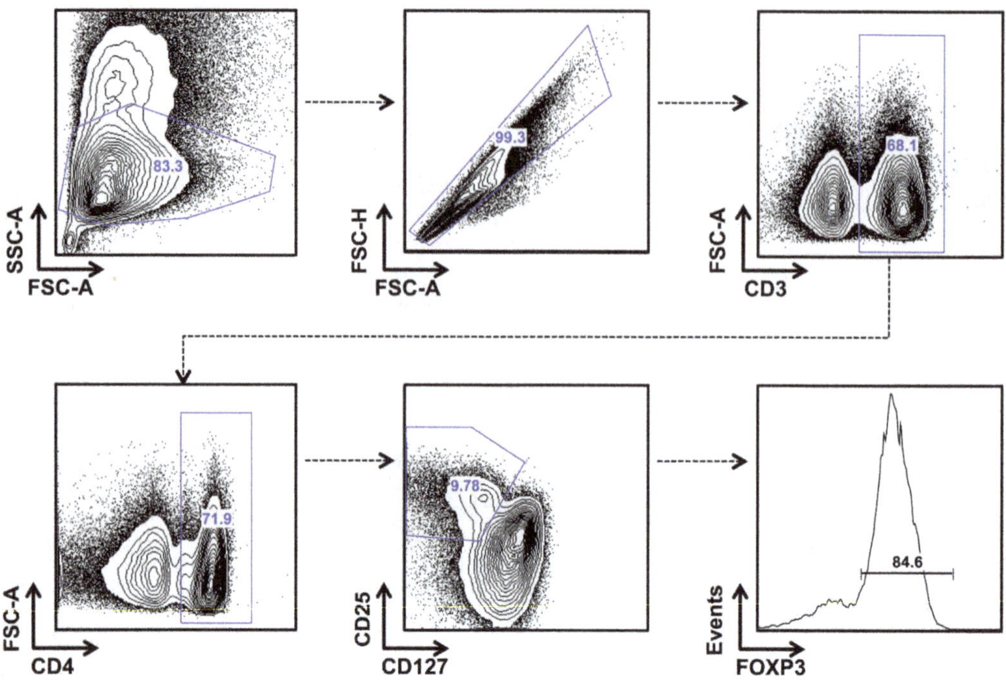

Figure 2. Gating strategy of T-reg. Lymphocytes and singlets were selected. Gates were then set up for CD3+ cells and CD4+. To identify the T-regs, a gate was set up to select CD25+CD127 $^{lo/-}$ and T-regs were defined as CD25+CD127 $^{lo/-}$ FOXP3+.

as age, sex and frailty, CD8+ T cells were not predictive of respiratory viral infection once all immune phenotypes with suspected association with respiratory viral infection were included in the model. This illustrates the need for a robust statistical approach, including adequate sample size allowing for adjustment for known confounders and other immune phenotypes when exploring associations between immune biomarkers and outcomes.

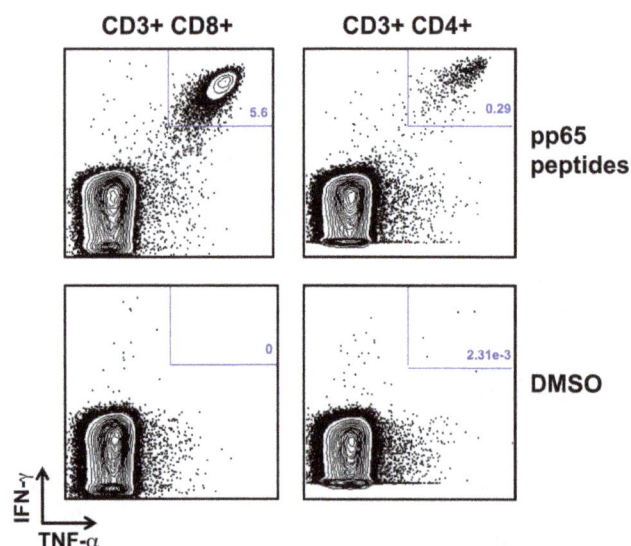

Figure 3. Gating strategy for CMV-reactive T cells. PBMC were stimulated with pp65 peptides to identify CMV-reactive T-cells. As a negative control, PBMC were stimulated with DMSO. Subsequently, the T-cells were stained for surface markers and intracellular cytokines. To define the CMV-reactive T-cells, the flow data was gated on singlet lymphocytes (as shown in Figures 1 and 2) and subsequently gated on CD3+CD8+ cells and CD3+CD4+. The plots show intracellular cytokine staining results for a single patient. CMV-reactive T-cells were defined as IFN-γ+ TNF-α+.

Frailty is a "state variable" which aims to capture a person's vulnerability to adverse health outcomes. The Clinical Frailty Scale used here has been previously validated in nursing home residents and has been shown to robustly predict outcomes including mortality, disability and cognitive decline [23]. Frailty influences health outcomes through a number of mechanisms, including overall burden of disease/comorbidity and reduced reserve to tolerate further insults. Frailty has also been associated with immunosenescence [44]. Because of its importance as a measure of overall health and its relevance to immune function, it was a relevant measure to include in this study.

Our analysis was greatly facilitated by an automated analysis approach which eliminated what would have otherwise been an extremely time-consuming process of manual gating over 1,000 FCS files using an approach that was unbiased relative to manual gating with variability as low or even lower than manual gating. This approach should help facilitate the efficiency of future large studies of immune biomarkers.

This study provides insights into the role of immunosenescence and the risk of respiratory viral infection in elderly nursing home residents. Although our study was designed to identify associations and not causation, our findings suggest the possibility that strategies to boost circulating T-regs [45] or vaccines to prevent infection with CMV [46] or prophylactic anti-viral therapy to prevent re-activation of CMV may reduce respiratory viral infections in this high-risk population. In addition, those identified at increased risk of respiratory viral infection could be offered alternative prevention strategies such as heightened surveillance during the highest risk periods, which could help prevent nursing home outbreaks and transmission to healthcare workers and their families.

Table 2. Respiratory viruses present in symptomatic elderly nursing home residents.

	Nasopharyngeal swabs positive for respiratory virus* n=87 n(%)
Influenza	21 (24)
Influenza A	16 (18)
Influenza B	5 (6)
RSV	12 (14)
RSV A	10 (11)
RSV B	2 (2)
Coronavirus	28 (32)
Coronavirus OC43	15 (17)
Coronavirus NL63/229E	9 (10)
Coronavirus HKU1	4 (5)
Rhinovirus	15 (17)
Human metapneumovirus	8 (9)
Parainfluenza	4 (5)
Parainfluenza 1	3 (3)
Parainfluenza 2	1 (1)

*One patient had mixed influenza A and rhinovirus.

Limitations of this study include lower than expected influenza viral infection. Although influenza is not necessarily the most common virus isolated in nursing homes, [1], we expected to see more than 21 cases in 1072 residents during the influenza season based on prior respiratory viral infection surveillance studies conducted in nursing homes [1,2]. We do not believe that cases were missed. Indeed, we performed prospective active surveillance for symptomatic respiratory viral infection, and approximately one third of the nasopharyngeal swabs were positive for virus, comparable to another study, which performed active surveillance

Table 3. Immune phenotype predictors of respiratory viral infection in univariable and multivariable analysis.

	HR (95% CI) Unadjusted	P-value	HR (95% CI) Final Model*	P-value
Age	0.99 (0.97–1.01)	0.35	0.99 (0.98–1.01)	0.30
Sex				
Male	Reference		Reference	
Female	1.13 (0.65–1.98)	0.66	1.03 (0.58–1.84)	0.92
Clinical Frailty Scale				
4	Reference		Reference	
5	1.44 (0.34–6.17)	0.62	2.68 (0.58–12.47)	0.21
6	1.99 (0.59–6.70)	0.27	3.67 (1.06–12.67)	0.04
7 or 8	1.41 (0.39–5.07)	0.60	2.45 (0.55–10.86)	0.24
CD8+ T-cell				
Low naïve CD8+ T-cell%	0.69 (0.51–0.95)	0.02		
High terminally differentiated CD8+ T-cell%	1.57 (1.10–2.24)	0.01		
High senescent CD8+ T-cell%	1.55 (1.11–2.17)	0.01		
High CMV-reactive CD8+ T-cell%	1.15 (0.65–2.03)	0.64		
CD4+ T-cell				
Low naïve CD4+ T-cell%	0.85 (0.61–1.18)	0.33		
High terminally differentiated CD4+ T-cell%	0.96 (0.60–1.55)	0.88		
High senescent CD4+ T-cell%	1.08 (0.71–1.64)	0.73		
High CMV-reactive CD4+ T-cell%	1.82 (1.13–2.94)	0.01	1.69 (1.03–2.78)	0.04
T-reg				
High T-reg%	0.47 (0.26–0.85)	0.01	0.41 (0.20–0.81)	0.01

*Final model adjusted for age, sex, frailty, high T-reg% and high CMV-reactive CD4+ T-cell%.

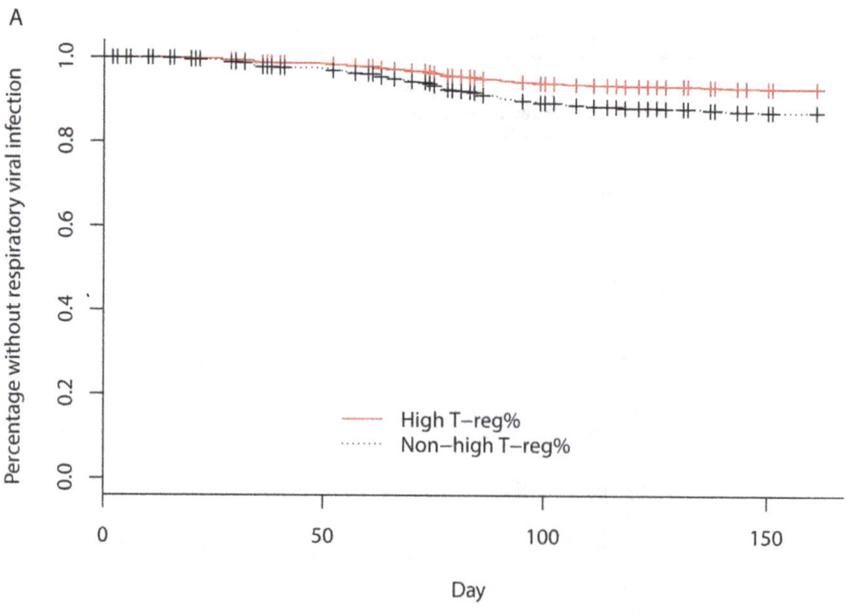

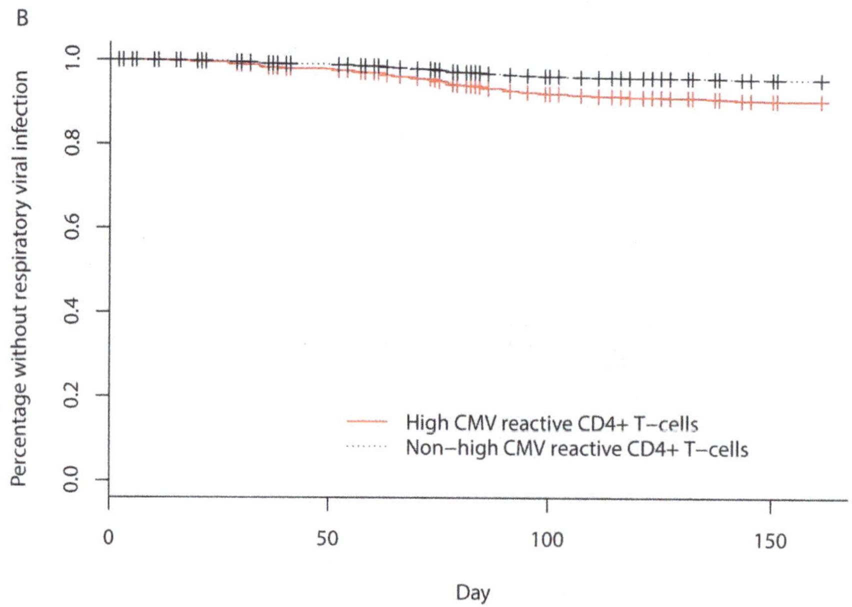

Figure 4. Time to respiratory viral infection stratified by a) T-reg%, adjusted for age, sex, frailty and CMV-reactive CD4+ T-cell%) and b) CMV-reactive CD4+ T-cell%, adjusted for age, sex, frailty and T-reg%.

for respiratory infections in nursing homes in Canada [2]. Instead, we believe the lower numbers were due to circulation of pandemic H1N1, an influenza strain that had less impact on older people during the 2009–2010 influenza season than pre-pandemic years and the relatively low incidence of influenza during 2010-2011 influenza season [47]. In addition, the lower numbers could have been due to the fact that we only included residents who had been vaccinated against influenza. We felt that influenza vaccination status was too important a confounder to manage statistically, both because of its potential ability to prevent influenza infection and because of its association with the healthy user bias [48,49]. It remains possible that there are different immune predictors for each of the different respiratory viruses in this vaccinated cohort and combining the respiratory viruses together in one combined endpoint limited its generalizability; however we chose *a priori* to combine the respiratory viruses together in a combined endpoint based on the fact they result in similar outcomes in this population [1,3–7]. The low number of participants with influenza precluded our ability to perform a sensitivity analysis, looking at immune phenotypes predictive of influenza infection.

An additional limitation was that we were unable to include immune phenotypes as continuous variables in the analysis. In general, maintaining data as continuous is preferred over categorizing data [50]; however an analysis including immune phenotype data as continuous was not feasible as it led to estimates with wide confidence intervals. Thus, the analysis was performed using categorized variables, similar to other aging studies [51–55]. Although seventy-three participants died prior to developing a respiratory viral infection, we do not believe this competing risk introduced significant bias. Competing risks are unlikely to bias the result when the follow-up is short, or the proportion of participants experiencing a competing risk is less than the proportion of participants experiencing the outcome [56]. In this study, the follow-up was short (only one influenza season) and the proportion of participants who died was less than those who developed a respiratory viral infection. Last, these results were obtained in a frail elderly population and may not be generalizable to community dwelling elderly.

In conclusion, in elderly nursing home residents, high CMV-reactive CD4+ T-cells were predictive of increased risk of respiratory viral infection and high T-regs were predictive of reduced risk during the ensuing respiratory viral season. These findings provide insights into immunosenescence and risk of infection and may help guide future prevention strategies.

Supporting Information

Figure S1 Comparison of automated versus manual gating for T-cell phenotypes. The same gating hierarchy was used for manual (top row) and automated (bottom row) approaches for the T-cell panel as described in the text. Similar results were obtained for both methods.

Acknowledgments

We wish to acknowledge the hard work and dedication of the clinical research staff on this project including Chenai Muzamhindo, Diane Dakers, Ashley Chin, Louise Rochon, Eliette Théberge, Sarah DeCoutere and Gale Tedder as well as the Canada's Michael Smith Genome Sciences Centre, Vancouver, Canada for high performance computing support. Dr. Jennie Johnstone receives salary support from CIHR. Mark Loeb holds the Michael G. DeGroote Chair in Infectious Diseases at McMaster University. Jonathan Bramson holds a Canadian Research Chair in Translational Cancer Immunology and the John Bienenstock Chair in Molecular Medicine.

Author Contributions

Conceived and designed the experiments: JJ SM TF J. McElhaney MA JB ML. Performed the experiments: RP FB J. Millar MM RB JM JB. Analyzed the data: JJ SW PD JB ML. Contributed reagents/materials/analysis tools: RB J. Mahony JB. Wrote the paper: JJ RP FB J. Millar SM TF J. McElhaney MA SW PD MM RB J. Mahoney JB ML.

References

1. Falsey A, Dallal G, Formica M, Andolina G, Hamer D, et al. (2008) Long-term care facilities: a cornucopia of viral pathogens. J Am Geriatr Soc 56: 1281–1285.
2. Loeb M, McGeer A, McArthur M, Peeling RW, Petric M, et al. (2000) Surveillance for outbreaks of respiratory tract infections in nursing homes. CMAJ 162: 1133–1137.
3. Drinka P, Gravenstein S, Langer E, Krause P, Shult P (1999) Mortality following isolation of various respiratory viruses in nursing home residents. Infect Control Hosp Epidemiol 20: 812–815.
4. Louie J, Yagi S, Nelson F, Kiang D, Glaser C, et al. (2005) Rhinovirus outbreak in a long-term care facility for elderly persons associated with unusually high mortality. Clin Infect Dis 41: 262–265.
5. Hicks L, Shepard C, Britz P, Erdman D, Fischer M, et al. (2006) Two outbreaks of severe respiratory disease in nursing homes associated with rhinovirus. J Am Geriatr Soc 54: 284–289.
6. Falsey A, McCann R, Hall W, Criddle M, Formica M, et al. (1997) The "common cold" in frail older person: impact of rhinovirus and coronavirus in a senior daycare center. J Am Geriatr Soc 45: 706–711.
7. Boivin G, De Serres G, Hamelin M, Côté S, Argouin M, et al. (2007) An outbreak of severe respiratory tract infection due to human metapneumovirus in a long-term care facility. Clin Infect Dis 44: 1152–1158.
8. Smith P, Bennett G, Bradley S, Drinka P, Lautenbach E, et al. (2008) SHEA/APIC Guideline: Infection prevention and control in the long-term care facility; Society for Healthcare Epidemiology of America (SHEA); Association for Professionals in Infection Control and Epidemiology (APIC). Am J Infect Control 36: 504–535.
9. Fulop T, Pawelec G, Castle S, Loeb M (2009) Immunosenescence and vaccination in nursing home residents. Clin Infect Dis 48: 443–448.
10. Johnstone J, Millar J, Lelic A, Verschoor C, Walter S, et al. (2014) Immunosenescence in the nursing home elderly. BMC Geriatrics 14: 50.
11. Saule P, Trauet J, Dutriez V, Lekeux V, Dessaint J, et al. (2006) Accumulation of memory T cells from childhood to old age: central and effector memory cells in CD4+ versus effector memory and terminally differentiated memory cells in CD8+ compartment. Mech Ageing Dev 127: 274–281.
12. Fahey J, Schnelle J, Boscardin J, Thomas J, Gorre M, et al. (2000) Distinct categories of immunologic changes in frail elderly. Mech Ageing Dev 115: 1–20.
13. Effros R, Boucher N, Porter V, Zhu X, Spaulding C, et al. (1994) Decline in CD28+ T cells in centenarians and in long-term T cell cultures: a possible cause for both in vivo and in vitro immunosenecence. Exp Gerontol 29: 601–609.
14. Boucher N, Dufeu-Duchesne T, Vicaut E, Farge D, Effros R, et al. (1998) CD28 expression in T cell aging and human longevity. Exp Gerontol 33: 267–282.
15. Wikby A, Johansson B, Olsson J, Löfgren S, Nilsson B, et al. (2002) Expansion of peripheral blood CD8 T-lymphocyte subpopulations and an association with cytomegalovirus seropositivity in the elderly: the Swedish NONA immune study. Exp Gerontol 37: 445–453.
16. Looney R, Falsey A, Campbell D, Torres A, Kolassa J, et al. (1999) Role of cytomegalovirus in the T-cell changes seen in elderly individuals. Clin Immunol 90: 213–219.
17. Fulop T, Larbi A, Wikby A, Mocchegiani E, Hirokawa K, et al. (2005) Dysregulation of T-cell function in the elderly: scientific basis and clinical implications. Drugs Aging 22: 589–603.
18. Goronzy J, Fulbright J, Crowson C, Poland G, O'Fallon W, et al. (2001) Value of immunological markers in predicting responsiveness to influenza vaccination in elderly individuals. J Virol 75: 12182–12187.
19. Saurwein-Teissl M, Lung T, Marx F, Gschösser C, Asch E, et al. (2002) Lack of antibody production following immunization in old age: association with CD8+ CD28- T cell clonal expansions and an imbalance in the production of Th1 and Th2 cytokines. J Immunol 168: 5893–5899.
20. Trzonkowski P, Mysliwska J, Szmit E, Wieckiewicz J, Lukaszuk K, et al. (2003) Association between cytomegalovirus infection, enhanced proinflammatory response and low level of anti-hemagglutinins during the anti-influenza vaccination – an impact of immunosenescence. Vaccine 21: 3826–3836.
21. Wang L, Xie Y, Zhu L, Chang T, Mao Y, et al. (2010) An association between immunosenescence and CD4+CD25+ regulatory T-cells: a systematic review. Biomed Environ Sci 23: 327–332.
22. Rowe J, Ertelt J, Way S (2012) Foxp3+ regulatory T-cells, immune stimulation and host defence against infection. Immunology 136: 1–10.
23. Rockwood K, Abeysundera M, Mitnitski A (2007) How should we grade frailty in nursing home patients? J Am Med Dir Assoc 8: 595–603.
24. Langley J, Warshawsky B, Ismail S, Crowcroft N, Hanrahan A, et al. (2009) Statement on seasonal trivalent inactivated influenza vaccine for 2009–2010. CCDR 35: ACS-6.
25. Langley J, Warshawsky B, Ismail S, Crowcroft N, Hanrahan A, et al. (2010) Statement on seasonal trivalent inactivated influenza vaccine for 2010–2011. CCDR 36: ACS-6.
26. Langley J, Warshawsky B, Cooper C, Crowcroft N, Hanrahan A, et al. (2011) Statement on seasonal trivalent inactivated influenza vaccine for 2011–2012. CCDR 37: ACS-5.
27. Disis M, dela Rosa C, Goodell V, Kuan L, Chang J, et al. (2006) Maximizing the retention of antigen specific lymphocyte function after cryopreservation. J Immunol 308: 13–18.
28. Lelic A, Verschoor C, Ventresca M, Parsons R, Evelegh C, et al. (2012) The polyfunctionality of human memory CD8+ T cells elicited by acute and chronic virus infections is not influenced by age. PLoS Pathog 8: e1003076.
29. Verschoor C, Johnstone J, Millar J, Dorrington M, Habibagahi M, et al. (2013) Blood CD33(+)HLA-DR(-) myeloid-derived suppressor cells are increased with age and a history of cancer. J Leukoc Biol 93: 633–637.
30. Submitted as an R package in Bioconductor: An open source, open development software project to provide tools for the analysis and comprehension of high-throughput genomic data.
31. Marshall A, Altman D, Holder R (2010) Comparison of imputation methods for handling missing covariate data when fitting a Cox proportional hazards model: a resampling study. BMC Med Res Methodol 31: 112.
32. Fulop T, Larbi A, Witkowski J, McElhaney J, Loeb M, et al. (2010) Aging, frailty and age-related disease. Biogerontology 11: 547–563.

33. Wei L, Lin D, Weissfeld L (1989) Regression-analysis of multivariate incomplete failure time data by modeling marginal distributions. J Am Stat Assoc 84: 1065–1073.
34. R Core Team (2013) R: A language and environment for statistical computing. R Foundation for Statistical Computing, Vienna, Austria. ISBN 3-900051-07-0. Available: http://www.R-project.org/.
35. Keynan Y, Card C, McLaren P, Dawood M, Kasper K, et al. (2008) The role of regulatory T-cells in chronic and acute viral infections. Clin Infect Dis 46: 1046–1052.
36. Lages C, Suffia I, Velilla P, Huang B, Warshaw G, et al. (2008) Functional regulatory T cells accumulate in aged hosts and promote chronic infectious disease reactivation. J Immunol 181: 1835–1848.
37. Betts R, Prabhu N, Ho A, Lew F, Hutchinson P, et al. (2012) Influenza A virus infection results in a robust, antigen-responsive, and widely disseminated Fox3+ regulatory T cell response. J Virol 86: 2817–2825.
38. Fulton R, Meyerholz D, Varga S (2010) Foxp3+ CD4 regulatory T cells limit pulmonary immunopathology by modulating the CD8 T cell response during respiratory syncytial virus infection. J Immunol 185: 2382–2392.
39. Williams-Bey Y, Jiang J, Murasko D (2011) Expansion of regulatory T cells in aged mice following influenza infection. Mech Ageing Dev 132: 163–170.
40. Koch S, Larbi A, Ozcelik D, Solana R, Gouttefangeas C, et al. (2007) Cytomegalovirus: A driving force in human T-cell immunosenescence. Ann NY Acad Sci 1114: 23–25.
41. Pawelec G, Derhovanessian E, Larbi A, Strindhall J, Wikby A, et al. (2009) Cytomegalovirus and human immunosenescence. Rev Med Virol 19: 47–56.
42. den Elzen W, Vossen A, Cools H, Westendorp R, Kroes A, et al. (2011) Cytomegalovirus infection and responsiveness to influenza vaccination in elderly residents of long-term care facilities. Vaccine 29: 4869–4874.
43. Derhovanessian E, Theeten H, Hahnel K, Van Damme P, Cools N, et al. (2013) Cytomegalovirus-associated accumulation of late-differentiated CD4 T-cells correlates with poor humoral response to influenza vaccination. Vaccine 31: 685–690.
44. McElhaney J, Zhou X, Talbot H, Soethout E, Bleackley R, et al. (2012) The unmet need in the elderly: How immunosenescence, CMV infection, co-morbidities and frailty are a challenge for the development of more effective influenza vaccines. Vaccine 30: 2060–2067.
45. Sehrawat S, Rouse B (2011) Tregs and infections: on the potential value of modifying their function. J Leukoc Biol 90: 1079–1087.
46. Krause P, Bialek S, Boppana S, Griffiths PD, Laughlin C, et al. (2013) Priorities for CMV vaccine development. Vaccine 32: 4–10.
47. Mitchell R, Taylor G, McGeer A, Frenette C, Suh K, et al. (2013) Understanding the burden of influenza infection among adults in Canadian hospitals: a comparison of the 2009–2010 pandemic season with the prepandemic and postpandemic seasons. Am J Infect Control 41: 1032–1037.
48. Jackson L, Jackson M, Nelson J, Neuzil K, Weiss N (2006) Evidence of bias in estimates of influenza vaccine effectiveness in seniors. Int J Epidemiol 35: 337–344.
49. Jackson L, Nelson J, Benson P, Neuzil K, Reid R, et al. (2006) Functional status is a confounder of the association of influenza vaccine and risk of all cause mortality in seniors. Int J Epidemiol 35: 345–352.
50. Bennette C, Vickers A (2012) Against quantiles: categorization of continuous variables in epidemiologic research, and its discontents. BMC Med Res Methodol 12: 21.
51. Izaks G, Remarque E, Becker S, Westendorp R (2003) Lymphocyte count and mortality risk in older persons. The Leiden 85-plus study. J Am Geriatr Soc 51: 1461–1465.
52. Leng S, Xue Q, Tian J, Huang Y, Yeh S, et al. (2009) Associations of neutrophil and monocyte counts with frailty in community-dwelling disabled older women: results from the Women's Health and Aging Studies I. Experimental Gerontol 44: 511–516.
53. Collerton J, Martin-Ruiz C, Davies K, Hilkens C, Isaacs J, et al. (2012) Frailty and the role of inflammation, immunosenescence and cellular ageing in the very old: cross-sectional findings from the Newcastle 85+ study. Mech Ageing Dev 133: 456–466.
54. Wang G, Kao W, Murakami P, Xue Q, Chiou R, et al. (2010) Cytomegalovirus infection and the risk of mortality and frailty in older women: a prospective observational cohort study. Am J Epidemiol 171: 1144–1152.
55. Mathei C, Vaes B, Wallemacq P, Degryse J (2011) Associations between cytomegalovirus infection and functional impairment and frailty in the BEFRAIL cohort. J Am Geriatr Soc 59: 2201–2208.
56. Berry S, Ngo L, Samelson E, Kiel D (2010) Competing risk of death: an important consideration in studies of older adults. J Am Geriatr Soc 58: 783–787.

20

Mortality among People with Severe Mental Disorders Who Reach Old Age: A Longitudinal Study of a Community-Representative Sample of 37892 Men

Osvaldo P. Almeida[1,2,3*], **Graeme J. Hankey**[4,5], **Bu B. Yeap**[4,6], **Jonathan Golledge**[7,8], **Paul E. Norman**[9], **Leon Flicker**[2,4,10]

1 School of Psychiatry & Clinical Neurosciences, University of Western Australia, Perth, Australia, **2** WA Centre for Health & Ageing, Centre for Medical Research, Perth, Australia, **3** Department of Psychiatry, Royal Perth Hospital, Perth, Australia, **4** School of Medicine and Pharmacology, University of Western Australia, Perth, Australia, **5** Department of Neurology, Sir Charles Gairdner Hospital, Perth, Australia, **6** Department of Endocrinology, Fremantle Hospital, Fremantle, Australia, **7** Queensland Research Centre for Peripheral Vascular Disease, School of Medicine and Dentistry, James Cook University, Townsville, Australia, **8** Department of Vascular and Endovascular Surgery, The Townsville Hospital, Townsville, Australia, **9** School of Surgery, University of Western Australia, Perth, Australia, **10** Department of Geriatric Medicine, Royal Perth Hospital, Perth, Australia

Abstract

Background: Severe mental illnesses are leading causes of disability worldwide. Their prevalence declines with age, possibly due to premature death. It is unclear, however, if people with severe mental disorders who reach older age still have lower life expectancy compared with their peers and if their causes of death differ.

Methods and Findings: Cohort study of a community-representative sample of 37892 Australian men aged 65–85 years in 1996–1998. Follow up was censored on the 31st December 2010. Lifetime prevalence of schizophrenia spectrum, bipolar, depressive and alcohol-induced disorder was established through record linkage. A subsample of 12136 consented to a face-to-face assessment of sociodemographic, lifestyle and clinical variables. Information about causes of death was retrieved from the Australian Death Registry. The prevalence of schizophrenia spectrum, bipolar, depressive and alcohol-induced disorders was 1.2%, 0.3%, 2.5% and 1.8%. The mortality hazard for men with a severe mental disorder was 2.3 and their life expectancy was reduced by 3 years. Mortality rates increased with age, but the gap between men with and without severe mental disorders was not attenuated by age. Cardiovascular diseases and cancer were the most frequent causes of death. The excess mortality associated with severe mental disorders could not be explained by measured sociodemographic, lifestyle or clinical variables.

Conclusions: The excess mortality associated with severe mental disorders persists in later life, and the causes of death of younger and older people with severe mental disorders are similar. Hazardous lifestyle choices, suboptimal access to health care, poor compliance with treatments, and greater severity of medical comorbidities may all contribute to this increased mortality. Unlike young adults, most older people will visit their primary care physician at least once a year, offering health professionals an opportunity to intervene in order to minimise the harms associated with severe mental disorders.

Editor: James D. Clelland, The Nathan Kline Institute, United States of America

Funding: This work was supported by the National Health and Medical Research Council of Australia (NHMRC) project grant numbers 279408, 379600, 403963, 513823 and 634492 (URL: www.nhmrc.gov.au). The funders had no role in study design, data collection and analysis, decision to publish, or preparation of the manuscript.

Competing Interests: The authors have declared that no competing interests exist.

* Email: osvaldo.almeida@uwa.edu.au

Introduction

Mental and substance use disorders are leading causes of years lived with disability worldwide [1]. There is also evidence that the life expectancy of people with severe mental illnesses is ten to fifteen years lower than that of the general population [2], mainly because of a high number of deaths due to cardiovascular events (myocardial infarctions and strokes), respiratory diseases and suicide [3,4,5,6]. While suicide could be considered a direct consequence of severe mental illness [7], the underlying reasons for the excessive mortality due to cardiovascular and respiratory diseases are less clear. Unhealthy lifestyle practices commonly associated with psychiatric disorders, such as smoking, might play a role [8,9,10,11], as may some medications used to treat these conditions. Second generation antipsychotics have been associated with the metabolic syndrome and cardiovascular events [12], certain antidepressants with cardiovascular complications [13], and anxiolitics and hypnotics with accidental injuries and premature death [14].

Premature mortality may explain, at least in part, the lower prevalence of severe mental disorders such as schizophrenia, mood and alcohol-induced disorders, in late compared with early adult life [15,16], as the number of new older people affected is lower than the number of prevalent cases who die early. Consequently, older people with severe mental disorders consist of a group of survivors and a relatively small number of new cases [17]. Old survivors could, conceivably, have had a more benign course of illness or healthier lifestyle than those who died early, whereas new cases would have had only limited exposure to the potentially detrimental effects associated with their illness. Thus, there may be no excess mortality among people with severe mental disorders who reach old age. Clarifying whether or not this is the case is important because the number of older people living with severe mental disorders will continue to increase as the population ages [18], and policy makers need to know whether to target this population with interventions that promote health and increase survival.

The Health In Men Study (HIMS) is a longitudinal investigation of a community-representative sample of about 38000 men aged 65–85 years at study entry. Past mental health history was retrieved via health record linkage and mortality data monitored until the end of 2010 [19]. These data were used to determine: (1) the prevalence of severe mental disorders in older men at the start of the study, (2) the 14-year cause-specific mortality of older men with and without severe mental disorders, (3) differences in the life expectancy of older men with and without severe mental disorders, (4) the clinical and lifestyle characteristics of participants with and without severe mental disorders who consent to assessment. We hypothesised that: (1) the prevalence of alcohol-induced, mood and schizophrenia spectrum disorders (severe mental disorders) would be lower than that reported for younger adults, (2) the mortality hazard, causes of death and life expectancy of older men with and without severe mental disorders would be similar, and that (3) men with and without severe mental disorders would have similar lifestyle and clinical characteristics.

Methods

Study design and setting

HIMS is a cohort study of a community-representative sample of older Western Australian men that started in 1996–1998. Follow up data were censored on the 31st December 2010.

Participants

Men aged 65–85 years were identified using an electronic copy of the Western Australian electoral roll (enrolment to vote is compulsory for all Australian adults). We received a list with the contact details of 49801 men. Of those, 1839 had already died at the time the study started and another 9482 did not receive an invitation to participate because they were living outside the immediate Perth metropolitan region. Of the remaining 38480 men, 588 were excluded from further follow up because they had a recorded diagnosis of dementia (International Classification of Diseases 9th edition, ICD-9 code 290). Hence, the study sample for this study consisted of 37892 older men free of dementia at study entry who were recruited between the 2nd April 1996 and the 18th November 1998. Of these, a random sample of 18968 received an invitation to complete a face-to-face assessment: 12136 accepted.

This study followed the principles of the Declaration of Helsinki and was approved by the Ethics Committees of the University of Western Australia and of the Department of Health of Western Australia. The 12136 men who completed the face-to-face assessment provided written informed consent to participate. The remaining 25756 men were not asked to provide written informed consent. For this reason, their data were anonymised and de-identified by the Data Linkage Unit of the Department of Health of Western Australia prior analysis. The procedures for data extraction and analysis followed the regulations for privacy and security of Western Australia (http://www.datalinkage-wa.org.au/privacy-and-security), and were approved by the Human Research Ethics Committee of the Department of Health and by the Legal Data Custodian of the Department of Health of Western Australia.

Healthy participant bias

This study used exposure and outcome data for the entire population, so that no participation bias is involved. However, only 12136 of the 18968 participants invited completed the assessment for HIMS. For this reason, we examined the prevalence of mental disorders and mortality among non-invited men (n = 18924), HIMS participants who completed the assessment (n = 12136), and invited men who did not provide a response to our invitation (n = 6832).

Outcomes

The primary outcome of interest in this study was all-cause mortality, which we measured using the Western Australian Data Linkage System (WADLS).[19] WADLS retrieves information from the Australian Bureau of Statistics about all deaths in Australia, including information about the reported causes of death (http://www.abs.gov.au/ausstats/abs@.nsf/mf/3303.0). We used the International Classification of Diseases codes (ICD-9 until 30/06/2008 and ICD-10 from 01/07/2008) to group the causes of mortality into the following categories: infections (ICD-9 codes ranging from 001 to 139; ICD-10 codes starting with 'A' or 'B'), cancers (ICD-9 codes ranging from 150 to 165, 185 to 192, 200 to 208; ICD-10 codes starting with 'C', D00 and D48), cardiovascular diseases (ICD-9 codes 410 to 414, 430 to 438; ICD-10 codes starting with 'I'), chronic respiratory diseases (ICD-9 codes 490 to 496; ICD-10 codes starting with 'J'), substance-induced or mental diseases (ICD-9 codes 290 to 329; ICD-10 codes starting with 'F'), diseases of the nervous system (ICD-9 codes 330–339; ICD-10 codes starting with 'G'), suicide (ICD-9 codes E950 to E959, E960 to E969; ICD-10 codes X60 to X84), and accidents (ICD-9 codes E800 to E899, E910; ICD-10 codes starting with 'V' or W00 to W19). Deaths due to other causes were placed in a separate group.

Exposures at study entry

We retrieved information about past diagnosis of mental disorders from the WADLS, which connects together all death records, acute hospital admissions (including psychiatry), hospital movements, cancer registry and psychiatric outpatient contacts. The mental health records go back to 1966 (i.e., 30 years before the starting date for this study) [19]. In this study, we were interested in the effect of severe mental disorders that would require input from specialist mental health services: schizophrenia spectrum disorders, bipolar disorder, depressive disorder, and alcohol-induced disorders. Schizophrenia spectrum disor-

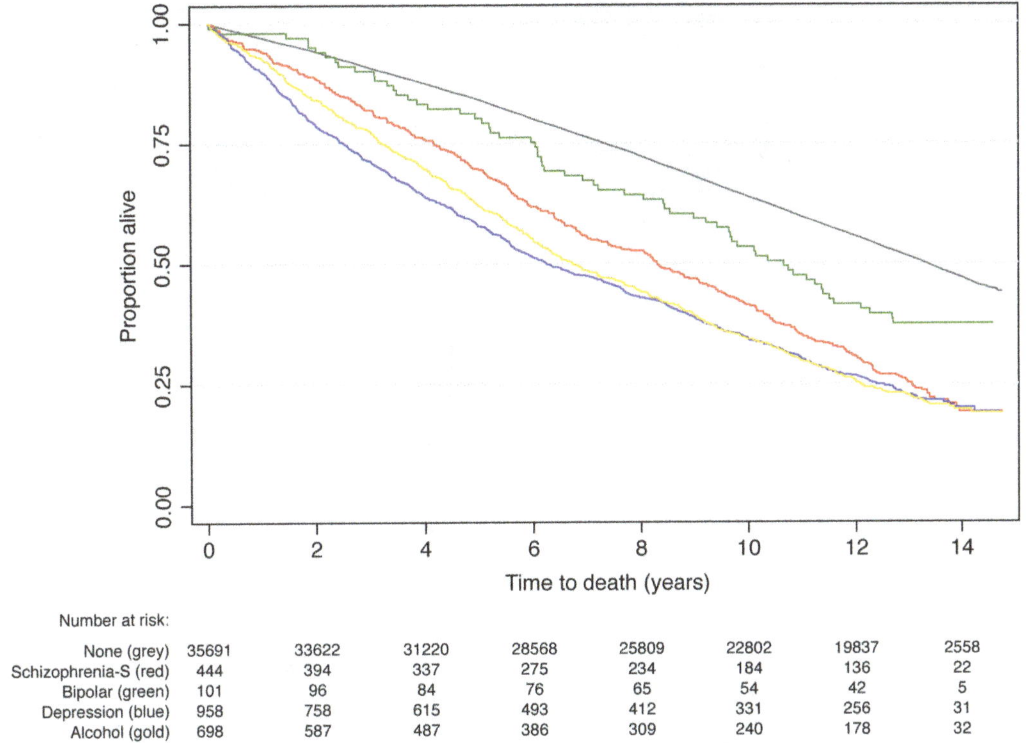

Figure 1. Survival over a follow up period of up to 14.7 years of a community-representative sample of older men with and without serious mental health disorders. The age-adjusted mortality hazard was 2.0 (95%CI = 1.8,2.2), 1.5 (95%CI = 1.2,1.9), 2.3 (95%CI = 2.1,2.5) and 2.6 (95%CI = 2.4,2.8) for men with a past diagnosis of schizophrenia spectrum disorder (Schizophrenia-S), bipolar disorder, depression and alcohol-induced disorders.

ders included schizophrenia, schizophreniform and schizoaffective disorders (ICD-9 codes 295), delusional disorders (ICD-9 codes 297), other schizophrenia spectrum disorders (ICD-9 codes 298.8 and 298.9), and schizotypal disorder (ICD-9 code 301.22). A diagnosis of bipolar disorder was assigned to men who had a recorded ICD-9 code 296.0, 296.4, 296.5, 296.6, 296.7, and 296.80 or 296.89. Men with the following ICD-9 codes were deemed to have had depression before joining the study: 296.2, 296.3, 296.82, 296.90, 298.0, 311. Men with a past recorded ICD-9 code 291 or 303 were identified as having a alcohol-induced disorder. The diagnosis of schizophrenia spectrum disorder took precedence over all other diagnosis, followed by bipolar disorder, depressive disorder and, finally, alcohol-induced disorder. We grouped all other men under the label 'no severe mental disorder'. Previous studies have shown that WADLS yields accurate diagnoses for severe mental disorders [20].

Other study measures at study entry and at the face-to-face assessment

We calculated the age of participants as the difference, in years, between the date of study entry and the date of birth. We then grouped men in 5-year blocks: 65–69, 70–74, 75–79 and 80 or more years. In addition, the 12136 men who completed the clinical assessment provided information about their place of birth (Australia or overseas), marital status, education (high school completed or not), and past self-reported medical history of strokes, angina or heart attacks or bypass surgery, bronchitis or asthma, diabetes and hypertension. We also measured the blood pressure of participants using standardised procedures, and reclassified as hypertensive men with a systolic blood pressure ≥140 mmHg or diastolic blood pressure>90 mmHg.

We measured the height of participants in centimetres (without shoes) and their weight in Kilograms (to 0.2 Kg, light clothing). The body mass index (BMI) was calculated in Kg/m^2 and was used to assign men to the following groups: underweight (BMI<18.5), normal (18.5≤BMI<25), overweight (25≤BMI<30) and obese (BMI≥30). We also asked men how many minutes they spent in a usual week doing vigorous exercise (that made them breathe hard or puff and pant) and considered those who reported 150 minutes or more of weekly activity to be physically active. We inquired whether they had ever smoked (yes/no) and to men who answered 'yes', we asked whether they were still smoking (yes/no). We used this information to group men into never smokers, past smokers and current smokers. Finally, participants answered the following questions about their use of alcohol: 'Have you ever drunk alcohol?' (yes/no), 'Have you drunk alcohol in the last year?' (yes/no), 'If yes, how many standard drinks do you have each day in a usual week?' A standard drink is equivalent to 10 grams of alcohol. We provided guidelines to assist participants calculate the number of drinks consumed.

Study size

A study of this size (n = 37892) would be expected to include at least 150 men with schizophrenia spectrum disorder [21], 150 with bipolar disorder [22], and 750 each with major depression and alcohol-induced disorders [23,24]. We would expect about 50% of older men without a severe mental disorder to die during follow up. If an additional 5% of those

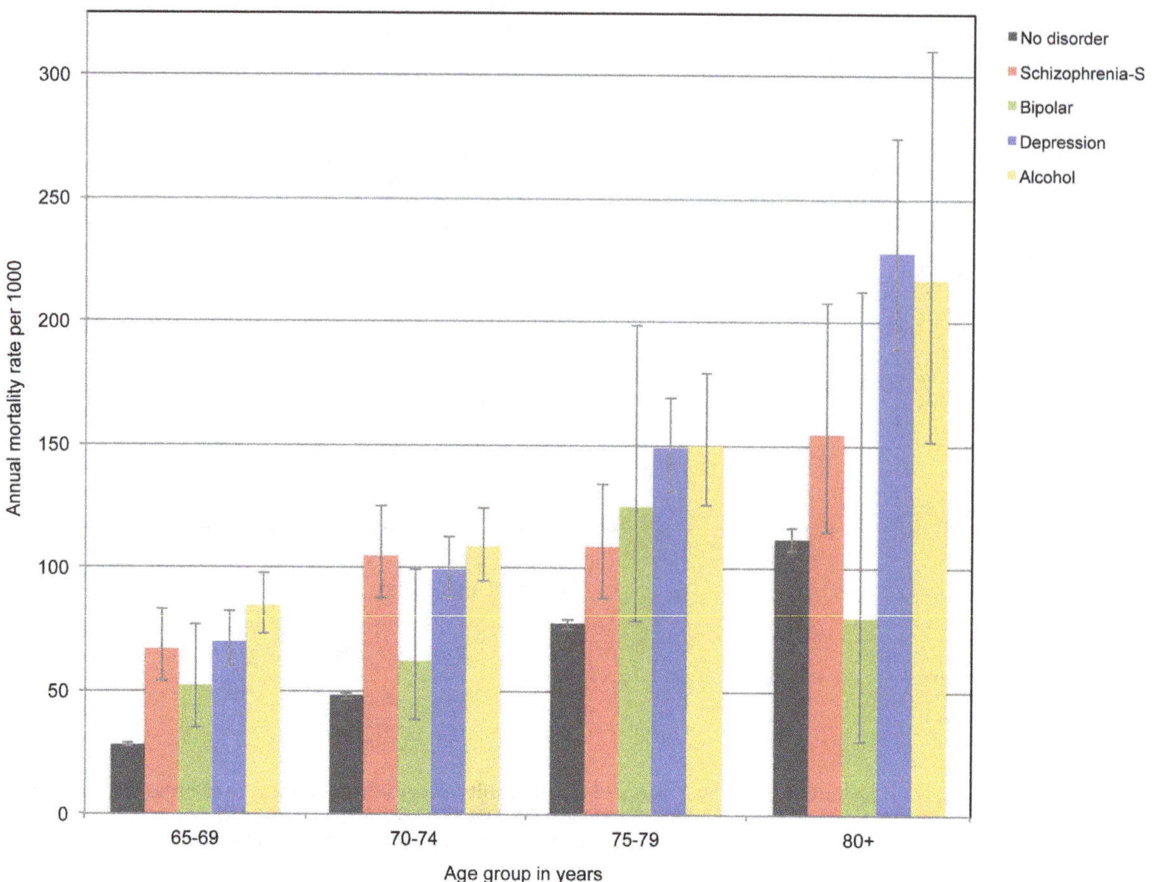

Figure 2. The bars show the mortality rate per 1000 person-years for older men with and without severe mental disorders according to their age group at the time of enrollment. The whiskers indicate the 95% confidence limits of the mean rate. Schizophrenia-S: schizophrenia spectrum disorders. Mean time to event (death or end of follow up) was 10.1 years (standard deviation =4.2; range 1 day to 14.7 years).

with a severe mental disorder die during the same period, this study would have over 95% power to declare this difference as significant for a two-tailed alpha of 5%.

Statistical methods

We used the statistical package Stata/IC 13.1 to manage and analyse the data (StataCorp LP, 2013). Descriptive statistics summarised categorical data as count and proportions (%), and continuous variables as mean, range, and standard deviation of the mean (SD). Of the 37892 men included in the study, a random sample of 18,968 received an invitation for assessment, and 12136 attended their appointment. Details about the selection procedure have been described elsewhere [25].

We used the proportion command of Stata to estimate the prevalence of severe mental disorders (95% confidence intervals were calculated using a logit transformation that allows for the estimation of the standard error of the proportion). We subsequently employed Cox regression to estimate the mortality hazard ratio (HR) of older men with past recorded history of severe mental disorders, and set the origin on the participants' date of birth, the beginning of follow up as the date of randomisation, and the date of death as the time of the event. Data were censored on the 31st December 2010. Survival data were plotted using the Kaplan-Meier survivor function. We calculated the mortality rate of people with and without severe mental disorders per-thousand person-years using the strate command of Stata. A similar Cox regression model was used to estimate the mortality hazard of the 12136 men who completed the assessment for HIMS.

Analysis of the risk of specific causes of death according to the four severe mental disorder groups (schizophrenia spectrum, bipolar, depression and alcohol-induced) was based on competing risks regression models. These models investigate the event of interest (e.g., death from cardiovascular disease) when competing events are present and impede the occurrence of the event of interest (e.g., death by cancer or by a respiratory disease, etc.). The risk estimates, in this case, are expressed as sub-hazard ratio (SHR).

We used Pearson's chi-square statistic to compare the distribution of severe mental disorders, age, and death during the subsequent follow up of these three samples (i.e., controls not invited, invited participants who underwent assessment, and invited participants who did not respond to our invitation for assessment). The age distribution of these three groups was also compared using oneway analysis of variance. Logistic regression was applied to determine the odds ratio (OR) of having a severe mental disorder of HIMS participants and non-responders compared with controls, as well as their odds of death.

We calculated the 95% confidence interval (95%CI) for all risk estimates, rates, differences and proportions. Alpha was set at 0.05 and all testes reported were two-tailed.

Table 1. Causes of death over a 14-year period among older men with and without severe mental disorders.

	No severe mental disorder	Schizophrenia-S	Bipolar	Depression	Alcohol
	N = 35691	**N = 444**	**N = 101**	**N = 958**	**N = 698**
	n (%)	**n (%)**	**n (%)**	**n (%)**	**n (%)**
Causes of death:	**1 (Reference)**	**SHR (95%CI)**	**SHR (95%CI)**	**SHR (95%CI)**	**SHR (95%CI)**
Alive	17750 (49.7)	101 (22.7)	38 (37.6)	211 (22.0)	148 (21.2)
Infection	222 (0.6)	7 (1.6)	0	9 (0.9)	9 (1.3)
		2.4 (1.1, 5.1)	–	1.5 (0.8, 2.9)	**2.0 (1.0, 3.9)**
Cancer	5976 (16.7)	61 (13.7)	11 (10.9)	185 (19.3)	143 (20.5)
		0.8 (0.6, 1.0)	0.6 (0.3, 1.1)	**1.2 (1.0, 1.4)**	**1.2 (1.0, 1.5)**
Cardiovascular diseases	6160 (17.3)	118 (26.6)	23 (22.8)	254 (26.5)	185 (26.5)
		1.6 (1.3, 1.9)	1.4 (0.9, 2.1)	**1.6 (1.4, 1.9)**	**1.6 (1.4, 1.9)**
Chronic respiratory diseases	1634 (4.6)	44 (9.9)	10 (9.9)	102 (10.6)	86 (12.3)
		2.1 (1.6, 2.9)	**2.2 (1.2, 4.1)**	**2.4 (2.0, 2.9)**	**2.8 (2.2, 3.4)**
Substance induced, mental disorders	432 (1.2)	22 (4.9)	5 (4.9)	14 (1.5)	13 (1.9)
		3.7 (2.4, 5.7)	**4.2 (1.7, 10.4)**	1.1 (0.7, 1.9)	1.5 (0.9, 2.6)
Nervous system, including dementia	702 (2.0)	33 (7.4)	1 (1.0)	44 (4.6)	14 (2.0)
		3.7 (2.6, 5.2)	0.5 (0.1, 3.5)	**2.3 (1.7, 3.1)**	1.0 (0.6, 1.7)
Suicide	78 (0.2)	0	2 (2.0)	7 (0.7)	1 (0.1)
		–	**8.6 (2.1, 35.0)**	**3.6 (1.7, 7.9)**	0.6 (0.1, 4.4)
Accidents	249 (0.7)	5 (1.1)	1 (1.0)	7 (0.7)	7 (1.0)
		1.5 (0.6, 3.7)	1.4 (0.2, 10.0)	1.0 (0.5, 2.2)	1.4 (0.7, 2.9)
Other	2488 (7.0)	53 (11.9)	10 (9.9)	125 (13.0)	92 (13.2)
		1.7 (1.3, 2.2)	1.4 (0.8, 2.7)	**2.0 (1.6, 2.4)**	**1.9 (1.5, 2.4)**

Schizophrenia-S: schizophrenia spectrum disorders.
SHR: sub-hazard ratio derived from competing-risks regression. 95%CI: 95% confidence interval of the sub-hazard ratio.
Bold print denotes statistically significant association.

Results

The study sample consisted of 37892 men aged 65 to 85 years at study entry (mean = 72.4, SD = 4.6). Of these, 444 had a recorded diagnosis in WADLS of schizophrenia spectrum (1.2%, 95%CI = 1.1%, 1.3%), 101 of bipolar (0.3%, 95%CI = 0.2%, 0.3%), 958 of depression (2.5%, 95%CI = 2.4%, 2.7%), and 698 of alcohol-induced disorder (1.8%, 95%CI = 1.7%, 2.0%). Oneway analysis of variance showed that men with a past diagnosis of alcohol-induced disorder were 0.5, 1.2 and 1.8 years younger than men without a severe mental disorder, schizophrenia spectrum and depression respectively ($p<0.05$ after Scheffe correction for multiple comparisons). Men with depression were 1.3, and 2.0 years older than their counterparts with no diagnosis and with diagnosis of bipolar disorder ($p>0.05$ after Scheffe correction for multiple comparisons).

By 31st December 2010, 19644 men had died (51.8%), of whom 343 had a schizophrenia spectrum disorder, 63 bipolar, 747 depression and 550 an alcohol-induced disorder. Figure 1 shows the proportion of participants alive during follow up according to the presence of a severe mental disorder. The age-adjusted mortality hazard ratio for men with a severe mental disorder was 2.3 (95%CI = 2.2, 2.4) and their life expectancy was reduced by 2.8 years (95%CI = 2.6, 3.0) compared with their peers. Age-adjusted life expectancy was reduced, on average, 2.0 (95%CI = 1.6, 2.3), 1.1 (95%CI = 0.4, 1.9), 2.8 (95%CI = 2.6, 3.1) and 3.1 (2.8, 3.4) years for men with schizophrenia spectrum, bipolar, depressive and alcohol-induced disorder, respectively. We then completed a sensitivity analysis by excluding from the sample men who died within the first two years of follow up: the mortality hazard associated with any severe mental disorder remained largely unchanged (HR = 2.1, 95%CI = 2.0, 2.2 after the sensitivity analysis).

We stratified participants by age groups (65–69, 70–74, 75–79, 80+) to ascertain their mortality rate. Figure 2 shows the results of these analyses according to the presence of a severe mental disorder before randomisation. The annual mortality rate of men increased with increasing age and was consistently higher amongst those with than without a severe mental disorder. The mortality rate estimate for men with bipolar disorder was imprecise for those aged over 80 years because there were only 6 people in this group.

Table 1 shows the causes of death of participants with and without a severe mental disorder. Men with past diagnosis of schizophrenia spectrum disorders showed excess mortality due to infections, cardiovascular diseases, chronic respiratory diseases, substance-induced or mental disorders, diseases of the nervous system and other. These were no suicides in this group. Men with past diagnosis of bipolar disorder died more frequently than controls of chronic respiratory diseases, suicide, and mental disorders (including substance-induced). Men with depression showed evidence of excess mortality due to cancer, cardiovascular events, chronic respiratory diseases and diseases of the central nervous system, as well as suicide and other causes of death. Finally, men with a past diagnosis of alcohol-induced disorder died more frequently than men without a severe mental disorder of infections, cancer, cardiovascular and respiratory diseases.

Table 2 shows the characteristics of men according to their randomisation assignment: not-invited and invited HIMS participants. Men who joined HIMS were 0.4 and 1.1 years younger than non-invited participants and those who did not respond. In addition, HIMS non-responders were 0.7 years older than men who were not invited (p<0.05 for all analyses, after Scheffe correction for multiple comparisons). There was also an excess of men with severe mental disorders among non-responders than among non-invited men or those included in HIMS. Compared with non-invited men, men included in HIMS had a lower odds of severe mental disorder (OR = 0.7, 95%CI = 0.6, 0.8), whereas non-responder had 43% greater odds of having a severe mental disorder (OR = 1.4, 95%CI = 1.3, 1.6). Similarly, HIMS participants had lower odds of death than non-invited men (OR = 0.8, 95%CI = 0.7,0.8), whereas non-responders had higher chance of dying (OR = 1.5, 95%CI = 1.4, 1.5). Compared with non-invited men, HIMS participants lived 0.7 years longer (95%CI = 0.6, 0.8), whereas non-responders died 1.1 (95%CI = 1.0, 1.2) years earlier than non-invited men and 1.8 (95%CI = 1.6, 1.9) years earlier than HIMS participants.

The sociodemographic, lifestyle and clinical characteristics of men who completed the HIMS assessment are summarised in table 3. Men with schizophrenia spectrum, depression and alcohol-induced disorders were less likely to be married than men with no severe mental disorder, whereas those with depression and alcohol-induced disorders were less likely to have completed high school education. Men with history of alcohol-induced disorders were less physically active than controls without a severe mental disorder. More people with schizophrenia spectrum and alcohol induced disorders were underweight, whereas more people with bipolar disorder were obese. There were more past and current smokers among men with history of schizophrenia spectrum and alcohol-induced disorder, and more current smoking among those with bipolar disorder. Regular alcohol use was less frequent in men with history of depression, but much more frequent among those with a history of alcohol-induced disorder. Two men with history of alcohol-induced disorder denied having previously consumed alcohol. Chronic respiratory illnesses were more prevalent in men with schizophrenia spectrum disorders, coronary heart disease in men with past bipolar, depression and alcohol-induced disorder, and strokes in men with schizophrenia spectrum, depression and alcohol induced disorder. Cox regression showed that the mortality hazard associated with a past severe mental disorder was 2.3 (95%CI = 1.8, 2.9) for schizophrenia spectrum, 1.8 (95%CI = 1.2, 2.8) for bipolar, 1.9 (95%CI = 1.7,2.3) for depression and 2.7 (95%CI = 2.2,3.2) for alcohol-induced disorder. After adjusting the analyses for all the variables listed in the table 3, the respective mortality hazards were 1.9 (95%CI = 1.5, 2.4), 1.5 (95%CI = 0.9, 2.4), 1.6 (95%CI = 1.4, 1.9) and 1.9 (95%CI = 1.6, 2.3). If alcohol use is excluded from the model, the mortality hazards were 2.0 (95%CI = 1.5, 2.5) for schizophrenia spectrum, 1.4 (95%CI = 0.9, 2.3) for bipolar, 1.7 (95%CI = 1.4, 1.9) for depression, and 2.0 (95%CI = 1.7, 2.5) for alcohol-induced disorder.

Discussion

The recorded prevalence of severe mental disorders in this large community-representative sample of older men was 5.8%. Schizophrenia spectrum disorders affected 1.2% of the population, bipolar 0.3%, depression 2.5%, and alcohol-induced disorders 1.8%. The mortality hazard ratio for men with a severe mental disorder was 2.3 times greater than for men free of significant mental health problems, and this excess mortality occurred across all four diagnostic groups under investigation.

Table 2. Basic characteristics of participants according to their random assignment to the control or Health In Men Study (HIMS) group.

		Controls	HIMS			
			Included	No response		
		N = 18924	N = 12136	N = 6832		
		n (%)	n (%)	n (%)	Chi-square statistic (df)	p-value
Age in years:	65–69	6768 (35.8)	4731 (39.0)	2150 (31.5)	264.94 (4)	<0.001
	70–74	6549 (34.6)	4210 (34.7)	2213 (32.4)		
	75–79	4224 (22.3)	2502 (20.6)	1748 (25.6)		
	80+	1383 (7.3)	693 (5.7)	721 (10.5)		
Schizophrenia spectrum		228 (1.2)	97 (0.8)	119 (1.7)	132.54 (8)	<0.001
Bipolar disorder		49 (0.3)	28 (0.2)	24 (0.3)		
Depressive disorder		479 (2.5)	236 (1.9)	243 (3.6)		
Alcohol induced disorder		366 (1.9)	154 (1.3)	178 (2.6)		
Died during follow up		9849 (52.0)	5608 (46.2)	4187 (61.3)	398.54 (2)	<0.001

df: number of degrees of freedom.
HIMS participants were, on average, 0.4 years younger than controls (95% confidence interval of the mean difference, 95%CI = 0.3,0.5; p<0.001) and 1.1 (95%CI = 0.9,1.2; p<0.001) years younger than men who did not respond to the invitation to join the study. Non-invited men were 0.7 years (95%CI = 0.5,0.8; p<0.001) younger than participants who did not respond to the invitation to take part in HIMS.

Table 3. Characteristics of older men according to recorded diagnoses of severe mental disorders before the clinical assessment for HIMS.

		No disorder	Schizophrenia-S		Bipolar		Depression		Alcohol	
		N=11619	N=97		N=28		N=236		N=154	
Characteristics at assessment:		n (%)	n (%)	OR (95%CI)	n (%)	OR (95%CI)	n (%)	OR (95%CI)	n (%)	OR (95%CI)
Age in years:	65–69	4448 (38.3)	33 (34.0)	Reference	14 (50.0)	Reference	77 (32.6)	Reference	65 (42.2)	Reference
	70–74	4058 (34.9)	39 (40.2)	1.3 (0.8,2.1)	5 (17.9)	0.4 (0.1,1.1)	86 (36.4)	1.2 (0.9,1.7)	58 (37.7)	1.0 (0.7,1.4)
	75–79	2435 (21.0)	17 (17.5)	0.9 (0.5,1.7)	8 (28.6)	1.0 (0.4,2.5)	51 (21.6)	1.2 (0.8,1.7)	25 (16.2)	0.7 (0.4,1.1)
	80+	678 (5.8)	8 (8.3)	1.6 (0.7,3.5)	1 (3.6)	0.5 (0.1,3.6)	22 (9.3)	**1.9 (1.2,3.0)**	6 (3.9)	0.6 (0.3,1.4)
Australian born		5229 (45.0)	38 (39.2)	0.8 (0.6,1.2)	13 (46.4)	1.1 (0.5,2.2)	109 (46.2)	1.0 (0.8,1.4)	80 (51.9)	1.3 (1.0,1.8)
Marital status: married		9533 (82.1)	61 (62.9)	**0.4 (0.2,0.6)**	20 (71.4)	0.5 (0.2,1.2)	166 (70.3)	**0.5 (0.4,0.7)**	85 (55.2)	**0.3 (0.2,0.4)**
Education: high school or above		4698 (40.5)	37 (38.1)	0.9 (0.6,1.4)	14 (50.0)	1.5 (0.7,3.1)	74 (31.4)	**0.7 (0.5,0.9)**	50 (32.5)	**0.7 (0.5,1.0)**
Body mass index:	normal	3540 (30.5)	25 (25.8)	Reference	7 (25.0)	Reference	78 (33.0)	Reference	49 (32.0)	Reference
	underweight	74 (0.6)	3 (3.1)	**5.7 (1.7,19.4)**	0	–	3 (1.3)	1.8 (0.6,6.0)	5 (3.3)	**4.9 (1.9,12.6)**
	overweight	5913 (50.9)	56 (57.7)	1.3 (0.8,2.2)	8 (28.6)	0.7 (0.2,1.9)	109 (46.2)	0.8 (0.6,1.1)	72 (47.1)	0.9 (0.6,1.3)
	obese	2085 (18.0)	13 (13.4)	0.9 (0.4,1.7)	13 (46.4)	**3.1 (1.3,7.9)**	46 (19.5)	1.0 (0.7,1.4)	27 (17.6)	0.9 (0.6,1.5)
Physically active		1979 (17.0)	13 (13.4)	0.8 (0.4,1.4)	5 (17.9)	1.1 (0.4,2.8)	29 (12.3)	0.7 (0.5,1.0)	15 (9.7)	**0.5 (0.3, 0.9)**
Smoking history:	never	3438 (29.6)	16 (16.5)	Reference	9 (32.1)	Reference	68 (28.8)	Reference	18 (11.7)	Reference
	past	6965 (59.9)	65 (67.0)	**2.0 (1.2,3.5)**	9 (32.1)	0.5 (0.2,1.2)	135 (57.2)	1.0 (0.7,1.3)	83 (53.9)	**2.3 (1.4,3.8)**
	current	1216 (10.5)	16 (16.5)	**2.8 (1.4,5.7)**	10 (35.7)	**3.1 (1.3,7.7)**	33 (14.0)	1.4 (0.9,2.1)	53 (34.4)	**8.3 (4.9,14.3)**
Alcohol use:	never	694 (6.2)	6 (6.6)	Reference	0	–	23 (10.0)	Reference	2 (1.3)	Reference
	past	1238 (11.1)	15 (16.5)	1.4 (0.5,3.6)	3 (11.5)	Reference	54 (23.6)	1.3 (0.8,2.2)	41 (27.5)	**11.5 (2.8,47.7)**
	≤ 28 drinks/week	8732 (78.1)	64 (70.3)	0.8 (0.4,2.0)	23 (88.5)	1.1 (0.3,3.6)	145 (63.3)	**0.5 (0.3,0.8)**	75 (50.3)	3.0 (0.7,12.2)
	>28 drinks/week	522 (4.7)	6 (6.6)	1.3 (0.4,4.1)	0	–	7 (3.1)	**0.4 (0.2,0.9)**	31 (20.8)	**20.6 (4.9,86.5)**
Chronic respiratory illness		2520 (22.5)	34 (37.4)	**2.1 (1.3,3.1)**	10 (38.5)	2.1 (1.0,4.7)	56 (24.4)	1.1 (0.8,1.5)	36 (24.2)	1.1 (0.7,1.6)
Hypertension		9523 (82.0)	71 (73.2)	**0.6 (0.4,0.9)**	19 (67.9)	0.5 (0.2,1.0)	182 (77.1)	0.7 (0.5,1.0)	124 (80.5)	0.9 (0.6,1.4)
Diabetes		1322 (11.4)	12 (12.4)	1.1 (0.6,2.0)	5 (17.9)	1.7 (0.6,4.5)	38 (16.0)	**1.5 (1.1,2.1)**	27 (17.5)	**1.7 (1.1,2.5)**
Coronary heart disease		2016 (18.0)	20 (22.0)	1.3 (0.8,2.1)	9 (34.6)	**2.4 (1.1,5.4)**	80 (34.9)	**2.4 (1.9,3.2)**	39 (26.2)	**1.6 (1.1,2.3)**
Stroke		805 (7.2)	13 (14.3)	**2.1 (1.2,3.9)**	4 (15.4)	2.3 (0.8,6.8)	43 (18.8)	**3.0 (2.1,4.2)**	19 (12.7)	**1.9 (1.2,3.1)**
Died during follow up		5245 (45.1)	73 (75.3)	**3.7 (2.3,5.9)**	19 (67.9)	**2.6 (1.2,5.7)**	156 (66.1)	**2.4 (1.8,3.1)**	114 (74.0)	**3.5 (2.4,5.0)**

Schizophrenia-S: schizophrenia spectrum disorders. See text for information about the mortality hazard. OR: odds ratio, 95%CI: 95% confidence interval of the odds ratio.

The mortality rate increased with increasing age, and the gap in the rates between men with and without history of severe mental disorder remained more or less stable for the different age groups. Our data also showed that men with severe mental disorders who agreed to complete a clinical assessment had different educational, sociodemographic, lifestyle and clinical background, although these variables could not adequately explain the excess mortality of this population.

Strengths and limitations of the study design

This study has the merit of having assembled a large community-representative sample of older men, which allowed us to ascertain with precision the unbiased prevalence of relatively uncommon mental disorders of older age. Establishment of 'caseness of mental disorder' was based on data retrieved from the WADLS since 1966, which covers all inpatient and outpatient contacts with mental health services (but not primary care) [26]. We have treated our prevalence estimates as indicative of the lifetime presence of the disorder, although health contacts occurring exclusively before 1966 would have been missed. This could have generated 'false-negative' cases, although the chronic and recurring course of these disorders suggest this is unlikely to have been a source of bias. Even it that were the case, the potential inclusion of cases among men assigned to the 'no severe mental disorder' group would have minimised differences in mortality hazard when we compared people with and without severe mental disorders. Hence, the observed differences are most likely valid, although we cannot dismiss the possibility that the effect of severe mental disorders on mortality could be higher than our estimates suggest. We also acknowledge that case-ascertainment using record linkage may not be as accurate or as valid as structured systematic assessments that lead to a diagnosis according to accepted criteria. Existing data suggest that the WADLS diagnoses for severe mental disorders such as schizophrenia and bipolar disorder are valid [20]. The diagnosis of alcohol-induced disorder has some face-validity regarding mortality [7], and our finding that 1 in every 5 men who had received this diagnosis were still drinking heavily at the time of assessment for HIMS suggest that they had been, and perhaps some had continued to be, problem drinkers.

Every person deceased in Australia is entered in the death registry, which forms part of WADLS. The registry allows for the recording of the main cause of death, as well as up to 20 other secondary causes. In this study, we used only the code for the main cause of death and concede that there is a certain degree of subjectivity on how these diagnoses are assigned. For example, a person with schizophrenia might be admitted to hospital with a chest infection that eventually leads to death. Some doctors may record schizophrenia as the main cause of death (particularly if the chest infection is considered to have arisen as a result of poor mobility associated with the illness), while others might record infection. For this reason, we included substance-induced and other mental disorders as possible causes of death in this cohort. It is also conceivable that some of the men included in the study moved away from Australia and that their deaths were not recorded in the death registry. However, movements away from Australia are minimal in this older age group [27], suggesting that this would have had a negligible impact on our estimates. Importantly, our analysis of the causes of death took into account competing risks, and this approach to the analysis of the data provides a more accurate estimate of the risk of death due to a specified condition than Cox regression.

The inclusion of prevalent cases of dementia in the sample could have biased our results, as these patients may present psychiatric and behavioural symptoms that could be misdiagnosed as a psychotic or mood disorder. Such misclassification bias would have contributed to increase the mortality hazard of people with a severe mental disorder, as older people with dementia have lower life expectancy than those without [28]. We tried to minimise such a possibility by excluding from the study 588 people with a recorded diagnosis of dementia (known prevalent cases) and by completing a sensitivity analysis that excluded men who had died within the initial two years of follow up: the results remained virtually unchanged. This sensitivity analysis also aimed to decrease confounding due to severe prevalent medical morbidity when follow up started. For example, if the diagnosis of a severe mental disorder (e.g., depression) were made opportunistically at the time of admission to hospital because of a significant medical morbidity (e.g., stroke), then short-term survival ascribed to the mental disorder would have been confounded by the concurrent morbidity.

Moreover, we acknowledge that we did not have access to data about factors likely to mediate or facilitate the premature death of all older men with severe mental disorders. This limitation was partly circumvented by analysing the data from the 12136 HIMS participants, which showed that some socio-demographic, lifestyle and clinical factors could potentially attenuate the risk of death among these men. We concede, however, that HIMS was associated with healthy participant bias and that inferences drawn from this sample should be interpreted with caution. Finally, it is important to note that the results of this study were limited to men and may not be directly applicable to women, although the results of other investigations indicate that the life expectancy of women with severe mental disorders is similarly reduced [2].

Interpretation of the findings

The results of this study confirmed our prediction that the recorded lifetime prevalence of severe mental disorders in later life would be lower than that reported for younger age-groups. We found that the prevalence of severe mental disorders in this old cohort of men was 5.8%. The Health 2000 Study recruited 8028 people aged 30 years or older living in Finland [29]. After an initial screening for psychotic symptoms, eligible participants were interviewed with the Composite International Diagnostic Interview (CIDI) and lifetime psychiatric diagnoses followed the DSM-IV criteria. Non-affective psychosis (akin to our definition of schizophrenia spectrum disorder) was present in 2.3% of those aged 45–54, 55–64 and over 65 years [29]. The prevalence of bipolar disorder decreased from 0.4% among those aged 45–54 to 0.2% among those aged 55 to 64 and 0.1% among those older than 65 years, although confidence limits were wide and consistent with our results [29]. In the present study, it is conceivable that false positive cases were included in the group of schizophrenia spectrum disorders because of the hierarchical approach we used to ascribe diagnosis. The consequence of such a misclassification would be inflation in the prevalence of schizophrenia spectrum disorders relative to other diagnostic categories, such as bipolar disorder.

The prevalence of depressive disorders in our study was lower than the lifetime prevalence of 10.6% among those aged over 60 years reviewed by the National Comorbidity Survey Replication, which in turn was 1.5 to 2 times lower than in younger age-groups [30]. Such a discrepancy may be partly due to the fact that, among the severe mental disorders, major depression is the condition most commonly treated outside mental health specialist settings [31]. Consequently, depressive disorders recorded in the WADLS are most likely true cases (i.e., high specificity), although the system may lack sensitivity to identify uncomplicated depression managed successfully in the primary care sector. In addition, the hierarchical approach we used to ascribe diagnoses (schizophrenia spectrum then bipolar then depressive then alcohol-induced disorders) might have contributed to reduce the number of people identified as having a depressive disorder, and may further explain the relative low prevalence of depression in our sample.

Data from the Australian Survey of Mental Health and Well-Being showed that the 12-month prevalence of alcohol use disorders falls from 10.5% among those aged 18–34 years to 1.8% for people older than 55 years [32]. However, American data suggest that lifetime prevalence in later life may be as high as 16.1% [33]. As for depressive disorders, the hierarchical system that we used to assign diagnoses could have decreased the number of men with alcohol-induced disorders, as some of them might have been ascribed other diagnoses (schizophrenia spectrum, bipolar or depression) [34]. This, together with the limited sensitivity of the WADLS to record uncomplicated cases (for example, alcohol abuse), may have led to an underestimation of the true lifetime prevalence of alcohol-induced disorders in the present cohort. Notwithstanding these potential caveats, the WADLS identified cases of severe mental disorder that require assistance from specialist medical services. We acknowledge, though, that we did not have access to comparable data from other age groups and that our inferences about the decreasing prevalence of severe mental disorders in later life are indirect.

Our data also confirmed that people with recorded history of past severe mental disorders who reach old age have lower life expectancy and greater mortality hazard than men with no such history. As a group, men with a past severe mental disorder died 2.8 years earlier than their counterparts and were twice as likely to die during the subsequent 14 years of follow up. The underlying reasons for this excess mortality are not immediately apparent, although others have suggested that hazardous lifestyle (such as smoking) and poor physical health drive this process [10]. Using data from a subsample of this cohort (HIMS), we found that men with schizophrenia spectrum, bipolar, depression and alcohol-induced disorders differed from their counterparts on a number of lifestyle, medical, educational and sociodemographic variables, but that the excess mortality of those with mental disorders could not be explained entirely by these factors (although statistical adjustment for these factors did attenuate the hazard ratio). It is also possible that the severity of the medical comorbidities among those with mental disorders was different. For example, diabetes may be present in both groups, but may not be as well controlled in men with a severe mental disorder. There is evidence that people with severe mental disorders do not receive the same level of care for physical comorbidities as people without these disorders [35], and their compliance with medical treatments may be suboptimal [36]. Thus, people with severe mental disorders may have more frequent medical comorbidities which, when present, may be more severe than in the general population because of suboptimal access to services and compliance with treatments. This could explain why medical complications and death may occur earlier in older people with than without severe mental disorders. As a result, we have had to reject our hypothesis that men with severe mental disorders who reach older age do not have greater mortality than their peers. In fact, out data indicate that the unfavourable clinical outcomes seen in younger patients with severe mental disorders persist later in life. Whether appropriate treatment with psychotropic medications would decrease or increase the risk of death of older men with severe mental disorders cannot be determined from our data.

Cardiovascular diseases were the most frequent cause of death of older men with and without severe mental disorders, although there was a significant excess of cardiovascular events among cases. Infections, cardiovascular and respiratory diseases, mental disorders, and diseases of the central nervous system were more frequent causes of death among those with schizophrenia spectrum disorder than men without a severe mental disorder. Cancer was less frequent among the former than the latter (albeit not significantly), and there were no deaths by suicide in the schizophrenia spectrum group. Such a mortality pattern is similar to that observed among younger people with schizophrenia and related disorders: what kills people with schizophrenia spectrum disorders in early life continues to kill those who reach old age [10,21,37,38]. The exception, in the case of schizophrenia spectrum disorders, is suicide, which is not infrequent in early life [39]. The number of men with bipolar disorder in the sample was small, which contributed to the imprecision of the estimates for cause of mortality. Nonetheless, the excessive mortality due to respiratory diseases is noteworthy, particularly in light of the high prevalence of smoking [40]. Two men with bipolar disorder died by suicide, which is also a more frequent cause of death in younger people with bipolar disorder than in the general population [41]. Depression was associated with excessive mortality due to infections, cancer, cardiovascular and respiratory diseases, as well as other causes. These findings are consistent with those reported for younger people with depression [42]. Similarly, men with a recorded history of alcohol-induced disorder had higher risk of dying as a result of infections, cancer, cardiovascular and respiratory diseases [43]. Taken together, these results show the causes of death associated with schizophrenia spectrum, bipolar, depression and alcohol-induced disorders overlap, although differences in the distribution of deaths attributable to cancer and suicide seem to differ.

Conclusions

This study has shown that older men with severe mental disorders have greater mortality hazard and lower life expectancy than their peers. The underlying reasons for this increase in mortality are not entirely clear, but hazardous lifestyle choices, the presence of disabling medical comorbidities, poor compliance with treatment, and suboptimal access to health services may all play a part. There is now evidence that adoption of healthy lifestyle practices, even very late in life, is associated with measurable health benefits, so that smoking cessation, limited alcohol consumption and physical activity should become an integral part of the management of older adults with severe mental disorders [44,45]. Similarly, the management of chronic medical conditions, such as hypertension, can decrease the risk of adverse health events among octogenarians, which indicates that there is no reason to withhold effective treatments from older people when these are available.

As a community, we are yet to address successfully the excess mortality associated with severe mental disorders. Unlike young adults, most older people will be in contact with health services at least once a year [46], offering policy makers and health professionals a unique opportunity to intervene and improve the clinical outcomes of this segment of the population. Perhaps these older adults could teach us important lessons that would eventually guide the design of interventions that are effective at improving the clinical outcomes of people with severe mental disorders across the lifespan.

Acknowledgments

We thank participants and research staff for their kind contribution to this study. We also thank colleagues at the Data Linkage Unit of the Department of Health of Western Australia for data retrieval and ongoing support.

Author Contributions

Conceived and designed the experiments: OPA. Performed the experiments: OPA GJH BBY JG PEN LF. Analyzed the data: OPA. Contributed reagents/materials/analysis tools: OPA GJH BBY JG PEN LF. Wrote the paper: OPA GJH BBY JG PEN LF.

References

1. Whiteford HA, Degenhardt L, Rehm J, Baxter AJ, Ferrari AJ, et al. (2013) Global burden of disease attributable to mental and substance use disorders: findings from the Global Burden of Disease Study 2010. Lancet 382: 1575–1586.
2. Lawrence D, Hancock KJ, Kisely S (2013) The gap in life expectancy from preventable physical illness in psychiatric patients in Western Australia: retrospective analysis of population based registers. BMJ 346: f2539.
3. Joukamaa M, Heliovaara M, Knekt P, Aromaa A, Raitasalo R, et al. (2001) Mental disorders and cause-specific mortality. Br J Psychiatry 179: 498–502.
4. Druss BG, Zhao L, Von Esenwein S, Morrato EH, Marcus SC (2011) Understanding excess mortality in persons with mental illness: 17-year follow up of a nationally representative US survey. Med Care 49: 599–604.
5. Osborn DP, Levy G, Nazareth I, Petersen I, Islam A, et al. (2007) Relative risk of cardiovascular and cancer mortality in people with severe mental illness from the United Kingdom's General Practice Rsearch Database. Arch Gen Psychiatry 64: 242–249.
6. Lawrence D, Jablensky AV, Holman CD, Pinder TJ (2000) Mortality in Western Australian psychiatric patients. Soc Psychiatry Psychiatr Epidemiol 35: 341–347.
7. Lawrence D, Almeida OP, Hulse GK, Jablensky AV, Holman CD (2000) Suicide and attempted suicide among older adults in Western Australia. Psychol Med 30: 813–821.
8. Almeida OP, Alfonso H, Pirkis J, Kerse N, Sim M, et al. (2011) A practical approach to assess depression risk and to guide risk reduction strategies in later life. Int Psychogeriatr 23: 280–291.
9. Almeida OP, Hankey GJ, Yeap BB, Golledge J, McCaul K, et al. (2013) A risk table to assist health practitioners assess and prevent the onset of depression in later life. Prev Med 57: 878–882.
10. Brown S, Inskip H, Barraclough B (2000) Causes of the excess mortality of schizophrenia. Br J Psychiatry 177: 212–217.
11. Morgan VA, McGrath JJ, Jablensky A, Badcock JC, Waterreus A, et al. (2013) Psychosis prevalence and physical, metabolic and cognitive co-morbidity: data from the second Australian national survey of psychosis. Psychol Med: 1–14.
12. Correll CU, Frederickson AM, Kane JM, Manu P (2006) Metabolic syndrome and the risk of coronary heart disease in 367 patients treated with second-generation antipsychotic drugs. J Clin Psychiatry 67: 575–583.
13. Weeke P, Jensen A, Folke F, Gislason GH, Olesen JB, et al. (2012) Antidepressant use and risk of out-of-hospital cardiac arrest: a nationwide case-time-control study. Clin Pharmacol Ther 92: 72–79.
14. Weich S, Pearce HL, Croft P, Singh S, Crome I, et al. (2014) Effect of anxiolytic and hypnotic drug prescriptions on mortality hazards: retrospective cohort study. BMJ 348: g1996.
15. Andrews G, Henderson S, Hall W (2001) Prevalence, comorbidity, disability and service utilisation. Overview of the Australian National Mental Health Survey. Br J Psychiatry 178: 145–153.
16. Regier DA, Farmer ME, Rae DS, Myers JK, Kramer M, et al. (1993) One-month prevalence of mental disorders in the United States and sociodemographic characteristics: the Epidemiologic Catchment Area study. Acta Psychiatr Scand 88: 35–47.
17. Meesters PD, de Haan L, Comijs HC, Stek ML, Smeets-Janssen MM, et al. (2012) Schizophrenia spectrum disorders in later life: prevalence and distribution of age at onset and sex in a dutch catchment area. Am J Geriatr Psychiatry 20: 18–28.
18. Salomon JA, Wang H, Freeman MK, Vos T, Flaxman AD, et al. (2012) Healthy life expectancy for 187 countries, 1990–2010: a systematic analysis for the Global Burden Disease Study 2010. Lancet 380: 2144–2162.
19. Holman CD, Bass AJ, Rosman DL, Smith MB, Semmens JB, et al. (2008) A decade of data linkage in Western Australia: strategic design, applications and benefits of the WA data linkage system. Aust Health Rev 32: 766–777.
20. Jablensky AV, Morgan V, Zubrick SR, Bower C, Yellachich LA (2005) Pregnancy, delivery, and neonatal complications in a population cohort of women with schizophrenia and major affective disorders. Am J Psychiatry 162: 79–91.
21. Saha S, Chant D, Welham J, McGrath J (2005) A systematic review of the prevalence of schizophrenia. PLoS Med 2: e141.
22. Almeida OP, Fenner S (2002) Bipolar disorder: similarities and differences between patients with illness onset before and after 65 years of age. Int Psychogeriatr 14: 311–322.
23. Pirkis J, Pfaff J, Williamson M, Tyson O, Stocks N, et al. (2009) The community prevalence of depression in older Australians. J Affect Disord 115: 54–61.
24. Hirata ES, Almeida OP, Funari RR, Klein EL (2001) Validity of the Michigan Alcoholism Screening Test (MAST) for the detection of alcohol-related problems among male geriatric outpatients. Am J Geriatr Psychiatry 9: 30–34.
25. Norman PE, Flicker L, Almeida OP, Hankey GJ, Hyde Z, et al. (2009) Cohort Profile: The Health In Men Study (HIMS). Int J Epidemiol 38: 48–52.
26. Holman CD, Bass AJ, Rouse IL, Hobbs MS (1999) Population-based linkage of health records in Western Australia: development of a health services research linked database. Aust N Z J Public Health 23: 453–459.
27. ABS (2011) 3401.0 – Overseas arrivals and departures, Australia. Australian Bureau of Statistics.
28. Lee M, Chodosh J (2009) Dementia and life expectancy: what do we know? J Am Med Dir Assoc 10: 466–471.
29. Perala J, Suvisaari J, Saarni SI, Kuoppasalmi K, Isometsa E, et al. (2007) Lifetime prevalence of psychotic and bipolar I disorders in a general population. Arch Gen Psychiatry 64: 19–28.
30. Kessler RC, Berglund P, Demler O, Jin R, Merikangas KR, et al. (2005) Lifetime prevalence and age-of-onset distributions of DSM-IV disorders in the National Comorbidity Survey Replication. Arch Gen Psychiatry 62: 593–602.
31. Almeida OP, Pirkis J, Kerse N, Sim M, Flicker L, et al. (2012) A randomized trial to reduce the prevalence of depression and self-harm behavior in older primary care patients. Ann Fam Med 10: 347–356.
32. Hall W, Teesson M, Lynskey M, Degenhardt L (1999) The 12-month prevalence of substance use and ICD-10 substance use disorders in Australian adults: findings from the National Survey of Mental Health and Well-Being. Addiction 94: 1541–1550.
33. Lin JC, Karno MP, Grella CE, Warda U, Liao DH, et al. (2011) Alcohol, tobacco, and nonmedical drug use disorders in U.S. Adults aged 65 years and older: data from the 2001–2002 National Epidemiologic Survey of Alcohol and Related Conditions. Am J Geriatr Psychiatry 19: 292–299.
34. Grant BF, Stinson FS, Dawson DA, Chou SP, Dufour MC, et al. (2004) Prevalence and co-occurrence of substance use disorders and independent mood and anxiety disorders: results from the National Epidemiologic Survey on Alcohol and Related Conditions. Arch Gen Psychiatry 61: 807–816.
35. Lawrence DM, Holman CD, Jablensky AV, Hobbs MS (2003) Death rate from ischaemic heart disease in Western Australian psychiatric patients 1980–1998. Br J Psychiatry 182: 31–36.
36. DiMatteo MR, Lepper HS, Croghan TW (2000) Depression is a risk factor for noncompliance with medical treatment: meta-analysis of the effects of anxiety and depression on patient adherence. Arch Intern Med 160: 2101–2107.
37. Barak Y, Achiron A, Mandel M, Mirecki I, Aizenberg D (2005) Reduced cancer incidence among patients with schizophrenia. Cancer 104: 2817–2821.
38. Nordentoft M, Wahlbeck K, Hallgren J, Westman J, Osby U, et al. (2013) Excess mortality, causes of death and life expectancy in 270,770 patients with recent onset of mental disorders in Denmark, Finland and Sweden. PLoS One 8: e55176.
39. Osby U, Correia N, Brandt L, Ekbom A, Sparen P (2000) Mortality and causes of death in schizophrenia in Stockholm county, Sweden. Schizophr Res 45: 21–28.
40. Diaz FJ, James D, Botts S, Maw L, Susce MT, et al. (2009) Tobacco smoking behaviors in bipolar disorder: a comparison of the general population, schizophrenia, and major depression. Bipolar Disord 11: 154–165.
41. Dalton EJ, Cate-Carter TD, Mundo E, Parikh SV, Kennedy JL (2003) Suicide risk in bipolar patients: the role of co-morbid substance use disorders. Bipolar Disord 5: 58–61.
42. Lemogne C, Nabi H, Melchior M, Goldberg M, Limosin F, et al. (2013) Mortality associated with depression as compared with other severe mental disorders: a 20-year follow-up study of the GAZEL cohort. J Psychiatr Res 47: 851–857.
43. Eliasen M, Becker U, Gronbaek M, Juel K, Tolstrup JS (2014) Alcohol-attributable and alcohol-preventable mortality in Denmark: an analysis of which

intake levels contribute most to alcohol's harmful and beneficial effects. Eur J Epidemiol 29: 15–26.

44. Almeida OP, Garrido GJ, Alfonso H, Hulse G, Lautenschlager NT, et al. (2011) 24-month effect of smoking cessation on cognitive function and brain structure in later life. Neuroimage 55: 1480–1489.

45. Lautenschlager NT, Cox KL, Flicker L, Foster JK, van Bockxmeer FM, et al. (2008) Effect of physical activity on cognitive function in older adults at risk for Alzheimer disease: a randomized trial. JAMA 300: 1027–1037.

46. Britt H, Miller GC, Charles J, Henderson J, Bayram C, et al. (2009) General practice actiivity in Australia 1999-00 to 2008-09. Canberra: AIHW.

21

Is There Still Room for Novel Viral Pathogens in Pediatric Respiratory Tract Infections?

Blanca Taboada[1], Marco A. Espinoza[1], Pavel Isa[1], Fernando E. Aponte[1], María A. Arias-Ortiz[2], Jesús Monge-Martínez[2], Rubén Rodríguez-Vázquez[2], Fidel Díaz-Hernández[2], Fernando Zárate-Vidal[2], Rosa María Wong-Chew[3], Verónica Firo-Reyes[4], Carlos N. del Río-Almendárez[5], Jesús Gaitán-Meza[6], Alberto Villaseñor-Sierra[7], Gerardo Martínez-Aguilar[8], Ma. del Carmen Salas-Mier[8], Daniel E. Noyola[9], Luis F. Pérez-Gónzalez[10], Susana López[1], José I. Santos-Preciado[3], Carlos F. Arias[1]*

1 Instituto de Biotecnología, Universidad Nacional Autónoma de México, Cuernavaca, Morelos, Mexico, **2** Colegio de Pediatría del Estado de Veracruz, Veracruz, Mexico, **3** Facultad de Medicina, Universidad Nacional Autónoma de México, México D.F., Mexico, **4** Hospital General de México, México D.F., Mexico, **5** Hospital Pediátirco de Coyoacán, México D.F., Mexico, **6** Nuevo Hospital Civil de Guadalajara "Dr. Juan I. Menchaca", Guadalajara, Jalisco, Mexico, **7** Centro de Investigación Biomédica de Occidente, IMSS, Guadalajara, Jalisco, Mexico, **8** Unidad de Investigación Biomédica IMSS, Durango, Durango, Mexico, **9** Universidad Autónoma de San Luis Potosí, San Luis Potosí, Mexico, **10** Hospital Central "Dr. Ignacio Morones Prieto", San Luis Potosí, Mexico

Abstract

Viruses are the most frequent cause of respiratory disease in children. However, despite the advanced diagnostic methods currently in use, in 20 to 50% of respiratory samples a specific pathogen cannot be detected. In this work, we used a metagenomic approach and deep sequencing to examine respiratory samples from children with lower and upper respiratory tract infections that had been previously found negative for 6 bacteria and 15 respiratory viruses by PCR. Nasal washings from 25 children (out of 250) hospitalized with a diagnosis of pneumonia and nasopharyngeal swabs from 46 outpatient children (out of 526) were studied. DNA reads for at least one virus commonly associated to respiratory infections was found in 20 of 25 hospitalized patients, while reads for pathogenic respiratory bacteria were detected in the remaining 5 children. For outpatients, all the samples were pooled into 25 DNA libraries for sequencing. In this case, in 22 of the 25 sequenced libraries at least one respiratory virus was identified, while in all other, but one, pathogenic bacteria were detected. In both patient groups reads for respiratory syncytial virus, coronavirus-OC43, and rhinovirus were identified. In addition, viruses less frequently associated to respiratory infections were also found. Saffold virus was detected in outpatient but not in hospitalized children. Anellovirus, rotavirus, and astrovirus, as well as several animal and plant viruses were detected in both groups. No novel viruses were identified. Adding up the deep sequencing results to the PCR data, 79.2% of 250 hospitalized and 76.6% of 526 ambulatory patients were positive for viruses, and all other children, but one, had pathogenic respiratory bacteria identified. These results suggest that at least in the type of populations studied and with the sampling methods used the odds of finding novel, clinically relevant viruses, in pediatric respiratory infections are low.

Editor: Amit Kapoor, Columbia University, United States of America

Funding: This work was supported by grants 153639 (to JIS-P) and "Influenza 2009" (to CFA) from the National Council for Science and Technology—Mexico. www.conacyt.mx. FEA was recipient of a scholarship from the National Council for Science and Technology—Mexico. The funders had no role in study design, data collection and analysis, decision to publish, or preparation of the manuscript.

Competing Interests: The authors have declared that no competing interests exist.

* Email: arias@ibt.unam.mx

Introduction

Acute respiratory infections (ARIs) are the most common illnesses in humans and are associated with significant morbidity and mortality in young children in developing countries and elderly people in developed countries. In children, 156 million episodes of pneumonia are recorded annually worldwide, of which more than 95% are reported in developing countries [1,2]. In 2008, 1.6 million children younger than 5 years died from pneumonia [3]. To try to reduce child mortality due to ARIs, is important to perform a more accurate diagnosis of the pathogens associated with those deaths in children younger than 5 years of age [1].

Introduction of PCR-based diagnostic methods has increased the ability to detect respiratory viruses, which are responsible for most ARIs in young children [4,5,6]. Several respiratory viruses, such as influenza, parainfluenza virus, adenovirus, respiratory syncytial virus (RSV) and coronavirus (HCoV) have been known for some time as etiological agents of lower tract respiratory infections (LRTI). More recently, with the improvement of diagnostic methods, rhinovirus (RV), which had been thought to be mostly associated with mild-to-moderate upper respiratory tract infections (URTI) was also found to be associated with severe respiratory infections [7,8] and, in the last decade, several new respiratory viruses have been identified, such as human metapneumovirus (hMPV), HCoV-NL63 and -HKU1, human bocavirus (HBoV), parechovirus (HPeV), polyomavirus KI and WU, and enterovirus 104 and 109 [9,10,11,12,13,14,15]. In this regard, the fact that even with state-of-the-art diagnostic tools in most studies a virus is detected in only 50% to 80% of upper and lower ARIs [4,5,6,16,17,18,19] a wonder is if there are more respiratory viruses associated to ARIs than those currently known [20].

In this work, we analyzed by next generation sequencing (NGS) nasopharyngeal samples from children with LRTI and URTI that had been found negative for a panel of 21 respiratory pathogens (15 viruses and 6 bacteria) using commercial multiplex PCR methods. This study contributes to the description of the viral and bacterial populations present in nasopharyngeal samples from children with lower and upper ARIs using a metagenomic approach, which so far has been employed in limited studies [21,22,23], and suggests that the current diagnostic methods likely miss known respiratory pathogens, which might explain the relatively high proportion of undiagnosed cases.

Materials and Methods

Study populations and clinical samples

Two pediatric populations with symptomatic respiratory tract infections were included in this study. The first consisted of children with LTRI that required hospital admission due to clinical or radiological signs or symptoms of pneumonia in four different states of Mexico. Nasal washings with 1.5 ml of saline solution were collected from 250 children (male:female ratio, 1.43; age range, 1–76 months) between March 2010 and April 2011. The second population was composed of patients with symptomatic URTI that attended the private consult in five different cities of the state of Veracruz, Mexico. Nasopharyngeal swabs (rayon-tipped, BD BBL) were collected from 526 children (male:female ratio, 1.27; age range, 0–191 months) from September 2011 to April 2012. All samples were placed in vials containing viral transport medium (1:1 in the case of nashal washings; Microtest M4-RT, Remel) and sent frozen in blue ice either to the Institute of Biotechnology in Cuernavaca (URTI samples) or to the School of Medicine in Mexico City (LRTI samples) and stored at −70°C until analyzed. All children were previously healthy, not diagnosed with tuberculosis or signs of malnutrition, and not immunocompromised. Administration of antibiotics before hospital admission was not registered; in outpatients no antibiotics were administered before sample collection. The children included in the study were those that arrived consecutively at the collection places during the study period, with no further selection. The study (project 186) was approved by the institutional review boards of the School of Medicine and the Institute of Biotechnology of the National University of Mexico and from the institutional review board and ethics committee of each participant hospital. Written informed consent was obtained from each parent or guardian prior to enrollment.

Pathogen detection

The respiratory specimens from hospitalized and outpatient children were previously screened for viruses using the xTAG Bioplex respiratory Viral Panel (Abbott, Rungis, France) (JI Santos et al., in preparation) and the Seeplex RV15 ACE detection kit (Seegene, Seoul, Korea) (Wong-Chew et al., in preparation), respectively. The virus-negative samples from both groups of patients were screened in this work by a multiplex PCR (Seeplex Pneumobacter ACE detection kit, Seegene, Seoul, Korea) for the presence of six bacteria commonly associated to respiratory infections: *Streptococcus pneumoniae, Haemophilus influenzae, Chlamydophila pneumoniae, Legionella pneumophila, Bordetella pertussis*, and *Mycoplasma pneumoniae*.

Nucleic acid extraction, amplification and barcode labeling

Genetic material from clinical samples was extracted with the PureLink Viral RNA/DNA kit according to the manufacturer's instructions (Invitrogen, Waltham, MA). Before extraction, samples (200 μl) were treated with Turbo DNAse (Ambion, Waltham, MA) and RNAse (Sigma, St. Louis, MO) for 30 min at 37°C and immediately chilled on ice. Nucleic acids were eluted in nuclease-free water, aliquoted, quantified in NanoDrop ND-1000 (NanoDrop Technologies, Waltham, MA), and stored at −70°C until further use. Sample random primer-amplification of nucleic acids was performed essentially as described previously [24]. Briefly, reverse transcription was done using SuperScript III Reverse Transcriptase (Invitrogen, Waltham, MA) and primer-A (5'-GTTTCCCAGTAGGTCTCN_9-3'). Complementary DNA (cDNA) strand was generated by two rounds of synthesis with Sequenase 2.0 (USB, USA). The cDNA obtained was then amplified with KlenTaq polymerase (Sigma, St. Louis, MO) using the primer-B (5'-GTTTCCCAGTAGGTCTC-3') and 20 cycles of the following program: 30 sec at 94°C, 1 min at 50°C, 1 min at 72°C. After cleaning the PCR products with the DNA Clean & Concentrator-5 kit (Zymo Research, Irvine, CA), DNA was digested with the GsuI restriction enzyme (Fermentas Waltham, MA) for 2 h at 30°C to remove sequences corresponding to PCR primers. After digestion, samples were purified again and used as starting material to prepare 300 bp-sized libraries using Illumina's Genomic DNA sample Prep Kit with multiplex primers as suggested by the manufacturer (Illumina, San Diego, CA). Libraries were loaded in a flow cell (4 or 5 libraries per lane) and sequencing was performed by 72 cycles of nucleotide extension followed by acquisition of multiplex code in a Genome Analyzer IIx. The datasets generated by the GAIIx were deposited in the European Nucleotide Archive, with study accession numbers PRJEB7390 and PRJEB7391 for URTI and LRTI samples respectively.

Deep sequencing and sequence analysis

Image analysis and base calling were performed with the Illumina GAPipeline program (version 1.3.0) using standard parameters. To separate the samples, the pooled data from each lane were binned by barcode. In-house scripts were developed for the sequence analysis, including the following steps:

i) Preprocessing. For each read, the adapter and 5' and 3' bases with no-call sites (N residues) and low-quality (Phred-like scores $<$ 20) were trimmed. Then, low complexity reads and less than 35 bases long were removed. Finally, identical reads were collapsed into a single representative sequence to optimize analysis time. Only reads passing the preprocessing step were considered valid.

ii) Removal of host sequences. The program SMALT (Wellcome Trust Sanger Institute, 2012) was used to align the reads against mitochondrial, human genome, and bacterial ribosomal RNA to remove them, using 90% coverage and 90% identity.

iii) Taxonomic identification. To minimize CPU time, valid reads were aligned to bacteria, fungi and viruses nt NCBI databases, using SMALT with 70% coverage and identity. Then, the reads that mapped were aligned with standalone BLASTn against the databases described above, using an E-value of 1e–03.

To avoid misclassification, the first 100 hits were obtained for each sequence. Reads that did not map were considered as unidentified.

iv) Taxonomic classification. To assign reads to the most appropriate taxonomic level the software MEGAN 4.70.4 was used, which assigns a read to the lowest common taxonomic ancestor of the organisms corresponding to the set of significant hits.

v) Assembly. Reads assigned to the same virus family level were subsequently used for *de novo* assembly with Velvet 1.1.04 to increase the accuracy of classification. Each assembly contig was aligned against BLASTn database.

vi) Detection of novel viruses. All unidentified sequences unaligned using SMALT nucleotide alignment were assembled *de novo* with Metavelvet modified by us to improve the assembly efficiency. First, we conducted exploratory assemblies of the reads using multiple hash lengths (k = 17–35). Then, additional assembly of all unused reads from the exploratory assemblies was done (k = 21). Finally, we assembled all contigs obtained from all exploratory assemblies and the unused reads assembly by using the program VelvetOptimiser. From this final assembly, contigs that were greater than 180 nt were directly compared with NCBI nr (non- redundant protein) database using BLASTx with an E-value of 100 in an attempt to identify novel viruses.

Phylogenetic tree inference

Metagenomic contigs from specific viruses that were at least 150 nt-long, were phylogenetically characterized. The analysis required a different approach compared to full-length genomes due to the fact that metagenomics sequences are fragmentary and not completely overlapping. Therefore, for each virus, a database of complete genomes was first created using all sequences available in GenBank until January 2014. Then, a reference alignment was done with sequences of this database by using MUSCLE method. Next, we combined metagenomics contigs into a single large alignment by using the software MAFFT with the option align fragment sequences to reference alignment. Finally, maximum likelihood trees were generated with 1000 repetitions bootstrap using the MEGA program.

Results

Pathogen detection

In previous studies we screened by RT-PCR the presence of 15 respiratory viruses in nasal washings from 250 hospitalized children with clinical diagnosis suggestive of viral pneumonia and in 526 nasopharyngeal samples from pediatric children with URTI (see Materials and Methods). Table 1 shows the frequency of the different viruses found in both types of samples. Among the viruses detected, considering both single and multiple infections, RSV-A and rhinovirus showed the highest frequency in both LRTI and URTI. At least one virus was detected in 71.2% (178/250) of LRTI (Santos et al., manuscript in preparation) and 71.5% (376/526) of URTI (Wong-Chew et al., manuscript in preparation). In 40 of the 250 LRTI samples (16%) a viral coinfection was found. Thirty-four of these samples had a dual infection, with the combination of RSV-A/RV and RSV-A/AdV being the more frequent, while 6 children had triple virus infections. In the case of URTI, 73 of the 526 samples (13.9%) showed a viral coinfection. Sixty-three of these samples had a dual infection, with the combination of AdV/EV and RV/CoV 229/N63 being the more frequent. Eight children had triple virus infections, and two were infected simultaneously with four viruses.

The virus-negative samples were screened by a multiplex PCR for the presence of six bacteria commonly associated to respiratory infections. In 64.7% (46/71, LRTI) and 68.7% (103/150, URTI) of the virus-negative samples at least one bacterial pathogen was found. The most frequent bacteria detected in children in both types of populations were *S. pneumoniae* (36 LRTI, 88 URTI) and *H. influenzae* (24 LRTI, 47 URTI); in a few cases *C. pneumoniae* (9 URTI) and *M. pneumoniae* (2 LRTI, 2 URTI) were also detected. In 37 children with URTI two different bacteria were found, and in 3 children 3 bacteria were detected. In the case of LRTI, 8 children had a mixed infection. It is important to have in mind that bacterial colonization, frequently at lower bacterial colony counts, may be detected by very sensitive laboratory tests, and even more frequently than viruses, these bacteria may not be associated with acute disease.

After screening for common respiratory viruses and bacteria, 90% of children with LRTI and 91.3% with URTI had at least one pathogen identified. The remaining 25 (10%) hospitalized and 46 (8.7%) outpatient children remained negative for all the tested pathogens and were then characterized by next-generation sequencing (NGS).

Next-generation sequencing of negative samples

To search for either known or novel respiratory pathogens in the double-negative (virus and bacteria) samples, the nucleic acids in these samples were isolated, amplified by PCR, and sequenced using the Illumina platform, as described in Materials and Methods. The 25 samples from children with LRTI were sequenced individually (listed in Table 2). In the case of the URTI samples, 9 were sequenced individually, while the amount of DNA isolated from the other 37 samples was too low to be analyzed independently, thus, they were used to prepare 16 pools for sequencing: 13 pools of two samples, 1 pool of three samples, and 2 pools of four samples (Table 3).

The total number of DNA reads and the valid unique reads obtained from each sample after passing the quality controls are shown in Tables 2 and 3. The valid reads were analyzed for the presence of sequences from human, bacterial, fungal, or viral origin. As expected, the most abundant reads were from human origin, representing 70% and 80% of LRTI and URTI patients, respectively (Fig. 1). Bacterial sequences made up the second largest data set, representing 15.2% of the sequence reads in LRTI and 8.5% in URTI. Viral sequences represented 0.56% and 0.57% of valid reads in LRTI and URTI, respectively, and only 0.05% of reads corresponded to fungi (Fig. 1). Finally, approximately 13% and 10% of the sequences in both LRTI and URTI could not be classified since no homolog was found (E-value 1e–03) or there were contradicting database hits. This category is referred to as 'undefined' in Figure 1. Of interest, despite the fact that the samples from LRTI and URTI were collected by different methods (nasal washings vs. swabs), and from children with different clinical syndromes and varying severity of respiratory disease, the proportion of sequences from different origins was very similar.

The undefined sequence reads from all samples were assembled, and contigs ≥180 nt were compared with non-redundant protein database of GenBank (E-value 100) to find sequences that could be distantly related to known viral sequences and could thus represent novel viruses. Indeed, short sequences are less likely than long sequences to retrieve statistically significant similarities in Blast searches, and sequence assembly into longer contigs is helpful to overcome this difficulty. As result of this, all filtered contigs aligned either to bacterial or human proteins during BLASTx runs. An analysis revealed that the contigs that map to bacteria showed only 60–80% nucleotide identity to their best-matching reference, indicating that they most likely represent novel species within their

Table 1. Frequency of viral pathogens in children with URTI and LRTI.

Virus	URTI (%) [a]	LRTI (%)
Respiratory syncytial virus-A	96 (18.3)	77 (30.8)
Rhinovirus	92 (17.5)	62 (24.8)
Influenza virus A	48 (9.1)	4 (1.6)
Adenovirus	38 (7.2)	14 (5.6)
Enterovirus	31 (5.9)	2 (0.8)
Metapneumovirus	28 (5.3)	19 (7.6)
Coronavirus 229E/NL63	28 (5.3)	2 (0.8)
Coronavirus OC43	18 (3.4)	4 (1.6)
Parainfluenza virus 3	18 (3.4)	27 (10.8)
Parainfluenza virus 1	15 (2.9)	8 (3.2)
Bocavirus	13 (2.5)	8 (3.2)
Parainfluenza virus 4	13 (2.5)	2 (0.8)
Parainfluenza virus 2	9 (1.7)	7 (2.8)
Influenza virus B	7 (1.3)	4 (1.6)
Respiratory syncytial virus-B	7 (1.3)	2 (0.8)

[a]The number of viruses include those present in single and mixed infections. The percentage refers to the total number of viruses detected.

Table 2. DNA reads obtained after NGS sequencing of LRTI samples.

Sample	No. of reads	[a]No. of valid reads (%)
11	7,336,101	6,243,183 (85.8)
17	13,118,032	10,877,350 (83.5)
24	8,522,571	580,599 (7.0)
28	4,210,763	3,400,829 (81.3)
47	9,051,977	1,474,628(16.3)
64	10,626,262	1,125,214 (10.7)
66	11,937,236	713,915 (6.1)
67	10,779,916	696,529 (6.6)
86	16,500,963	1,806,051 (11.1)
111	13,312,546	941,951 (7.3)
124	17,270,372	1,943,449 (11.4)
125	10,053,798	627,927 (6.4)
147	6,229,459	464,760 (7.5)
151	14,208,710	1,248,513(8.9)
206	2,881,815	137,274 (9.1)
210	16,684,541	9,969,067 (60.2)
211	10,784,070	1,099,819 (10.4)
213	9,137,653	775,688 (8.6)
214	11,503,832	4,321,038 (37.8)
225	18,787,796	1,534,587 (8.4)
227	19,294,597	1,483,230 (7.9)
233	14,731,213	3,628,367 (24.9)
236	13,712,286	974,744 (7.2)
237	17,095,111	2,780,835 (16.8)
238	12,373,402	3,277m334 (26.7)

[a]Valid DNA reads after discarding those that did not pass the quality filter, and removing repeated reads (see Methods).

Table 3. DNA reads obtained after NGS sequencing of URTI samples.

[a]Individual and pooled samples	No. of reads	[b]No. of valid reads (%)
C06, C55, T78, V24	4,323,309	1,707,160 (39.5)
C16, C61	2,113,065	1,134,387 (53.7)
C27, C01	2,951,784	1,474,233 (49.9)
C29, M40, T41, V39	3,325,315	1,235,867 (37.2)
C41, T50	3,765,099	1,708,531 (45.4)
C46, P54	4,289,979	2,278,068 (53.1)
M23, M44	3,607,011	1,982,487 (55.0)
M28	7,294,104	3,292,828(45.1)
P06, P150	5,010,364	2,387,550 (47.7)
P108	4,609,150	1,021,900 (22.2)
P147, P191	3,454,018	1,540,283 (44.6)
P149, P153	4,381,981	2,534,733 (57.8)
P151, P181	4,638,675	2,207,800 (47.6)
P173	2,974,252	613,487 (20.6)
P176, P186, P213	4,210,620	2,176,224 (51.7)
P183	1,654,081	272,720 (16.5)
P19, P88	8,727,411	5,067,242 (58.1)
P69	3,072,261	631,373 (20.6)
T33, T39	4,863,936	3,308,371 (68.0)
T36	1,228,687	446,932 (36.4)
T38	3,309,781	1,420,555 (42.9)
T43, T44	3,183,181	2,325,025 (73.0)
T65	78,467	30,443 (38.8)
V26	3,469,556	1,496,608 (43.1)
P131, V61	3,939,137	2,288,528 (58.1)

[a]The samples that were pooled for sequencing are indicated.
[b]Valid DNA reads after discarding those that did not pass the quality filter, and removing repeated reads (see Methods).

corresponding genera and thus could not be classified during alignments with BLASTn. Nonetheless, the vast majority of reads (50% to 90%) were not assembled into contigs. The unassembled reads were low complexity sequences or library artifacts as adapter chimeras, suggesting that it is unlikely that they correspond to novel viruses. A remaining small amount of sequences could not be assembled due to non-uniform read depth because of a non-uniform species abundance distribution.

Viruses detected by NGS in double-negative samples

DNA sequence reads from at least one virus commonly associated to respiratory infections was found in 20 out of the 25 double-negative samples of LRTI patients (Table 4): 5 samples were positive for RSV reads, 11 samples for HCoV-OC-43, and 9 for RV. In addition, 5 samples contained HBoV and in 12 samples anelloviruses (torque teno -TTV-, torque teno mini -TTMV-, or torque teno midi viruses -TTMDV) were also detected; rotavirus, papillomavirus, and herpesvirus sequences were identified once in the samples, and reads from several viruses from both animal (bat picornavirus, bovine viral diarrheal virus, bovine kobovirus) and plant origin (potato virus Y, pepper mild mottle virus), as well as various bacteriophages were also found (Table 4). Regarding bacteria, DNA sequence reads from *S. pneumoniae* were the most frequent, being present in all but one of the 25 samples sequenced, and *M. catarrhalis, L. pneumoniae*, and *H. influenzae* were less frequently found. DNA reads from other bacteria less commonly associated with respiratory infections were also detected (Table 4). Some of the samples had sequence reads corresponding to up to 8 different viruses or 15 different bacteria. Of interest, including the NGS results, 79.2% (198/250) of the samples had a respiratory virus detected, and in the remaining 52 samples at least one bacteria was found, such that all 250 samples from children with LRTI had a respiratory pathogen identified.

DNA reads from one to five typical respiratory viruses were detected in 22 of the 25 sequenced double-negative individual and/or pooled samples from children with URTI (Table 5): The virus most frequently detected was RV, which was found in 19 of the pooled and/or individual samples; some of the samples had more than one type of virus, such that we found sequence reads from 4 RV subtype A, 4 subtype B, and 19 subtype C. One sample was positive for RSV, 3 for HCoV-OC43, 3 for human enterovirus A71, and 3 samples had HBoV. Of interest, 5 of the samples had DNA reads from Saffold virus, a virus recently described to be associated to respiratory infections. Also, among these samples we identified 3 containing herpesvirus, 5 papillomavirus, 2 human astrovirus, 4 rotavirus, and 10 anelloviruses (TTV, TTMV, TTMDV). Similar to what was found in LRTI, in children with URTI DNA reads of viruses from animal (white spot syndrome and bat picornavirus) and plant origin (Okra mosaic virus, capsicum chlorosis virus, cucumber mosaic virus, pepper

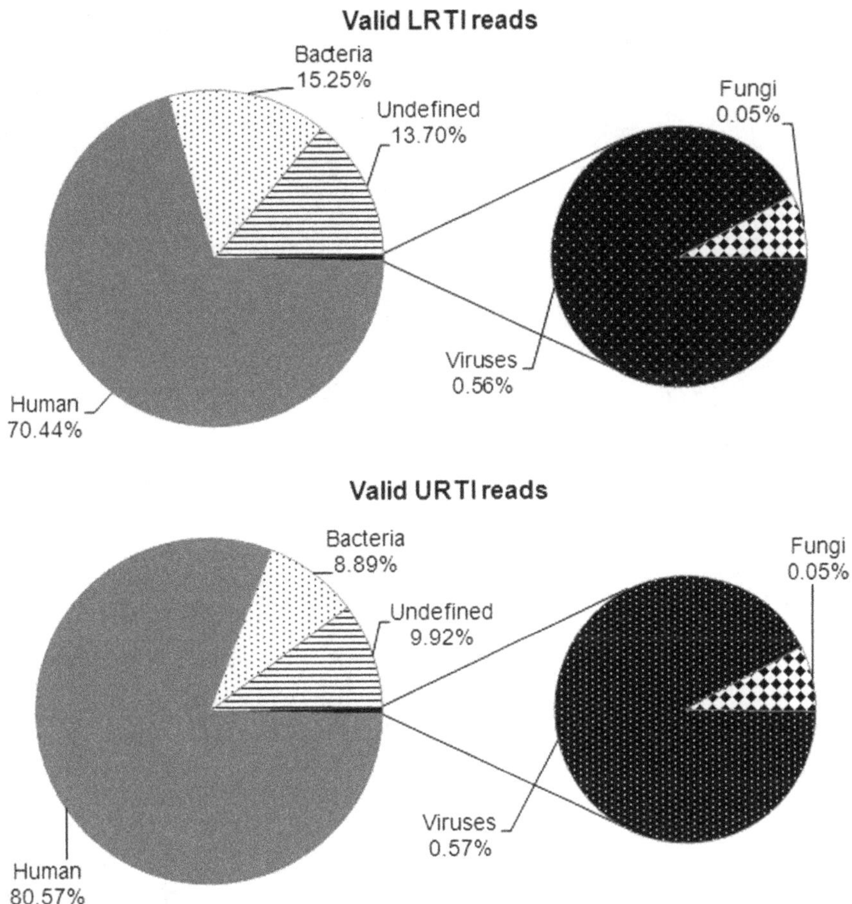

Figure 1. Taxonomic classification of the generated DNA sequencing reads. Valid DNA reads obtained by NGS of LRTI and URTI clinical samples were split into human, bacterial, fungal, and viral origin. Those reads not present in the four previous categories were classified as "undefined". Average values for all LRTI and URTI samples are shown.

mild mottle virus, and tomato mosaic virus) were also detected. In the majority of samples bacteriophages were found. After NGS, all pooled samples had DNA sequences from at least one respiratory virus, while three individual (not pooled) samples remained negative for common respiratory viruses (Table 5). In two of these samples (P183 and T38) *M. catarrhalis* was detected and *S. pneumoniae* was additionally present in one of them. The third sample (T65) remained negative for both viruses (including phages) and bacteria. Some of the samples from URTI had sequence reads corresponding to up to 11 different viruses or 18 different bacteria. Considering the NGS results, and assuming that in the pooled samples the identified viruses were each present in a different sample, 76.6% (403/526) of the children had a common respiratory virus detected, while in all but one of the other 129 children a respiratory bacteria was identified.

Genome assembly and phylogenetic analyses

To estimate the sequence coverage of the NGS-identified viruses, the sequence reads were assembled *de novo*, and all contigs were used to estimate the extent of the virus genome coverage. A significant coverage was obtained for several of the detected viruses. In patients with LRTI, the genome of 14 viruses was assembled with coverage higher than 20% (Table 6). As indication of the sensitivity of NGS and of the relative abundance of some viruses not detected by the conventional PCR, we could assemble more than 95% of the genome of two RV strains, 98% of one HBoV, and 99.8% of one HCoV-OC43 strain. In the case of children with URTI, at least 50% of the genome was covered for 15 viruses, including RV, HEV, Saffold virus, and TTV (Table 7), with 8 of them having a genome coverage of more than 90%. For the DNA reads of the animal viruses identified in both types of children populations the coverage ranged between 0.57 and 4.9%, and for plant viruses between 0.13 and 7.15% in the case of tomato mosaic virus (Tables 5A and B).

The assembled sequences from HCoV-OC43, RV, HBoV, Saffold, and anelloviruses were used to construct phylogenetic trees to determine the genetic similarity of the viruses characterized in this work with those in databases (see Materials and Methods). All viruses from LRTI and URTI grouped with clades formed by previously reported virus sequences (not shown). Anelloviruses could be readily classified as TTV, TTMV, or TTMDV, with some samples containing the three genera (Tables 4 and 5). All HCoV detected belong to species HCoV-OC43 and grouped with other known betacoronaviruses. HBoVs were all genotype 1, while the Saffold viruses detected in this work belonged to either genotype 2 or 3. Of interest, in the case of some RV, HBoV, Saffold, and anelloviruses, different contigs mapped to different clades, suggesting that recombination events are common in this type of viruses, as has been reported for RV [25].

Table 4. Pathogens identified by NGS in children with lower respiratory tract infections.

	Samples																								
Pathogen detected	**47**	**86**	**124**	**111**	**28**	**206**	**210**	**211**	**213**	**214**	**225**	**227**	**233**	**236**	**237**	**238**	**17**	**24**	**11**	**125**	**147**	**151**	**64**	**66**	**67**
VIRUSES																									
Respiratory syncytial virus	3[a]	372	-	-	-	-	-	-	-	-	-	-	-	-	-	-	12	-	-	-	-	7	-	318	-
Coronavirus OC43	-	-	-	-	5	-	45	4	3	1222	-	-	-	-	-	239049	1672	2	392	600	-	-	-	-	3
Rhinovirus A	5	-	66	-	2	-	-	16009	-	-	-	3	206	-	16	-	-	-	-	-	-	3	-	-	-
Rhinovirus C	-	-	121	-	-	-	-	63	-	-	3	-	38475	-	39	-	-	-	-	-	-	-	-	-	-
Human bocavirus	-	-	-	-	-	-	162	-	-	87209	6	-	-	-	-	322	483	-	46	-	-	-	-	-	-
Torque teno virus (TTV)	-	-	-	-	-	-	5	3	616	7	-	1007	125	-	-	15	7	32	-	-	2	-	9	160	-
Torque teno mini virus (TTMV)	-	-	-	-	-	-	46	-	6	-	-	-	-	-	-	3	-	7	-	-	-	-	2	54	-
Torque teno midi virus (TTMDV)	-	-	-	-	-	-	-	-	-	-	-	-	9	-	-	-	-	-	-	-	-	-	-	6	-
Human herpes virus	-	-	-	-	-	-	-	-	-	-	-	-	-	-	-	-	-	-	2	-	-	-	-	-	-
Human papilloma virus	-	-	-	-	-	-	-	-	-	-	-	31	-	-	-	-	-	-	-	-	-	-	-	-	-
Rotavirus	-	-	-	-	-	-	-	3	-	-	-	-	-	-	-	-	-	-	-	-	-	-	-	-	-
Bat picornavirus	-	-	-	-	-	-	-	4	-	-	-	-	-	-	-	-	-	-	-	-	-	-	-	-	-
Bovine kobuvirus	-	-	-	-	-	-	6	130	-	-	-	-	-	-	-	-	-	-	-	-	-	-	-	-	-
Bovine viral diarrhea virus	-	-	-	-	-	-	5	20	-	-	-	-	-	-	-	-	-	-	-	-	-	-	-	-	-
Pepper mottle virus	-	-	-	-	-	-	-	-	-	-	-	-	8	-	-	-	-	-	-	-	-	-	-	-	-
Potato virus Y	-	-	-	7	-	-	-	-	-	-	-	-	-	-	-	-	-	-	-	-	-	-	-	-	-
Phages	-	236	294	955	-	-	33	109	83	9	82	394	32	117	25	17	-	335	2	2384	569	383	67	1201	1345
BACTERIA																									
Streptococcus pneumoniae	3	10	14	7	-	57	4	34	25	37	3	22	25	6	94	418	4	25	23	27	420	48	186	104	3,964
Haemophilus influenzae	4	130	41	210	-	-	-	5	35	17	-	13	-	-	-	-	-	41	-	-	-	-	105	-	-
Moraxella catarrhalis	110	11,845	380	-	-	-	-	23	2,213	12	1,237	3	1,909	5	70	-	58	6	-	10	-	3	-	6	13
Legionella pneumophila	-	5	5	-	-	-	3	21	-	-	3	24	-	4	-	-	-	-	-	-	-	118	-	-	-
Klebsiella pneumoniae	-	-	-	37	-	5	-	5	6	-	2	-	-	4	-	-	-	-	3	-	-	-	-	-	-
Staphylococcus aureus	-	-	14	31	-	-	64	12	85	2	248	-	17	322	5	-	-	52	-	43	4	-	31	-	22
Rahnella	-	14	-	2,239	-	-	-	-	5	-	3	3	-	-	-	-	-	906	-	8	-	-	-	15	4
Burkholderia cepacia	3	228	242	1,753	-	133	29	475	236	22	420	1,135	98	148	16	-	-	325	-	25	163	15	255	1,168	106
Acinetobacter baumannii	67	1,419	1,092	4,622	-	685	152	1,491	1,660	57	1,252	1,793	579	46	37	54	-	2,248	-	2,210	180	350	347	783	2,425
Pseudomonas aeruginosa	14	398	222	1,044	-	531	61	282	430	9	719	1,525	123	914	26	10	1	-	-	965	63	199	307	1,175	369
Mycobacterium tuberculosis	-	7	-	11	-	-	-	-	3	-	7	-	-	-	-	-	-	-	-	-	-	-	-	-	-
Actinomycetales	15,563	25	52	316	-	38	-	61	161	16	77	151	17	19	32	-	-	-	-	33	-	10	15	-	-
Burkholderia gladioli	22	3,716	3,897	36,947	-	174	320	7,756	2,264	439	10,157	13,733	1,661	2,473	235	127	5	107	-	645	355	355	3,143	460	500
Malassezia globosa	35	154	270	-	447	-	1,554	48	-	785	208	146	848	-	214	620	1,915	-	1,062	21	102	392	141	142	87

Table 4. Cont.

Pathogen detected	Samples 47	86	124	111	28	206	210	211	213	214	225	227	233	236	237	238	17	24	11	125	147	151	64	66	67
Pseudomonas mendocina	-	98	67	359	-	154	12	112	86	-	291	430	27	90	10	-	-	63	-	623	19	74	93	50	75
Staphylococcus epidermidis	-	88	-	2681	-	-	5,007	-	1,341	-	-	-	-	-	88	-	-	-	-	15	-	210	-	40	111
Leifsonia xyli	2,494	-	-	-	-	-	-	-	-	-	-	-	-	-	-	-	-	-	-	-	-	-	-	-	-
Acidovorax	69	1,280	885	6,704	-	808	222	1,325	2,042	106	3,814	5,079	543	551	59	40	17	7,074	-	7,704	2,057	995	771	5,345	5,061

[a]Number of valids DNA reads in the sample por the corresponding pathogen.

Discussion

Improvements in diagnostic methods have increased the rate of identification of viral pathogens in different clinical conditions, such as gastrointestinal, respiratory, or neurologic infections. However, despite these advances there are still a significant number of cases (20–50%), in which the etiologic agents are believed to be viruses, but the agent is not identified [26]. Previously, we reported the presence of a respiratory virus in about 71% of nasal samples obtained from children with LRTI and URTI (Aponte et al., manuscript in preparation; see also the Pathogen Detection section above), using a PCR method able to detect 15 different respiratory viruses. After PCR screening the virus-negative samples for the presence of respiratory bacteria, 89.6% of children with LRTI and 91.1% with URTI had at least one potential pathogen identified. These percentages were raised to levels close to 80% for viruses in both patient populations after NGS analysis of the double-negative samples, and essentially 100% of the samples had either a common respiratory virus or bacteria identified (in only one of 526 URTI samples DNA reads from a potential pathogen was not identified). It is interesting that 6 of the 8 samples from both LRTI and URTI that were negative for viruses after NGS had less than one million valid reads (Tables 2 and 3). Since the number of sequence reads directly correlates with the amount of nucleic acids present in the original sample [21], the absence of virus detection in these samples could represent false-negative results; it is likely that with a larger amount of sample, or deeper sequencing, respiratory viruses could have also been detected.

The samples that resulted negative for viruses by PCR, and subsequently determined as PCR-positive for respiratory bacterial pathogens, were not characterized by NGS, but it is reasonable to assume that a high percentage of them could have also been positive for viruses by deep sequencing. It is difficult, however, to determine with confidence, which, if any, of the detected pathogens could be responsible for the clinical respiratory symptoms observed. The virus or bacteria detected by these methods could be present in the patient as an asymptomatic carrier state or as causal agents of asymptomatic infections. Studies comparing the presence of respiratory pathogens in nasal specimens from healthy children will help to resolve this issue. In addition, PCR and NGS are such sensitive techniques that the presence of small amounts of viral targets may not necessarily have clinical relevance. An additional limitation of this study is the limited number of samples analyzed. Exploring the possibility to define cutoff levels represents the next necessary step for diagnosing viral respiratory infections using molecular tests [27]. It is important to mention, however, that for several of the RV and HCoV detected in this study high genome sequence coverages were achieved. This observation indicates that a high number of DNA reads, and probably also of virus particles, were present in the samples. These viruses could have been undetected by PCR due to mismatches in the diagnostic primers used.

Of interest, the classes of viruses found by NGS in patients with LRTI and URTI were very similar, although their frequencies were different in the two study populations. RV was more frequently found in URTI (19 of 25 samples) vs. LRTI (9 of 25 samples), while coronavirus was more represented in LRTI (11/25) than in URTI (3/25). Only one of the 46 samples of children with URTI was positive for RSV, while in 5 of 25 samples from children with LRTI RSV was detected. Saffold viruses, members of the picornaviridae family and cardiovirus genus, were found only in children with URTI. Since their initial description in 2007, these viruses have been shown to circulate worldwide, occur early

Table 5. Pathogens identified by NGS in children with upper respiratory tract infections.

Pathogen detected	Samples[a] C06, C55, T78, V24	C16, C61	C27, C01	C29, M40, M41, V39	C41, T50	C46, P54	M23, M44	M28	P06, P150	P108	P131, V61	P147, P191	P14,9 P153	P151, P181	P173	P176, P186, P213	P183	P19, P88	T69	T33, T39	T36	T38	T43, T44	T65	V26
VIRUSES																									
Respiratory syncytial virus	-	-	-	-	-	-	-	-	-	-	-	-	-	-	-	-	-	-	-	3	-	-	-	-	-
Coronavirus OC43	-	-	-	-	-	-	-	-	-	-	-	3	24	-	38	-	-	-	-	-	-	-	-	-	-
Rhinovirus A	-	-	-	-	-	-	-	-	-	-	49	59	-	1,052	-	-	-	-	2	-	-	-	-	-	-
Rhinovirus B	-	-	-	-	-	-	-	-	14	-	3,995	12	-	8	-	-	-	-	-	-	-	-	-	-	-
Rhinovirus C	8418[b]	15	59	3,667	115,617	44	65,889	2	11,233	-	702	46	55	54	-	66	-	11,026	-	1,395	41	-	14,561	-	207
Human enterovirus A	-	-	-	-	15	-	-	-	15,236	-	78	-	-	-	-	-	-	-	-	-	-	-	-	-	-
Human bocavirus	-	-	-	-	-	-	-	-	-	12	8	-	-	-	-	-	-	-	-	-	-	-	-	-	98
Saffold virus	182	-	-	183	-	-	-	-	-	-	10	-	2,672	-	-	9,891	-	-	-	-	-	-	-	-	-
Torque teno virus (TTV)	-	-	9	-	7	187	-	-	12	-	212	14	-	7	-	-	-	-	-	3	-	-	-	-	-
Torque teno mini virus (TTMV)	-	-	-	3	5	100	-	-	22	-	3,408	9	-	17	-	-	-	-	-	-	-	-	-	-	-
Torque teno midi virus (TTMDV)	3	-	-	8	12	11	-	-	-	-	2,711	5	-	7	-	-	-	11	-	-	-	-	-	-	-
Human herpes virus	-	-	-	-	-	3	-	-	-	36	-	-	-	-	-	-	-	53	-	-	-	-	-	-	-
Human papilloma virus	-	-	3	-	-	-	6	-	-	-	3	-	-	118	-	-	-	5	-	-	-	-	-	-	-
Rotavirus	-	-	-	3	-	27	-	-	-	-	-	-	-	-	-	3	-	-	-	4	-	-	-	-	-
Human astrovirus	6	-	-	-	3	-	-	-	-	-	-	-	-	-	-	-	-	-	-	-	-	-	-	-	-
Bat picornavirus	-	-	-	-	-	-	-	-	-	-	4	-	-	-	-	-	-	-	-	-	-	-	7	-	-
Capsicum chlorosis virus	-	-	-	-	-	-	-	-	-	-	-	-	-	-	-	2	-	-	-	-	-	-	-	-	-
Cucumber mosaic virus	12	18	-	-	-	-	6	-	-	-	-	-	-	-	-	-	-	-	-	-	-	-	-	-	-
Okra mosaic virus	-	-	-	-	-	-	-	-	-	-	-	-	-	-	-	-	-	2	-	-	-	-	-	-	-
Pepper mottle virus	-	-	2	-	-	-	-	-	-	-	-	-	-	-	-	-	-	-	-	-	-	-	-	-	-
Tomato mosaic virus	-	16	12	-	-	4	-	-	3	-	-	4	-	-	-	-	-	8	-	-	-	-	-	-	-
White spot syndrome virus	-	-	-	-	-	-	-	-	-	-	-	-	-	-	-	31	-	-	-	-	-	-	-	-	-
Phages	10	28	31	54	46	102	60	6	12	11	16	327	36	139	10	568	6	21	8	43	4	-	8	-	6
BACTERIA																									
Streptococcus pneumoniae	13	80	103	14	3	180	12	51	42	3	15	21	51	83	-	20	-	274	9	-	4	-	-	-	-
Haemophilus influenzae	15	-	4	4	3	47	15	-	4	-	-	173	10	41	-	288	47	6	-	-	-	-	-	-	-
Moraxella catarrhalis	235	8	15	4	34	172	22	6,192	26	10	446	-	11	6	-	6	-	142	-	76	11	8	-	-	-
Legionella pneumophila	8	22	-	14	-	-	22	4	-	-	15	-	-	-	-	-	-	-	-	-	-	-	-	-	-
Klebsiella pneumoniae	-	9	-	3	-	-	-	-	-	-	-	-	-	-	-	-	-	3	-	-	-	-	-	-	-
Staphylococcus aureus	9	13	4	24	16	-	36	-	-	-	-	-	20	10	-	12	-	21	-	5	-	-	288	-	-

Table 5. Cont.

	Samples[a]																								
Pathogen detected	**C06, C55, T78, V24**	**C16, C61**	**C27, C01**	**C29, M40, M41, V39**	**C41, T50**	**C46, P54**	**M23, M44**	**M28**	**P06, P150**	**P108**	**P131, V61**	**P147, P191**	**P14,9 P153**	**P151, P181**	**P173**	**P176, P186, P213**	**P183**	**P19, P88**	**T69**	**T33, T39**	**T36**	**T38**	**T43, T44**	**T65**	**V26**
Rahnella	5	-	-	-	-	-	-	-	-	-	-	-	15	-	-	-	-	-	-	-	-	-	-	-	-
Burkholderia cepacia	65	46	16	9	7	-	-	14	-	-	-	-	4	-	-	-	-	-	-	-	-	-	-	-	-
Acinetobacter baumannii	1,783	1,754	825	1,301	778	2,390	5,204	402	202	-	654	2,107	208	1,544	-	1,347	17	556	-	179	-	-	179	-	50
Pseudomonas aeruginosa	81	37	32	134	16	115	97	29	131	-	61	167	163	211	-	196	-	274	17	16	-	-	7	-	-
Mycobacterium tuberculosis	6	-	4	-	-	-	-	-	-	-	-	-	-	-	-	-	-	-	-	-	-	-	-	-	-
Actinomycetales	1,017	410	2,283	1,141	7,369	575	692	357	1,600	64	482	1,049	1,106	779	13	753	122	13,679	201	2,159	13	-	341	-	117
Burkholderia gladioli	-	4	-	9	-	-	-	-	-	-	-	-	-	-	-	-	-	-	-	-	-	-	-	-	-
Malassezia globosa	21	10	87	17	145	103	34	267	-	43	578	12	111	48	123	102	-	136	31	77	11	75	57	-	42
Pseudomonas mendocina	124	106	53	242	56	109	160	46	146	-	73	201	137	205	-	214	-	370	50	17	-	-	3	-	-
Rhodotorula glutinis	265	396	74	202	134	69	510	11	-	-	-	-	10	-	-	8	-	19	-	7	-	-	-	-	-
Staphylococcus epidermidis	27	110	62	19	149	27	57	9	52	-	18	-	50	205	-	62	-	-	29	6	-	-	3	-	-
Lysinibacillus sphaericus	115	301	539	29	84	117	568	234	-	-	-	-	-	-	-	-	-	18	-	-	-	-	-	-	-
Acidovorax	508	190	117	356	76	80	315	124	30	-	163	136	-	189	-	207	-	58	-	31	-	-	9	-	12
Fervidobacterium nodosum	278	677	519	345	320	999	1,152	164	349	-	270	681	1,487	1,094	-	590	-	41	93	208	-	-	121	-	-

[a]When more than one sample were pooled for sequencing, the code for the various samples is mentioned.
[b]Number of valids DNA reads in the sample por the corresponding pathogen.

Table 6. Genome coverage for viruses present in LRTI samples.

Sample	Virus[a]	No. of Contigs	No. of reads incorporated into contigs	Genome size	Genome Coverage (%)
86	RSV	22	213	15,191	6.75
124	RV-A	6	47	7,129	7.43
	RV-C	10	96	7,107	24.34
111	PVY	1	7	9,704	1.75
210	HBoV	16	74	5,299	33.97
	HCoV	3	10	30,578	5.89
	TTMV	2	14	2,912	8.24
	BKV	1	4	8,374	1.07
	BVDV	1	3	12,230	0.57
211	RV-A	1	13,418	7,129	94.60
	RV-C	11	47	7,107	17.03
	BatPV	1	3	7,753	0.97
	BKV	5	83	8,374	4.90
	BVDV	1	9	12,230	0.61
	RV	1	3	17,360	0.40
213	TTV	12	407	3,725	32.48
214	HBoV	4	53,548	5,299	97.62
	HCoV	80	848	30,578	39.96
	TTMV	1	3	2,912	2.40
225	HBoV	1	3	5,299	1.51
	RV-C	1	2	3,725	2.01
227	TTV	8	777	3,725	34.90
	HPV	1	12	7,466	0.94
233	RV-A	16	127	7,129	26.65
	RV-C	2	30712	7,107	97.88
	TTV	16	75	3,725	52.35
237	RV-A	1	3	7,129	0.98
	RV-C	6	35	7,107	7.46
238	HBoV	22	202	5,299	38.69
	HCoV	5	85766	30,578	99.81
	TTV	1	4	3,725	2.01
17	HBoV	32	279	5,299	61.80
	HCoV	112	1,021	30,578	20.52
	RSV	1	3	15,191	0.49
24	TTV	12	1	3,725	1.88
11	HBoV	6	45	5,299	12.08
	HCoV	15	291	30,578	5.72
125	HCoV	32	382	30,578	11.28
151	RSV	1	4	15,191	0.46
66	RSV	24	274	15,191	15.40
	TTV	3	107	3,725	9.93
	TTMV	2	23	2,912	4.46

[a]RSV, respiratory syncytial virus; RV-A, rhinovirus species A, RV-C; rhinovirus species C; HBoV, human bocavirus, HCoV, human coronavirus OC43; TTV, torque teno virus; TTMV, torque teno mini virus; BKV, bovine kobuvirus; BVDV, bovine viral diarrhea virus; BatPV, bat picornavirus; HPV, human papillomavirus; PVY, potato virus Y.

in life, and involve the respiratory and gastrointestinal tracts. The association of these viruses with clinical symptoms is under investigation and requires additional epidemiological studies to clarify their pathogenicity [28]. Anelloviruses (TTV, TTMV, TTMDV) were found in both LRTIs and URTIs. Members of this family ubiquitously infect humans and establish persistent infections, although causal disease associations are currently lacking [10]. It is interesting to note that common gastrointestinal viruses such as astrovirus and rotavirus were found in some of the samples. It is not surprising though, since rotaviruses have long being

Table 7. Genome coverage for viruses present in URTI samples.

Sample	Virus[a]	No. of Contigs	No. of reads incorporated into contigs	Genome size	Genome Coverage (%)
C27, C01	ToMV	2	12	6,383	1.88
	TTMDV	2	5	3256	4.45
	HPV	1	2	7466	0.94
	RV-C	9	45	7107	11.3
C41, T50	TTMV	2	5	2912	3.78
	TTMDV	2	10	3256	3.22
	TTV	1	3	3725	2.28
	RV-C	1	92130	7107	95.40
C16, C61	CMV	4	10	3356	7.15
	ToMV	3	15	6386	2.98
	RV-C	2	10	7107	2.74
M23, M44	CMV	1	3	3356	5.36
	RV-C	1	39840	7107	97.20
P108	HHV	5	12	116114	0.28
	HBoV	2	5	5299	2.64
P06, P150	HEV-A	2	12352	7,413	97.88
	TTMV	1	6	2912	4.12
	RV-C	4	8798	7107	92.74
P149, P153	HCoV	3	11	30,578	0.78
	SAFV	5	1909	8,115	83.03
	RV-C	4	26	7107	4.50
P173	HCoV	3	9	30,578	0.69
P151, P181	RV-A	7	943	7,129	50.78
	RV-B	1	4	7,215	0.97
	HPV	9	45	7466	12.46
	TTMV	2	7	2912	4.98
	TTV	1	3	3725	0.87
	RV-C	5	17	7107	6.33
P147, P191	RV-A	3	12	7,129	4.35
	RV-B	1	4	7,215	1.25
	ToMV	1	3	6,384	1.25
	TTMV	1	3	2912	3.43
	TTMDV	1	3	3256	2.15
	TTV	1	5	3725	2.01
	RV-C	5	15	7107	6.26
P176, P186, P213	WSSV	6	31	292,967	0.13
	SAFV	5	8023	8,115	90.92
	RV-C	8	37	7107	9.01
C46, P54	RV	3	12	17360	1.09
	TTMV	6	73	2912	15.45
	TTMDV	1	11	3256	2.15
	TTV	13	150	3725	50.74
	RV-C	3	9	7107	2.25
P19, P88	HHV	3	12	116114	0.18
	HPV	0	0	7466	0.00
	ToMV	1	7	6,384	1.25
	TTMDV	1	6	3256	3.38
	RV-C	10	8726	7107	62.77
T36	RV-C	5	21	7107	4.43
T33, T39	RV-C	12	1319	7107	68.74

Table 7. Cont.

Sample	Virus[a]	No. of Contigs	No. of reads incorporated into contigs	Genome size	Genome Coverage (%)
T43, T44	RV-C	3	14165	7107	92.92
C06, C55, T78, V24	HASTV	2	5	6,759	2.52
	CMV	1	6	3356	2.09
	SAFV	2	126	8,115	2.42
	RV-C	3	7989	7107	92.66
V26	HBoV	8	77	5299	15.30
	RV-C	7	143	7107	15.06
C29, M40, M41, V39	SAFV	8	135	8,115	8.76
	TTMV	1	5	2912	2.75
	RV-C	11	3061	7107	63.89
P131, V61	BatPV	1	2	7,753	0.90
	HBoV	1	4	5299	2.08
	RV-A	3	14	7,129	3.23
	RV-B	4	3145	7,215	90.33
	HEV A	3	13	7,413	3.10
	TTMV	9	1531	2912	47.12
	TTMDV	4	1881	3256	29.67
	TTV	13	126	3725	42.31
	RV-C	4	618	7107	19.77

[a]RSV, respiratory syncytial virus; RV-A, rhinovirus species A; RV-B; rhinovirus species B; RV-C; rhinovirus species C; HBoV, human bocavirus, HCoV, human coronavirus OC43; TTV, torque teno virus; TTMV, torque teno mini virus; TTMDV, torque teno midi virus; BKV, bovine kobuvirus; BVDV, bovine viral diarrhea virus; BatPV, bat picornavirus; HPV, human papillomavirus; PVY, potato virus Y, ToMV, tomato mosaic virus; CMV, cucumber mosaic virus; HHV, human herpes virus; HVE-A, human enterovirus A; SAFV, Saffold virus; WSSV, white spot syndrome virus; HASTV, human astrovirus.

suspected to reach the gastrointestinal tract via mouth and nose. In fact, some rotavirus infections have been associated with respiratory symptoms [29]. Finally, we found low amounts of DNA reads corresponding to animal and plant viruses. The number of these types of viruses is larger than previously reported in respiratory samples [21], although plant viruses have been found more abundantly in human feces [30]. Both, plant and animal viruses are thought to be derived either from consumed food or acquired from the environment.

The search for new viruses using NGS technologies in mammalian, avian, and in particular, human samples, has contributed to the identification of new viruses in animal reservoirs and in different conditions of disease [31]. However, the important effort invested in mammal and avian virus detection has only resulted in the discovery of variants of virus species, sister species to known viruses, and rarely genera. These observations contrast with the recent efforts to discover arthropod viruses, which have yielded widely divergent taxa that sometimes have even defined novel families [32]. Altogether, these observations and the presence of DNA sequence reads from common respiratory viruses or bacteria in essentially 100% of the samples collected from children with LRTI and URTI, suggest there is limited potential for the discovery of so far undescribed, clinically relevant, viruses associated to pediatric respiratory disease at least in the type of populations studied and with the sampling and diagnostic methods employed.

Acknowledgments

We thank Miguel L. García-León for his help in handling and organizing all pneumonia samples. We also thank the Instituto de Biotecnologia-UNAM for giving us access to its computer cluster and Jerome Verleyen for his computer support. This work was supported by grants 153639 (to JI Santos) and "Influenza 2009" (to CF Arias) from the National Council for Science and Technology-Mexico (CONACYT). F.E.A. is recipient of a scholarship from CONACYT.

Author Contributions

Conceived and designed the experiments: BT PI CFA. Performed the experiments: BT MAE FEA PI. Analyzed the data: BT CFA. Contributed reagents/materials/analysis tools: MAA-O JM-M R-RV FD-H FZ-V RMW-C VF-R CNR-A JG-M AV-S GM-A MCS-M DEN LFP-G JIS-P. Wrote the paper: CFA BT SL JIS-P DEN GM-A RMW-C AV-S.

References

1. Rudan I, O'Brien KL, Nair H, Liu L, Theodoratou E, et al. (2013) Epidemiology and etiology of childhood pneumonia in 2010: estimates of incidence, severe morbidity, mortality, underlying risk factors and causative pathogens for 192 countries. J Glob Health 3: 010401.
2. Ruuskanen O, Lahti E, Jennings LC, Murdoch DR (2011) Viral pneumonia. Lancet 377: 1264–1275.
3. Black RE, Cousens S, Johnson HL, Lawn JE, Rudan I, et al. (2010) Global, regional, and national causes of child mortality in 2008: a systematic analysis. Lancet 375: 1969–1987.
4. Chiu CY, Urisman A, Greenhow TL, Rouskin S, Yagi S, et al. (2008) Utility of DNA microarrays for detection of viruses in acute respiratory tract infections in children. J Pediatr 153: 76–83.
5. Ruohola A, Waris M, Allander T, Ziegler T, Heikkinen T, et al. (2009) Viral etiology of common cold in children, Finland. Emerg Infect Dis 15: 344–346.
6. van Gageldonk-Lafeber AB, Heijnen ML, Bartelds AI, Peters MF, van der Plas SM, et al. (2005) A case-control study of acute respiratory tract infection in general practice patients in The Netherlands. Clinical infectious diseases: an official publication of the Infectious Diseases Society of America 41: 490–497.

7. Gern JE (2010) The ABCs of rhinoviruses, wheezing, and asthma. J Virol 84: 7418–7426.
8. Heikkinen T, Jarvinen A (2003) The common cold. Lancet 361: 51–59.
9. Debiaggi M, Canducci F, Ceresola ER, Clementi M (2012) The role of infections and coinfections with newly identified and emerging respiratory viruses in children. Virol J 9: 247.
10. Jartti T, Jartti L, Ruuskanen O, Soderlund-Venermo M (2012) New respiratory viral infections. Curr Opin Pulm Med 18: 271–278.
11. Allander T, Tammi MT, Eriksson M, Bjerkner A, Tiveljung-Lindell A, et al. (2005) Cloning of a human parvovirus by molecular screening of respiratory tract samples. Proc Natl Acad Sci U S A 102: 12891–12896.
12. Harvala H, Simmonds P (2009) Human parechoviruses: biology, epidemiology and clinical significance. J Clin Virol 45: 1–9.
13. van den Hoogen BG, de Jong JC, Groen J, Kuiken T, de Groot R, et al. (2001) A newly discovered human pneumovirus isolated from young children with respiratory tract disease. Nat Med 7: 719–724.
14. van der Hoek L, Pyrc K, Jebbink MF, Vermeulen-Oost W, Berkhout RJ, et al. (2004) Identification of a new human coronavirus. Nat Med 10: 368–373.
15. Woo PC, Lau SK, Chu CM, Chan KH, Tsoi HW, et al. (2005) Characterization and complete genome sequence of a novel coronavirus, coronavirus HKU1, from patients with pneumonia. J Virol 79: 884–895.
16. Erdman DD, Weinberg GA, Edwards KM, Walker FJ, Anderson BC, et al. (2003) GeneScan reverse transcription-PCR assay for detection of six common respiratory viruses in young children hospitalized with acute respiratory illness. J Clin Microbiol 41: 4298–4303.
17. Gruteke P, Glas AS, Dierdorp M, Vreede WB, Pilon JW, et al. (2004) Practical implementation of a multiplex PCR for acute respiratory tract infections in children. J Clin Microbiol 42: 5596–5603.
18. Murdoch DR, Jennings LC, Bhat N, Anderson TP (2010) Emerging advances in rapid diagnostics of respiratory infections. Infect Dis Clin North Am 24: 791–807.
19. Syrmis MW, Whiley DM, Thomas M, Mackay IM, Williamson J, et al. (2004) A sensitive, specific, and cost-effective multiplex reverse transcriptase-PCR assay for the detection of seven common respiratory viruses in respiratory samples. J Mol Diagn 6: 125–131.
20. Hustedt JW, Vazquez M (2010) The changing face of pediatric respiratory tract infections: how human metapneumovirus and human bocavirus fit into the overall etiology of respiratory tract infections in young children. Yale J Biol Med 83: 193–200.
21. Lysholm F, Wetterbom A, Lindau C, Darban H, Bjerkner A, et al. (2012) Characterization of the viral microbiome in patients with severe lower respiratory tract infections, using metagenomic sequencing. PloS One 7: e30875.
22. Willner D, Furlan M, Haynes M, Schmieder R, Angly FE, et al. (2009) Metagenomic analysis of respiratory tract DNA viral communities in cystic fibrosis and non-cystic fibrosis individuals. PloS One 4: e7370.
23. Wylie KM, Mihindukulasuriya KA, Sodergren E, Weinstock GM, Storch GA (2012) Sequence analysis of the human virome in febrile and afebrile children. PloS One 7: e27735.
24. Sorber K, Chiu C, Webster D, Dimon M, Ruby JG, et al. (2008) The long march: a sample preparation technique that enhances contig length and coverage by high-throughput short-read sequencing. PloS One 3: e3495.
25. Waman VP, Kolekar PS, Kale MM, Kulkarni-Kale U (2014) Population structure and evolution of Rhinoviruses. PloS One 9: e88981.
26. Tang P, Chiu C (2010) Metagenomics for the discovery of novel human viruses. Future Microbiol 5: 177–189.
27. Jansen RR, Wieringa J, Koekkoek SM, Visser CE, Pajkrt D, et al. (2011) Frequent detection of respiratory viruses without symptoms: toward defining clinically relevant cutoff values. J Clin Microbiol 49: 2631–2636.
28. Himeda T, Ohara Y (2012) Saffold virus, a novel human Cardiovirus with unknown pathogenicity. J Virol 86: 1292–1296.
29. Estes MK, Greenberg HB (2013) Rotaviruses. In: Knipe DM, Howley, P.M., editor. Fields Virology. 6th ed. Philadelphia: Wolters Kluwer/Lippincott Williams & Wilkins. pp. 1347–1401.
30. Zhang T, Breitbart M, Lee WH, Run JQ, Wei CL, et al. (2006) RNA viral community in human feces: prevalence of plant pathogenic viruses. PLoS Biology 4: e3.
31. Chiu CY (2013) Viral pathogen discovery. Curr Opin Microbiol 16: 468–478.
32. Junglen S, Drosten C (2013) Virus discovery and recent insights into virus diversity in arthropods. Curr Opin Microbiol 16: 507–513.

c-di-GMP Enhances Protective Innate Immunity in a Murine Model of Pertussis

Shokrollah Elahi[1]*, Jill Van Kessel[2], Tedele G. Kiros[3], Stacy Strom[2], Yoshihiro Hayakawa[4], Mamoru Hyodo[4], Lorne A. Babiuk[1], Volker Gerdts[2,3]*

1 Faculty of Medicine and Dentistry, University of Alberta, Edmonton, Alberta, Canada, **2** Vaccine and Infectious Disease Organization, International Vaccine Centre, University of Saskatchewan, Saskatoon, Saskatchewan, Canada, **3** Department of Veterinary Microbiology, Western College of Veterinary Medicine, University of Saskatchewan, Saskatoon, Saskatchewan, Canada, **4** Faculty of Engineering, Department of Applied Chemistry, Aichi Institute of Technology, Toyota, Japan

Abstract

Innate immunity represents the first line of defense against invading pathogens in the respiratory tract. Innate immune cells such as monocytes, macrophages, dendritic cells, NK cells, and granulocytes contain specific pathogen-recognition molecules which induce the production of cytokines and subsequently activate the adaptive immune response. c-di-GMP is a ubiquitous second messenger that stimulates innate immunity and regulates biofilm formation, motility and virulence in a diverse range of bacterial species with potent immunomodulatory properties. In the present study, c-di-GMP was used to enhance the innate immune response against pertussis, a respiratory infection mainly caused by *Bordetella pertussis*. Intranasal treatment with c-di-GMP resulted in the induction of robust innate immune responses to infection with *B. pertussis* characterized by enhanced recruitment of neutrophils, macrophages, natural killer cells and dendritic cells. The immune responses were associated with an earlier and more vigorous expression of Th1-type cytokines, as well as an increase in the induction of nitric oxide in the lungs of treated animals, resulting in significant reduction of bacterial numbers in the lungs of infected mice. These results demonstrate that c-di-GMP is a potent innate immune stimulatory molecule that can be used to enhance protection against bacterial respiratory infections. In addition, our data suggest that priming of the innate immune system by c-di-GMP could further skew the immune response towards a Th1 type phenotype during subsequent infection. Thus, our data suggest that c-di-GMP might be useful as an adjuvant for the next generation of acellular pertussis vaccine to mount a more protective Th1 phenotype immune response, and also in other systems where a Th1 type immune response is required.

Editor: Eliane Namie Miyaji, Instituto Butantan, Brazil

Funding: This study was funded through a grant from the Bill and Melinda Gates Foundation through the Grand Challenges in Global Health Program, and the Canadian Institutes of Health Research. The funders had no role in study design, data collection and analysis, decision to publish, or preparation of the manuscript.

Competing Interests: The authors have declared that no competing interests exist.

* Email: elahi@ualberta.ca (SE); volker.gerdts@usask.ca (VG)

Introduction

Pertussis is one of the most serious childhood diseases responsible for hundreds of thousands of deaths every year. The disease is primarily caused by infection with the Gram-negative bacterium *Bordetella pertussis and* occasionally by *Bordetella parapertussis*. More recently, cases of *Bordetella holmesii* have been identified during pertussis outbreaks that have mainly affected adolescents [1]. Pertussis is characterized by severe respiratory symptoms including paroxysmal cough and apnea. The infection is mediated via inhalation of aerosol droplets and typically remains localized in the respiratory tract [2]. However, in immunosuppressed subjects the disease can progress to generalized bacteremia [3].

Over the past two decades, a resurgence of pertussis in infants and a shift of cases from children to adolescents/adults have been reported worldwide [4,5]. The immune response against *B. pertussis* relies on both specific and innate immune responses. Although specific correlates of protection have not yet been fully established, the use of vaccines over decades has proven to be highly effective in reducing the disease. Both acelluar pertussis vaccines (Pa) and the whole-cell pertussis vaccines (Pw) are currently available and various studies have demonstrated the importance of vaccine-induced antibodies against *B. pertussis* virulence factors including pertussis toxin (Ptx), fimbria (fim 2 and fim 3) and pertactin [6–10]. However, it has been difficult to establish a direct correlation between antibody titers and protection from disease [11,12]. Cell-mediated immunity, and in particular $CD4^+$ T cells are involved in protection, especially when using Pw vaccines [13,14]. Other reports have shown that the secretion of IFN-γ is critical for effective control of bacterial spread in the lung. For example, IFN-$\gamma^{-/-}$ or IFN-γ defective mice developed disseminating lethal infections following challenge [2,15]. Furthermore, protection may also be associated with the induction of IL-12 [16] and TNF-α required for effective phagocytosis of the bacteria [17,18]. More recently, Th-17 cells and the secretion of IL-17 have also been implicated in cell-mediated protection from *B. pertussis* [19].

The innate immune response against pertussis involves various immune cells including macrophages, neutrophils, dendritic cells, γδ-T cells, NK cells and NKT cells [20]. The two main phagocytic cell populations that constitute pulmonary innate immunity are resident alveolar macrophages and recruited neutrophils [21]. In addition, local and rapidly recruited lung dendritic cells have been demonstrated to internalize bacteria and promote the expression of type 1 cytokines by NK cells, T cells, and NKT cells [22–26], which then directly impact specific immune responses. Here, we evaluated the potential of cyclic diguanylate (c-di-GMP; 3′, 5′-cyclic diguanylate) to act as innate immune stimulator.

C-di-GMP was first identified in Gluconacetobacter xylinum and Agrobacterium tumefaciens. The molecule is involved in various intracellular signaling pathways including cellulose biosynthesis [27–29], bacterial growth, cellular adhesion, cell-surface interactions and biofilm formation [30–34]. c-di-GMP is found at concentrations of 5–10 μM in many bacterial species, but not in eukaryotes [35–37]. Recently, a number of studies have shown that the innate immune response elicited by c-di-GMP is a potent immunomodulator for the treatment of bacterial infections and can act as an immune modulator and immunostimulatory molecule [32,38]. For example, intramammary administration of c-di-GMP has been shown to prevent colonization and biofilm formation by *Staphylococcus aureus* in a murine model of mastitis [39]. In another study, intranasal or subcutaneous administration of c-di-GMP stimulated a robust innate immune response characterized by increased recruitment of immune cells into the lung which resulted in protection against intratracheal challenge with *Klebsiella pneumonia* in mice [32]. Furthermore, intranasal administration of c-di-GMP significantly reduced nasopharyngeal *Streptococcus pneumoniae* colonization by induction of a robust but transient proinflammatory response characterized by production of cytokines, chemokines and recruitment of pulmonary DCs [40]. Intraperitoneal administration of c-di-GMP in mice enhanced monocyte and granulocyte recruitment [38]. Interestingly, stimulation of human immature dendritic cells with c-di-GMP resulted in an increase in the expression of costimulatory molecules CD80/CD86 and maturation marker CD83, MHC class II, cytokines, chemokines and chemokine receptors [38]. More recently, STING has been identified as a direct detector of cyclic dinucleotides, provides more insight into the fundamental mechanisms by which the innate immune system can detect bacterial infection [41]. Here, we demonstrate that intranasal administration of c-di-GMP in mice resulted in induction of protective immune responses against bacterial challenge with *B. pertussis*. These results also confirm previous observations that innate immunity plays an important role in disease protection against *B. pertussis* infection.

Materials and Methods

Mice

Female specific pathogen free BALB/c mice were obtained at 5–7 weeks of age from the Charles River Institute. All animals were maintained under specific pathogen free conditions within the animal care unit of VIDO until the day of sacrifice. This study was carried out in strict accordance with the recommendations in the Guide for the Care and Use of Laboratory Animals of the Canadian Council for Animal Care. The protocol was approved by the Committee on the Ethics of Animal Experiments of the University of Saskatchewan. All surgery was performed under sodium pentobarbital anesthesia, and all efforts were made to minimize suffering.

c-di-GMP

The c-di-GMP used in our study was chemically synthesized and prepared as described previously [42]. The purity of the c-di-GMP used in this study was>98% and was confirmed by HPLC, ^{31}P-NMR, and ESI-TOF Mass Spectophotometrical analysis. The peptides used in this study were free of endotoxin contamination as determined by the Limulus assay. Control c-GMP (Sigma) or c-di-GMP was reconstituted at a concentration of 200 μM in 30 μl of sterile saline for treatment of mice.

Bacterial culture

Bacterial suspensions of strain Tohama I were stored at −70°C in Casamino acid plus 10% glycerol. Organisms were grown on the surface of Charcoal agar (Becton Dickinson and Company, USA) containing 10% (vol/vol) defibrinated sheep blood and 40 μg/ml of Cephalexin (Sigma-Aldrich, USA) at 37°C for 48 hr. Bacteria were harvested from plates by scraping off and resuspending bacteria in Stainer-Scholte (SS) medium. Bacteria were washed by centrifugation at 2500 g for 10 min. The pellets were resuspended in phosphate buffered saline (PBS; pH 7.2) and adjusted to the indicated optical density (OD) at 600 nm using a spectrophotometer (Ultrospec 3000, Pharmacia Biotech, U.K). The bacterial suspension was kept on ice until it was used for the challenge. The corresponding viable counts of these suspensions were determined by plating serial dilutions of the bacterial suspension onto Charcoal agar plates and incubation at 37°C for 4–5 days.

Respiratory challenge

Mice were lightly anaesthetized while a single drop of 30 μl c-di-GMP, the nucleotide control c-GMP or PBS (0.1 M, pH 7,2) was administered intranasally (i.n.) 24 hr prior to bacterial challenge. For challenge mice were anaesthetized and an inoculum containing 1–3×10^7 *B. pertussis* was carefully placed on the top of each nostril, and allowed to be inhaled [43]. After the challenge at days 2, 4 and 6, lungs were removed from mice and placed in SS medium or PBS (0.1 M, pH 7,2) containing 0.4 mM of irreversible serine protease inhibitor APMSF (4-Amidinophenyl-methanesulfonyl fluoride; Roche Diagnostics GmbH, Germany).

Whole lung homogenization for bacterial and cytokine determination

The whole lung from each mouse was homogenized in 2 ml of SS medium. Bacterial counts were assessed by plating serial dilutions of the homogenate onto Charcoal agar plates and incubation at 37°C for 4–5 days. For assessment of cytokine levels the whole lungs were homogenized in 2 ml of PBS containing APMSF for cytokine determination and flow cytometric analysis. The lung homogenates in PBS with protease inhibitor were then centrifuged at 1200xg for 10 min. Supernatants were collected and stored at −20°C for measurement of cytokine levels.

Detection of cytokine levels by ELISA

Concentrations of murine IFN-γ, TNF-α, IL-4, IL-6, IL-12, IL-17, IL-23 and MCP-1 were measured in serum and lung homogenate supernatants using an Endogen, Opteia or capture Duoset ELISA development system. Immunolon 2-HB 96-well plates were coated with anti-mouse IFN-γ (4 μg/ml), anti-mouse TNF-α (0.8 μg/ml), anti-mouse IL-4 (4 μg/ml), anti-mouse IL-6 (2 μg/ml), anti-mouse IL-12p70 (4 μg/ml), anti-mouse IL-23 (2 μg/ml; R & D Systems), anti-mouse IL-17 (2 μg/ml; eBioscience) and anti-mouse MCP-1 (1:250; BD Biosciences) overnight at 4°C. Prior to use, the plates were blocked with PBS

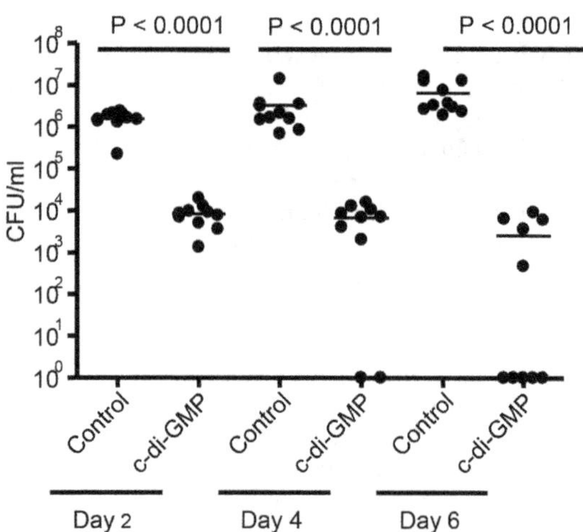

Figure 1. Pretreatment with c-di-GMP reduces the bacterial load in the lungs of mice challenged with *B. pertussis*. Mice were intranasally treated with c-di-GMP or control (PBS) at 24 hr prior to challenge. Bacterial counts were determined at day 2, 4 and 6 post challenge. The results are expressed as the mean values ± the standard deviations per lung, as counted from individual lungs of 10 mice per group from three separate experiments. *, P<0.0001 in lung homogenates versus the control group.

and 1% bovine serum albumin (BSA) for 1 h at room temperature (RT). Samples were added to the wells in a volume of 50 µl plus 50 µl of PBS-1% BSA and incubated for 2 h at RT. The reaction was amplified with biotinylated monoclonal antibodies to murine IFN- γ (0.4 µg/ml), TNF-α (0.2 µg/ml), IL-4 (0.4 µg/ml), IL-6 (0.2 µg/ml), IL-8 (25 µg/ml), IL-10 (50 µg/ml), IL-12p70 (0.4 µg/ml), IL-23 (Quantikine kit; all from R & D Systems), IL-17 (0.5 g/ml; eBioscience) and MCP-1 (1:250; BD Biosciences). Plates were incubated for 1 h at RT. Detection was carried out with peroxidase-conjugated streptavidin (1:5000; Jackson Laboratories) following 60 min incubation at RT and reaction was visualized with p-nitrophenylphospate (Sigma-Aldrich). Standard curves were generated using recombinant murine IFN- γ, TNF-α, IL-4, IL-6, IL-12, IL-17, IL-23 and MCP-1.

Quantification of nitric oxide (NO) in the lung

Lung homogenates were collected and centrifuged down at 10000 g for 20 min before the assay. The production of NO was determined by measuring the accumulation of nitrite, the stable metabolite of NO, in homogenate supernatants using the Griess reaction (Colorimetric assay kit, Alexis Biomedicals, Switzerland) as previously described [44]. A standard nitrite curve was generated in the same fashion using $NaNO_2$.

Lung leukocyte isolation

To remove intraepithelial lymphocytes (IEL) lung tissues were treated with 20 ml PBSA-buffer (0.1 M, pH 7,2) with 2 mM EDTA, pH 7.3 for 45 min on stir at 37°C. To remove lamina propria lymphocytes (LPL), lung tissues were enzymathically digested in digestion buffer (20 mM PBS containing 5% fetal bovine serum, 1% Hepes, 1% antibiotic/antimycotic and 250 U/ml collagenase type V) for 45 min on stir at 37°C. The total lung cell (IEL and LPL) suspension was, pooled, pelleted, resuspended, and centrifuged through a 30%, 40% and 60% percoll gradient to enrich for leukocytes for flow analysis. Cell counts and viability were determined on a hemocytometer using trypan blue exclusion.

Messenger RNA expression analysis using real-time PCR

The whole lung was removed at different time points and immediately snap frozen in liquid nitrogen and then stored at 70°C for further RNA extraction. Total RNA was extracted from 30 to 50 mg of tissue using the RNeasy Mini kit (Qiagen, Mississauga, Canada). Total RNA quantity and purity were determined by optical density (OD) at 260 and 280 nm wavelengths using a spectrophotometer (Ultrospec 2000, Pharmacia Biotech, Baie d'Urfe, PQ). RNA samples were treated with DNAse I Amp Grade (Invitrogen) (1 U/µg of RNA). The absence of genomic DNA contamination was validated by use of treated RNA as template directly in PCR. One microgram of total RNA was used for a reverse transcription reaction (total 21 µl) with $Oligo(dt)_{12-18}$ primers and SuperScript II reverse transcriptase (SuperScript first strand synthesis system for RT-PCR (Invitrogen) for evaluation of relative expression. Negative controls were made by replacing the reverse transcriptase with diethyl pyrocarbonate-treated water. The resulting single-stranded cDNA was then used in for real-time PCR (qPCR) analysis (iCycler iQ Real-Time PCR detection system, Bio-Rad, Hercules, CA) for evaluation of relative expression. cDNA was combined with primer/probe sets and IQ SYBR Green Supermix (Bio Rad) according to the manufacturer's recommendations. Primers for mouse beta defensin 3 (mBD3) forward (5′-TCTGTTTGCATTTCTCCTGGTG-3′), reverse (5′-TAAACTTCCAACAGCTGG-AGTGG-3′) and mBD4 forward (5′-TCTGTTTGCATTTCTCCTGGTG-3′), reverse (5′-TTTGCTAAAAGCTGCAGGTGG-3′) and mouse macrophage-inflammatory protein (mMIP-2), forward, 5′-GAA CAT CCA GAG CTT GAG TGT GA-3′, reverse, 5′-CCT TGA GAG TGG CTA TGA CTT CTG T-3′, respectively. The PCR conditions were 95°C for 3 min, followed by 45 cycles with denaturation at 95°C for 15 s, annealing temperature for 30 s, and elongation at 72°C for 30 s. The specificity of the PCR reactions was assessed by the analysis of the melting curves of the products, size verification and sequencing of the amplicons. Samples were normalized by using the average cycle threshold (CT) of glyceraldehyde-3-phosphate dehydrogenase (GAPDH) as a reference in each tissue. The suitability of GAPDH as a reference was confirmed by the lack of variation observed between animals from a same group. Relative quantitation of mRNA levels was plotted as fold-increase compared to untreated control lungs.

Flow cytometric analysis

Using FITC or PE-labeled antibodies (BD Pharmingen, San Diego, CA), isolated cells were stained with anti-CD4, anti-CD8, anti-αß-Tcr, anti-γδ-Tcr, anti-DX5 (NK cell marker), anti-CD11c, CD40, CD83, CD86 and their isotype controls. Cells were collected on a FACS Calibur cytometer (BD) using Cell Quest software (BD).

In vitro growth inhibition assays

The sensitivity of *B. pertussis* to c-di-GMP was compared with synthetically derived porcine cathelicidin protegrin 1 (PG1) and human cathelicidin LL-37 by co-culturing appropriate concentrations of c-di-GMP, PG1 and LL-37 in 20 mM PBSA (280 µl) with $5–7\times10^6$ CFU (10 µl) bacteria as previously described [45]. Plates were incubated at 37°C for 2 hrs. Supernatants were plated onto Charcoal agar plates to evaluate the number of viable bacteria.

Statistical analysis

All outcome data from this study followed non-normal distributions. To account for this, outcome data were ranked and then an ANOVA or a Student's t-test was used to detect

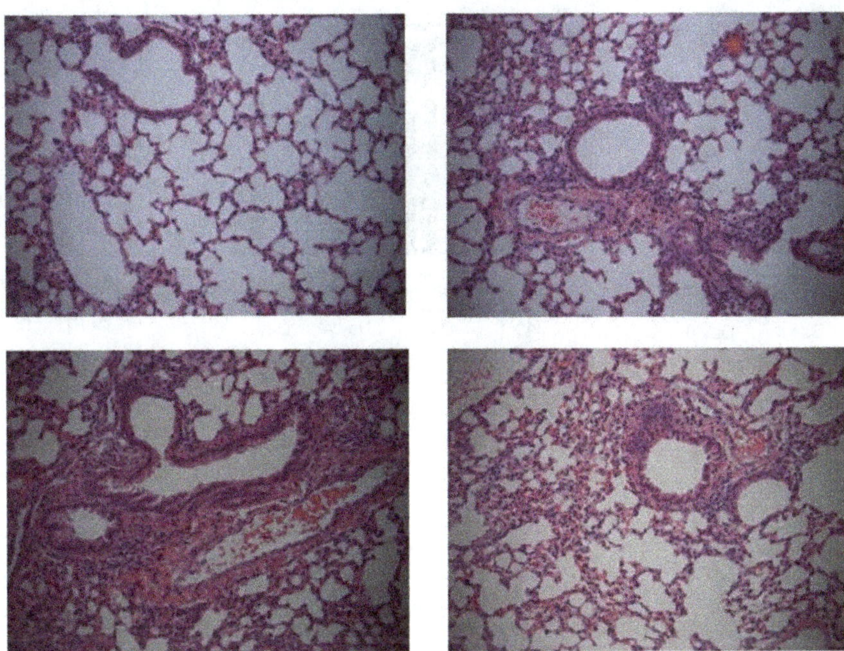

Figure 2. Infiltration of neutrophils and macrophages in c-di-GMP treated animals. (A) Photomicrograph of lung biopsies taken from a control mouse at 24 hr post treatment with c-GMP, obtained with a 10 X objective plus digital zoom. (B-D) Photomicrographs of lung biopsies taken from three different mice at 24 h post treatment with c-di-GMP (10 X objective plus digital zoom).

differences amongst the experimental groups. The distributions of the ranked data and the residuals from each ANOVA were consistent with the assumptions of procedure. If there were more than two experimental groups in the analysis and the ANOVA was significant, the means of the ranks were compared using Tukey's test. Probabilities less than or equal to 0.05 were considered significant.

Results

c-di-GMP pretreatment reduces bacterial load in lungs of infected mice

Balb/c mice were either treated intranasally with c-di-GMP (200 nM) or PBS and 24 hr later intranasally challenged with $1–3\times10^7$ CFU *B. pertussis*, strain Tohama I. Bacterial counts were determined at days 2, 4 and 6 post challenge. As shown in Fig. 1, intranasal treatment with c-di-GMP resulted in a significant reduction of bacterial counts in lungs of infected mice at 2, 4 and 6 days post challenge ($p<0.0001$). In some experiments C-GMP instead of PBS used as control but no effects on *B. pertussis* colonization was noted (data not shown).

c-di-GMP treatment increases cell recruitment to the lung

To address whether treatment with c-di-GMP enhanced recruitment of immune cells to the lung, mice were intranasally treated with either c-di-GMP or equal concentrations of nucleotide control c-GMP. 24 hr later their lungs were removed and cell recruitment into the lung was assessed by histology using H& E staining. As shown in Figure 2, administration of c-di-GMP resulted in increased numbers of neutrophils and macrophages recruited into alveolar walls and spaces, as well as perivascular lymphoid infiltrations. Flow cytometry at 1, 2, 4 and 6 days post challenge revealed that c-di-GMP administration resulted in a fivefold increase of CD11c+ cells and about a fivefold increase of NK cells expressing DX5 compared to control mice (Table 1). No differences in the number of total αß-T cells or γδ-T cells were observed between the two groups (data not shown).

Enhanced cytokine and chemokine production following treatment with c-di-GMP

To define the potential mechanisms of enhanced dendritic and NK cell recruitment, we assessed the induction of cytokines and chemokines following treatment with c-di-GMP and challenge

Table 1. The effects of c-di-GMP on cellular recruitment and activation in the lung following c-di-GMP treatment.

Cell population	c-di-GMP-treated	Control
DX5+ (NK)	29.1%	6.2%
CD11c	10.2%	2.0%
γδ TCR	6.0%	2.0%
CD86	54.4%	33.0%

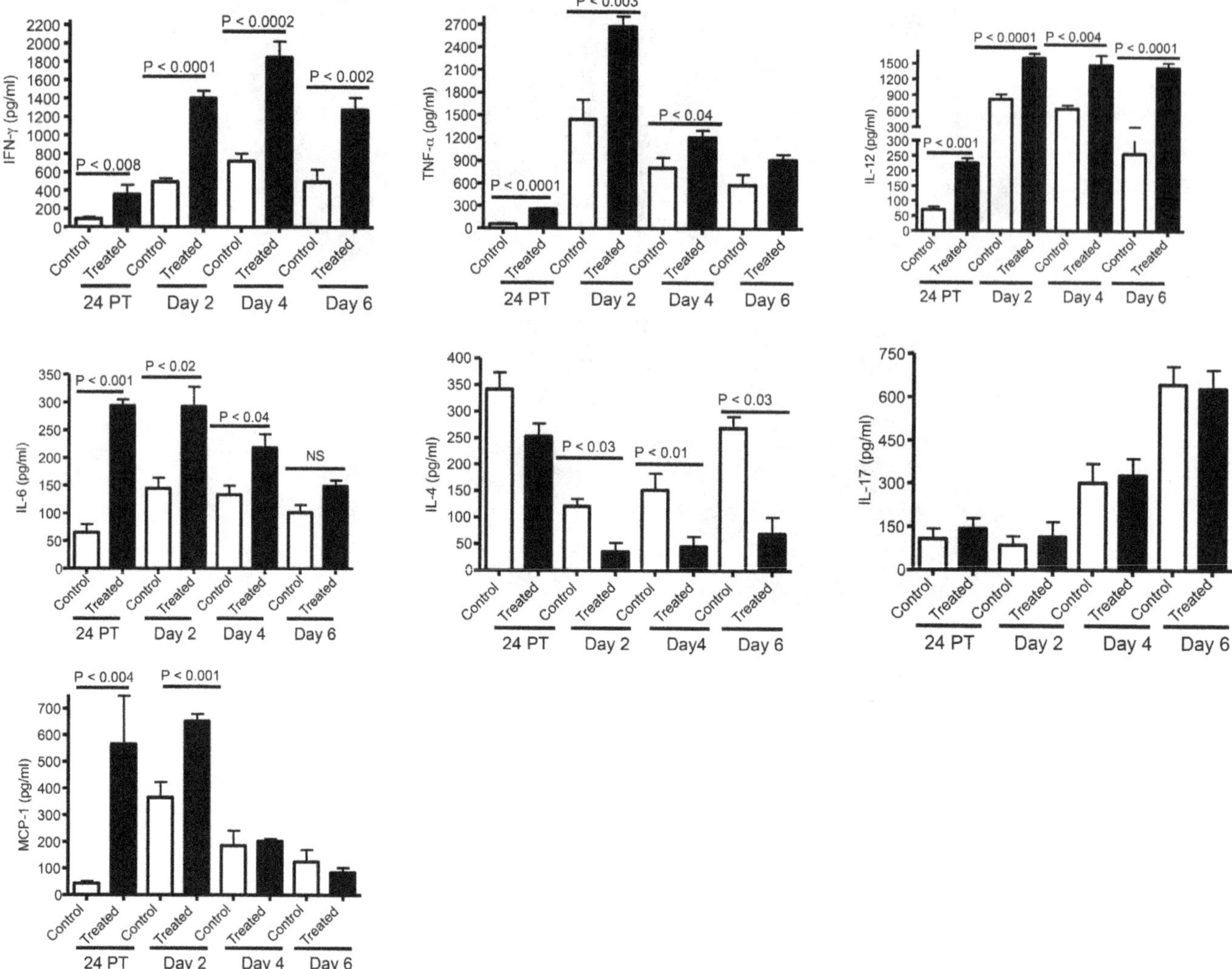

Figure 3. Cytokine (IFN-γ, TNF-α, IL-12p70, IL-6, IL-4 and IL-17) and chemokine (MCP-1) concentrations in whole lung homogenates following c-di-GMP treatment and intranasal challenge infection with *B. pertussis*. Mice were treated with c-di-GMP (black bars) or control c-GMP (white bars) at 24 hr prior to challenge infection. Whole lungs were removed and cytokine concentrations determined in lung homogenate supernatants at 24 hr post treatment (24PT) and days two, four and six post challenge (Day 2–6). The results shown are as the means ± SD of cytokine and chemokine concentrations detected by ELISA from 3 separate experiments and nine to twelve animals per group.

infection with *B. pertussis*. Administration of c-di-GMP resulted in significant production of IFN-γ, TNF-α, IL-12p70 and IL-6 in the lungs of mice 24 hr post treatment ($p \leq 0.008$) and at days 2, 4 and 6 post challenge ($P \leq 0.004$; Fig. 3). In contrast, pretreatment with c-di-GMP reduced IL-4 production ($P \leq 0.03$) at days 2, 4 and 6 post infection, but did not significantly alter the expression of either IL-17 or IL-23 (Fig. 3 and data not shown). However, pretreatment with c-di-GMP significantly enhanced the production of MCP-1 prior to and at 24 hr post infection ($P < 0.004$; Fig. 3) as well as the expression of MIP-2, mRNA levels (>3 fold increase; Fig. 4) at days 2 and 4 post challenge ($P < 0.005$ and $P < 0.05$ respectively). No changes in the expression of beta defensin 3 (BD-3) and beta defensin 4 (BD-4) were observed.

c-di-GMP treatment enhances the production of nitric oxide in vivo

Nitric oxide has been shown to be a necessary component of effective innate immunity against bacterial and fungal agents [44,46]. To investigate whether the enhanced clearance of bacteria observed in c-di-GMP treated mice was associated, in part, to increased production of NO, we assessed the presence of nitrite, the stable metabolite of NO, in c-di-GMP treated or control mice at 24 and 48 hr post intranasal infection with *B. pertussis*. As shown in Fig. 5, mice treated with c-di-GMP produced significantly more NO in their lungs at 24 hr post treatment ($P < 0.005$) and at 24 hr post challenge as compared to control animals ($P < 0.034$). In some experiments C-GMP instead of PBS used as control but no effects on NO production observed (data not shown).

Disease protection is not mediated by direct antimicrobial activity

The direct inhibitory effects of c-di-GMP were compared with known antimicrobial peptides (AMPs) *in vitro*. AMPs have both direct, broad-spectrum antimicrobial activity and the ability to modulate immune responses against a wide range of pathogens [47,48]. The antimicrobial activity of c-di-GMP against *B. pertussis* was tested and compared with protegrin-1 (PG1)

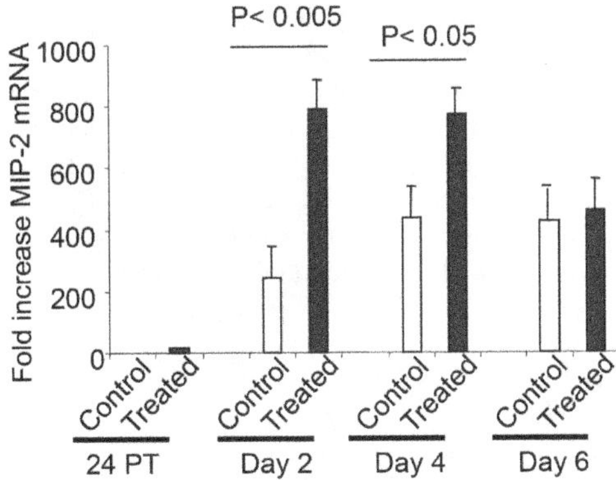

Figure 4. MIP-2 mRNA levels in lung tissues following c-di-GMP treatment. Mice were treated intranasally with c-di-GMP or control c-GMP at 24 hr prior to challenge infection. MIP-2 mRNA levels in lung were determined prior to challenge and at days 2, 4 and 6 post challenge by real-time PCR. Values shown represent the fold increase of the mean compared to non-infected control mice (five to eight animals per group).

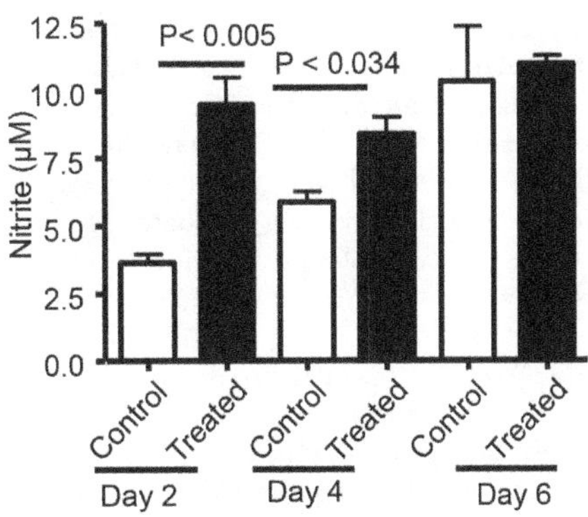

Figure 5. Nitric oxide production following c-di-GMP treatment. Nitrite production, as a measure of NO expression, was assessed at 24 hr after treatment with c-di-GMP and 24 hr after infection with *B. pertussis* in lungs of mice. Control animals were treated with PBS. Values shown represent the means ± SD from two independent experiments (10 animals per group).

and LL-37, previously tested in our lab, using inhibition assays [45]. c-di-GMP was used at 5 and 150 µg/ml and PG1 and LL-37 were used at concentrations of 5–10 µg/ml. As shown in Fig. 6, *B. pertussis* was completely resistant to killing by c-di-GMP while both the porcine PG-1 and the human cathelicidin LL-37 displayed strong antimicrobial activities resulting in 1000 to 10,000,000 fold reduction of bacterial numbers ($p = 0.009$). Interestingly, even higher concentrations of c-di-GMP as well as prolonged incubation did not increase its inhibitory effect against *B. pertussis* (data not shown).

Discussion

In the present study we demonstrated that intranasal treatment of mice with c-di-GMP resulted in the induction of strong respiratory immune responses against infections with *B. pertussis*. These responses were characterized by an early expression of MIP-2, a potent neutrophil recruiter, and MCP-1, a chemokine involved in the recruitment of monocytes, NK, iDCs and B cells. The immune responses were skewed towards a Th1-type response, which was further enhanced by challenge infection with *B. pertussis*. In contrast, c-di-GMP treatment reversed the induction of IL-4 production after bacterial infection. These findings are in line with previous studies indicating that Th1-helper T cells and their cytokines are necessary for effective clearance of *B. pertussis* [2,20,49–51]. Our results are consistent with recent studies in mice showing that treatment with c-di-GMP stimulates protective innate immune response and provides protection against *Klebsiella pneumoniae* and *Streptococcus pneumoniae* challenge infections [32,40]. c-di-GMP was also proven efficacious in enhancing bacterial clearance of *S. aureus* in mice [33]. In addition, treatment with c-di-GMP resulted in enhancement of MCP-1 production, which may have contributed to increased recruitment of monocyte, macrophage, neutrophil, NK cell and DCs into the lungs of c-di-GMP treated animals. These cells have all been implicated in providing protection against bacterial pathogens including *B. pertussis* [51]. For example, NK cells are potent producers of innate IFN-γ in response to extracellular signals including the cytokines IL-12 and TNF-α [52]. NK cells provide resistance to *B. pertussis* by activating IL-12-mediated production of IFN-γ, which enhances the antibacterial activity of monocytes/macrophages, but also promotes the differentiation of Th1 cells [20]. The ability of c-di-GMP to enhance Th1 type immune response supports the direct priming of DCs [38,40]. It has been shown that c-di-GMP activates p38 mitogen-activated protein kinase and results in enhanced IL-12 expression by DCs [32,38]. Although, immune cells other than DCs could contribute to enhanced IL-12 production including macrophages, we propose that direct priming of DCs by c-di-GMP induces IL-12 production which stimulates IFN-γ secretion possibly from NKs. *B. pertussis* infection is more severe in IFN-$\gamma^{-/-}$ mice [2], whereas *B. pertussis* disseminates from the lungs and causes organ failure in IFN-γ $R^{-/-}$ mice [15]. Although the precise role of NK cells in this study has not been investigated in details, based upon similar studies its possible to suggest that NK cells through secretion of IFN-γ might play a significant role in bacterial dissemination, pathology and bacterial clearance in mouse lungs, possibly via activated macrophages [2,15]. In addition, other studies have shown that NK cells confer resistance to *B. pertussis* by IL-12 mediated production of IFN-γ, suggesting a role for IFN-γ early in

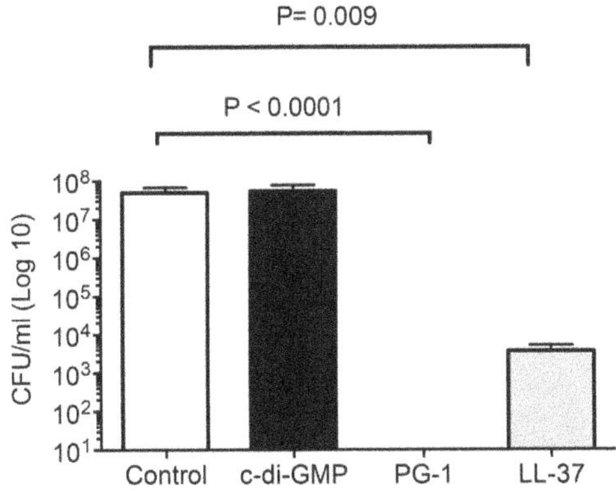

Figure 6. Sensitivity of *B. pertussis* to c-di-GMP in comparison to the human and porcine cathelicidins LL-37 and PG1. A total of 5×10^6 to 7×10^6 CFU *B. pertussis* were co-cultured in duplicates with 10 µg/ml of the respective peptide in 20 mM PBS for 2 h. Bacterial numbers were determined by plate counts. Results are form three separate experiments and expressed as the means ± SD.

infection [20]. Moreover, a defective TNF-α response has been shown as a potential risk factor for infection with *B. pertussis* [18]. Taken together, these results indicate that clearance of infection is dependent on a combination of innate immune responses mediated by IFN-γ, IL-12, TNF-α and other Th1 type cytokines. Although, most recent findings demonstrate that both Th1 and Th17 cells contribute to the clearance of infection with *B. pertussis* in mice [53], in our studies c-di-GMP did not induce significant levels of IL-17 or IL-23.

Treatment with c-di-GMP also resulted in enhanced recruitment and activation of DCs and macrophages, possibly through increased release of chemoattractants such as MCP-1. Furthermore, the induction of enhanced Th 1 type cytokines in response to c-di-GMP treatment indicates that c-di-GMP can act directly on DCs which is in agreement with recent studies showing that c-di-GMP stimulated DC mediated immune responses by induction of cytokines, chemokines and increases the cell surface expression of maturation markers, leading to an overall Th1 type response [38].

The recruitment and/or activation of innate immune cells into the lungs prior to challenge infection likely contribute to improved bacterial clearance in c-di-GMP treated animals. Both macrophages and neutrophils have been shown to kill *B. pertussis in vitro*, however their mechanisms of killing, which may involve oxygen or nitrogen intermediates, are still not known [51]. It has been shown that NO is produced *in vitro* by alveolar macrophages stimulated with *B. pertussis* and by peritoneal macrophages following immunization with Pw or by alveolar macrophages following respiratory infection with *B. pertussis* [54–56]. IFN-γ can augment NO production by macrophages infected with *B. pertussis* [57]. Purified pertussis toxin has been shown to stimulate IFN-γ secretion through direct activation of T cells and subsequent NO production [58]. Moreover, production of NO by peritoneal macrophages from mice immunized with Pw has been shown to correlate with efficacy in the intra-cerebral (i.c.) challenge model of pertussis [59]. In addition, protection induced with Pw is compromised in NO synthase-deficient mice [60], which indicates reactive nitrogen intermediates may function in intracellular killing of *B. pertussis*. Therefore, enhanced production of nitric oxide in the treated mice with c-di-GMP, possibly by alveolar macrophages, and Th1 type cytokines such as IFN-γ, as inducer of iNOS may play a protective role in clearance of *B. pertussis*.

Introduction of the Pw in the 1950s significantly reduced the incidence of pertussis but was replaced by Pa in most developed countries [11]. Although, Pa is a safer vaccine, the resurgence of pertussis might be associated with suboptimal or waning immunity induced by Pa [61]. Analysis of immune responses in children demonstrated that Pa promote a Th2 type, whereas Pw preferentially induce a Th1 type immune response [62,63]. Pa vaccines are delivered to children using alum as the adjuvant which preferentially promotes a Th2 type immune response. In the current study we have shown that c-di-GMP pretreatment increases IFN-γ expression and reduces IL-4 expression following *B. pertussis* challenge. This suggest that utilizing a Th1 type inducing adjuvant such as c-di-GMP with Pa instead of alum-adjuvant could provide more effective and protective immune response against pertussis. Therefore, it would be very advantageous to determine whether c-di-GMP could be used as an adjuvant with the Pa to induce a more protective Th1 type immune response against pertussis. Because our findings demonstrate that priming the innate immune system by c-di-GMP is capable to further skew the immune response towards a Th1 type and away from a Th2 type immune response during subsequent infection with *B. pertussis*.

Taken together, in the present study, we demonstrated that chemically derived c-di-GMP, while having no direct antimicrobial activity against *B. pertussis*, acted as an innate immune stimulator resulting in the expression of various cytokines and chemokines and activation of monocytes, granulocytes and DCs. This resulted in enhanced Th1 type immune response and improved clearance of bacteria from the lung. We suggest that c-di-GMP with such a broad biological activity can be utilized for clinical purposes in human and animals as an immunomodulator, immunoenhancer or vaccine adjuvant where a Th1 type immune response is needed. Our study also highlights the importance of the innate immune response and Th1 type cytokines in induction of protection against *B. pertussis* infection.

Acknowledgments

We are thankful to the VIDO Animal Care Staff for their assistance with housing, challenging and monitoring the animals. We are especially thankful to Dr. Don Wilson and Barry Carroll. The manuscript was published with permission of the Director of VIDO as manuscript # 539.

Author Contributions

Conceived and designed the experiments: SE LAB VG. Performed the experiments: SE JVK TGK SS. Analyzed the data: SE VG. Contributed reagents/materials/analysis tools: YH MH. Wrote the paper: SE VG.

References

1. Rodgers L, Martin SW, Cohn A, Budd J, Marcon M, et al. (2013) Epidemiologic and Laboratory Features of a Large Outbreak of Pertussis-Like Illnesses Associated With Cocirculating Bordetella holmesii and Bordetella pertussis-Ohio, 2010–2011. Clinical Infectious Diseases 56: 322–331.
2. Barbic J, Leef MF, Burns DL, Shahin RD (1997) Role of gamma interferon in natural clearance of Bordetella pertussis infection. Infect Immun 65: 4904–4908.
3. Kenyon C, Miller C, Ehresmann K (2004) Fata case of umsuspected pertussis diagnosed from a blood culture. MMWR 53: 131–132.
4. Cherry JD (2012) Epidemic pertussis in 2012–the resurgence of a vaccine-preventable disease. N Engl J Med 367: 785–787.
5. Zepp F, Heininger U, Mertsola J, Bernatowska E, Guiso N, et al. (2011) Rationale for pertussis booster vaccination throughout life in Europe. Lancet Infect Dis 11: 557–570.
6. Halperin SA, Issekutz TB, Kasina A (1991) Modulation of Bordetella pertussis infection with monoclonal antibodies to pertussis toxin. J Infect Dis 163: 355–361.
7. Mountzouros KT, Kimura A, Cowell JL (1992) A bactericidal monoclonal antibody specific for the lipooligosaccharide of Bordetella pertussis reduces colonization of the respiratory tract of mice after aerosol infection with B. pertussis. Infect Immun 60: 5316–5318.
8. Redhead K, Watkins J, Barnard A, Mills KH (1993) Effective immunization against Bordetella pertussis respiratory infection in mice is dependent on induction of cell-mediated immunity. Infect Immun 61: 3190–3198.
9. Shahin RD, Brennan MJ, Li ZM, Meade BD, Manclark CR (1990) Characterization of the protective capacity and immunogenicity of the 69-kD outer membrane protein of Bordetella pertussis. J Exp Med 171: 63–73.
10. Shahin RD, Hamel J, Leef MF, Brodeur BR (1994) Analysis of protective and nonprotective monoclonal antibodies specific for Bordetella pertussis lipooligosaccharide. Infect Immun 62: 722–725.
11. Greco D, Salmaso S, Mastrantonio P, Giuliano M, Tozzi AE, et al. (1996) A controlled trial of two acellular vaccines and one whole-cell vaccine against pertussis. Progetto Pertosse Working Group. N Engl J Med 334: 341–348.
12. Gustafsson L, Hallander HO, Olin P, Reizenstein E, Storsaeter J (1996) A controlled trial of a two-component acellular, a five-component acellular, and a whole-cell pertussis vaccine. N Engl J Med 334: 349–355.
13. Mills KH, Barnard A, Watkins J, Redhead K (1993) Cell-mediated immunity to Bordetella pertussis: role of Th1 cells in bacterial clearance in a murine respiratory infection model. Infect Immun 61: 399–410.
14. Mahon BP, Brady MT, Mills KH (2000) Protection against Bordetella pertussis in mice in the absence of detectable circulating antibody: implications for long-term immunity in children. J Infect Dis 181: 2087–2091.

15. Mahon BP, Sheahan BJ, Griffin F, Murphy G, Mills KH (1997) Atypical disease after Bordetella pertussis respiratory infection of mice with targeted disruptions of interferon-gamma receptor or immunoglobulin mu chain genes. J Exp Med 186: 1843–1851.
16. Mahon BP, Ryan MS, Griffin F, Mills KH (1996) Interleukin-12 is produced by macrophages in response to live or killed Bordetella pertussis and enhances the efficacy of an acellular pertussis vaccine by promoting induction of Th1 cells. Infect Immun 64: 5295–5301.
17. Mobberley-Schuman PS, Weiss AA (2005) Influence of CR3 (CD11b/CD18) expression on phagocytosis of Bordetella pertussis by human neutrophils. Infect Immun 73: 7317–7323.
18. Wolfe DN, Mann PB, Buboltz AM, Harvill ET (2007) Delayed Role of Tumor Necrosis Factor- alpha in Overcoming the Effects of Pertussis Toxin. J Infect Dis 196: 1228–1236.
19. Higgins SC, Jarnicki AG, Lavelle EC, Mills KH (2006) TLR4 mediates vaccine-induced protective cellular immunity to Bordetella pertussis: role of IL-17-producing T cells. J Immunol 177: 7980–7989.
20. Byrne P, McGuirk P, Todryk S, Mills KH (2004) Depletion of NK cells results in disseminating lethal infection with Bordetella pertussis associated with a reduction of antigen-specific Th1 and enhancement of Th2, but not Tr1 cells. Eur J Immunol 34: 2579–2588.
21. Toews GB, Gross GN, Pierce AK (1979) The relationship of inoculum size to lung bacterial clearance and phagocytic cell response in mice. Am Rev Respir Dis 120: 559–566.
22. Banchereau J, Steinman RM (1998) Dendritic cells and the control of immunity. Nature 392: 245–252.
23. Ferlazzo G, Morandi B, D'Agostino A, Meazza R, Melioli G, et al. (2003) The interaction between NK cells and dendritic cells in bacterial infections results in rapid induction of NK cell activation and in the lysis of uninfected dendritic cells. Eur J Immunol 33: 306–313.
24. Hellwig SM, Rodriguez ME, Berbers GA, van de Winkel JG, Mooi FR (2003) Crucial role of antibodies to pertactin in Bordetella pertussis immunity. J Infect Dis 188: 738–742.
25. Kradin RL, Sakamoto H, Preffer FI, Dombkowski D, Springer KM, et al. (2000) Accumulation of macrophages with dendritic cell characteristics in the pulmonary response to Listeria. Am J Respir Crit Care Med 161: 535–542.
26. Liu CH, Fan YT, Dias A, Esper L, Corn RA, et al. (2006) Cutting edge: dendritic cells are essential for in vivo IL-12 production and development of resistance against Toxoplasma gondii infection in mice. J Immunol 177: 31–35.
27. Ross P, Weinhouse H, Aloni Y, Michaeli D, Weinberger-Ohana P, et al. (1987) Regulation of cellulose synthesis in Acetobacter xylinum by cyclic diguanylic acid. Nature 325: 279–281.
28. Ross P, Mayer R, Weinhouse H, Amikam D, Huggirat Y, et al. (1990) The cyclic diguanylic acid regulatory system of cellulose synthesis in Acetobacter xylinum. Chemical synthesis and biological activity of cyclic nucleotide dimer, trimer, and phosphothioate derivatives. J Biol Chem 265: 18933–18943.
29. Valla S, Coucheron DH, Fjaervik E, Kjosbakken J, Weinhouse H, et al. (1989) Cloning of a gene involved in cellulose biosynthesis in Acetobacter xylinum: complementation of cellulose-negative mutants by the UDPG pyrophosphorylase structural gene. Mol Gen Genet 217: 26–30.
30. Jenal U (2004) Cyclic di-guanosine-monophosphate comes of age: a novel secondary messenger involved in modulating cell surface structures in bacteria? Curr Opin Microbiol 7: 185–191.
31. Jenal U, Malone J (2006) Mechanisms of cyclic-di-GMP signaling in bacteria. Annu Rev Genet 40: 385–407.
32. Karaolis DK, Newstead MW, Zeng X, Hyodo M, Hayakawa Y, et al. (2007) Cyclic di-GMP stimulates protective innate immunity in bacterial pneumonia. Infect Immun 75: 4942–4950.
33. Karaolis DK, Rashid MH, Chythanya R, Luo W, Hyodo M, et al. (2005) c-di-GMP (3'-5'-cyclic diguanylic acid) inhibits Staphylococcus aureus cell-cell interactions and biofilm formation. Antimicrob Agents Chemother 49: 1029–1038.
34. Hecht GB, Newton A (1995) Identification of a novel response regulator required for the swarmer-to-stalked-cell transition in Caulobacter crescentus. J Bacteriol 177: 6223–6229.
35. Romling U, Amikam D (2006) Cyclic di-GMP as a second messenger. Curr Opin Microbiol 9: 218–228.
36. Romling U, Gomelsky M, Galperin MY (2005) C-di-GMP: the dawning of a novel bacterial signalling system. Mol Microbiol 57: 629–639.
37. Ross P, Mayer R, Benziman M (1991) Cellulose biosynthesis and function in bacteria. Microbiol Rev 55: 35–58.
38. Karaolis DK, Means TK, Yang D, Takahashi M, Yoshimura T, et al. (2007) Bacterial c-di-GMP is an immunostimulatory molecule. J Immunol 178: 2171–2181.
39. Brouillette E, Hyodo M, Hayakawa Y, Karaolis DK, Malouin F (2005) 3',5'-cyclic diguanylic acid reduces the virulence of biofilm-forming Staphylococcus aureus strains in a mouse model of mastitis infection. Antimicrob Agents Chemother 49: 3109–3113.
40. Yan HB, KuoLee R, Tram K, Qiu HY, Zhang JB, et al. (2009) 3 ',5 '-Cyclic diguanylic acid elicits mucosal immunity against bacterial infection. Biochemical and Biophysical Research Communications 387: 581–584.
41. Burdette DL, Monroe KM, Sotelo-Troha K, Iwig JS, Eckert B, et al. (2011) STING is a direct innate immune sensor of cyclic di-GMP. Nature 478: 515–518.
42. Kawai R, Nagata R, Hirata A, Hayakawa Y (2003) A new synthetic approach to cyclic bis(3'–>5')diguanylic acid. Nucleic Acids Res Suppl: 103–104.
43. Halperin SA, Heifetz SA, Kasina A (1988) Experimental respiratory infection with Bordetella pertussis in mice: comparison of two methods. Clin Invest Med 11: 297–303.
44. Elahi S, Pang G, Ashman RB, Clancy R (2001) Nitric oxide-enhanced resistance to oral candidiasis. Immunology 104: 447–454.
45. Elahi S, Buchanan R, Attah-Poku S, Townsend H, Babiuk LA, et al. (2005) The host defense peptide beta-defensin 1 confers protection against Bordetella pertussis in newborn piglets. Infect Immun Submitted.
46. Tsai WC, Strieter RM, Zisman DA, Wilkowski JM, Bucknell KA, et al. (1997) Nitric oxide is required for effective innate immunity against Klebsiella pneumoniae. Infect Immun 65: 1870–1875.
47. Rollins-Smith LA, Doersam JK, Longcore JE, Taylor SK, Shamblin JC, et al. (2002) Antimicrobial peptide defenses against pathogens associated with global amphibian declines. Dev Comp Immunol 26: 63–72.
48. Zasloff M (2002) Antimicrobial peptides of multicellular organisms. Nature 415: 389–395.
49. Brady MT, Mahon BP, Mills KH (1998) Pertussis infection and vaccination induces Th1 cells. Immunol Today 19: 534.
50. Greenberger MJ, Kunkel SL, Strieter RM, Lukacs NW, Bramson J, et al. (1996) IL-12 gene therapy protects mice in lethal Klebsiella pneumonia. J Immunol 157: 3006–3012.
51. Mills KH (2001) Immunity to Bordetella pertussis. Microbes Infect 3: 655–677.
52. Ye J, Ortaldo JR, Conlon K, Winkler-Pickett R, Young HA (1995) Cellular and molecular mechanisms of IFN-gamma production induced by IL-2 and IL-12 in a human NK cell line. J Leukoc Biol 58: 225–233.
53. Ross PJ, Sutton CE, Higgins S, Allen AC, Walsh K, et al. (2013) Relative contribution of Th1 and Th17 cells in adaptive immunity to Bordetella pertussis: towards the rational design of an improved acellular pertussis vaccine. PLoS Pathog 9: e1003264.
54. Torre D, Pugliese A, Speranza F, Fiori GP, Perversi L, et al. (1993) Interferon-gamma levels in serum and bronchoalveolar lavage fluid of mice infected with Bordetella pertussis. J Infect Dis 167: 762–765.
55. Torre D, Ferrario G, Bonetta G, Perversi L, Speranza F (1996) In vitro and in vivo induction of nitric oxide by murine macrophages stimulated with Bordetella pertussis. FEMS Immunol Med Microbiol 13: 95–99.
56. Xing DK, Canthaboo C, Corbel MJ (2000) Effect of pertussis toxin on the induction of nitric oxide synthesis in murine macrophages and on protection in vivo. Vaccine 18: 2110–2119.
57. Mahon BP, Mills KH (1999) Interferon-gamma mediated immune effector mechanisms against Bordetella pertussis. Immunol Lett 68: 213–217.
58. Sakurai S, Kamachi K, Konda T, Miyajima N, Kohase M, et al. (1996) Nitric oxide induction by pertussis toxin in mouse spleen cells via gamma interferon. Infect Immun 64: 1309–1313.
59. Canthaboo C, Xing D, Corbel M (1999) Development of a nitric oxide induction assay as a potential replacement for the intracerebral mouse protection test for potency assay of pertussis whole cell vaccines. Dev Biol Stand 101: 95–103.
60. Canthaboo C, Xing D, Wei XQ, Corbel MJ (2002) Investigation of role of nitric oxide in protection from Bordetella pertussis respiratory challenge. Infect Immun 70: 679–684.
61. Klein NP, Bartlett J, Rowhani-Rahbar A, Fireman B, Baxter R (2012) Waning protection after fifth dose of acellular pertussis vaccine in children. N Engl J Med 367: 1012–1019.
62. Ausiello CM, Urbani F, La Sala A, Lande R, Piscitelli A, et al. (1997) Acellular vaccines induce cell-mediated immunity to Bordetella pertussis antigens in infants undergoing primary vaccination against pertussis. Dev Biol Stand 89: 315–320.
63. Ryan M, Murphy G, Ryan E, Nilsson L, Shackley F, et al. (1998) Distinct T-cell subtypes induced with whole cell and acellular pertussis vaccines in children. Immunology 93: 1–10.

23

Real-Time Bioluminescence Imaging of Mixed Mycobacterial Infections

MiHee Chang[1], Katri P. Anttonen[1], Suat L. G. Cirillo[1], Kevin P. Francis[2], Jeffrey D. Cirillo[1]*

1 Department of Microbial Pathogenesis and Immunology, Texas A&M Health Science Center, Bryan, Texas, United States of America, 2 PerkinElmer, Alameda, California, United States of America

Abstract

Molecular analysis of infectious processes in bacteria normally involves construction of isogenic mutants that can then be compared to wild type in an animal model. Pathogenesis and antimicrobial studies are complicated by variability between animals and the need to sacrifice individual animals at specific time points. Live animal imaging allows real-time analysis of infections without the need to sacrifice animals, allowing quantitative data to be collected at multiple time points in all organs simultaneously. However, imaging has not previously allowed simultaneous imaging of both mutant and wild type strains of mycobacteria in the same animal. We address this problem by using both firefly (*Photinus pyralis*) and click beetle (*Pyrophorus plagiophthalamus*) red luciferases, which emit distinct bioluminescent spectra, allowing simultaneous imaging of two different mycobacterial strains during infection. We also demonstrate that these same bioluminescence reporters can be used to evaluate therapeutic efficacy in real-time, greatly facilitating our ability to screen novel antibiotics as they are developed. Due to the slow growth rate of mycobacteria, novel imaging technologies are a pressing need, since they can they can impact the rate of development of new therapeutics as well as improving our understanding of virulence mechanisms and the evaluation of novel vaccine candidates.

Editor: Yung-Fu Chang, Cornell University, United States of America

Funding: This work was supported by grant 48523 from the Bill and Melinda Gates Foundation and grant AI104960 from the National Institutes of Health. The funders had no role in study design, data collection and analysis, decision to publish, or preparation of the manuscript.

Competing Interests: KPF is employed by PerkinElmer. JDC is also a founder of and consultant for Global BioDiagnostics Corp. and owns significant stock in the company. There are no patents, products in development or marketed products to declare.

* Email: jdcirillo@medicine.tamhsc.edu

Introduction

Tuberculosis (TB) is a major public health problem, with over eight million new cases and 1.3 million deaths attributed to TB in 2012 [1]. Tuberculosis is a pulmonary infection that is acquired through inhalation of bacteria arising from infected individuals. The absence of a candidate with clearly superior efficacy to the current vaccine [2], an attenuated form of *Mycobacterium bovis*, bacillus Calmette-Guérin (BCG), and the unsatisfactory results of a recent anti-tuberculosis vaccine trial [3] demonstrate that additional strategies for rapid evaluation of vaccines are greatly needed. Vaccine efficacy trials would be facilitated by the ability to evaluate the challenge dose in real-time, as could be accomplished with imaging, rather than waiting the one month required for determination of bacterial load by colony forming units (cfu) with *M. tuberculosis*. Due to the difficulty of clearing *M. tuberculosis* from an infected host, successful treatment requires multiple antibiotics that must be taken for six months or more [1]. Such a long treatment time leads to patient non-compliance and has resulted in emergence of multi-drug and extensively drug resistant *M. tuberculosis* strains. The slow growth rate of *M. tuberculosis* [4,5] makes virulence studies extremely slow in comparison to other pathogens, resulting in limited availability of information regarding mechanisms of disease establishment and progression. New tools for the study of TB in animal models are needed to facilitate development of TB prevention and treatment strategies.

Our group has been developing imaging technologies to analyze the dynamics of *M. tuberculosis* infections. We have found that tdTomato fluorescent protein labelled *M. tuberculosis* can be detected in the lungs of infected mice, but not green fluorescent protein (GFP) labelled bacteria, most likely due to the shorter emission wavelength of GFP [6,7]. The number of bacteria required for detection by tdTomato is 10^5 cfu, a relatively high number as compared to the infectious dose of 1–10 cfu. Interestingly, we have also used tdTomato labelled BCG infected mice to assess the efficacy of microendoscopy for detection [8], significantly improving limits of detection. In the case of *M. tuberculosis*, secreted β-lactamase BlaC can be used in reporter enzyme fluorescence (REF) to cleave fluorogenic substrates made using fluorescent dyes linked to quenchers via a β-lactam ring [9,10]. REF allows the detection of *M. tuberculosis* in live animals without the need to genetically modify the bacteria, enabling it to be used to detect *M. tuberculosis* in clinical samples [11]. Although fluorescence systems have shown great promise, bioluminescence has the potential to allow rapid evaluation of bacterial viability and avoids the need for removal of autofluorescence normally seen in mammalian tissues.

Bacterial and eukaryotic bioluminescence systems have been used as reporters in bacteria [12–31]. The bacterial bioluminescence reporter systems are based on expression of the bacterial *luxCDABE* operon to produce a light signal [32]. No exogenous substrate is required, since the *luxCDE* genes code for substrate synthesis enzymes [33]. The *Photorhabdus luminescens* luciferase system [34] has been expressed from a plasmid in many different genera of bacteria, including strains of *Salmonella* that were first used to demonstrate non-invasive optical imaging in vivo [35]. Modified versions of this lux operon have been used in mycobacteria [16]. Expression of only the enzymatically active luciferase, *luxAB*, from *Vibrio harveyi*, has also been used in mycobacteria to study bacterial dissemination and antibiotic treatment efficacy, but requires delivery of an aldehyde that is poorly membrane permeable [19,30,31]. The eukaryotic bioluminescence systems take advantage of luciferases from insects, including the North American firefly *Photinus pyralis* and the click beetle *Pyrophorus plagiophthalamus* [24], and use a luciferin substrate that has good membrane permeability. Expression of firefly luciferase in mycobacteria has been used *in vitro* to study antibiotic resistance in different strains [12–16,27,36,37], as well as *in vivo* [15,18,19,30,38]. Possibly the reasons that luciferases are commonly used for antimicrobial studies is their rapid loss of signal due to the requirement of ATP for light production, in contrast to fluorescent proteins that are very stable and fluorogenic probes that depend on the pharmacokinetics of the fluorescent product for signal loss [9]. The emission spectra of the insect luciferases are usually in the yellow-red range, compared to the bacterial luciferases that emit in the green to blue range [24]. Light at shorter wavelengths (e.g., blue-green) is more problematic for *in vivo* imaging, since animal tissues absorb more light at wavelengths below 600 nm [39]. Light produced by the bacteria is absorbed by the surrounding tissues and is highly attenuated [40]. Use of bioluminescence in mycobacteria has concentrated on evaluating antibiotic resistance *in vitro* [12–16,27,31,36,37] or *in vivo* [15,18,19,30,38].

We have developed optimized bioluminescence systems to study mycobacterial infection kinetics in real-time. We chose two luciferases, click beetle red luciferase (CBRlux) and firefly luciferase (FFlux) that have large proportions of their emission spectra in the far red wavelengths of light [40] making them good optical reporters for *in vivo* imaging. We optimized the codon usage of these genes for mycobacteria, and expressed both CBRlux and FFlux from plasmids in BCG. These bioluminescent mycobacterial strains were then used to quantify bacterial burden, both *in vitro* and in animals using non-invasive optical imaging. We show that these constructs can be used for subcutaneous detection of 10^3 cfu *in vivo*. Moreover, the different spectra maxima of the two luciferases allow use of mixed cultures and quantitative differentiation of bacterial numbers expressing them, both *in vitro* and *in vivo*, permitting simultaneous imaging of both CBRlux and FFlux. We also demonstrate detection of these bioluminescent bacteria in the lungs of intratracheally infected mice and found that the signal is sensitive to antibiotic treatment. These observations demonstrate feasibility for simultaneous detection of multiple mycobacterial strains during infection, as well as rapid evaluation of novel intervention strategies and virulence assessment in animal models.

Materials and Methods

Bacterial strains and growth conditions

Strains and plasmids used in this study are listed in table 1. BCG was grown in M-OADC-Tw made with 7H9 broth (Difco, Detroit, MI) supplemented with 0.5% glycerol, 10% OADC (oleic acid dextrose complex without catalase), and 0.05% Tween 80 or Middlebrook 7H9 supplemented with 10% OADC and 15 g/liter Bacto agar (M-OADC agar) or on 7H11 selective agar (Difco) medium supplemented with 80 μg ml^{-1} hygromycin. The composition of the OADC supplement used was as described in the Difco manual [41] with the exception that it does not contain catalase. A stock solution of 1% (wt/vol) oleic acid is made in 0.2 N NaOH prior to adding 5 ml of the stock solution per 100 ml final volume of OADC supplement.

In the case of growth curves, mycobacteria were inoculated at OD_{600} of 0.02 into 96-well plates with or without different concentrations of both isoniazid (INH) plus rifampin (RIF) and incubated at 37°C. Luminescence and OD_{600} readings were taken every 2 days up to 28 post inoculation with a Mithras multimode reader (Berthold Technologies, TN). To measure luminescence of mixed cultures, strains were inoculated at an OD_{600} of 0.02 and incubated at 37°C for 10 to 14 days. The bacteria were diluted to 2×10^8 cfu ml^{-1} and the two strains were mixed at rations of 1:1, 10:1, 1:10, 100:1 and 1:100. Dilutions of bacterial cultures were plated on M-OADC agar and incubated at 37°C for 3–4 weeks to obtain cfu.

Construction of luciferase expression plasmids

CBRlux and FFlux expression plasmids were constructed by cloning each luciferase gene between the *Nhe*I and *Pac*I sites of pJDC89 [42] or a derivate of pJDC89 where the P_{hsp60} had been replaced by the P_{L5} promoter [43–45]. This vector uses the mycobacterial pAL5000 low-copy number origin of replication, that is stable in mycobacteria [46,47]. CBRlux and FFlux codon sequences were optimized for expression in mycobacteria (GenScript, NJ) and the resulting genes were also inserted into pJDC89 vector via the *Nhe*I and *Pac*I sites. Codon optimized sequences have been submitted to Genbank (accession numbers: JQ031640 for CBRlux and JQ031641 for FFlux). Expression strains were constructed by transforming the plasmids into BCG by electroporation and plating the bacteria on M-OADC agar supplemented with 80 μg ml^{-1} hygromycin to select for the presence of plasmid. The presence of plasmid was confirmed in all strains by selecting multiple colonies and screening for those that produced maximal luminescence in the presence of 2 mM luciferin. In all cases, less than 10-fold variation was observed between individual colonies selected from transformants with a single construct. Luminescence was measured in white 96-well plates containing 50 μl of each bacteria suspended in culture medium and 50 μl of 2 mM luciferin added to each well and luminescence measured at 10 s post-addition and every 10 s thereafter.

Cell lines, culture conditions and macrophage infection assays

Murine macrophage cell line J774A.1 (ATCC TIB67) was maintained in high glucose Dulbecco's Modified Eagle Medium (DMEM, Gibco) supplemented with 10% heat inactivated FBS (Gibco) and 2 mM L-glutamine at 37°C in the presence of 5% CO_2. Cell infection assays were performed as described previously [48]. Briefly, 5×10^4 J774A.1 cells were seeded in white 96-well plates for 20 h to allow formation of a monolayer. Mycobacteria were added at multiplicities of infection (MOI) of 100, 10, 1 and 0.1 bacteria per macrophage, incubated for 30 min to allow

Table 1. Strains and Plasmids.

Strain	[a]Genotype	Source or Reference
E. coli ***XL1 Blue***	*recA1 endA1 gyrA96 thi-1 hsdR17 supE44 relA1 lac* [F' *proAB lacI^q ZΔM15 Tn10 (Tet^r)*]	Stratagene
BCG	*Mycobacterium tuberculosis* var. *bovis* bacillus Calmette-Guérin strain Pasteur	Statens Serum Institute, Copenhagen, Denmark
BCG16	BCG::pJDC134	Current study
BCG18	BCG::pJDC89	Current study
BCG26	BCG::pJDC132	Current study
BCG47	BCG::pJDC181	Current study
BCG48	BCG::pJDC182	Current study
BCG51	BCG::pJDC178	Current study
BCG52	BCG::pJDC179	Current study
Plasmid	**Characteristics**	
pJDC89	P_{hsp60} Hyg^r oriM	[42]
pJDC132	pJDC89 CBRlux	Current study
pJDC134	pJDC89 FFlux	Current study
pJDC178	pJDC89 P_{L5} optCBRlux	Current study
pJDC179	pJDC89 P_{L5} optFFlux	Current study
pJDC181	pJDC89 optCBRlux	Current study
pJDC182	pJDC89 optFFlux	Current study

[a]Hyg = hygromycin, Tet = tetracycline, oriM = mycobacterial pAL5000 origin of replication [47,62], P_{hsp60} = promoter from 60 kDa heat shock protein [63], P_{L5} = promoter from the L5 mycobacteriophage [45,64], CBRlux = click beetle red luciferase, FFlux = firefly luciferase, optCBRlux = click beetle red luciferase with all amino acid codons modified to the optimal codons for mycobacteria, optFFlux = firefly luciferase with all amino acid codons modified to be optimal for mycobacteria.

internalization, washed twice with pre-warmed PBS to remove extracellular bacteria, 50 µl of complete DMEM added to each well and luminescence was measured at 1, 2 and 7 d post-infection in the same manner as for bacteria in culture.

Animal infections

Five- to seven-week old female BALB/C mice were used in all experiments. Mice were housed in groups of less than five in polycarbonate cages in a temperature, humidity and light controlled environment and provided commercial chow and tap water *ad libitum*. Mice were allowed to acclimate to the facilities for one week prior to studies. Subcutaneous infections were carried out by shaving the backs of mice and injecting dilutions of bacteria subcutaneously at specific sites in the back of each mouse. The mice were then imaged at 24 h post-infection and necropsied to determine cfu present at the site of inoculation. Alternatively, mice were infected intratracheally with 1×10^6 bacteria, as described previously [25,26]. Two mice per group, randomly allocated, were imaged and sacrificed for necropsy to determine thresholds of detection, correlate luminescence with cfu and compare different luminescence constructs. Antibiotic treatment was carried out with four mice per group, randomly allocated, by administration of RIF plus INH intraperitoneally daily at 10 mg kg^{-1} animal body weight. At each time point a group of animals in each treatment category were imaged, necropsied, lungs imaged and homogenized for cfu determination by plating dilutions of tissue homogenates. Animal use protocols were reviewed and approved by the Institutional Animal Care and Use Committee of Texas A&M University under AUP#2011-67.

Imaging mycobacterial infections

Imaging was performed essentially as described previously [25,26]. Briefly, mice were anesthetized using isoflurane and imaged using the IVIS Spectrum imaging system (PerkinElmer). Luciferin was injected intraperitoneally between 10 and 15 min prior to imaging to measure luminescence. Luciferin was injected at 150 mg/kg of animal body weight. Images were acquired with up to 5 min exposures and analysed with Living Image Software v3.1. For some experiments, spectral algorithms were used to differentiate signals from the two different luciferases. Images were acquired using different emission filters from 520 nm to 720 nm and signal quantified at each wavelength.

Statistical Analyses

All experiments were carried out in triplicate and repeated at least two times, with similar results obtained. Data shown are for a representative experiment. The significance of the results were determined using the Student's t test for pairwise comparisons or ANOVA with the Tukey-Kramer post-hoc pairwise t test for comparisons of three or more groups. GraphPad Prism 5 software was used to facilitate statistical analyses. $P<0.05$ was considered significant.

Results

Expression of luciferases does not impact mycobacterial growth

Bioluminescence from luciferases can be used to track both eukaryotic cells for cancer studies and bacterial pathogens in animal models [15,18–26,28–30,35,49–52]. Luciferases have great potential for tracking pathogenic mycobacteria in animal models for rapid quantitative analysis of bacterial loads in all organs during disease, vaccine efficacy studies and evaluation of novel therapeutics. Firefly luciferase (FFlux, from *P. pyralis*) and click beetle red luciferase (CBRlux, from *P. plagiophthalamus*) were cloned into mycobacterial expression vector pJDC89 under the control of two different constitutively active promoters; the P_{hsp60} promoter or the P_{L5} promoter [43–45]. The resulting constructs were transformed into BCG and evaluated for growth rate and light production over 18 days (Figure 1). Luminescence correlates well with bacterial numbers during the exponential phase of growth (Figure 1C). During exponential growth, the amount of light produced increases along with bacterial numbers and plateaus at around 8 days, which is approximately the same time the cultures reach stationary phase. After reaching stationary phase, light production remains relatively constant until 20 days post inoculation. Constant light production, despite increasing bacterial numbers, is most likely a reflection of the metabolic state of stationary phase mycobacteria, since light production by coleopteran luciferases is dependent on ATP [32]. Neither luciferase had an impact on the growth rate of BCG and light production was very similar overall for both luciferases. During log phase there was a higher level of light production from FFlux as compared to CBRlux (Figure 1B), which could be due to a number of factors, including FFlux having less of a metabolic impact on mycobacteria, allowing greater light production or improved translation of the FFlux gene due to preferred codon usage. These data demonstrate that expression of both CBRlux and FFlux are well tolerated by mycobacteria and light production correlates with bacterial numbers under most conditions, suggesting that these reporters will be valuable for tracking mycobacteria during infections.

Luciferases allow quantification of intracellular mycobacteria

Mycobacteria are primarily considered intracellular pathogens that can readily infect and replicate within macrophages [53,54]. Since metabolic changes could impact expression of luciferase by mycobacteria, we examined whether a similar correlation with bacterial numbers was observed when the bacteria are growing within macrophages to that observed in culture. Using bacteria to cell ratios of 0.1 to 100 in murine macrophages, we found that both CBRlux and FFlux produced signal above background that correlated very well ($r^2 = 0.96$ for CBRlux, $r^2 = 0.92$ for FFlux) with bacterial numbers (Figure 2). This correlation is sufficient to allow accurate quantification of bacterial numbers by luminescence in the place of cfu. The level of luminescence produced was stable out to 7 days post-infection of macrophages and both CBRlux and FFlux produce similar levels of luminescence. We show that intracellular growth does not significantly impact levels of light produced by CBRlux or FFlux, allowing these reporters to be used during macrophage infection to quantify bacterial numbers present.

Thresholds of detection for mycobacteria during mouse infection

Since both CBRlux and FFlux allow quantification of intracellular mycobacteria, we examined their limits of detection for mycobacteria during infection in animals. We infected mice subcutaneously with 10^2 to 10^7 cfu of BCG expressing CBRlux or FFlux to determine effects of infection on light production (Figure 3). Although somewhat difficult to distinguish in whole body images due to higher numbers of bacteria saturating the dynamic range of the imager, the threshold of bacteria detected ($p<0.05$) using this imaging system is 10^3 cfu for CBRlux and 10^4 cfu for FFlux. The number of bacteria present at each site was confirmed after imaging by plating homogenized tissue for cfu and correlates well with luminescence from 10^3 to 10^7 cfu (Figure 3B). CBRlux displayed significantly higher luminescence than FFlux

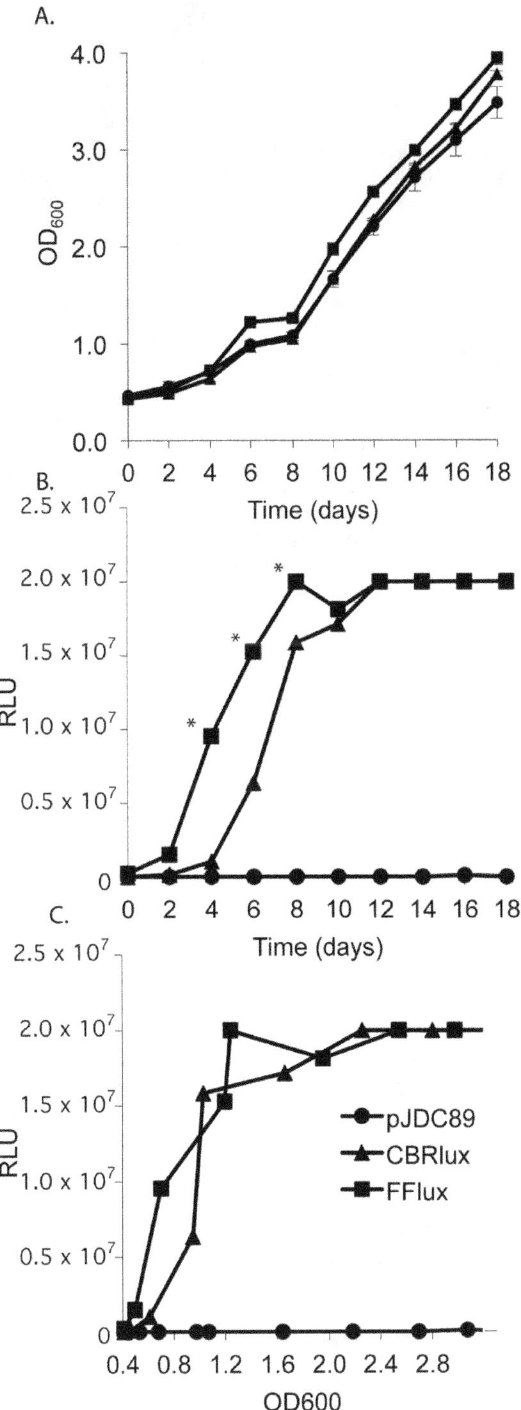

Figure 1. Luminescence of mycobacteria during growth in bacteriological media. Luminescent (FFlux and CBRlux) and non-luminescent (pJDC89) BCG carrying the vector backbone display similar growth rates in M-ADC-TW plus hygromycin (80 µg/ml) laboratory medium (A). Luminescence for both firefly (FFlux) and click beetle red (CBRlux) luciferase expressing BCG (BCG16 and BCG26) increases steadily over time until approximately 12 days post-inoculation (B). The correlation between luminescence and optical density of BCG cultures expressing FFlux, CBRlux or the vector (pJDC89) alone (C). Data and error bars represent the means and standard deviations, respectively, of triplicate samples. Error bars are often too small to be visible around the marker for the mean. RLU = relative light units. * indicate data points with P<0.05 for FFlux vs. CBRlux.

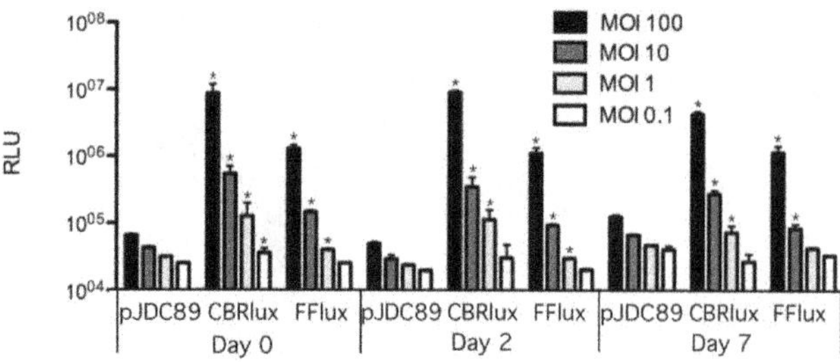

Figure 2. Luminescence from mycobacteria within macrophages. Luminescence detected from firefly (FFlux) and click beetle red (CBRlux) luciferase expressing BCG (BCG16 and BCG26) or BCG carrying the vector (pJDC89) alone within J774A.1 macrophages. Infections in macrophages were carried out with various multiplicities of infection (MOI) from 0.1 to 100 bacteria per cell for 30 min and washed to remove extracellular mycobacteria. Luciferin was added immediately after infection (day 0) and on days 2 and 7 post-infection ~15 min before luminescence measurements. Data and error bars represent the means and standard deviations, respectively, of triplicate samples. RLU = relative light units. * indicate data points with $P<0.05$ for luciferase vs. pJDC89 expressing BCG at the same time point and same MOI.

for most bacterial numbers during subcutaneous infection. This observation combined with the lower threshold of detection observed with CBRlux suggests that luminescence produced by CBRlux penetrates mammalian tissue more readily than FFlux, most likely due to the longer wavelength of luminescence produced by CBRlux as compared to FFlux [24,40].

Luciferases allow imaging of pulmonary infections in mice

Most mycobacterial infections occur through the respiratory route, which is a more difficult site to image optically due to the greater tissue depth than for subcutaneous infections. Although a 10^3 cfu threshold of detection is promising to allow sensitive tracking of mycobacteria during pulmonary infections, it is unclear whether such low numbers could be detected in deeper tissues. We tested this possibility by imaging mice infected intratracheally with BCG expressing CBRlux and FFlux (Figure 4). We found that both luciferases allowed the detection of 10^6 cfu of BCG in the lungs of mice with short exposures of 1 min resulting in 100-fold higher p/sec luminescence than background (Figure 4B). Although both dorsal and ventral images could be used to detect the presence of bacteria, ventral imaging resulted in higher luminescence for both CBRlux and FFlux. Moreover, despite bacterial numbers in the lungs for both CBRlux and FFlux strains being comparable (~10^6 in both cases) luminescence was nearly 10-fold higher for CBRlux than FFlux in both dorsal and ventral images. The location of the source of luminescence was confirmed post-mortem by collecting images after opening the chest cavities of the mice (Figure 4C). All of the observed luminescence originated from the lungs at 24 h post-infection. These observations indicate that ventral imaging is more sensitive for tracking mycobacterial pulmonary infections with imaging and luminescence produced by CBRlux being greater than FFlux, making CBRlux a more sensitive reporter for tracking pulmonary infections with mycobacteria.

Spectral characteristics of CBRlux and FFlux allow simultaneous imaging

Since both CBRlux and FFlux can be used to track mycobacterial infections in mice and they produce luminescence that is maximal at different wavelengths, we tested whether their signals could be separated using available algorithms for spectral unmixing. Spectral unmixing involved first capturing multiple images of the same animals, infected by both CBRlux and FFlux subcutaneously, using a range of different emission filters on a whole body optical imager (Figure 5A). We captured images of infected mice in this manner using filters from 500 to 740 nm and found that the maximum luminescence for FFlux is 540 to 600 nm and for CBRlux is 600 to 620 nm (Figure 5C). Furthermore, between 500 and 520 nm, there is almost no luminescence from CBRlux and signal obtained for FFlux is near maximal, suggesting that the spectral characteristics of these two luciferases will allow their signal to be separated and quantified.

We examined the kinetics of light production for the luciferases in mixed cultures to determine whether they competed differently for the substrate, luciferin or their presence together would interfere with levels of signal produced. We mixed cultures of CBRlux and FFlux expressing strains in 1:1, 1:10 and 1:100 ratios and measured luminescence in 96-well plates (Figure 5D). After a rapid increase in light production to the maximum value within 10 s after addition of luciferin, there is a rapid decrease in the amount of luminescence for the FFlux expressing BCG strain. Light production continues to decrease over 2 minutes. Conversely, light produced by CBRlux takes slightly longer (20–30 s) to reach maximum values and stays at the maximum value for at least 2 minutes. We found that the mixing of the two luciferase emissions results in a slight increase in overall light production but that the kinetics of the light production were similar to that of the major luciferase present. However, when the two luciferases were mixed at a 1:1 ratio, the light production resembled a combination of the two kinetic curves for each luciferase, with a lower initial maximum as compared to FFlux alone, but an extended plateau comparable to CBRlux. These results indicate that each luciferase contributes relatively equally to the total luminescence produced by mixed cultures and there is little interference between them or competition for substrate when mixed together.

CBRlux and FFlux can be imaged simultaneously during mixed infections

The ability to independently quantify two mycobacteria expressing different luciferases during mixed infections would be extremely valuable for evaluating competition assays with mutant and wild type bacteria. We evaluated this theory by infecting mice subcutaneously with mixtures of 10:1, 1:1 and 1:10 FFlux to CBRlux expressing bacteria. At 24 h post-infection, infected mice were imaged at a range of different wavelengths from 500 to 740 nm (Figure 6A) and the resulting signal at each infection site spectrally unmixed to quantify the number of FFlux and CBRlux bacteria present (Figure 6B, C). After spectral unmixing, infections with FFlux and CBRlux expressing bacteria can be differentiated and the luminescence observed at each site of infection correlated with the numbers of each bacteria present. Composite images were constructed to display the intensity of signal for each luciferase at equally infected sites (1:1 ratio of FFlux:CBRlux) on the animal as a combination of the luminescence present at that site; whereas sites where there is a 10:1 ratio of bacteria (10:1 FFlux:CBRlux or 1:10 FFlux:CBRlux), the second luciferase is observed as a smaller sector within the zone displaying luminescence for the primary luciferase present. These observations suggest that CBRlux and FFlux allow simultaneous quantification of two strains of mycobacteria, even when the two strains are in a mixed infection in mice. Two luminescence markers for imaging have numerous applications in pathogenesis studies to follow mutant and wild type strains, analysis of antimicrobial resistance

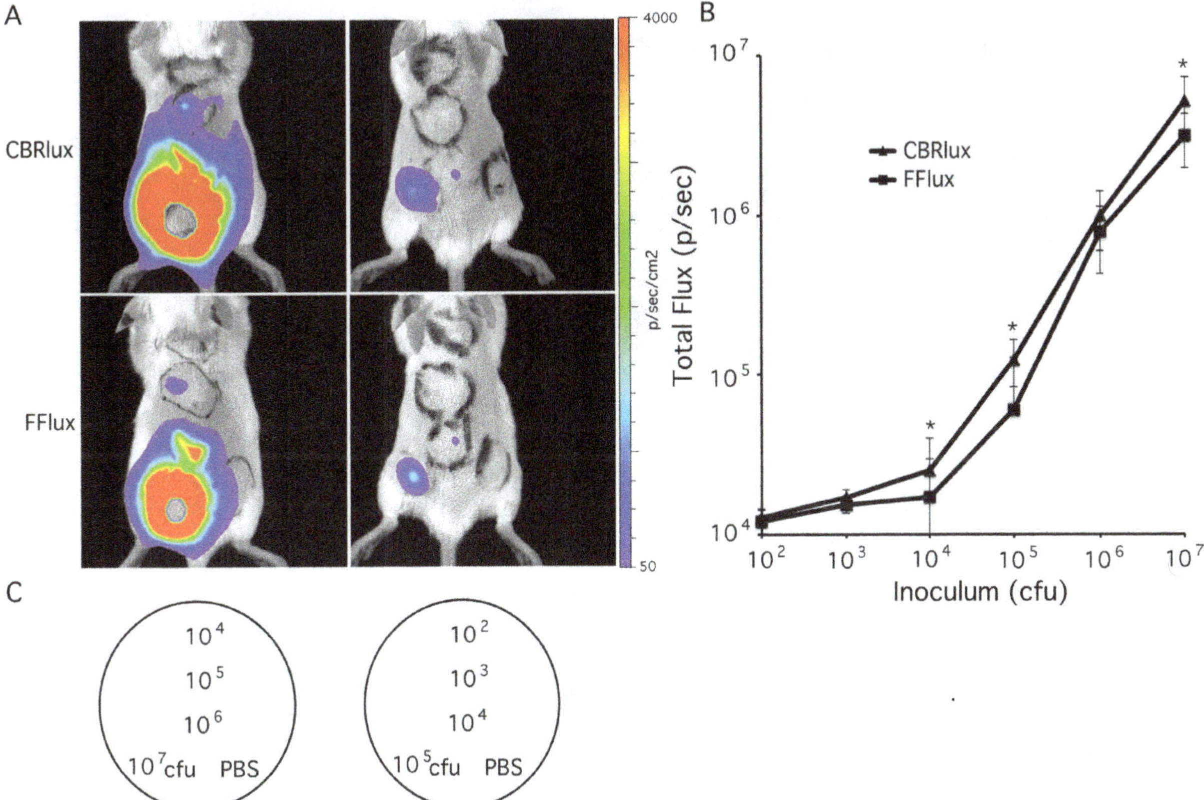

Figure 3. Correlation of bacterial numbers with luminescence. Whole body images of luminescence from BALB/C mice (2/group) inoculated subcutaneously with 10^2 to 10^7 colony forming units (cfu) of BCG expressing click beetle red (CBRlux) or firefly (FFlux) luciferase (A) at 24 h post-inoculation. After imaging, mice were sacrificed and cfu determined by plating homogenates of skin region from injection site. Bioluminescence from each inoculation site correlates well with the number of bacteria present for both CBRlux and FFlux (B). Template for injection sites using different numbers of cfu or PBS control (C). Data and error bars represent the means and standard deviations, respectively, of duplicate samples. Data are expressed as total Flux in photons per second (p/sec). * indicate data points with $P<0.05$ for CBRlux vs. FFlux expressing BCG at the same inoculum.

when two populations are present differing in susceptibility, and evaluation of both vaccine and challenge dose in vaccine efficacy studies.

Optimization of luciferases for spectral imaging of co-infections

The importance of CBRlux and FFlux for real-time analysis of mycobacterial infections makes it a high priority to further optimize their sensitivity to achieve the best thresholds of detection possible. Two different versions of each CBRlux and FFlux gene were used; one with the original DNA sequence and a second with the amino acid codon usage optimized to mycobacterial preferred amino acids (accession number JQ031640 for CBRlux and JQ031641 for FFlux). We also utilized two promoters, the mycobacteriaophage L5 promoter and the *hsp60* promoter, both of which are thought to drive high levels of transcription [42–45]. There was a significant increase in light production for both CBRlux and FFlux in the strains where these genes were codon optimized (Figure 7). In addition, *hsp60* promoter expression produced a stronger signal than expression from the L5 promoter. Consistent with our observation that FFlux produced higher luminescence than CBRlux in its native form, which might be due to the presence of several rare codons in CBRlux, optimization of CBRlux codon usage had a greater impact on light production than optimization of FFlux. Similar to our *in vitro* results, codon optimized CBRlux with optimized codon usage and expressed from the *hsp60* promoter resulted in higher luminescence than CBRlux expressed from the L5 promoter (Figure 7C). Overall, the optimized luciferase constructs and particularly the optimized CBRlux display significantly higher luminescence than non-optimized luciferases, suggesting that use of optimized luciferases can improve thresholds of detection beyond that observed with native luciferases.

CBRlux allows rapid evaluation of therapeutic efficacy

Since coleopteran luciferases require ATP for the production of light, antimicrobial treatment of mice infected with luminescent mycobacteria, resulting in reduced metabolic activity or death of the bacteria, should result in a decrease in bioluminescence. Having a rapid readout for effectiveness of candidate antimicrobials would greatly facilitate development of therapeutics against mycobacterial infections, since obtaining results normally takes over a month due to the time necessary for formation of colonies on media to demonstrate a decrease in bacterial load. The ability of antibiotics to reduce signal in CBRlux expressing mycobacteria was examined by treating 10^4 BCG in culture medium with INH+RIF for two days and comparing the inhibition of luminescence to loss of cfu (Figure 8A, B). We found that inhibition of luminescence was very similar to the level of killing observed by cfu assays, though the percent was somewhat greater with cfu, suggesting that luminescence may be a more sensitive measure of viable bacteria persisting in a population than cfu. We evaluated the utility of

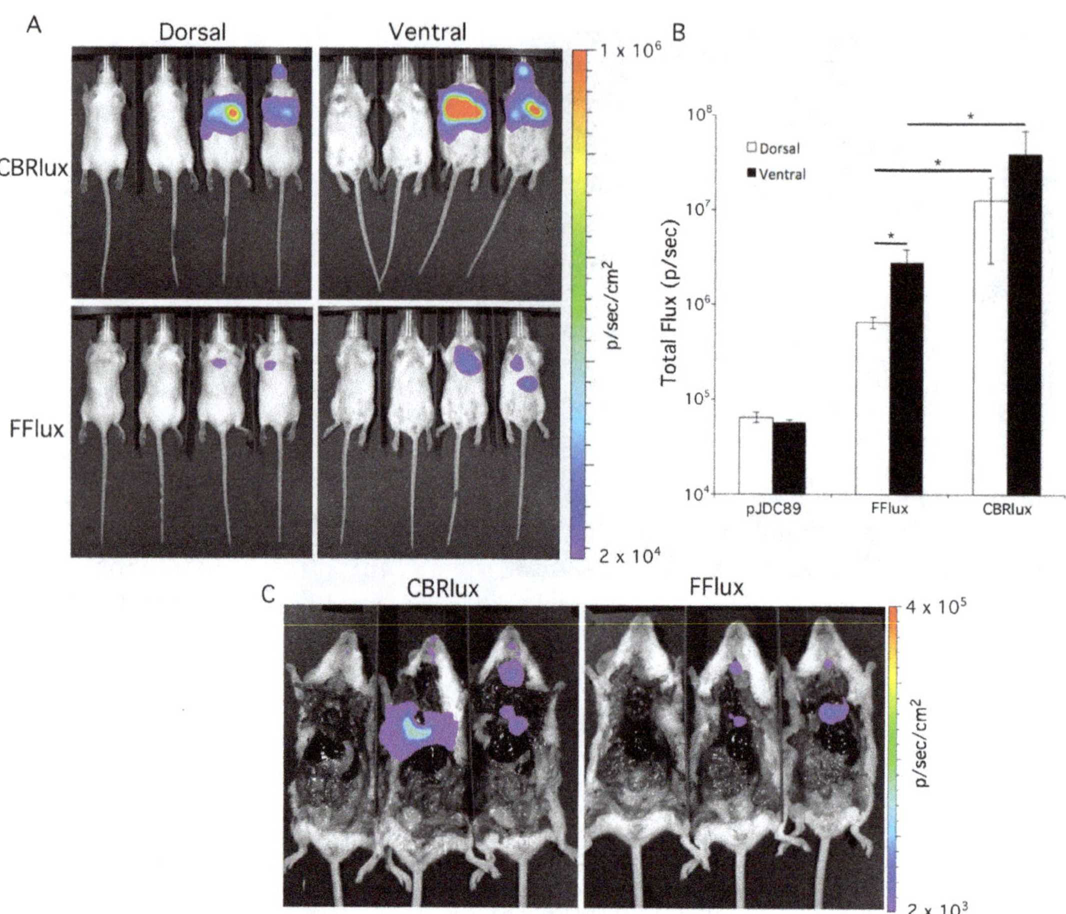

Figure 4. Luminescence allows imaging during pulmonary infection. Whole body dorsal and ventral images of luminescence from click beetle red (CBRlux) and firefly (FFlux) luciferase expressing BCG inoculated intratracheally into BALB/C mice (2/group) at 10^6 cfu (A). Two vector only (pJDC89) control mice were imaged along with each set of two CBRlux or FFlux mice (vector controls on left). Data are expressed as total Flux in photons per second (p/sec). Luminescence is greater with CBRlux than with FFlux and ventral imaging is more sensitive than dorsal imaging (B). Imaging of mice post-mortem with open chest cavities demonstrates the luminescence signal originates from the lungs (C). Data and error bars represent the means and standard deviations, respectively, of duplicate samples. * indicate data points with $P<0.05$ between data indicated by horizontal bars.

CBRlux for evaluating therapeutics by infecting mice with 10^6 cfu of BCG via the intratracheal route followed by treatment with INH+RIF for six days post-infection (Figure 8C–F). We found that luminescence was significantly lower in treated than untreated animals from 24 h post-treatment. Since BCG does not replicate in mice, the bacterial load decreased throughout the experiment, as expected. However, the treated group displayed lower luminescence at all time points and lower cfu at most time points. Similar to observations in vitro, reductions in cfu appeared to be more dramatic than luminescence, but the remaining luminescence is likely due to the presence of bacteria that are not killed by treatment. These observations demonstrate that CBRlux can be used to evaluate therapeutic efficacy more rapidly than conventional cfu-based assays both in vitro and during mycobacterial infections in mice, suggesting that this reporter may be a more sensitive measure of only partial sterilization than cfu in therapeutic efficacy studies.

Discussion

Despite decades of study into TB and *M. tuberculosis*, little is known regarding many aspects of mycobacterial disease progression and dissemination. Dissemination from the lung to pulmonary lymph nodes and other organs is thought to be required for the establishment of acquired immunity [55] but whether mycobacteria disseminate within host cells or extracellularly remains controversial. Traditional methods for quantification of bacterial burden in different organs requires sacrificing animals and plating tissue homogenates for cfu determination, which is both time consuming and costly due to the large number of animals required and the one month or more required for colonies to form on media. A growing body of literature suggests that photonic imaging can now be utilized to estimate mycobacterial burdens during infections in animals more rapidly [6,7,9,10,14,17–19,25,26,30,56]. We have used FFlux and CBRlux to label pathogenic mycobacteria and visualize infection in live animals. Although the current study utilized BCG, the same vectors can be used in *M. tuberculosis*, without any expected change in signal produced, since these organisms are part of the tuberculosis-complex and very closely related [57–59]. This strategy enables us to follow the infection in individual mice throughout the entire experiment, reducing the number of animals needed to conduct statistically significant experiments. Each animal serves as its own control, since each individual can be followed throughout the

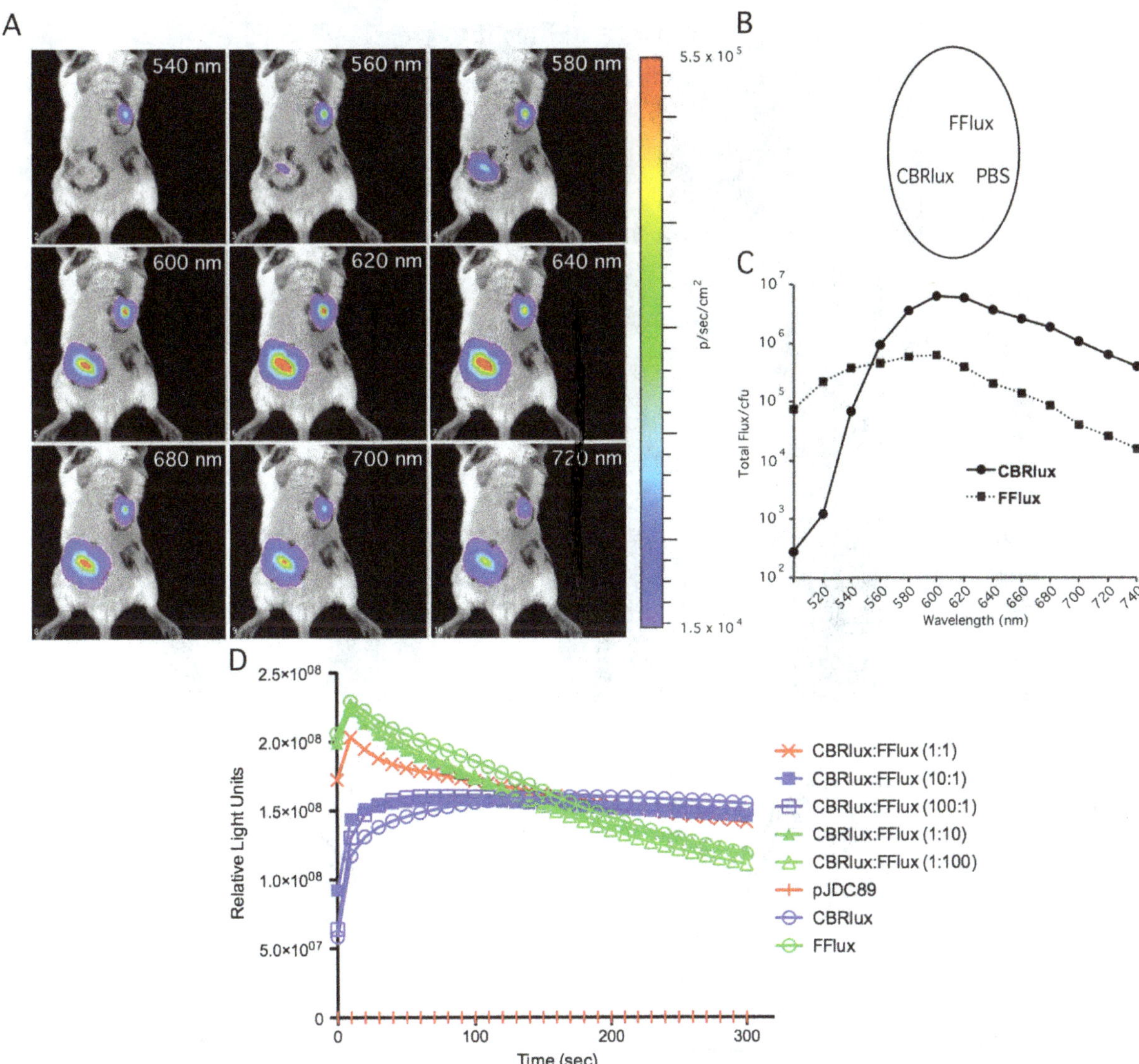

Figure 5. Spectral characteristics of firefly and click beetle red luciferase. Collection of whole body images of BALB/C mice (2/group) infected subcutaneously with 10^6 cfu of BCG expressing click beetle red (CBRlux) or firefly (FFlux) luciferase at defined wavelengths between 540 nm and 720 nm demonstrates that very little luminescence is obtained from CBRlux at short wavelengths and, similarly, less is obtained for FFlux at longer wavelengths (A). Template map for subcutaneous inoculation of BCG strains and PBS control (B). Quantitation of total Flux (p/sec) at different wavelengths for areas with CBRlux of FFlux indicates that luminescence from each reporter can be spectrally separated (C). Comparing luminescence kinetics obtained with mixed cultures of 10^4 total cfu CBRlux and FFlux expressing BCG at ratios from 1:1 to 1:100 shows that the kinetic curve of a mixed culture resembles that of the luciferase that is at higher numbers in the culture. Furthermore, at the similar numbers (1:1) the kinetic curve appears to be a mix between the two curves for the luciferases. Since the kinetic curves are directly relates to the numbers of each strain present, it is likely that these luciferases compete similarly for available substrate (D). Luminescence was measured using a plate reader after injecting 50 µl of 2 mM luciferin. Measurements began 10 s after adding luciferin and were taken every 10 s up to 5 min.

entire experiment, reducing the experimental variability usually due to animal-to-animal differences. Theoretically, imaging could ultimately obviate the need to sacrifice animals unless localization to specific tissues must be confirmed, cellular level analyses are needed or interpretation is complicated by a change in the correlation between cfu and signal. Animals can be monitored over time with imaging and only sacrificed at key time points for more detailed analyses.

We took advantage of existing luminescent markers, CBRlux and FFlux, to label BCG by expressing the luciferases from plasmids. The two promoters used in this study show little difference in luminescence but we were able to greatly increase the signal by optimizing the codon usage in the CBRlux and FFlux genes for that preferred by mycobacteria, similar to codon optimization of luciferases described in other studies [17,18]. Expression of either luciferase does not appear to cause growth defects in these bacteria and signal production remains at a relatively constant level up to seven days in the absence of the selective marker for the expression plasmid, even when bacteria are grown in a macrophage culture. These findings show that our constructs offer robust expression systems for CBRlux and FFlux and they have little or no detrimental effect on mycobacterial growth. Interestingly, background luminescence is extremely low with bacteria containing vector alone, but in both macrophages and mouse tissues, background with vector alone is higher, decreasing the signal-to-noise ratios and, thereby, increasing the

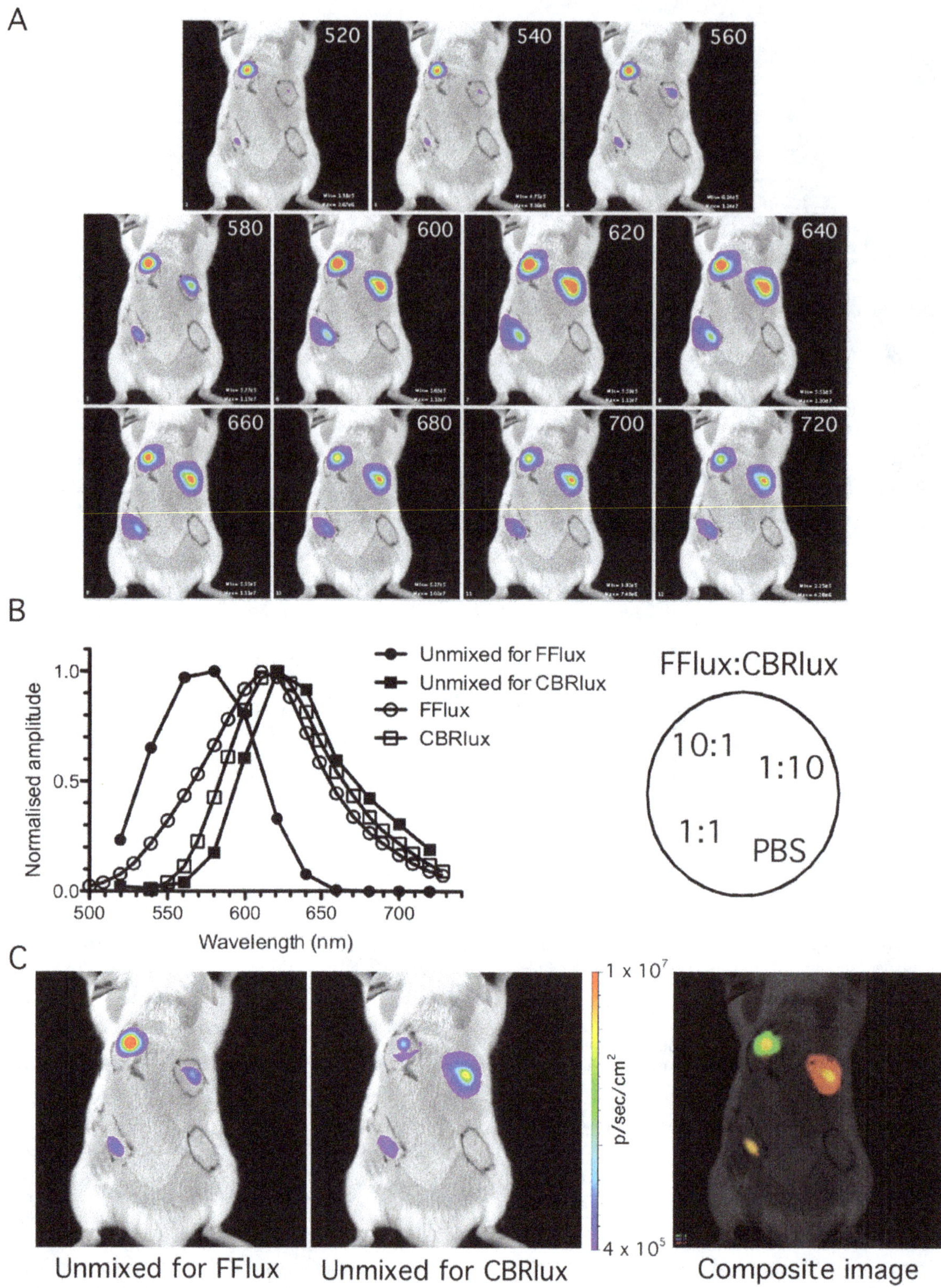

Figure 6. Spectral unmixing of luminescence allows quantitation of mixed bacterial infections. Whole body images were obtained from BALB/C mice (2/group) subcutaneously infected with a total of 10^7 cfu BCG mixed at different ratios from 1:10 to 1:1 expressing click beetle red (CBRlux) or firefly (FFlux) luciferase at defined wavelengths from 520 nm to 720 nm demonstrates ability to quantitatively separate signal from CBRlux and FFlux in mixed infections, similar to those seen in mixed cultures (A). Normalized quantification of signal at defined wavelengths after spectral unmixing for FFlux or CBRlux (left panel) and map of subcutaneous inoculation sites on mice (right panel) for imaging (B). After unmixing signal at each injection site correlates with the number of FFlux or CBRlux bacteria present (C). The composite image (on the right) shows green for quantitative FFlux signal, red for CBRlux signal and orange at positions of co-localization of both CBRlux and FFlux signals.

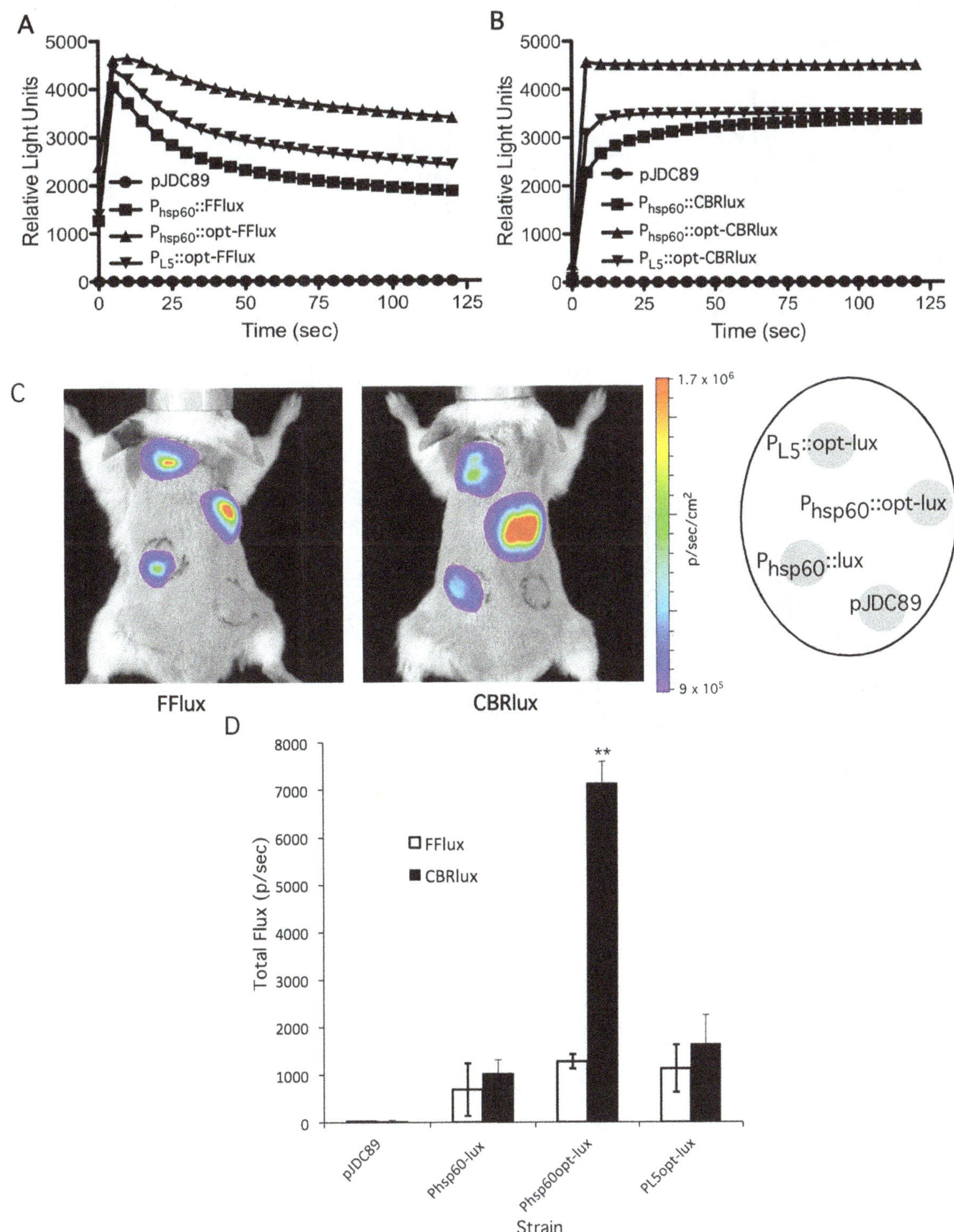

Figure 7. Codon optimized luciferases produce more light than non-optimized luciferases. BCG (10^4 cfu) expressing wild type click beetle red (CBRlux) or firefly (FFlux) luciferases or the same luciferases synthetically optimized for mycobacterial codon usage (opt) were examined in liquid culture for light production over time in the presence of 2 mM luciferin (A, B). Results shown are for the individual strains of each type selected for maximal luminescence as described in the methods. BCG containing the vector alone (pJDC89) was used as a control. Both the L5 and hsp60 promoters were examined with the codon optimized luciferases to evaluate which promoter results in the greatest light production. Whole body images of BALB/C mice (2/group) subcutaneously infected with 10^6 cfu of the same BCG strains show similar results to those found in liquid culture where codon optimized luciferases produce greater luminescence (C). A map of subcutaneous inoculation sites on mice is shown in the right panel. Quantitation of each inoculation site for total Flux photons per second (p/sec) indicates that the codon optimized CBRlux expressed from hsp60 emits the most light (D). Data and error bars represent the means and standard deviations, respectively, of two mice. ** indicates $p<0.01$ as compared to FFlux in the same construct.

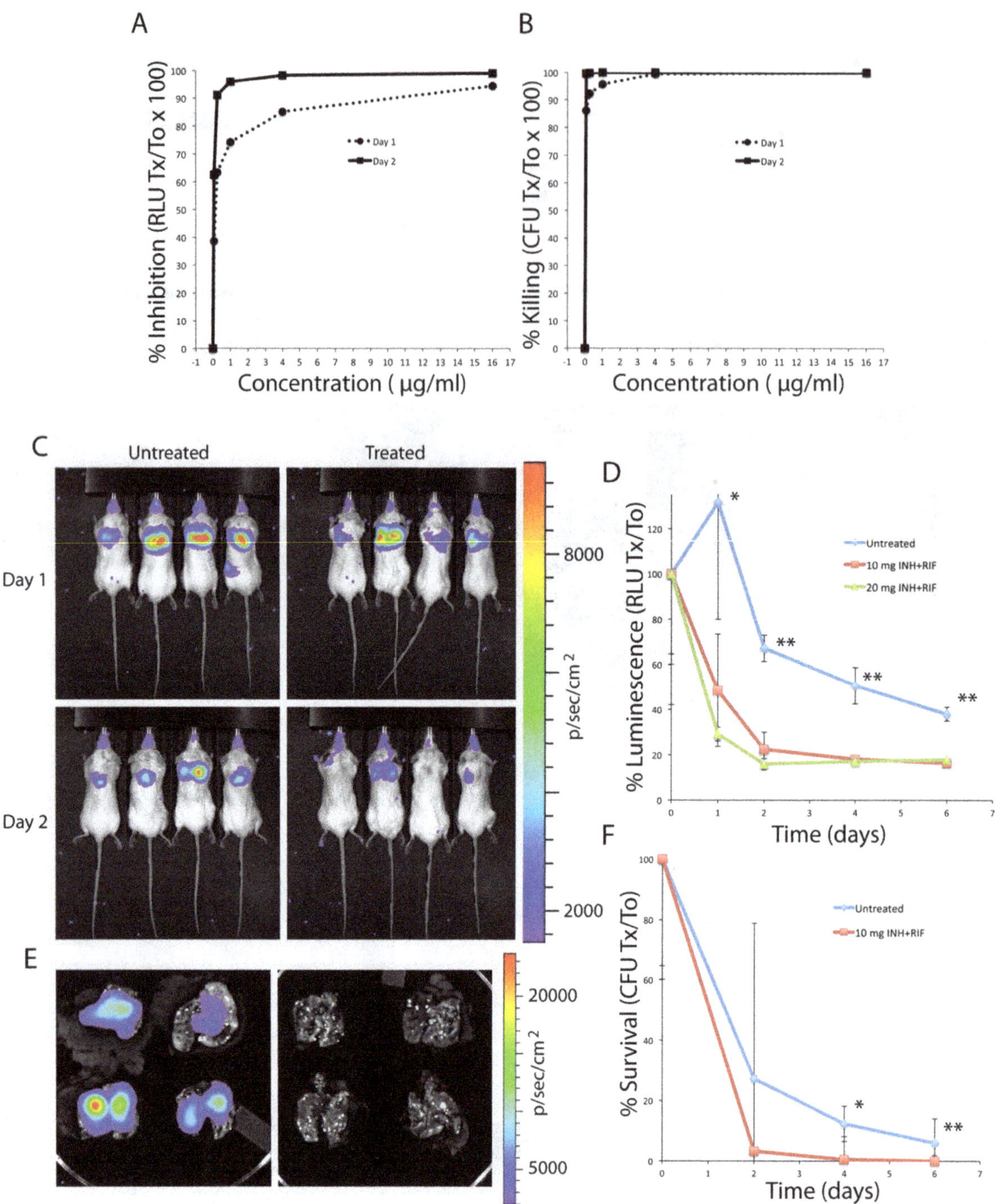

Figure 8. Codon optimized click beetle red luciferase (CBRlux) allows rapid therapeutic evaluation. Percent inhibition of light production (A) and bacterial killing (B) for 10^4 of BCG expressing codon optimized CBRlux (optCBRlux) in the presence of different concentrations of isoniazid (INH) plus rifampin (RIF) during culture in bacterial media after 24 (day 1) or 48 h (day 2) as compared to the absence of antimicrobials. Whole body imaging during pulmonary infection in BALB/C mice (4/group) with 4×10^6 cfu of BCG expressing optCBRlux after 24 and 48 hr treatment with 10 mg/kg INH+RIF results in a reduction in luminescence (C). Quantitation of the percentage of the initial luminescence as compared to each time point out to six days post-treatment confirms the reduced luminescence in treated animals (D). Similarly, ex-vivo imaging of lungs at 2 days to confirm luminescence observed in whole body images is derived from the lungs and is reduced after antibiotic treatment (E). Untreated and treated panels for lung images are indicated in panel C. Correlation of luminescence with cfu present was confirmed by plating homogenates from the same animals at each time point (F). Data and error bars represent the means and standard deviations, respectively, of four mice. * indicates $p<0.05$ and ** indicates $p<0.01$ as compared to treated group at the same time point.

number of bacteria required to obtain significant signal, in the presence of mammalian cells. Despite this issue, we can detect as few as 10^3 cfu during mouse subcutaneous infection significantly above background, a very promising threshold of detection. Theoretically, these constructs should be expressed well in any mycobacterial species, including different mutant backgrounds, offering a simple method to label mycobacteria for use of *in vivo* imaging in pathogenesis, as well as vaccine and therapeutic studies.

Two different luminescence reporters, CBRlux and FFlux, with different emission spectra, allow dual bioluminescent labeling to study mycobacterial infections *in vivo*, similar to the system described for Escherichia coli [60]. The luminescence from BCG expressing FFlux or CBRlux can be localized to the site of infection with detection limits as low as 10^3 bacteria by subcutaneous inoculation. Thus, the lower limits of detection using bioluminescence are lower than those found for *in vivo* imaging of mycobacteria using fluorescent markers [6]. This improvement in limits of detection reduces the number of bacteria required for detection, thus facilitating the use of more clinically relevant infectious doses, which is particularly important for infections with *M. tuberculosis*. However, since subcutaneous inoculations were used to determine this threshold of detection, it is likely that pulmonary infections with *M. tuberculosis* will require somewhat higher inocula to produce similar signal due to attenuation from increased mammalian tissue depth. Overall, CBRlux and FFlux, with emission maxima in the far red window, offer less signal loss due to light absorption and scattering in tissue, making them more compatible with *in vivo* imaging [39]. Furthermore, because these two luciferases use the same luciferin substrate, they can be imaged and discriminated simultaneously. We are able separate the two signals spectrally, allowing the strains that express them to be tracked and quantified. These luciferases will allow us to perform competition assays between mutant and wild type strains in the same animal. Dual color luminescence has been described with red and a green luciferases that can be spectrally separated in other systems [60,61], but have not been used in mycobacteria. Our study supports the potential for multiple luciferases to be imaged simultaneously *in vitro* and *in vivo* using unmixing algorithms. A study dissecting the role of the adaptive immune response described the use *luxAB* labelled BCG in a RAG-$2^{-/-}/\gamma_c R^{-/-}$ mouse background [30]. In this study, wild type $CD90^+$ T-cells were used to complement the mutant mice and reduce luminescence to undetectable levels by 10 weeks. Our dual luciferase system could be used to analyze immunological events during bacterial infection in real time by labeling a subset of immune cells in conjunction with bioluminescent bacteria. This strategy will allow us to dissect both the bacterial and host pathways involved in mycobacterial pathogenesis. Analysis of multiple mycobacterial strains or both the pathogen and host in the same animal are only possible using multiple luminescent reporters that can be spectrally separated. It is important to remember that, due to the overlap in the wavelengths of detection for CBRlux and FFlux, it may be challenging to always accurately and sensitively discriminate them, particularly when signal levels are extremely low for one or the other of these luciferases. Further studies are needed to identify additional luciferases that may be used in this manner, possibly with more easily separated spectral characteristics, allowing analysis of at least three strains or multiple host elements during infection.

We used our luminescent mycobacterial strains to determine the effect of antibiotic treatment on light production both *in vitro* and during infection. Similar to previous studies [12–16,18,27,31,36–38], the level of bioluminescence is sensitive to increased amounts of antibiotics, suggesting that our constructs could be used to rapidly screen for efficacy of new antibiotics in high-throughput studies. Also, using *in vivo* imaging for infections and antibiotic treatment, we can verify the efficacy of antimicrobials that are effective *in vitro*, consistent with studies from other groups [38]. One caveat of the current study is that plasmids were used, which, although we observed a good correlation with cfu for seven days in the absence of selection, may not allow longer-term studies in vivo due to plasmid loss. This issue could be overcome through the use of integrating plasmids that are much more stable or placement of the constructs into specific sites in the chromosome by allelic exchange. Despite these caveats, these data demonstrate that luciferases can be exceedingly valuable for analysis of novel prevention and treatment strategies for mycobacterial infections.

We found that CBRlux and FFlux serve as highly sensitive luminescent reporters for mycobacteria, allowing determination of spatio-temporal distribution of bacteria within mice during infection. CBRlux and FFlux signals can be spectrally separated for simultaneous quantitative analysis of two different bacterial strains or bacteria along with a host cell type or marker. These luciferases can be used to sensitively detect of bacteria in pulmonary infections and can be used to evaluate therapeutic efficacy in real time. Moreover, this approach provides a novel strategy to facilitate dissecting mycobacterial pathogenesis, as well as improved understanding of therapeutic and vaccine studies.

Acknowledgments

We thank Tonya Shepherd for useful comments on the manuscript.

Author Contributions

Conceived and designed the experiments: MC KPA SLGC KPF JDC. Performed the experiments: MC KPA SLGC. Analyzed the data: MC KPA SLGC KPF JDC. Contributed reagents/materials/analysis tools: MC KPA SLGC KPF JDC. Wrote the paper: MC KPA SLGC KPF JDC.

References

1. WHO (2013) Global tuberculosis report 2013. Geneva, Switzerland: World Health Organization. 1–289 p.
2. Evans TG, Brennan MJ, Barker L, Thole J (2013) Preventive vaccines for tuberculosis. Vaccine 31 Suppl 2: B223–226.
3. Tameris MD, Hatherill M, Landry BS, Scriba TJ, Snowden MA, et al. (2013) Safety and efficacy of MVA85A, a new tuberculosis vaccine, in infants previously vaccinated with BCG: a randomised, placebo-controlled phase 2b trial. Lancet 381: 1021–1028.
4. Cole ST, Brosh R, Parkhill J, Garnier T, Churcher C, et al. (1998) Deciphering the biology of *Mycobacterium tuberculosis* from the complete genome sequence. Nature 393: 537–544.
5. Cole ST (2002) Comparative and functional genomics of the Mycobacterium tuberculosis complex. Microbiology 148: 2919–2928.
6. Kong Y, Subbian S, Cirillo SL, Cirillo JD (2009) Application of optical imaging to study of extrapulmonary spread by tuberculosis. Tuberculosis (Edinb) 89 Suppl 1: S15–17.
7. Kong Y, Akin AR, Francis KP, Zhang N, Troy TL, et al. (2011) Whole-body imaging of infection using fluorescence. Curr Protoc Microbiol Chapter 2: Unit2C 3.
8. Mufti N, Kong Y, Cirillo JD, Maitland KC (2011) Fiber optic microendoscopy for preclinical study of bacterial infection dynamics. Biomed Opt Express 2: 1121–1134.
9. Kong Y, Yao H, Ren H, Subbian S, Cirillo SL, et al. (2010) Imaging tuberculosis with endogenous {beta}-lactamase reporter enzyme fluorescence in live mice. Proc Natl Acad Sci U S A.
10. Kong Y, Cirillo JD (2010) Reporter enzyme fluorescence (REF) imaging and quantification of tuberculosis in live animals. Virulence 1: 558–562.
11. Xie H, Mire J, Kong Y, Chang M, Hassounah HA, et al. (2012) Rapid point-of-care detection of the tuberculosis pathogen using a BlaC-specific fluorogenic probe. Nat Chem 4: 802–809.
12. Bartzatt R, Sule P, Cirillo SLG, Cirillo JD (2014) Novel tuberculostatic agents suitable for treatment of *Mycobacterium tuberculosis* infections of the central nervous system. Brit J Pharm Res 4: 1535–1551.
13. Kapoor R, Eimerman PR, Hardy JW, Cirillo JD, Contag CH, et al. (2011) Efficacy of Antimicrobial Peptoids against Mycobacterium tuberculosis. Antimicrob Agents Chemother 55: 3058–3062.

14. Singh V, Biswas RK, Singh BN (2014) Double recombinant Mycobacterium bovis BCG strain for screening of primary and rationale-based antimycobacterial compounds. Antimicrob Agents Chemother 58: 1389–1396.
15. Zhang T, Li SY, Nuermberger EL (2012) Autoluminescent Mycobacterium tuberculosis for rapid, real-time, non-invasive assessment of drug and vaccine efficacy. PLoS One 7: e29774.
16. Andreu N, Fletcher T, Krishnan N, Wiles S, Robertson BD (2012) Rapid measurement of antituberculosis drug activity in vitro and in macrophages using bioluminescence. J Antimicrob Chemother 67: 404–414.
17. Andreu N, Zelmer A, Fletcher T, Elkington PT, Ward TH, et al. (2010) Optimisation of bioluminescent reporters for use with mycobacteria. PLoS One 5: e10777.
18. Andreu N, Zelmer A, Sampson SL, Ikeh M, Bancroft GJ, et al. (2013) Rapid in vivo assessment of drug efficacy against Mycobacterium tuberculosis using an improved firefly luciferase. J Antimicrob Chemother 68: 2118–2127.
19. Zhang T, Li SY, Converse PJ, Almeida DV, Grosset JH, et al. (2011) Using bioluminescence to monitor treatment response in real time in mice with Mycobacterium ulcerans infection. Antimicrob Agents Chemother 55: 56–61.
20. Dothager RS, Flentie K, Moss B, Pan MH, Kesarwala A, et al. (2009) Advances in bioluminescence imaging of live animal models. Curr Opin Biotechnol 20: 45–53.
21. Campbell-Valois FX, Sansonetti PJ (2014) Tracking bacterial pathogens with genetically-encoded reporters. FEBS Lett 588: 2428–2436.
22. Andreu N, Zelmer A, Wiles S (2011) Noninvasive biophotonic imaging for studies of infectious disease. FEMS Microbiol Rev 35: 360–394.
23. Hutchens M, Luker GD (2007) Applications of bioluminescence imaging to the study of infectious diseases. Cell Microbiol 9: 2315–2322.
24. Contag CH, Bachmann MH (2002) Advances in in vivo bioluminescence imaging of gene expression. Annu Rev Biomed Eng 4: 235–260.
25. Kong Y, Shi Y, Chang M, Akin AR, Francis KP, et al. (2011) Whole-body imaging of infection using bioluminescence. Curr Protoc Microbiol Chapter 2: Unit2C 4.
26. Chang MH, Cirillo SL, Cirillo JD (2011) Using luciferase to image bacterial infections in mice. J Vis Exp.
27. Sharma S, Gelman E, Narayan C, Bhattacharjee D, Achar V, et al. (2014) A simple and rapid method to determine antimycobacterial potency of compounds using autoluminescent Mycobacterium tuberculosis. Antimicrob Agents Chemother.
28. Hyde JA, Weening EH, Chang M, Trzeciakowski JP, Hook M, et al. (2011) Bioluminescent imaging of Borrelia burgdorferi in vivo demonstrates that the fibronectin-binding protein BBK32 is required for optimal infectivity. Mol Microbiol 82: 99–113.
29. Lee J, Attila C, Cirillo SLG, Cirillo JD, Wood TK (2009) Indole and 7-hydroxyindole diminish Pseudomonas aeruginosa virulence. Microbial Biotechnol 2: 75–90.
30. Heuts F, Carow B, Wigzell H, Rottenberg ME (2009) Use of non-invasive bioluminescent imaging to assess mycobacterial dissemination in mice, treatment with bactericidal drugs and protective immunity. Microbes Infect 11: 1114–1121.
31. Andrew PW, Roberts IS (1993) Construction of a bioluminescent mycobacterium and its use for assay of antimycobacterial agents. J Clin Microbiol 31: 2251–2254.
32. Waidmann MS, Bleichrodt FS, Laslo T, Riedel CU (2011) Bacterial luciferase reporters: the Swiss army knife of molecular biology. Bioeng Bugs 2: 8–16.
33. Meighen EA (1994) Genetics of bacterial bioluminescences. Annu Rev Genet 28: 117–139.
34. Frackman S, Anhalt M, Nealson KH (1990) Cloning, organization, and expression of the bioluminescence genes of Xenorhabdus luminescens. J Bacteriol 172: 5767–5773.
35. Contag CH, Contag PR, Mullins JI, Spilman SD, Stevenson DK, et al. (1995) Photonic detection of bacterial pathogens in living hosts. Mol Microbiol 18: 593–603.
36. Cooksey RC, Crawford JT, Jacobs WR Jr, Shinnick TM (1993) A rapid method for screening antimicrobial agents for activities against a strain of Mycobacterium tuberculosis expressing firefly luciferase. Antimicrob Agents Chemother 37: 1348–1352.
37. Arain TM, Resconi AE, Hickey MJ, Stover CK (1996) Bioluminescence screening in vitro (Bio-Siv) assays for high-volume antimycobacterial drug discovery. Antimicrob Agents Chemother 40: 1536–1541.
38. Hickey MJ, Arain TM, Shawar RM, Humble DJ, Langhorne MH, et al. (1996) Luciferase in vivo expression technology: use of recombinant mycobacterial reporter strains to evaluate antimycobacterial activity in mice. Antimicrob Agents Chemother 40: 400–407.
39. Rice BW, Cable MD, Nelson MB (2001) In vivo imaging of light-emitting probes. J Biomed Opt 6: 432–440.
40. Zhao H, Doyle TC, Coquoz O, Kalish F, Rice BW, et al. (2005) Emission spectra of bioluminescent reporters and interaction with mammalian tissue determine the sensitivity of detection in vivo. J Biomed Opt 10: 41210.
41. Difco (1984) Difco Manual: Dehydrated Culture Media and Reagents for Microbiology. Detroit, MI: Difco Laboratories.
42. Mehta PK, Pandey AK, Subbian S, El-Etr SH, Cirillo SL, et al. (2006) Identification of Mycobacterium marinum macrophage infection mutants. Microb Pathog 40: 139–151.
43. Miltner E, Daroogheh K, Mehta PK, Cirillo SLG, Cirillo JD, et al. (2005) Identification of Mycobacterium avium genes that affect invasion of the intestinal epithelium. Infect Immun 73: 4214–4221.
44. Cirillo SLG, Lum J, Cirillo JD (2000) Identification of novel loci involved in entry by *Legionella pneumophila*. Microbiology 146: 1345–1359.
45. Barletta RG, Kim DD, Snapper SB, Bloom BR, Jacobs WR Jr (1992) Identification of expression signals of the mycobacteriophages Bxb1, L1, and TM4 using *Escherichia-Mycobacterium* shuttle plasmids pYUB75 and pYUB76 designed to create translational fusions to the *lacZ* gene. J Gen Microbiol 138: 23–30.
46. Park B, Subbian S, El-Etr SH, Cirillo SL, Cirillo JD (2008) Use of gene dosage effects for a whole-genome screen to identify Mycobacterium marinum macrophage infection loci. Infect Immun 76: 3100–3115.
47. Stolt P, Stoker NG (1996) Functional definition of regions necessary for replication and incompatibility in the *Mycobacterium fortuitum* plasmid pAL5000. Microbiol 142: 2795–2802.
48. Subbian S, Mehta PK, Cirillo SL, Bermudez LE, Cirillo JD (2007) A *Mycobacterium marinum mel2* mutant is defective for growth in macrophages that produce reactive oxygen and reactive nitrogen species. Infect Immun 75: 127–134.
49. Luker KE, Luker GD (2010) Bioluminescence imaging of reporter mice for studies of infection and inflammation. Antiviral Res 86: 93–100.
50. Branchini BR, Ablamsky DM, Davis AL, Southworth TL, Butler B, et al. (2010) Red-emitting luciferases for bioluminescence reporter and imaging applications. Anal Biochem 396: 290–297.
51. Hardy J, Francis KP, DeBoer M, Chu P, Gibbs K, et al. (2004) Extracellular replication of Listeria monocytogenes in the murine gall bladder. Science 303: 851–853.
52. Francis KP, Yu J, Bellinger-Kawahara C, Joh D, Hawkinson MJ, et al. (2001) Visualizing pneumococcal infections in the lungs of live mice using bioluminescent Streptococcus pneumoniae transformed with a novel gram-positive lux transposon. Infect Immun 69: 3350–3358.
53. Janagama HK, Hassounah HA, Cirillo SL, Cirillo JD (2011) Random inducible controlled expression (RICE) for identification of mycobacterial virulence genes. Tuberculosis (Edinb) 91 Suppl 1: S66–68.
54. Danelishvili L, Wu M, Stang B, Harriff M, Cirillo SL, et al. (2007) Identification of Mycobacterium avium pathogenicity island important for macrophage and amoeba infection. Proc Natl Acad Sci U S A 104: 11038–11043.
55. Chackerian AA, Alt JM, Perera TV, Dascher CC, Behar SM (2002) Dissemination of Mycobacterium tuberculosis is influenced by host factors and precedes the initiation of T-cell immunity. Infect Immun 70: 4501–4509.
56. Zelmer A, Carroll P, Andreu N, Hagens K, Mahlo J, et al. (2012) A new in vivo model to test anti-tuberculosis drugs using fluorescence imaging. J Antimicrob Chemother 67: 1948–1960.
57. Wayne LG, Gross WM (1968) Base composition of deoxyribonucleic acid isolated from mycobacteria. J Bacteriol 96: 1915–1919.
58. Wayne LG, Kubica GP (1986) Mycobacteria. In: Sneath PHA, Mair NS, Sharpe ME, Holt JG, editors. Bergey's Manual of Systematic Bacteriology. Baltimore: Williams & Wilkins. 1436–1457.
59. Imaeda T (1985) Deoxyribonucleic acid relatedness among selected strains of *Mycobacterium tuberculosis*, *Mycobacterium bovis*, *Mycobacterium bovis* BCG, *Mycobacterium microti*, and *Mycobacterium africanum*. Int J Syst Bacteriol 35: 147–150.
60. Foucault ML, Thomas L, Goussard S, Branchini BR, Grillot-Courvalin C (2010) In vivo bioluminescence imaging for the study of intestinal colonization by Escherichia coli in mice. Appl Environ Microbiol 76: 264–274.
61. Mezzanotte L, Que I, Kaijzel E, Branchini B, Roda A, et al. (2011) Sensitive dual color in vivo bioluminescence imaging using a new red codon optimized firefly luciferase and a green click beetle luciferase. PLoS One 6: e19277.
62. Ranes MG, Rauzier J, Lagranderie M, Gheorghiu M, Gicquel B (1990) Functional analysis of pAL5000, a plasmid from *Mycobacterium fortuitum*: construction of a "mini" Mycobacterium-*Escherichia coli* shuttle vector. J Bacteriol 172: 2793–2797.
63. Stover CK, de la Cruz VF, Fuerst TR, Burlein JE, Benson LA, et al. (1991) New use of BCG for recombinant vaccines. Nature 351: 456–460.
64. Lee MH, Pascopella L, Jacobs WR Jr, Hatfull GF (1991) Site-specific integration of mycobacteriophage L5: integration-proficient vectors for *Mycobacterium smegmatis*, BCG, and *M. tuberculosis*. Proc Natl Acad Sci USA 88: 3111–3115.

Permissions

All chapters in this book were first published in PLOS ONE, by The Public Library of Science; hereby published with permission under the Creative Commons Attribution License or equivalent. Every chapter published in this book has been scrutinized by our experts. Their significance has been extensively debated. The topics covered herein carry significant findings which will fuel the growth of the discipline. They may even be implemented as practical applications or may be referred to as a beginning point for another development.

The contributors of this book come from diverse backgrounds, making this book a truly international effort. This book will bring forth new frontiers with its revolutionizing research information and detailed analysis of the nascent developments around the world.

We would like to thank all the contributing authors for lending their expertise to make the book truly unique. They have played a crucial role in the development of this book. Without their invaluable contributions this book wouldn't have been possible. They have made vital efforts to compile up to date information on the varied aspects of this subject to make this book a valuable addition to the collection of many professionals and students.

This book was conceptualized with the vision of imparting up-to-date information and advanced data in this field. To ensure the same, a matchless editorial board was set up. Every individual on the board went through rigorous rounds of assessment to prove their worth. After which they invested a large part of their time researching and compiling the most relevant data for our readers.

The editorial board has been involved in producing this book since its inception. They have spent rigorous hours researching and exploring the diverse topics which have resulted in the successful publishing of this book. They have passed on their knowledge of decades through this book. To expedite this challenging task, the publisher supported the team at every step. A small team of assistant editors was also appointed to further simplify the editing procedure and attain best results for the readers.

Apart from the editorial board, the designing team has also invested a significant amount of their time in understanding the subject and creating the most relevant covers. They scrutinized every image to scout for the most suitable representation of the subject and create an appropriate cover for the book.

The publishing team has been an ardent support to the editorial, designing and production team. Their endless efforts to recruit the best for this project, has resulted in the accomplishment of this book. They are a veteran in the field of academics and their pool of knowledge is as vast as their experience in printing. Their expertise and guidance has proved useful at every step. Their uncompromising quality standards have made this book an exceptional effort. Their encouragement from time to time has been an inspiration for everyone.

The publisher and the editorial board hope that this book will prove to be a valuable piece of knowledge for researchers, students, practitioners and scholars across the globe.

List of Contributors

Michael Owusu, Augustina Annan and Richard Larbi
Kumasi Centre for Collaborative Research in Tropical Medicine, Kwame Nkrumah University of Science and Technology, Kumasi, Ghana

Victor Max Corman, Jan Felix Drexler and Christian Drosten
Institute of Virology, University of Bonn Medical Centre, Bonn, Germany

Olivia Agbenyega and Priscilla Anti
Institute of Renewable and Natural Resources, Kwame Nkrumah University of Science and Technology, Kumasi, Ghana

Yaw Adu-Sarkodie
Department of Clinical Microbiology, Kwame Nkrumah University of Science and Technology, Kumasi, Ghana

Robin Wood, Carl Morrow, Elizabeth Piccoli, Darryl Kalil and Angelina Sassi
Desmond Tutu HIV Centre, Institute of Infectious Diseases and Molecular Medicine, and Department of Medicine, University of Cape Town Faculty of Health Sciences, Cape Town, South Africa

Samuel Ginsberg
Department of Electrical Engineering, Faculty of Engineering and the Built Environment, University of Cape Town, Cape Town, South Africa

Rochelle P. Walensky
Center for AIDS Research, Harvard Medical School, Boston, Massachusetts, United States of America

Jason R. Andrews
Division of Infectious Diseases and Geographic Medicine, Stanford University School of Medicine, Stanford, California, United States of America

Junguo Chen
Third Military Medical University, Chongqing, China

Feng Zhou
Third Military Medical University, Chongqing, China
Beijing Center for Disease Prevention and Control, Beijing Research Center of Preventive Medicine, Beijing, China

Li Zhang and Ying Deng
Beijing Center for Disease Prevention and Control, Beijing Research Center of Preventive Medicine, Beijing, China

Lei Gao, Xiangwei Li and Yu Yang
MOH Key Laboratory of Systems Biology of Pathogens, Institute of Pathogen Biology, Chinese Academy of Medical Sciences and Peking Union Medical College, Beijing, China

Yibin Hao
Zhengzhou Central Hospital, Zhengzhou, China

Xianli Zhao and Jianmin Liu
Henan Provincial Infectious Disease Hospital, Zhengzhou, China

Jie Lu
School of Public Health, Zhengzhou University, Zhengzhou, China

Moses Chapa Kiti, Dorothy Chelagat Koech and Patrick Kiio Munywoki
KEMRI-Wellcome Trust Research Programme, Kilifi, Kenya

Timothy Muiruri Kinyanjui
KEMRI-Wellcome Trust Research Programme, Kilifi, Kenya
Mathematics and WIDER, University of Warwick, Coventry, United Kingdom

David James Nokes
KEMRI-Wellcome Trust Research Programme, Kilifi, Kenya
School of Life Sciences and WIDER, University of Warwick, Coventry, United Kingdom

Graham Francis Medley
School of Life Sciences and WIDER, University of Warwick, Coventry, United Kingdom

Jae-Kwang Yoo
Inflammation Research, Amgen Inc., Seattle, Washington, United States of America
Beirne B. Carter Center for Immunology Research, University of Virginia, Charlottesville, Virginia, United States of America

Thomas J. Braciale
Beirne B. Carter Center for Immunology Research, University of Virginia, Charlottesville, Virginia, United States of America
Department of Microbiology, University of Virginia, Charlottesville, Virginia, United States of America
Department of Pathology, University of Virginia, Charlottesville, Virginia, United States of America

Céline Colin and Madeleine Decoin
INSERM U897 and CIC-EC7, Université de Bordeaux, Institut de Santé Publique Epidémiologie et Développement (ISPED), Bordeaux, France

Mathias Bruyand, François Dabis and Geneviève Chêne
INSERM U897 and CIC-EC7, Université de Bordeaux, Institut de Santé Publique Epidémiologie et Développement (ISPED), Bordeaux, France
Centre Hospitalier Universitaire (CHU) Bordeaux, Coordination Régionale de la lutte contre l'infection à VIH (COREVIH) Aquitaine, Bordeaux, France

Mojgan Hessamfar, Fabrice Bonnet and Philippe Morlat
INSERM U897 and CIC-EC7, Université de Bordeaux, Institut de Santé Publique Epidémiologie et Développement (ISPED), Bordeaux, France
Centre Hospitalier Universitaire (CHU) Bordeaux, Coordination Régionale de la lutte contre l'infection à VIH (COREVIH) Aquitaine, Bordeaux, France
CHU Bordeaux, Service de Médecine Interne et Maladies Infectieuses, Bordeaux, France

Patrick Mercié
INSERM U897 and CIC-EC7, Université de Bordeaux, Institut de Santé Publique Epidémiologie et Développement (ISPED), Bordeaux, France
Centre Hospitalier Universitaire (CHU) Bordeaux, Coordination Re´gionale de la lutte contre l'infection à VIH (COREVIH) Aquitaine, Bordeaux, France
CHU Bordeaux, Service de Médecine Interne et Immunologie Clinique, Bordeaux, France

Jean-Luc Pellegrin
Centre Hospitalier Universitaire (CHU) Bordeaux, Coordination Régionale de la lutte contre l'infection à VIH (COREVIH) Aquitaine, Bordeaux, France
CHU Bordeaux, Service de Médecine Interne et Maladies Infectieuses, Bordeaux, France
Université de Bordeaux, Bordeaux, France

Didier Neau and Charles Cazanave
Centre Hospitalier Universitaire (CHU) Bordeaux, Coordination Régionale de la lutte contre l'infection à VIH (COREVIH) Aquitaine, Bordeaux, France
CHU de Bordeaux, Fédération des Maladies Infectieuses et Tropicales, Bordeaux, France
Université de Bordeaux, Bordeaux, France

Julian W. Tang
Alberta Provincial Laboratory for Public Health, University of Alberta Hospital, Edmonton, Canada
Department of Medical Microbiology and Immunology, University of Alberta, Edmonton, Canada
Department of Laboratory Medicine, National University Hospital, Singapore, Singapore

Andre D. Nicolle and Christian A. Klettner
Department of Laboratory Medicine, National University Hospital, Singapore, Singapore

Evelyn S. C. Koay
Department of Laboratory Medicine, National University Hospital, Singapore, Singapore
Department of Pathology, Yong Loo Lin School of Medicine, National University of Singapore, Singapore, Singapore

Yuguo Li
Department of Mechanical Engineering, The University of Hong Kong, Hong Kong SAR, China

Caroline X. Gao
Department of Mechanical Engineering, The University of Hong Kong, Hong Kong SAR, China
Turning Point Alcohol and Drug Centre, Eastern Health, Melbourne, Australia
Eastern Health Clinical School, Monash University, Melbourne, Australia

Cherie Heilbronn and Belinda Lloyd
Turning Point Alcohol and Drug Centre, Eastern Health, Melbourne, Australia
Eastern Health Clinical School, Monash University, Melbourne, Australia

J. S. Malik Peiris, Benjamin J. Cowling and Daniel Chu
School of Public Health, The University of Hong Kong, Hong Kong SAR, China

Gerald C. Koh
Saw Swee Hock School of Public Health, National University of Singapore, Singapore, Singapore

Jovan Pantelic
Department of Mechanical Engineering, University of Maryland, Baltimore, Maryland, United States of America

Chandra Sekhar, David K. W. Cheong and Kwok Wai Tham
Department of Building, School of Design and Environment, National University of Singapore, Singapore, Singapore

Wendy Tsui and Alfred Kwong
Department of Family Medicine and Primary Healthcare, Hong Kong West Cluster, Hospital Authority, Hong Kong SAR, China

Kitty Chan
University Health Service, The University of Hong Kong, Hong Kong SAR, China

Douglas S. Goodin
Department of Neurology, University of California San Francisco, San Francisco, California, United States of America

David Kaufman
Slone Epidemiology Center at Boston University, Boston, Massachusetts, United States of America

Michael Corwin
Slone Epidemiology Center at Boston University, Boston, Massachusetts, United States of America
Care-Safe, Boston, Massachusetts, United States of America

Howard Golub
Care-Safe, Boston, Massachusetts, United States of America

Shoshana Reshef and Mark J. Rametta
Bayer HealthCare Pharmaceuticals, Whippany, New Jersey, United States of America

Volker Knappertz
Teva Pharmaceuticals, Frazer, Pennsylvania, United States of America, Department of Neurology, Heinrich Heine University, Dusseldorf, Germany

Gary Cutter
University of Alabama School of Public Health, Birmingham, Alabama, United States of America

Dirk Pleimes
Myelo Therapeutics GmbH, Berlin, Germany

Ramy A. Fodah and Tia L. Pfeffer
Department of Microbiology and Immunology, University of Louisville, Louisville, Kentucky, United States of America

Jonathan M. Warawa
Department of Microbiology and Immunology, University of Louisville, Louisville, Kentucky, United States of America
Center for Predictive Medicine, University of Louisville, Louisville, Kentucky, United States of America

Jacob B. Scott
Dental School, University of Louisville, Louisville, Kentucky, United States of America
College of Dentistry, Ohio State University, Columbus, Ohio, United States of America

Hok-Hei Tam
Department of Chemical Engineering, Massachusetts Institute of Technology, Cambridge, Massachusetts, United States of America

Pearlly Yan and Ralf Bundschuh
The Comprehensive Cancer Center and The James Cancer Hospital and Solove Research Institute, Division of Hematology, Department of Internal Medicine, Ohio State University, Columbus, Ohio, United States of America
Departments of Physics and Chemistry and Biochemistry and Center for RNA Biology, Ohio State University, Columbus, Ohio, United States of America

Maela Tebon, Valentino Bezzerri, Valentina Lovato, Cinzia Cantù, Silvia Munari, Giulio Cabrini and Maria Cristina Dechecchi
Laboratory of Molecular Pathology, Department of Pathology and Diagnostics, University Hospital of Verona, Verona, Italy

Sandro Sonnino, Nicoletta Loberto, Massimo Aureli and Rosaria Bassi
Department of Medical Biotechnology and Translational Medicine, University of Milano, Milano, Italy

Roberto Gambari and Ilaria Lampronti
Department of Life Sciences and Biotechnology, Section of Biochemistry and Molecular Biology, University of Ferrara, Ferrara, Italy

Alberto Cavazzini and Nicola Marchetti
Department of Chemistry and Pharmaceutical Sciences, University of Ferrara, Ferrara, Italy

Maria Grazia Giri
Medical Physics Unit, Department of Pathology and Diagnostics, University Hospital of Verona, Verona, Italy

Seng H. Cheng
Genzyme, a Sanofi Company, Framingham, Massachusetts, United States of America

Du Luping and Sun Bing
Institute of Veterinary Medicine, Jiangsu Academy of Agricultural Sciences, Key Laboratory of Veterinary Biological Engineering and Technology, Ministry of Agriculture, Nanjing, Jiangsu Province, China

Li Bin, Yu Zhengyu, Liu Maojun, Feng Zhixin, Wei Yanna, Wang Haiyan, Shao Guoqing and He Kongwang
Institute of Veterinary Medicine, Jiangsu Academy of Agricultural Sciences, Key Laboratory of Veterinary Biological Engineering and Technology, Ministry of Agriculture, Nanjing, Jiangsu Province, China

Jiangsu Co-innovation Center for Prevention and Control of Important Animal Infectious Diseases and Zoonoses, Yangzhou, China

Caroline Bidot
UR341 MIA, INRA, Jouy-en-Josas, France

Natacha Go
UR341 MIA, INRA, Jouy-en-Josas, France
LUNAM Université, Oniris, INRA UMR 1300 BioEpAR, Nantes, France

Catherine Belloc
LUNAM Université, Oniris, INRA UMR 1300 BioEpAR, Nantes, France

Suzanne Touzeau
UMR1355 ISA, INRA, Université Nice Sophia Antipolis, CNRS, Sophia Antipolis, France
BIOCORE, Inria, Sophia Antipolis, France

Hongyu Miao, Le Zhang, Jeanne Holden-Wiltse and Hulin Wu
Department of Biostatistics and Computational Biology, University of Rochester Medical Center, Rochester, New York, United States of America

Mark Y. Sangster, Alexandra M. Livingstone, David J. Topham and Tim R. Mosmann
David H. Smith Center for Vaccine Biology and Immunology, Department of Microbiology and Immunology, University of Rochester Medical Center, Rochester, New York, United States of America

Martin S. Zand and Shannon P. Hilchey
Department of Medicine, University of Rochester Medical Center, Rochester, New York, United States of America

Alan S. Perelson
Theoretical Biology and Biophysics, Los Alamos National Laboratory, Los Alamos, New Mexico, United States of America

Elske van den Berg, Reinout A. Bem, Albert P. Bos and Job B. M. van Woensel
Pediatric Intensive Care Unit, Emma Children's Hospital, Academic Medical Center, Amsterdam, The Netherlands

Rene Lutter
Department of Respiratory Medicine and Experimental Immunology, Academic Medical Center, Amsterdam, The Netherlands

Linda Fritts and Michael B. McChesney
Center for Comparative Medicine, University of California Davis, Davis, California, United States of America

Huma Qureshi, Meritxell Genescà and Christopher J. Miller
Center for Comparative Medicine, University of California Davis, Davis, California, United States of America
California National Primate Research Center, University of California Davis, Davis, California, United States of America

Marjorie Robert-Guroff
Vaccine Branch, National Cancer Institute, National Institutes of Health, Bethesda, Maryland, United States of America

Trong-Neng Wu and Chiu-Ying Chen
Department of Public Health, China Medical University, Taichung, Taiwan,

Kuang-Hsi Chang
Department of Public Health, China Medical University, Taichung, Taiwan
Department of Medical Research, Taichung Veterans General Hospital, Taichung, Taiwan

Mei-Yin Chang
Department of Medical Laboratory Science and Biotechnology, School of Medical and Health Sciences, Fooyin University, Kaohsiung, Taiwan

Chih-Hsin Muo
Management Office for Health Data, China Medical University Hospital, Taichung, Taiwan

Chia-Hung Kao
Graduate Institute of Clinical Medical Science, College of Medicine, China Medical University, Taiwan
Department of Nuclear Medicine and PET Center, China Medical University Hospital, Taichung, Taiwan

Can Li, Chuangen Li and Andrew C. Y. Lee
Department of Microbiology, The University of Hong Kong, Hong Kong, China

Hazel W. L. Wu
Department of Microbiology, The University of Hong Kong, Hong Kong, China
State Key Laboratory of Emerging Infectious Diseases, The University of Hong Kong,
Hong Kong, China

Anna J. X. Zhang, Kelvin K. W. To and Jasper F. W. Chan
Department of Microbiology, The University of Hong Kong, Hong Kong, China
State Key Laboratory of Emerging Infectious Diseases, The University of Hong Kong, Hong Kong, China
Research Centre of Infection and Immunology, The University of Hong Kong, Hong Kong, China

Honglin Chen and Kwok-Yung Yuen
Department of Microbiology, The University of Hong Kong, Hong Kong, China
State Key Laboratory of Emerging Infectious Diseases, The University of Hong Kong, Hong Kong, China
Research Centre of Infection and Immunology, The University of Hong Kong, Hong Kong, China
Collaborative Innovation Center for Diagnosis and Treatment of Infectious Diseases, Hangzhou, China
Zhejiang University, Hangzhou, China

Ivan F. N. Hung
Research Centre of Infection and Immunology, The University of Hong Kong, Hong Kong, China
Department of Medicine, The University of Hong Kong, Hong Kong, China

Houshun Zhu
Department of Medicine, The University of Hong Kong, Hong Kong, China

Lanjuan Li
State Key Laboratory for Diagnosis and Treatment of Infectious Diseases, the First Affiliated Hospital, College of Medicine, Zhejiang University, Hangzhou, China
Collaborative Innovation Center for Diagnosis and Treatment of Infectious Diseases, Hangzhou, China
Zhejiang University, Hangzhou, China

Lu Wang, Fangfang Chen, Ruixue Yan, Lin Ge, Qianqian Qin, Liyan Wang, Zhengwei Ding, Wei Guo and Ning Wang
National Center for AIDS/STD Control and Prevention, Chinese Center for Disease Control and Prevention, Beijing, China

Jiannan Xing
National Center for AIDS/STD Control and Prevention, Chinese Center for Disease Control and Prevention, Beijing, China
Beijing Human Resources and Social Security Bureau, Beijing, China

Benjamin J. Cowling, Dennis K. M. Ip, Vicky J. Fang and Gabriel M. Leung
School of Public Health, Li Ka Shing Faculty of Medicine, The University of Hong Kong, Hong Kong Special Administrative Region, China

J. S. Malik Peiris
School of Public Health, Li Ka Shing Faculty of Medicine, The University of Hong Kong, Hong Kong Special Administrative Region, China
Centre for Influenza Research, Li Ka Shing Faculty of Medicine, The University of Hong Kong, Hong Kong Special Administrative Region, China

Piyarat Suntarattiwong and Tawee Chotpitayasunondh
Queen Sirikit National Institute of Child Health, Bangkok, Thailand

Jens Levy
Influenza Program, Thailand MOPH-US CDC Collaboration, Nonthaburi, Thailand

Sonja J. Olsen
Influenza Program, Thailand MOPH-US CDC Collaboration, Nonthaburi, Thailand
Influenza Division, US Centers for Disease Control and Prevention, Atlanta, Georgia, United States of America

Timothy M. Uyeki
Influenza Division, US Centers for Disease Control and Prevention, Atlanta, Georgia, United States of America

Hiroshi Nishiura
Graduate School of Medicine, The University of Tokyo, Bunkyo-ku, Tokyo, Japan

J. Mark Simmerman
Epidemiology and Medical Affairs, Sanofi Pasteur, Bangkok, Thailand

Loredana Guida and Ilaria Morelli
Internal Medicine and Critical Subacute Care Unit, Parma University Hospital, Parma, Italy

Antonio Nouvenne, Andrea Ticinesi, Erminia Ridolo, Loris Borghi and Tiziana Meschi
Internal Medicine and Critical Subacute Care Unit, Parma University Hospital, Parma, Italy
Department of Clinical and Experimental Medicine, University of Parma, Parma, Italy

Marcello Maggio
Department of Clinical and Experimental Medicine, University of Parma, Parma, Italy

Fulvio Lauretani
Geriatrics Unit, Parma University Hospital, Parma, Italy

Giuseppe Lippi
Laboratory of Clinical Chemistry and Hematology, Parma University Hospital, Parma, Italy

Emmanuel Serrano
Centre for Environmental and Marine Studies (CESAM), Departamento de Biología, Universidade de Aveiro, Aveiro, Portugal
Servei d'Ecopatologia de Fauna Salvatge (SEFaS), Departament de Medicina I Cirurgia Animals, Universitat Auto`noma de Barcelona, Bellaterra, Spain

Roser Velarde
Servei d'Ecopatologia de Fauna Salvatge (SEFaS), Departament de Medicina I Cirurgia Animals, Universitat Autònoma de Barcelona, Bellaterra, Spain

Joaquím Segalés
Centre de Recerca en Sanitat Animal (CReSA), Universitat Autònoma de Barcelona - I0Institut de Recerca i Tecnologia Agroalimentàries, Bellaterra, Spain
Departament de Sanitat i Anatomia Animals, Universitat Autònoma de Barcelona, Bellaterra, Spain

Jennie Johnstone and Stephen D. Walter
Department of Clinical Epidemiology and Biostatistics, McMaster University, Hamilton, Ontario, Canada

P. J. Devereaux
Department of Clinical Epidemiology and Biostatistics, McMaster University, Hamilton, Ontario, Canada
Department of Medicine, McMaster University, Hamilton, Ontario, Canada

Mark Loeb
Department of Clinical Epidemiology and Biostatistics, McMaster University, Hamilton, Ontario, Canada
Department of Medicine, McMaster University, Hamilton, Ontario, Canada
Department of Pathology and Molecular Medicine, McMaster University, Hamilton, Ontario, Canada
Institute for Infectious Disease Research, McMaster University, Hamilton, Ontario, Canada

Robin Parsons, Fernando Botelho and Jamie Millar
McMaster Immunology Research Centre, McMaster University, Hamilton, Ontario, Canada

Jonathan Bramson
McMaster Immunology Research Centre, McMaster University, Hamilton, Ontario, Canada
Department of Pathology and Molecular Medicine, McMaster University, Hamilton, Ontario, Canada
Institute for Infectious Disease Research, McMaster University, Hamilton, Ontario, Canada

Shelly McNeil
Canadian Center for Vaccinology, IWK Health Centre and Capital Health, Dalhousie University, Halifax, Nova Scotia, Canada

Tamas Fulop
Department of Medicine, Geriatrics Division, Research Center on Aging, University of Sherbrooke, Sherbrooke, Quebec, Canada

Janet McElhaney
Department of Medicine, Northern Ontario School of Medicine, Sudbury, Ontario, Canada

Melissa K. Andrew
Department of Medicine, Dalhousie University, Halifax, Nova Scotia, Canada

Mehrnoush Malekesmaeili
Terry Fox Laboratory, British Columbia Cancer Agency, Vancouver, British Columbia, Canada

Ryan R. Brinkman
Terry Fox Laboratory, British Columbia Cancer Agency, Vancouver, British Columbia, Canada
Department of Medical Genetics, University of British Columbia, Vancouver, British Columbia, Canada

James Mahony
Department of Pathology and Molecular Medicine, McMaster University, Hamilton, Ontario, Canada
Institute for Infectious Disease Research, McMaster University, Hamilton, Ontario, Canada

Osvaldo P. Almeida
School of Psychiatry and Clinical Neurosciences, University of Western Australia, Perth, Australia
WA Centre for Health and Ageing, Centre for Medical Research, Perth, Australia
Department of Psychiatry, Royal Perth Hospital, Perth, Australia

Leon Flicker
WA Centre for Health and Ageing, Centre for Medical Research, Perth, Australia
School of Medicine and Pharmacology, University of Western Australia, Perth, Australia
Department of Geriatric Medicine, Royal Perth Hospital, Perth, Australia

Graeme J. Hankey
School of Medicine and Pharmacology, University of Western Australia, Perth, Australia
Department of Neurology, Sir Charles Gairdner Hospital, Perth, Australia

Bu B. Yeap
School of Medicine and Pharmacology, University of Western Australia, Perth, Australia
Department of Endocrinology, Fremantle Hospital, Fremantle, Australia

Jonathan Golledge
Queensland Research Centre for Peripheral Vascular Disease, School of Medicine and Dentistry, James Cook University, Townsville, Australia
Department of Vascular and Endovascular Surgery, The Townsville Hospital, Townsville, Australia

Paul E. Norman
School of Surgery, University of Western Australia, Perth, Australia

Kevin Lahmers, Sudarvili Shanthalingam, Subramaniam Srikumaran and William J. Foreyt
Department of Veterinary Microbiology and Pathology, Washington State University, Pullman, Washington, United States of America

Thomas E. Besser, Kathleen A. Potter and J. Lindsay Oaks
Department of Veterinary Microbiology and Pathology, Washington State University, Pullman, Washington, United States of America
Washington Animal Disease Diagnostic Laboratory, Washington State University, Pullman Washington, United States of America

E. Frances Cassirer
Idaho Department of Fish and Game, Lewiston, Idaho, United States of America

Blanca Taboada, Marco A. Espinoza, Pavel Isa, Fernando E. Aponte, Susana López and Carlos F. Arias
Instituto de Biotecnología, Universidad Nacional Autónoma de México, Cuernavaca, Morelos, Mexico

María A. Arias-Ortiz, Jesús Monge-Martínez, Rubén Rodríguez-Vázquez, Fidel Díaz-Hernández and Fernando Zárate-Vidal
Colegio de Pediatría del Estado de Veracruz, Veracruz, Mexico

José I. Santos-Preciado and Rosa María Wong-Chew
Facultad de Medicina, Universidad Nacional Autónoma de México, México D.F., Mexico

Verónica Firo-Reyes
Hospital General de México, México D.F., Mexico

Carlos N. del Río-Almendárez
Hospital Pediátirco de Coyoacán, México D.F., Mexico

Jesús Gaitán-Meza
Nuevo Hospital Civil de Guadalajara "Dr. Juan I. Menchaca", Guadalajara, Jalisco, Mexico

Alberto Villaseñor-Sierra
Centro de Investigación Biomédica de Occidente, IMSS, Guadalajara, Jalisco, Mexico

Gerardo Martínez-Aguilar and Ma. del Carmen Salas-Mier
Unidad de Investigación Biomédica IMSS, Durango, Durango, Mexico

Daniel E. Noyola
Universidad Autónoma de San Luis Potosí, San Luis Potosí, Mexico

Luis F. Pérez-Gónzalez
Hospital Central "Dr. Ignacio Morones Prieto", San Luis Potosí, Mexico

Shokrollah Elahi and Lorne A. Babiuk
Faculty of Medicine and Dentistry, University of Alberta, Edmonton, Alberta, Canada

Jill Van Kessel and Stacy Strom
Vaccine and Infectious Disease Organization, International Vaccine Centre, University of Saskatchewan, Saskatoon, Saskatchewan, Canada

Volker Gerdts
Vaccine and Infectious Disease Organization, International Vaccine Centre, University of Saskatchewan, Saskatoon, Saskatchewan, Canada
Department of Veterinary Microbiology, Western College of Veterinary Medicine, University of Saskatchewan, Saskatoon, Saskatchewan, Canada

Tedele G. Kiros
Department of Veterinary Microbiology, Western College of Veterinary Medicine, University of Saskatchewan, Saskatoon, Saskatchewan, Canada

Yoshihiro Hayakawa and Mamoru Hyodo
Faculty of Engineering, Department of Applied Chemistry, Aichi Institute of Technology, Toyota, Japan

MiHee Chang, Katri P. Anttonen, Suat L. G. Cirillo and Jeffrey D. Cirillo
Department of Microbial Pathogenesis and Immunology, Texas A&M Health Science Center, Bryan, Texas, United States of America

Kevin P. Francis
PerkinElmer, Alameda, California, United States of America

Index

A
Acellular Pertussis Vaccine, 216, 223
Acute Respiratory Infections, 9, 202
Antibody-secreting Cell, 110
Antimicrobial Activity, 220
Avian Influenza, 146-147, 156-157

B
B-glucosidase Activity, 70, 74, 77
Bioluminescence, 224-226, 229, 235-236
Bordetella Pertussis, 216, 222-223
Bovine Kobuvirus, 208, 212, 214

C
Capsular Polysaccharide, 60, 62, 64-65, 67
Carbapenem, 69, 173, 179
Cardiovascular Disease, 194
Celecoxib, 146-147, 150, 153-155
Ceramide, 70-72, 75-77, 79-82
Coronavirus, 1, 6, 9, 181, 183, 187, 189, 202, 205, 208-210, 212, 214-215
Cystic Fibrosis, 70-71, 82, 215

D
Dementia, 138-145, 184, 192, 195, 198, 200

E
Endothelium, 124-125
Epithelial Cell, 66, 82-83, 149, 152, 154-155
Etiologic Agent, 11
Eukaryotic Initiation, 77

F
Flow Cytometry, 37, 40, 135-136, 181, 219
Follicular Helper Cell, 36, 38, 49, 121

G
Gaucher Disease, 76, 81
Glycoprotein, 89, 120
Glycosphingolipid Biosynthetic Pathway, 71
Glycosphingolipids, 81

H
Haematoxylin, 149, 151, 155
Hepatitis C Virus, 158, 164
Hexon Protein, 129, 131, 134, 136-137
Human Coronaviruses, 1, 9-10
Human Metapneumovirus, 9, 181, 183, 187, 189, 215

I
Immune Response, 83-85, 88-89, 91-94, 103, 105-109, 116, 119-120, 129, 136, 152, 156, 184, 216-217, 221-222, 235
Inflammatory Cytokine, 93, 147
Integrative Model, 92-93, 107
Intratracheal Infection, 61

K
Klebsiella Pneumonia, 217, 223

L
Latent Tuberculosis Infection, 19, 21, 23, 26
Legionella Pneumophila, 203, 208, 210, 236
Lung Leukocyte Isolation, 218
Lymphocyte, 49, 135-137, 182, 189-190

M
Macrophage Response, 83, 91, 109
Mammalian Respiratory Tract, 151
Miglustat, 70-77, 79, 81-82
Murine Respiratory Disease, 59, 62, 65-66
Mutant Adenovirus, 129
Mycoplasma Hyopneumoniae, 83, 91

N
Nasopharyngeal Swab, 52, 183
Necrotic Cell, 149
Nosocomial Pathogen, 59, 173

P
Parainfluenza, 1, 181, 183, 187, 202, 205
Pediatric Respiratory Tract, 202, 215
Pertussis, 203, 216-223
Phagocytosis, 67-69, 83, 93-95, 97, 99-103, 105-108, 216, 223
Phosphorylation, 77, 145
Pleiotropic Immuno-modulatory, 36
Pneumovirus, 122-125, 127-128, 215
Porcine Alveolar, 83, 89-91, 109
Porcine Respiratory, 83, 92-93, 109
Prophylactic Anti-viral Therapy, 186
Pseudomonas Aeruginosa, 70, 82, 208, 211, 236
Pulmonary Edema, 122-128
Pulmonary Virus Infection, 36, 47

R
Reproductive Syndrome Virus, 92-93, 109
Respiratory Pathogen, 35, 206

Respiratory Syncytial Virus, 1, 27, 35, 122, 127-128, 137, 172, 181, 190, 202, 205, 208, 210, 212, 214

Respiratory Tract Infections, 1-2, 8-10, 189, 202, 208, 210, 214-215

Respiratory Viral Infection, 181-189

Rhesus Macaques, 129, 131, 135, 137

Rhinovirus, 9-10, 181, 183, 187, 189, 202, 204-205, 208, 210, 212, 214

S

Spatial Analysis, 158-159, 161, 163

Sphingosine, 75, 80, 82

U

Uridine Triphosphate, 125

Z

Zanamivir, 58, 146-147, 150, 153-156

www.ingramcontent.com/pod-product-compliance
Lightning Source LLC
Chambersburg PA
CBHW080507200326
41458CB00012B/4112

* 9 7 8 1 6 3 2 4 1 7 5 5 8 *